"Feminine wisdom is the intelligence at the heart of creation. It is holistic, intuitive, contextual and functions as a field of infinite correlation. Dr. Northrup's book is an expression of this wisdom."
—Deepak Chopra, M.D., author of *Ageless Body, Timeless Mind*

"*Women's Bodies, Women's Wisdom* is a gateway to the deepest understanding of health and well-being. Women have an innate sense of spirituality, an ability to attune to the wisdom within themselves and the larger whole that has been systematically ignored in medicine. Dr. Northrup restores the spiritual to the medical, facilitating the understanding and confidence that every woman needs in order to create a healthy body and a fulfilled life."
—Joan Borysenko, Ph.D., author of *Minding the Body, Mending the Mind*

"While most male physicians seem hesitant even to use the word 'healing,' many women doctors—epitomized by Dr. Christiane Northrup—are demonstrating what genuine healing has always been about: the integration of the physical and the spiritual, psyche and soma, into a harmonious whole. This book demonstrates the reemergence of the feminine in healing, a force that has kept the inner pulse of healing beating for centuries. If you can't have Dr. Northrup for your doctor, read her book."
—Larry Dossey, M.D., author of *Healing Words, Meaning & Medicine,* and *Recovering the Soul*

"Dr. Chris Northrup's book is an outstanding collection of information and case histories that will benefit everyone who reads it. It lives up to the title and I certainly intend to share it with my wife and daughter. I could go on extolling its virtues but it will do more good if everyone just takes my advice and reads it."
—Bernie Siegel, M.D., author of *Love, Medicine, and Miracles*

"Dr. Christiane Northrup, founder of 'Women to Women,' a women-treating-women health clinic in Yarmouth, Maine, is truly a visionary for the '90s in women's health and wellness. Every topic a woman might ever wish to explore is covered within this ground-breaking medical guide."
            —*Body, Mind, Spirit* magazine

"At last a book that covers women's health that includes the broad areas of important medical and holistic knowledge we need to know to fully take care of ourselves. We are clearly led through basic physiological, medical, psychological, human-energy field, dietary, and physical-exercise information that will help us shift our personal health care into the new paradigm encompassed by women's wisdom."
            —Barbara Brennan, author of *Hands of Light* and
                        Light Emerging

"This is truly a remarkable book that will nourish the spirit as well as the body."
            —Ann Louise Gittleman, author of
                        Supernutrition for Women

"This book is outstanding in its concern and clarity of information about women's health issues."
            —Ondrea and Stephen Levine

Women's Bodies, Women's Wisdom

Creating Physical and Emotional

Health and Healing

Christiane Northrup, M.D.

BANTAM BOOKS

NEW YORK   TORONTO   LONDON   SYDNEY   AUCKLAND

This edition contains the complete text
of the original hardcover edition.
NOT ONE WORD HAS BEEN OMITTED.

WOMEN'S BODIES, WOMEN'S WISDOM
A Bantam Book
PUBLISHING HISTORY

Bantam hardcover edition published July 1994
Bantam trade paperback edition / July 1995

Bantam Books are published by Bantam Books, a division of Bantam
Doubleday Dell Publishing Group, Inc. Its trademark, consisting of the words
"Bantam Books" and the portrayal of a rooster, is Registered in U.S. Patent
and Trademark Office and in other countries. Marca Registrada. Bantam
Books, 1540 Broadway, New York, New York 10036.

PRINTED IN THE UNITED STATES OF AMERICA
BVG 10 9 8 7 6 5

This book is for all who believe that it is possible to live our lives fully regardless of our present or past circumstances.

It is for all who acknowledge the daily presence in our lives of mystery, uncertainty, and hope.

It is for those who yearn to be well and know that there is something more to healing than simply external substances or techniques.

This book is for every physician, nurse, healthcare practitioner, healer, or patient who has ever honestly acknowledged how much we don't know.

It is for those who know that our healing will not be complete until we bring the sacred back into our daily lives.

This book is dedicated with gratitude to the scientists and healers of the past, present, and future who have dared and continue to dare to go forward in faith despite the deadening effects of conventional thinking.

Contents

List of Figures   xiii

List of Tables   xv

Acknowledgments   xvii

Introduction: Physician, Heal Thyself   xxi
The Personal Is Political   xxiii
Women to Women   xxv
Creating Health   xxvii

PART ONE: FROM EXTERNAL CONTROL TO INNER GUIDANCE

1:   The Patriarchal Myth and the Addictive System   3
Our Cultural Inheritance   3
Patriarchy Results in Addiction   5
Fundamental Beliefs of the Addictive System   7
Reclaiming Our Own Authority   12

2:   Feminine Intelligence and a New Mode of Healing   25
Energy Fields and Energy Systems   25
Understanding the Bodymind   28
Feminine Intelligence: How Thoughts Are Embodied   32
Beliefs Are Physical   35
Healing Versus Curing   41

3:   Inner Guidance   50
Listening to Your Body and Its Needs   52
Emotional Cleansing: Healing from the Past   56
Dreams: A Doorway to the Unconscious   57
Intuition and Intuitive Diagnosis   58
How Inner Guidance Works   59

4: The Female Energy System   67
The Matter/Energy Continuum   67
Earth's Energy   72
The Chakras   73
The Lower Female Centers: Chakras One to Four   76
Other Chakra Issues   91

PART TWO: THE ANATOMY OF
WOMEN'S WISDOM

5: The Menstrual Cycle   95
Our Cyclical Nature   97
Our Cultural Inheritance   104
Menstrual Cramps (Dysmenorrhea)   113
Premenstrual Syndrome (PMS)   118
Irregular Periods   130
Excessive Buildup of the Uterine Lining (Endometrial
    Hyperplasia, Cystic and Adenomatous Hyperplasia)   131
Dysfunctional Uterine Bleeding (DUB)   133
Heavy Periods (Menorrhagia)   141
Healing Our Menstrual History: Preparing Our Daughters   144

6: The Uterus   149
Our Cultural Inheritance   151
Energy Anatomy   152
Chronic Pelvic Pain   155
Endometriosis   157
Fibroid Tumors   168

7: The Ovaries   194
Anatomy   196
Ovarian Cysts   201
Polycystic Ovaries (PCO)   204
Ovarian Cancer   215

8: Reclaiming the Erotic   225
We Are Sexual Beings   225
Finding Our True Sexuality   232
Women's Sexuality and Nature   234

9:   Vulva, Vagina, and Cervix   241
Our Cultural Inheritance   242
Anatomy   246
Human Papilloma Virus (HPV)   248
Herpes   256
Cervicitis   261
Cervical Dysplasia (Abnormal Pap Smears)   261
Cervical Cancer   272
Vaginal Infection (Vaginitis)   275
Sexually Transmitted Diseases   283

10:   Breasts   286
Our Cultural Inheritance   286
Anatomy   289
Breast Self-Exams   289
Benign Breast Symptoms: Breast Pain, Lumps, Cysts, and
     Nipple Discharge   293
Mammograms   298
Breast Cancer   303
Cosmetic Breast Surgery   314
Caring for Your Breasts   322

11:   Our Fertility   324
Abortion   325
Conscious Conception and Contraception   333
The Trauma of Infertility   350
Pregnancy Loss   362
Adoption   367
Fertility as Metaphor   371

12:   Pregnancy and Birthing   374
Our Cultural Inheritance: Pregnancy   375
The Transforming Power of Pregnancy   380
Our Cultural Inheritance: Labor and Delivery   384
Birth Technologies   390
My Personal Story   396
Turning Labor into Personal Power   403

13:   Motherhood: Bonding with Your Baby   414
Early Touching   414
Circumcision   418

Formula Versus Breast Milk   420
Mothering in the Addictive System: The Hardest Job
   in the World   425

14: Menopause   430
Our Cultural Inheritance   432
Kinds of Menopause   436
Symptoms of Menopause   442
Hot Flashes   444
Vaginal Dryness, Irritation, and Thinning   447
Osteoporosis   450
Sexuality in Menopause   457
Mood Swings and Depression   460
Fuzzy Thinking   461
Estrogen Replacement Therapy (ERT)   462
Phytoestrogens: Natural Hormones in Food   469
Estriol: An Estrogen That Deserves Attention   470
Deciding on Menopausal "Treatment"   472
Self-Care During Menopause   477

PART THREE: CHOICES FOR HEALING: CREATING YOUR PERSONAL PLAN

15: Steps for Healing   485
Step One: Get Your History Straight   485
Step Two: Sort Through Your Beliefs   494
Step Three: Respect and Release Your Emotions   506
Step Four: Learn to Listen to Your Body   509
Step Five: Learn to Respect Your Body   511
Step Six: Acknowledge a Higher Power or Inner Wisdom   514
Step Seven: Reclaim the Fullness of Your Mind   519
Step Eight: Get Help   525
Step Nine: Work with Your Body   530
Step Ten: Gather Information   531
Step Eleven: Forgive   532
Step Twelve: Actively Participate in Your Life   539

16: Getting the Most Out of Your Medical Care   544
Choosing a Health Care Provider   544
Healing the Pelvic Examination   548
Choosing a Treatment: From Surgery to Brown Rice   552
Creating Health Through Surgery   555

17: Nourishing Ourselves with Food   566
Our Cultural Inheritance   567
Reframing Self-Nourishment   572
Food and Energy   586
Grains, Beans, and Health: Macrobiotics   587
Getting Started   619
Food and Consciousness   624

18: The Power of Movement   627
Our Cultural Inheritance   628
Benefits of Exercise   629
Ways to Move the Body   630
Exercise and Addiction   633
Exercise, Amenorrhea, and Bone Loss   634
My Exercise Story: Making Peace   635
Getting Started   637

19: Healing Ourselves, Healing Our World   640
Our Mothers: Our Cells   642
A Ritual of Reclaiming   643
Conquering Our Fear of Our Shaman Past   646
Our Dreams: Earth's Dreams   648
Making the World Safe for Women: Start with Yourself   654

Appendix: Women to Women Guidelines for a Healthy
    Approach to Food   657

Resources   674

Notes   690

Index   737

List of Figures

Fig. 1: Earth's Energy Going Upward   74
Fig. 2: Chakra Diagram with Female Figure   77
Fig. 3: Menstrual Cycle (days)   99
Fig. 4: Lunar Chart for Menstrual Cycle   100
Fig. 5: The Female Mind/Body Continuum: Interactions
    Between the Brain and the Pelvis   107
Fig. 6: Uterus, Ovaries, and Cervix with Anatomic Labels   150
Fig. 7: Fibroid Diagram   169
Fig. 8: Breast Anatomy   290
Fig. 9: Breast Exam   291
Fig. 10: Fertility Awareness Charts   344–45
Fig. 11: Seeking Partnership (*Drawing by Whitney Oppersdorff*)   367
Fig. 12: (*Drawing by Whitney Oppersdorff*)   368
Fig. 13: Hormone-Producing Body Sites   437
Fig. 14: Currents of Wisdom   440
Fig. 15: The Energetics of Food   588
Fig. 16: Conventional American Approach to Calcium Intake   601
Fig. 17: Balanced Approach to Calcium Intake   603

List of Tables

Table 1: Characteristics of the Addictive System   16–17
Table 2: The Body as a Process vs. Medical World View   23
Table 3: External Guidance: Dominant Cultural View vs.
    Inner Guidance   51–52
Table 4: Energy Anatomy: Mental and Emotional Patterns,
    the Chakras, and the Physical Body   78–79
Table 5: The Anatomy of Women's Wisdom   96–97
Table 6: Comparing Contraceptive Methods   336–37
Table 7: Potential Risk Factors in Childbirth   388
Table 8: Benefits and Risks of Dietary Choices   592
Table 9: Nutritional Approaches for Women   596
Table 10: American Women's Need for, and Consumption
    of, Protein   597
Table 11: High Calcium Foods   604–5

Acknowledgments

Writing this book has been a long and difficult process. I could not have accomplished it without the support, guidance, and influence of many people.

I am grateful to the following people who have been instrumental in providing the structure within which I created this book:

Ned Leavitt, who called me at just the right moment in the Spring of 1990 and suggested that I write a book. Helen Rees, my agent, who intuitively understood this material from our first meeting—long before I had articulated my ideas fully. Leslie Meredith, my editor at Bantam, who believed in the importance of this book's message from the start. Brian Tart, also at Bantam, who provided support and kindness during the editing process. Sandi Gelles-Cole for her ability to refine and provide structure for my ideas. Judy Barrington, medical illustrator extraordinaire, who created the graphics in this book and supported me through the process of illustrating my ideas.

This book and the work that it documents would never have been possible if I had not learned to believe in my ability to create and live my dreams. Gail Straub, David Gershon, and Annie Gill O'Toole were instrumental in helping me do this.

I am grateful for the friendship and writing of Patricia Reis, MFA. Her in-depth work with my patients in the 1980s greatly helped me learn to trust my own intuition. Linda Trichter Metcalf, Ph.D., and Toby Simon, Ph.D., of the Proprioceptive Writing Center helped me find my writer's voice. Writing sessions with Judie Burwell helped me keep it alive. Through all of these individuals, plus the writings of Sonia Johnson, I learned the importance of a feminist perspective.

My colleagues at the Maine Medical Center and Mercy Hospital in Portland, Maine, including doctors, nurses, and supporting staff, have been open and accepting of my ideas for over a decade. The extended medical community in which I practice has provided quality healthcare and congenial support for both me and my patients for years. Dartmouth Medical School gave me excellent training as well as fresh air and pine trees. I especially acknowledge and thank Millard Simmons, M.D. He was (and continues to be, for today's students) a positive role model of an obstetrician/gynecologist who cares deeply for women. He supported my choice of OB/GYN as a career when few others did. I also thank Harriet Northrup, M.D., my aunt, whose presence in my life has borne witness to the history of women in medicine.

Michio Kushi and Annemarie Colbin showed me the importance of whole food in the creation of health. Their teaching gave me the means to change my own eating patterns and help my patients do the same.

My colleagues at the American Holistic Medical Association, including Norman Shealy, M.D., Ph.D., Gladys McGarey, M.D., Robert Anderson, M.D., and Bernie Siegel, M.D., have been role models of leading-edge physicians who have been pioneers in treating the whole patient, not just the patient's disease.

Patti Haladay, Fern Tsao, and Kathy McGonagle have skillfully nurtured my body after long hours of writing. Heidi and John at the Cafe at Fiddlehead Farm provided cheerful and personal service at many breakfasts where Mona Lisa Schulz and I pored over the manuscript.

My associates and staff at Women to Women have helped me co-create an honest and fulfilling way of practicing healthcare as well as working within a group. Thanks to Marcelle Pick, RNC, Mary Ellen Fenn, M.D., Bethany Hays, M.D., Susan Doughty, RNC, and everyone else at Women to Women. Together we keep learning what it means to "walk your talk." For this, along with the guidance of Joe Melnick, Ph.D., I will always be grateful.

For the past two years, Gina Barone has helped me keep the home fires burning as she supplied meals, transportation, help with the children, and friendship. Without her, I could not have completed this project. Before Gina joined us, Donna Mead and Jayne Quintal contributed their skills to keeping the family and household running smoothly and healthfully. My thanks for their presence in my life.

I honor and cherish the personal support and wisdom of Anne Wilson Schaef, whose ideas and friendship have been crucial for my recovery, both personally and professionally. Diane Fassel's sense of humor and perspective have been invaluable during my writing process. I also am grateful to the Wilson Schaef trainees for their honesty and perspective.

Diane Grover has been my nurse for fifteen years and is now the executive director of Women to Women. Her ability to transform ideas into physical reality is truly olympian. I cherish her constant support over the years and look forward to many more.

Brenda King Scheider, childhood friend and colleague, has continued to hold up a mirror and a camera that reflect me in the best light. We share a history and vision that nurtures and delights me. Her friendship has always been a gift in my life. I am especially grateful to have had it during this writing process.

My life has been truly blessed by the brilliance, generosity, and friendship of Caroline Myss, M.A. Her insight and ideas have nourished and inspired me greatly and have added enormously to my understanding of health and disease. I am grateful as well for her sense of humor, irreverence, and insight into the creative process.

Mona Lisa Schulz, M.D., PhD., showed up in my life, like an angel, completely unbidden, and then proceeded to become an invaluable contributor, researcher, graphic designer, inspiration, and friend. Without her rare perspective, research skills, personal presence, medical intuition, and outrageous sense of humor, my writing process would have been dull indeed. This book has been the beginning of what promises to be years of co-creation and research. For that I express great joy and thanks.

I wish to acknowledge the ongoing support, encouragement, and love of my immediate family. During this entire process, my husband Ken has been willing to move from the marriage archetype to the partnership archetype, all the while maintaining both a sense of humor and his own very demanding career. Our relationship has grown and matured through this not-so-easy process. My daughters, Ann and Kate, have enriched my life immeasurably. They have taught me that each child has her own destiny and style and that this must always be respected, regardless of the beliefs of her parents.

I give thanks for my extended family and the early support that set the stage for who I am today. My mother is the physical embodiment of the word strength. Her constant support of me has been a grounding tap root into the center of the Earth. She has been and continues to be a great gift in my life. My father's original thinking, enthusiasm, and approach to healing set the stage for my own life's work. Though no longer physically present, I feel his support daily.

My brothers, John and Bill, and my sisters, Penny and Cindy, have inspired me with their ability to create successful and full lives, despite going against conventional educational wisdom. Each has managed to listen to his or her inner wisdom and live from it.

My father once told me that I would not choose my patients, they would choose me. I am grateful for all the courageous women who chose me as their doctor over the years and helped me learn the material in this book.

Finally, I wish to acknowledge myself and the will that it took to keep on going through re-write after re-write, even long after I thought I was finished. I have learned about surrendering to a power much greater than myself. I have also learned that the power of my personal will and the process of surrender to a greater will are paradoxical and both necessary. Through the process of writing this book, I have reclaimed myself as a scientist and a writer.

Physician, Heal Thyself

*I*n 1981, while I was trying to breast-feed my first child full time and simultaneously work sixty or more hours a week, I developed a severe mastitis that eventually led to the loss of function of my right breast. Instead of taking a day or two off from work at the first sign of infection, which is what I would have told any patient to do, I neglected myself and continued to work, while getting sicker and sicker. I did this because I was torn in two directions. I believed then, and I still believe today, that breast milk is the best food for babies, and I was determined to feed my children optimally. I treated myself with antibodies because I was sure I'd be told to stop nursing if I went to another doctor. At the same time, I knew that women doctors had been accused by our male colleagues of being weak or incapable of pulling our weight, and I didn't want that label. At the time, I was working in a well-respected group OB/GYN practice. At the age of thirty-one I had made it in a male-dominated field of medicine, and I worked among colleagues I respected. I did not want to jeopardize my career path. So I neglected myself and continued working—and I got sicker and sicker.

Though I took medication, my infection was severe enough to be resistant to common antibodies. My condition progressed over several days until one night I began running a high fever and had shaking chills and delirium. During this time, I found out later, the infection was walling off in my body as an abscess deep in my breast. Even then, I went to work and continued to perform my duties.

Being both a mother and a doctor, I felt I had no choice. All my years of training had taught me to put my own needs last.

After several weeks of trying to treat myself, I finally called a surgeon who agreed to meet me in his office after I finished seeing patients (while popping Tylenol with codeine tablets throughout the day to fight off the pain). That same evening I ended up in surgery—the very thing that I had been determined to avoid.

The surgeon told my husband, who is also a doctor, that the abscess cavity under my breast was so large, it was penetrating into my chest wall—the worst he'd seen in thirty years of practice. He didn't know how I had managed to continue working in spite of it. I had ignored the age-old teaching "Physician, heal thyself." I was embarrassed that I had not successfully treated myself as a doctor, that I had myself become an ill person, a patient. I also felt my self-esteem as a mother was threatened if I could not breast-feed. (By this time my milk supply had dwindled significantly anyway from stress.) Yet I remember thinking that night in the hospital that I had to get back to work as soon as possible.

When my second child was born two years later, I assumed that the old damage had healed. Although I'd had to supplement the breast milk for my first child with formula, I figured I wouldn't have to do that again. But no milk could get out of my right breast for my new baby daughter, even though the milk came in on schedule. The prior infection had destroyed the duct structure of that breast. I was again afraid that I would be unable to nurse my baby. I had paid a price with my body for trying to prove myself two years earlier. Though I took full responsibility for this situation, I could see how I had learned to neglect myself. Ignoring my own physical needs and my own body was built right into the fabric of my life.

On the third postpartum day, in the depths of despair about my situation, I called LaLeche League International in Chicago to ask for advice. The woman who answered the phone had had the same problem as I had and informed me that I could nurse from only one side, as long as I nursed more frequently and didn't mind being lopsided! Following her advice, I was able to nurse enough to maintain my milk supply. Though I had to supplement with formula when I was away from my daughter at work, my milk was adequate for her needs whenever I was with her for long periods of time. I will be forever grateful to this grassroots organization of women, which was started in Chicago by a group of homemakers who wanted to nurse their babies in an era when the medical profession was less than supportive. (To this day, most OB/GYN residents are not given a formal course on breast-feeding and are therefore not as knowledgeable as they could be about this important function.)

Although I knew that the breasts are often the physical metaphor for giving, receiving, and nurturing, in my rush to nurture everyone else I had left myself out. My body, however, would not let me get away with my neglectful treatment of it and had communicated an important lesson to me: Our body symptoms have meaning beyond the immediate health problem they are warning us about. Carl Jung said that the gods visit us through illness, and I've come to believe that we can benefit emotionally, physically, and spiritually by paying attention to our body's messages.

While I had always believed this intellectually, to become effective as a healer I had to experience it personally. Only by living through a serious health problem did I become understanding of what other women with health and life problems are living through. As long as I was an overachieving, never-sick white female fully living out of the male-dominant worldview, I was not able to see the patterns that are so commonly associated with women's health problems. As long as I saw myself as separate from other women, I could never understand that these patterns were part of many women's struggles to be whole.

The Personal Is Political

Having babies and struggling to balance my work and my family changed me in ways that nothing else could. Instead of learning from books and professors, I was now learning from direct experience what feminists mean by "the personal is political." I learned that there is no such thing as a part-time mother. Once a woman has a baby, that child is a part of her twenty-four hours a day in ways that no one can explain until it happens to her. I was not prepared for the ache in my heart that occurred when I left my baby to go to work every day. I also began to question my longtime assumption that child care and motherhood were not real work.

I noticed right away that being at work was in many ways infinitely easier than being at home with two young children. I could get so much done! As a good daughter of patriarchy, I worshipped at the altar of efficiency and productivity. I began to rethink why it felt okay to care for other people's bodies but not for my own or my children's. Why did I feel so guilty whenever I rested? Even though I had a lot to do, why did I have trouble getting down on the rug and playing with my children for a half hour? Why did I feel that this was wasting time? I also wondered why this whole childcare thing was considered a women's issue—why were my children primarily *my* worry? My husband and I had had equal educations and equal incomes. Why hadn't his life changed much when the children were born?

As I noticed how my own and other women's well-being is affected by their family life, I had to step back and reassess everything I had ever believed about success, medicine, and myself. Up until my second child's birth, I had never considered myself a feminist. I had always been able to accomplish whatever I'd set my mind to. I didn't know what "those" women were talking about when they spoke of the injustices of society toward women. I didn't know that women and men were treated any differently, because I hadn't experienced (or more accurately, I hadn't noticed) those differences personally.

But my life became unglued when I was a doctor and a mother living in a society that suggests that a woman has to choose between those two roles if she wants to do at least one of them well. Nothing had prepared me for this. Superwoman was dying.

The insights catalyzed by my breast abscess affected not only my beliefs about my own health but my work as a doctor. I began to reassess my beliefs about and understanding of disease. I began to see that the PMS, pelvic pain, chronic vaginitis, and other problems that my patients had were often related to the contexts of their lives. Learning about their diets, work situations, and relationships often provided me with clues to the sources of their bodies' distress. I appreciated the life-patterns behind these conditions in ways that I had never even noticed before.

Over the years, as I developed more sensitivity to these patterns of health and illness in myself and my patients, I came to realize that without a commitment to looking at all aspects of one's life, improving habits and diet alone is not enough to effect a permanent cure for conditions that have been present for a long time. Over the last decade, I've worked with many women whose illnesses cannot be ascribed simply to what they eat and cannot be cured solely through medication or surgery. Following a macrobiotic diet or running three miles a day won't make a woman feel well if she's still living with an active alcoholic or workaholic, or if she has experienced incest and hasn't allowed herself to feel the emotions that are often associated with that history. Trying dietary changes and alternatives to drugs and surgery, however, can be first steps that open women to new ways of looking at their health. With a new outlook on their bodies and themselves, they often begin to heal mentally, emotionally, and spiritually as well as physically. Stories of such healings and spiritual awakenings are found throughout this book.

We can look at the illnesses in these women's stories, like my own breast abscess, as wake-up calls. Though these experiences were painful for the women involved, they brought us back to our bodies and grounded us again in a consciousness of what is important in life. My own illness showed me that my health is a process of balance and that, having ignored my body and inner self for so many years, I would have to look inward for the answers to the questions raised by my own and other women's health problems and challenges. Since Everywoman's problem occurs in part because of the nature of being female in this culture, which programs us to put the needs of others ahead of our own, we need to make radical changes in our minds and lives to get and stay healthy.

Women to Women

Because of these revelations, I left my group practice in 1985, determined to create a practice in which I could incorporate into treating my women patients not only medical care but what I knew about nutrition, lifestyle, and the experience of being female in this culture. Three other women and I decided to open a health care center for women that would value what it meant to be female. We knew there had to be alternatives to the conventional ways of creating health and treating women's health problems. We wanted to do more than just treat symptoms—we wanted to help women change the basic condition of their lives that had led to their health problems. For us, it would not be enough to "privatize" and isolate each woman's situation. We wanted to teach women that their wounding—physical, psychological, and spiritual—is part of a larger cultural wound that potentially affects all of us.

So the four of us—two nurse practitioners and two female OB/ GYNs—founded Women to Women in December 1985 in a small town in Maine. There were no models for what we had set out to do. We wanted to practice within the context of conventional medical care, which does have much to offer. I had watched far too many women make an entire career out of trying to heal a condition by avoiding conventional surgery, which could have been extremely helpful to them in making it easier for the physical body to regain and maintain health. (When a woman focuses too much on healing a condition, she often does so to avoid facing the issues that led to the condition in the first place. Thus, the healing process itself becomes addictive.) But we also wanted to reeducate our patients about health-enhancing behaviors. We all had experienced first-hand the power of thoughts and body symptoms to lead us to healing and to a deeper understanding of our bodies and ourselves. We wanted to lead our patients to this, too. In essence, that is also what I try to do in this book.

Women to Women has been a leap of faith from the beginning. Over the eight years of our practice there, we have learned that it is no small task to change our focus from "what can go wrong" to "what can go right" and to empower women to shift from destructive behaviors to those that are generally associated with health. Over the years we've had to acknowledge how entrenched our own habitual fears and health-destroying patterns have been. Our frustration with our patients' self-destructive habits has lessened as we have come to appreciate that we all shared these same patterns. The four of us found that we had to work on ourselves, on our own behaviors and ways of communicating, to become better caregivers and to keep ourselves open to the practice of medicine as a constant learning process. We worked to break down the hierarchical bar-

riers between ourselves and our patients so that the patients participated in their own healing in conscious ways, such as figuring out
the best diet or combination of holistic treatments. We would not
play Doctor God or Nurse God with them. Starting in 1986, we
enlisted the help of a skilled therapist who helped us be honest with
each other—instead of hiding our true feelings behind the veil of
"niceness" that most of us have been taught—when we would
discuss and decide on our business duties, shifts, on-call time, vacation, time off, and other necessary issues of practice and communication.

Creating Health

During the first five years of Women to Women, we learned that
our original instincts had been correct. The state of a woman's
health is indeed completely tied up with the culture in which she
lives and her position within it, as well as in the way she lives her life
as an individual. Our formal medical training had not acknowledged what now seems obvious to us.

But acknowledging that the cultural context of a woman's life
affects her health is only the first step in creating a new model for
women's wellness. The next step we took was to commit ourselves
to improving women's health by actively changing the circumstances of our and their lives.

In 1991 we formulated a credo for Women to Women: "We are
committed to living, creating, and enjoying health, balance, and
freedom on all levels, personally and professionally, while providing
educational and medical services which assist clients and patients in
using their own power to create the same in their lives." Whenever I
read this credo, my spirit is renewed. It is a vision that doesn't
require perfection. It requires that we do our best, remembering
that no one can fix our lives *for* us. Only we can do this for
ourselves, and we need to set out consciously to do it. I'm not
suggesting it is easy. Each of us needs support and guidance. Women
to Women has been a source of support and guidance for thousands
of women—a place where we tell our stories, heal our wounds, and
go forth to create health in our lives. And it is my goal that *Women's
Bodies, Women's Wisdom* also be a source of support and guidance,

as it presents healing stories of women who have been patients, colleagues, family, and friends. These women have found their voices and begun to heal and create health daily in their lives. Together these women are part of the greater women's consciousness—giving voice to our real identity and needs and reclaiming femininity and being female in our own way.

These stories are told in women's own words and images and depict women's often individually created but collectively valuable rituals. Most of the women are composite portraits. Though based on real people, their names and other identifying details of their stories have been changed. I hope that by reading these stories, you will be inspired to remember your own life history—not just your medical history—and will reflect on it in a new way. I hope that you will also be moved to write down your life and medical history—to see what patterns emerge, what links there are between the two. By examining, "naming," and then "reclaiming" your life, you too can heal.

You will also learn from these stories how to listen to your own body and trust its wisdom so that you can grow into wellness physically and spiritually. Medically speaking, this book addresses women's health issues, the care of our female systems and organs. I explore the diseases, discomforts, and dysfunctions of all the female systems and give suggestions on how to heal them. But beyond this explicit medical focus and advice, the most important guidance I hope to present—with the help of my advisers, my colleagues, and most of all my patients' examples—includes information that speaks to women's "insides." I want to awaken that still, small, wise intuitive voice in all of us, that voice of our own body that we have been forced to ignore through our culture's illness, misinformation, and dysfunction.

I've come to see that we're all in this together, and that women everywhere are birthing a new vision of women's health and wellness—and of identity. Central to this vision is that we trust what we know in our bones: that our bodies are our allies, and that they will always point us in the direction we need to go next.

May this book be a source of guidance, information, and support in your own healing journey.

PART ONE

From External
Control to
Inner Guidance

ONE

The Patriarchal Myth and the Addictive System

C onsciousness creates the body. Our bodies are made up of dynamic energy systems that are affected by our diets, relationships, heredity, and culture and the interplay of all these factors and activities. We're not even close to understanding how our bodily systems interact with each other, let alone how they interact with other people's. Yet over almost two decades of my practice, it has become clear to me that healing cannot occur for women until we have critically examined and changed some of the beliefs and assumptions that we all unconsciously inherit and internalize from our culture. We cannot hope to reclaim our bodily wisdom and inherent ability to create health without first understanding the influence of our society on how we think about and care for our bodies.

Our Cultural Inheritance

Western civilization has rested for the last five thousand years on the mythology of patriarchy, the authority of men and fathers. If, as Jamake Highwater says, "All human beliefs and activities spring from an underlying mythology," then it is easy to make the connection that if our culture is totally "ruled by the father," our view of our female bodies and even our medical system also follows male-oriented rules.[1] Yet patriarchy is only one of many systems of social organization.

Even so, we will not be able to create another kind of social organization until we heal ourselves in our own culture. I have been in the delivery room countless times when a female baby is born and the woman who has just given birth looks up at her husband and says "Honey, I'm sorry"—apologizing because the baby is not a son! The self-rejection of the mother herself, apologizing for the product of her own nine-month gestation period, labor, and delivery, is staggering to experience. Yet when my own second daughter was born, I was shocked to hear those very words of apology to my husband come right up into my brain from the collective unconscious of the human race. I never said them out loud, and yet they were there in my head—completely unbidden. I realized then how old and ingrained is this rejection of the female by men and women alike!

Our culture gives girls the message that their bodies, their lives, and their femaleness demand an apology. Have you noticed how often women apologize? I was walking down the street recently when a man ran into a woman who was walking by, causing her to drop a package. *She* apologized profusely. Somewhere deep inside many of us is an apology for our very existence. As Anne Wilson Schaef writes, "The original sin of being born female is not redeemable by works."[2] No matter how many degrees you get in college, no matter how many awards you earn, somehow you can never measure up. If we must apologize for our very existence from the day we are born, we can assume that our society's medical system will deny us the wisdom of our "second-class" bodies. In essence, patriarchy blares out the message that women's bodies are inferior and must be controlled.

Our culture habitually denies the insidiousness and pervasiveness of sex-related issues. I first learned in my medical practice that abuse against women is epidemic, whether subtle or overt. And I saw how abuse sets the stage for illness in our female bodies. Consider the following: A study by Dr. Gloria Bachmann estimates that up to 38 percent of adult women in the United States have been sexually abused as children. Because failure to report abuse is common, only 20 to 50 percent of these incidents ever come to the attention of authorities, so the percentage may be even higher. The FBI estimates that a woman living in the United States has a one-in-three chance of being raped in her lifetime, and 50 percent of all married women will be battered at least once in their marriages. The research of Dr. Leah Dickstein has documented that spousal abuse is the cause for one out of two suicide attempts among black women and one of four suicide attempts among white women. Research done by World Watch Institute's Lori Hesse points out that throughout the world, four times as many girls die of malnutrition as boys because food is given preferentially to boys. According to the United Nations Report on the Status of Women, women do two-thirds of the world's work for one-tenth of the world's wages, yet they own less than one one-hundredth of the world's property. The landmark study of gender bias in American schools by the American Association of University Women confirmed an earlier report by the Sadkers that compared to girls, boys are five times as likely to receive the most attention from teachers and eight times as likely to call out in class.[3]

Patriarchy Results in Addiction

The Judeo-Christian cosmology that informs Western civilization sees the female body and female sexuality in the person of Eve as responsible for the downfall of *man*kind. For thousands of years, women have been beaten, abused, burned at the stake, and blamed for all manner of evil simply because of their sex. We forget, in this era of rapid change, that women did not even win the right to vote until 1920!

In 1953 in her book *The Second Sex* Simone de Beauvoir wrote, "Man enjoys the great advantage of having a god endorse the code he writes. And since man exercises a sovereign authority over women it is especially fortunate that this authority has been vested in him by the Supreme Being. For the Jews, Mohammedans, and Christians among others, man is master by divine right; the fear of God will therefore repress any impulse towards revolt in the down-trodden female."[4] The belief that men are meant to be rulers of women runs deep in many Western traditions.

The patriarchal organization of our society demands that women, its second-class citizens, ignore or turn away from their hopes and dreams in deference to men and the demands of their families. This systematic stuffing or denying of our needs for self-expression and self-actualization causes us enormous emotional pain. To stay out of touch with our pain, women have commonly used addictive substances and developed addictive behaviors that have resulted in an endless cycle of abuse that we ourselves help perpetuate. Being abused or abusing ourselves, we become ill. When we become ill, we are treated by a patriarchal medical system that denigrates our bodies. Many of us are not given good medical care or even the same medical care that men receive for the same illnesses. So we often become sicker or develop chronic health problems, for which the medical establishment has no answers or treatments. This is the cycle that characterizes our current medical care.

Anne Wilson Schaef writes that "anything can be used addictively, whether it be substance (like alcohol) or a process (like work). This is because the purpose or function of an addiction is to put a buffer between ourselves and our awareness of our feelings. An addiction serves to numb us so that we are out of touch with what we know and what we feel."[5] Yet the good news is that when we acknowledge and release our emotional pain, we are put *immediately* in touch with our feelings, which can act as our inner guidance system. Clearly, we need a new kind of medical attitude and wisdom that helps put us in touch with our inner pain as the first step toward healing.

Seeing the connection between addiction and patriarchy has been key in my understanding of the patterns behind women's major health problems. The word *patriarchy*, unfortunately, is usually accompanied by blaming men, but blame is one of the key behaviors that keeps people stuck in systems that harm them. Neither women, nor men, nor society as a whole can move on and heal as long as one sex blames the other. We have to decide to move on, to leave blame behind us. Both men and women perpetuate the system in which we live with our daily addictive behaviors and attitudes. By renaming patriarchy the addictive system, Schaef has advanced our understanding of society's problems dramatically.[6] She demonstrates that the way our society functions is harmful to both men and women and that *both* genders participate fully in this system. I am grateful to her for her insights, on which I draw throughout this book. Renaming patriarchy the addictive system and seeing the ways in which this system is harmful to both men and women in no way undermines the importance of feminism and its insights. (See the Steps for Healing in Chapter 15.) I favor Sonia Johnson's definition of *feminism* because it contains a vision of healing within it: "Feminism is the articulation of the ancient, underground culture and philosophy based on the values that patriarchy has labeled 'womanly' but which are necessary for full humanity. Among the principles and values of feminism that are most distinct from those of patriarchy are universal equality, non-violent problem-solving, and cooperation with nature, one another, and other species."[7]

Fundamental Beliefs of the Addictive System

I encourage you to try to get a handle on how you participate in the addictive society. As you become more conscious of your own role in this feedback loop, both your health as an individual and our health as a society will improve. See if the following descriptions of our cultural attitudes toward women and health ring true for you. They may help you become more conscious of your own body and health issues.

Belief One: Disease Is the Enemy

Addictive systems have been properly described as societies that are either preparing for war or recovering from war. Such societies elevate the values of destruction and violence over values of nurturing and peace. We have only to look at what our society spends on defense to see where its values lie, since the amount of money this society spends on something is a measure of its worth in that society. The amount spent on weapons every minute could feed two thousand malnourished children for a year, while the price of one military tank could provide classrooms for thirty thousand students.[8]

As a result, the medical establishment describes our bodies not as natural systems homeostatically designed to tend toward health but rather as war zones. Military metaphors run rampant through the language of Western medical care. The disease or tumor is "the enemy," to be eliminated at all costs. It is rarely, if ever seen as a messenger trying to get our attention. Even the immune system, which works to keep us in balance, is described in militaristic terms, with its "killer" T-cells. Recently, at a conference on a tumor in our center, one of the radiologists said, "The previous bullets we've fired at that area [the pelvis, in this case] have failed to sterilize it from disease."

I believe that the modern medical preference for drugs and surgery as treatments is part of the aggressive patriarchal or addictive approach to disease. That which is natural and nontoxic is seen as inferior to the "big guns" of drugs, chemotherapy, and radiation. Drug-free, natural methods of treatment with well-studied, well-documented benefits, such as therapeutic touch, are ignored.[9] Treatments that offer complementary care are denigrated. Studies that demonstrate their worth are ignored as well. A classic example of a disregarded study—and there are many—is one on the effects of prayer. This study was truly double-blind: neither the doctors, the nurses, nor the patients knew who was being prayed for. But the patients in a coronary intensive care unit who were prayed for by a group who didn't know who they were praying for were far less likely to go into heart failure, need cardiopulmonary resuscitation (CPR), need artificial breathing (endotracheal intubation), develop infection or pneumonia, or require diuretics than the patients in the unit who were not prayed for.[10]

If a drug had shown an effect this striking, it would be considered unethical not to use it. Given these benefits and the total absence of side effects of prayers, a true scientist would be fascinated with this data and want to study the effects even further. Yet when Dr. Bernie Siegel posted this paper on the bulletin board in the doctor's lounge of his hospital, within a few hours a colleague had written "BULL-SHIT" across the front page!

The addictive system considers the body to be subordinate to the brain and its dictates of reason. It often teaches us to ignore fatigue, hunger, discomfort, or our need for caring and nurturing. It conditions us to see the body as an adversary, particularly when giving us messages that we don't want to hear. The culture often tries to kill the body-as-messenger along with its message. Yet our own body is the best health system we have—if we know how to listen to it.

Belief Two: Medical Science Is Omnipotent

We have been taught that our disease-care system is supposed to keep us healthy. We have been socialized to turn to doctors whenever we have concerns about our bodies and our health. We have been taught the myth of the medical gods—that doctors know more than we do about our bodies, that the expert holds the cure. It's no wonder that when I ask women to tell me what's going on in their bodies, they sometimes reply, "You tell me—you're the doctor!" Doctors are authority figures for some women, right up there with their husbands and priests. Yet each woman is more knowledgeable about herself than anyone else.

Women's ambivalence toward our bodies and our own judgment takes a toll on us psychologically. As one woman said to me recently, "I don't trust doctors. I don't like medicine. Yet I'm obsessed with them and am always drawn to looking at what's wrong with me. I go to a lot of doctors looking for answers, then I'm angry when they offer only drugs or surgery." Other women, when they are offered alternatives, reject them, firmly believing that only drugs or surgery will help. Either way, most women are trained to look outside themselves for answers because we live in a society in which so-called experts challenge and subordinate our own judgment and in which our ability to heal or stay healthy without constant outside help is not honored, encouraged, or even recognized.

As a physician, I was trained to be paternalistic, the all-knowing outside expert. The public, in turn, is conditioned to believe that doctors are the paragons for healthy behavior. My patients routinely expect, for example, that I will yell at them if they miss an annual Pap smear—something I've occasionally done myself! According to a report from the University of California, 50 percent of doctors do not have a personal physician—something that all doctors advocate for their patients. Twenty percent don't exercise, only 7 percent believe that they drink "too much" alcohol, and 50 percent of female physicians don't even do monthly breast self-exams![11] Yet people regularly give control of their health over to these imperfect models of unhealthy living.

Medicine itself has a very pathological focus. Scientists rarely study healthy people, and when people with chronic or terminal conditions manage to recover completely, defying the statistical medical prognosis, health professionals too often think that their initial diagnosis must have been wrong, instead of investigating why these people have done so well.[12] In medical school, I practiced on sick or dead people. I was trained in what could go wrong. I was taught to anticipate everything that could possibly go wrong and to plan for it. As an OB/GYN, I was taught that the normal process of labor and delivery was a "retrospective diagnosis" and that it could randomly become a disaster at any moment without warning. When this kind of training goes unquestioned by doctors, it creates self-fulfilling prophecies that lead to a high rate of forceps and cesarean deliveries.

Our culture and its addictive medical system believe that technology and testing will save us, that it is possible to control and quantify every variable, and that if we just had more data from more studies, we'd be able to improve our health, cure diseases, and live happily ever after. Americans and their doctors equate doing more with improving care. We also believe that we can "buy" an answer by throwing money at it. Again, we ignore or don't trust our inner guidance system and our own healing ability.

Physicians order lots of tests because they are uneasy about being uncertain. They are taught to behave as if it were intolerable to be uncertain. The more information physicians get, the more confidence they feel in the validity of their diagnoses, even when their confidence in the information is not justified. Health care consumers, for their part, are just as uncomfortable with uncertainty as their doctors are. They want to know things in absolute ways. When people ask me about genital herpes, for instance, they want to know "How did I get it?" "How do I know I won't give it to anyone else?" These questions are essentially unanswerable with absolute certainty.

Belief Three: The Female Body Is Abnormal

Because being male is considered the norm in the addictive system, most women internalize the idea that something is basically "wrong" with their bodies. They are led to believe that they must control many aspects of their bodies and that their natural odors and shapes are simply unacceptable. Women are socialized to think that their bodies are essentially dirty—requiring constant surveillance for "freshness" so that we don't "offend." Females naturally have more body fat than men, and because of better nutrition than in past decades, women today are also bigger than were their mothers and grandmothers. Yet the average fashion model, our cultural ideal, weighs 17 percent less than the average American woman. No wonder anorexia nervosa and bulimia are ten times more common in females than in males and are on the rise.[13]

This denigration of the female body has made many women either afraid of their bodies and their natural processes or else disgusted by them. Many never touch or get to know what their breasts feel like, for instance, because they're afraid of what they might find. They may feel guilty for touching them, equating this with masturbation, since breasts are erotic for men—another sign of how thoroughly we have turned our bodies over to men.

Health practitioners and women alike view even normal bodily functions such as menstruation, menopause, and childbirth as medical conditions requiring treatment. The attitude that our bodies are accidents waiting to happen seems to get internalized at a young age and sets the stage for women's future relationships with their bodies. Given what we are taught, it is no wonder that most of us feel ill prepared to deal with and trust ourselves. Our bodies have been "medicalized" since before we were born!

Our culture fears all natural processes: birthing, dying, healing, living. Daily, we are taught to be afraid. When my daughter was seven, she was out with her father chopping down some brush in our back yard. Suddenly she started to cry and came running into the house with a bleeding finger. She had cut herself on a blade of grass. As I calmly held her finger under some cold water and saw that it was only a tiny cut, she looked up at me and uttered what I consider a major healing principle: "It didn't hurt until I got scared."

Because our culture worships science and believes that it is "objective," we think that everything labeled "scientific" must be true. We believe that science will save us. But science as it is currently practiced is a cultural construct rife with all the biases of the addictive system in general. There is actually no such thing as completely objective data. Cultural bias determines which studies we believe and which we ignore. No one is immune to this behavior. We all have our sacred cows. A presenter at a medical conference once said,

"The human mind is an organ uniquely designed to create anti-bodies against new ideas."

Many procedures routinely performed on women's bodies in particular are not based on scientific data at all but are rooted in prejudice against the body's innate wisdom and healing power. Many procedures have their origins in emotional views of women handed down from previous generations. Routine episiotomies at delivery (cutting the tissue between the vagina and the rectum, which allegedly makes more room for the baby's head) are an example. Recent studies have shown that episiotomies increase blood loss, pain, and risk of long-term pelvic floor damage, something midwives have been saying for years. Episiotomy was and often still is done at delivery simply because obstetricians who do it are certain it *protects* the pelvic floor from injury. Obstetricians have only recently started to question the advisability of this routine procedure, as studies have shown that it is not helpful and can even be harmful.[14]

Reclaiming Our Own Authority

While true science is based on observation, experimentation, and continuous readjustment of thought processes and beliefs depending upon its empirical findings, the same is true for trusting our inner guidance. Ultimately, I've found it enormously empowering to realize that no scientific study can explain exactly how and why my own particular body acts the way it does. Only our connection with our own inner guidance and our emotions are reliable in the end. That is because we each comprise a multitude of processes that have never existed before and never will again. Science must acknowledge truthfully how much it doesn't know and leave room for mystery, miracles, and the wisdom of nature.

My father used to say, "Feelings are facts. Pay attention to them." Yet in my scientific training I quickly learned that feelings, intuition, spirituality, and all experiences of life that cannot be explained by the logical, rational parts of our minds or measured by our five senses are ignored or discounted. The addictive system fears emotional responses and highly values the control of emotions because it is so out of touch with them. Female bodies, long associated with cycles and subject to the ebb and flow of natural rhythms, are seen as especially emotional and in need of management. Our entire society functions in ways that keep us out of touch with what we know and feel.

In an addictive system, people in general and women especially are put on the defensive and act negatively. When I'm examining a pregnant woman and her blood sugar test comes back elevated, for example, she will almost invariably become very defensive about her eating habits. She will usually deny that she has consumed any nonnutritious or sweet foods at all, because she's ashamed that she's been "caught" sneaking sweets: a common enough impulse that pregnant women have. She gets defensive and feels that her body has betrayed her through her blood sugar. In order to educate her about how to give herself and her baby good nutrition and how to substitute healthy foods for junk, I first have to get through her defensiveness, which takes up time and energy that could be better spent in addressing her overall health.

Remaining unconscious about our acculturated habits takes an enormous emotional and physical toll on our bodies and spirits. These habits keep us from being connected with our inner guidance and our emotions. This disconnection, in turn, keeps us in a state of pain that increases the longer we deny it. It takes a lot of energy to stay out of touch with this pain, and we often turn to acculturated habits, such as addictive substances, to keep us from confronting that unhappiness and pain.

Almost everyone understands that physical destruction results from abusing alcohol and drugs. Fifty percent of the cases that my husband, an orthopedic surgeon, sees in the emergency room are related to alcohol abuse. As one of our staff surgeons says, "If it weren't for cigarettes and alcohol, I'd be out of a job!" What many people don't appreciate, however, is the enormous, and equally deadly toll taken by compulsive behaviors like overwork and over-eating, used to avoid or deny one's feelings.

Sexual and relationship addictions have gynecological implica-tions and result in the epidemics of sexually transmitted diseases, such as venereal warts, herpes, and cervical cancer. One of my patients was married to a recovering alcoholic and was suffering from chronic vaginitis, for which I could find no cause. She finally came to the realization that her husband had been "medicating himself through sex with me every day for years. I saw that my body was his bottle—he was using it and sex the same way he had used alcohol, and I thought it was my duty as a wife to comply."

My experiences in my own practice have led me to believe that health promotion and education won't do a thing to decrease health care expenses unless we as a society acknowledge the enormity of our own addictive behaviors and the personal pain hidden behind them. Only then can we begin to participate in our own recovery and create health. Every overweight woman I know is clear about what she "should" eat. She doesn't need more nutrition information. She needs first to *feel* the pain that the excess food is chronically pushing down. This can only happen when she takes control of her own health and allows her own inner guidance to prevail—when she learns, in essence, to trust her own body's wisdom.

The Power of Naming

A first step toward making a positive change in your life or your health is to name your current experience and allow yourself to feel it fully, emotionally, spiritually, and physically. Back in the 1980s, it was crucial for me to name my relationship addiction. Before I did so and began to make contact with my own inner guidance, I looked to others to affirm me and tell me that I was okay. I took their cues for how to act, feel, and look, and I was always seeing myself in terms of other people. I believed that if I said no to someone who needed me, I wouldn't be valued or loved.

I came to see that my tendency to rescue people in need, my acquiescence to others, and my saying yes to everyone came out of my attempt to exercise a form of control: I believed that if I said yes, I would earn their love. This wasn't good either for me or for them, since by putting myself in the position of being someone's rescuer, a substitute for their own higher power or inner guidance, I allowed them to remain out of touch with their own strengths. My behavior actually helped to create victims who needed me. Now, I can see and name this behavior as a relationship addiction. Now, when someone says they need me, I wait, check out the situation, and see what my inner guidance tells me before I decide how to respond.

One of the most common characteristics of people in our addictive society is dependency. "Dependency is a state in which you assume that someone or something outside you will take care of you because you cannot take care of yourself," writes Schaef. "Dependent persons rely on others to meet their emotional, psychological, intellectual, and spiritual needs."[15] For centuries women have relied on men to meet their economic needs (not that they were given much choice, since they were owned like property for centuries), while men have relied on women to meet their emotional needs. As one patient of mine said about her former marriage, "Our agreement was, he would make the money and I would do the emotions." Clarissa Pinkola Estes points out that one of the reasons women have not been more in touch with their creative instincts is that they have spent so much time succoring others who have been at war— either on the battlefield or in corporate America.[16]

The problem with this way of relating to others is that it prevents true intimacy. Intimacy can only take place in a partnership relationship, not one based on intersecting dependencies. My parents once cautioned me, "If a man ever says, 'I need you,' run the other way." It's good advice.

Naming the addictive characteristics in our daily life offers us a way out of the culturally induced trance that affects all women— the culture's definition of what it means to be a "good" woman as one who meets everyone's needs but her own. When you name an experience intellectually, be aware of how that experience feels in your body. Allow yourself to feel it physically. Otherwise, your own behavior—and your health—will not change. *Once an experience is consciously named and internalized, physically and emotionally, it can no longer influence us unconsciously.* We then begin to see how we have been influencing and perpetuating our own problems. Naming something that has affected us adversely is part of freeing ourselves from its continued influence. Many times healing cannot begin until we allow ourselves to *feel how bad things are* (or were in the past). Doing this frees emotional and physical energy that has been stuffed, stuck, denied, or ignored for many years. When we can allow ourselves to feel exactly how we feel without judgment, we begin to free our energy. Only then can we move toward what we want. Table 1 can help you name your addictive characteristics.

TABLE 1
CHARACTERISTICS OF THE ADDICTIVE SYSTEM

Characteristic	Definition	Examples
Blame	Believing that someone or something outside of yourself is the cause of whatever is happening to you	"I can't help the way I am. My mother was an alcoholic." "I married a man who is completely incapable of having an intimate relationship."
Denial	Being out of touch with your feelings, needs, or other information	"My parents weren't alcoholics, they were heavy social drinkers." "There's a fine line between drinking too much and being an alcoholic." "I don't know why I've gained 20 pounds. I never eat a thing that isn't healthy."
Confusion	Lacking clarity about a situation or your emotions	"Nobody ever tells me anything." "I never know what's going on around here."
Forgetfulness	Putting out of your mind, ceasing to notice	Forgetting appointments, car keys, personal belongings, bodily needs.
The Scarcity Model (Zero-Sum Model)	Believing that there's a limited amount of everything that's desirable: love, money, men, happiness	"If I am successful, someone else has to suffer." "It is not okay to acknowledge spending time or money on oneself."
Perfectionism	Having an extreme need for external order to cover internal chaos	Relentless pursuit of a perfect body, home, mate, job.

Characteristic	Definition	Examples
The Illusion of Control or Objectivity	Fearing your needs and feelings, and creating an illusion that you can somehow control yourself; separating yourself from your emotions, and believing that it is possible to be completely objective and unemotional	"If I could find the right drug, I could get rid of these panic attacks." "Premenstrually I become a different person. I'm like Dr. Jekyll and Mr. Hyde. I'm not myself." "The ozone level is high today. Please stay inside."
Negativism	Seeing life from a lackful viewpoint	"I always catch whatever is going around." "Now that I'm forty, everything is starting to fall apart." "You can't have that, it costs too much."
Dependency	Believing that someone or something outside of you will take care of you because you can't do it for yourself	"I can't leave my husband. Who would support me?" "I can't live without him."
Crisis Orientation	Using and creating an external crisis as a socially acceptable way to distract yourself from your feelings	"There's no question that we really look forward to the next multiple trauma. It gets the juices flowing." —Emergency Room Nurse
Defensiveness	Being unable to accept feedback and make positive adjustments	"Who are you to tell me that my PMS is related to my family? My childhood was perfect."
Dishonesty	Not telling the truth	"Do I need a break? No, I'm fine." "It wasn't that bad. I can handle it."
Dualistic Thinking	Believing that there are only two choices: one is right or good, the other is wrong or bad	"Vitamins and herbs are good. Drugs and surgery are bad."

Sources: Anne Wilson Schaef, *When Society Becomes an Addict* (New York: Harper and Row, 1987), p. 72; Anne Wilson Schaef and Diane Fassel, *The Addictive Organization* (New York: Harper and Row, 1988).

One of my patients had a chronic and painful vaginal and vulvar herpes condition that didn't respond to conventional drug therapy or even to alternatives such as dietary changes. After three years of unsuccessfully searching for a way to stop her recurrent outbreaks, she came to the following conclusion: "Maybe I just need to walk around for a while saying that my vagina hurts. I was never able to say that to my mother when I was little." From the moment she spoke this truth out loud, she began to heal. She told me that her father had sexually abused her for years and her mother hadn't believed her. Layer by layer, she began to uncover her wounds, name them, and heal. With great compassion for herself, she acknowledged the pain of her past and moved beyond judgment of herself and her parents. As she did this, her pain gradually decreased while her creative life as a writer began to blossom. Today, she no longer has herpes outbreaks.

Naming our society the addictive system and naming our behaviors within this system as addictions have been a major force for creating health both in my own life and in the lives of my patients.[17] The addictive system in general could not continue if enough people came to understand how it operates in their lives, named it, and then changed their behaviors accordingly. The addictive system as a whole operates with the same characteristics as each individual within the system. Thus, the addict mirrors the system and the system mirrors the addict.[18] I notice addictive system characteristics in myself, in my patients, at my workplace, and in my profession. But the degree to which one notices these characteristics within oneself, names them, then chooses to change this behavior is the degree to which she is healthy. As individuals do this work, society as a whole can become healthier.

If I hadn't created a life in which my family, colleagues, and loved ones shared this view, I'd forgo my personal needs regularly and burn out because of what I call my relationship addiction—what society calls being a good person (or doctor, mother, nurse, wife, or sister). I have surrounded myself with business colleagues and friends who are themselves committed to living in balance. We run our office with the intent that everyone takes responsibility for her own feelings and her own life—giving and receiving support as they need it. That means that my colleagues call my attention to behavior that is destructive—for instance, when I am being dishonest in saying I'm willing to be on call on a holiday (just to be nice) when I've already made personal plans to be away.

Part of creating health is allowing others to go through their own learning processes. No one can create health for another person. I have realized that I don't have the answers for everyone—and neither does anyone else. Only the individual herself can gain access to her inner guidance when she is ready. After years of feeling that I was responsible for having all the answers for others at the expense of myself, I no longer try to convince anyone of anything.

Many women are not in jobs and families that fully support their health. But if enough of us learn to value ourselves deeply, name our addictive behaviors, and commit to living our lives fully and joyfully, our jobs and circumstances will begin to change. Thoughts and consciousness influence our personal lives profoundly.

Naming and Healing Emotional Pain and Its Physical Consequences

Our emotions and thoughts have such profound effects on us because they are physically linked to our bodies via our immune, endocrine, and central nervous systems. All emotions, even those that are suppressed and unexpressed, have physical effects. Unexpressed emotions tend to "stay" in the body like small ticking time bombs—they are illnesses in incubation.

A culture that is unsupportive of women sets the stage early on for health problems because the context of a woman's life contributes greatly to the state of her health. Millions of women suffer from chronic pelvic pain, vaginitis, ovarian cysts, genital warts, endometriosis, and cervical dysplasia (or, abnormal cells caught by a Pap smear)—all diseases of organs that are unique to females. These conditions are the language through which our bodies speak to us. Through these our bodies are telling us that we need to heal from a deeper, often unconscious wounding—that we are never enough and that we are somehow tainted.

A forty-one-year-old executive came to see me because she was having uncomfortable hot flashes. She was on four times the normal dose of estrogen and was still getting no relief. In addition to being related to decreased estrogen levels, hot flashes are a neuroendocrine problem and increase with stress. When a woman feels that she is under stress, the frequency and severity of her hot flashes increases both objectively and subjectively. My patient had already had a hysterectomy and removal of her ovaries for uncontrollable pelvic pain as a result of severe endometriosis two years before. Now she seemed beyond relief. It took this patient two years to tell me that when she was six, she had been sexually molested in the basement of a candy store by the man who ran the store. While this was happening to her, she had felt frozen, unable to speak. She said, "I just went numb. He told me never to tell anyone, because if I did they'd never like me. I felt completely ashamed." On the day she did tell me, she still felt that she had done something wrong and that she was bad. She later said that she drove away from the office certain that once I knew the truth about her, I'd never like her again.

My patient attributes her medical history to this abuse as a child. Her pain got worse and worse into her adult life until she had her hysterectomy. The hysterectomy was actually a blessing for her, she later told me, because it was the beginning of her inner journey and deeper healing. The body often tries to bring our attention back to the "scene of the crime" to help us heal it.

This patient, trying to redeem "the original sin of being female" and the emotional pain that stemmed from it, had continually worked two jobs since high school and earned an MBA, and she is very successful in her work. She had used work, constant striving, and earning more degrees as a way to "prove herself" and to stay out of touch with that early emotional pain and feeling that she was unworthy and bad. Her beliefs stemmed directly from the addictive system and were reinforced by it. She still hasn't been able to shed a tear about her experience, an emotional release that I feel will help her once she's ready.

I agree with my patient that the seeds for her physical problems were planted by her emotional traumas. I am not saying that her childhood sexual abuse "caused" the endometriosis or chronic pelvic pain. What I am suggesting is that her early abuse, common to so many of my patients, set a pattern of discomfort in her bodymind. And the only way for her to begin her healing was to go back to the experience and expiate it, exorcise it from her life experience.

Only by tuning in to how we feel in our bodies can we appreciate our inner guidance. Yet we look to our schools to tell us what is worth learning, our governments to take care of our communities, and our doctors to immunize us against the latest germ. We learn that we will be okay if we follow the rules. One of our patients who recently developed vulvar cancer said, "I can't understand how this happened. I've come in for an exam every year, had normal Pap smears, and yet I still got cancer." Like this patient, we often believe that the tests themselves will prevent us from getting ill.

In first grade my daughter was told on the first day of school what were the acceptable times for students to go to the bathroom. I went in and told her teacher that in my practice I regularly see adult women with constipation and urinary problems who cannot move their bowels in public rest rooms because early "rules" from home and school like these had damaged their ability to know when their bodies need to perform a normal function. I didn't want this to happen to my daughter. I made sure she heard my conversation with her teacher so that she felt supported in going to the bathroom when she needed to go.

Healing Means Leaving Wounding Behind

We can't make a new world for ourselves as long as the addictive system lives within us. If we fail to notice the ways in which we daily cooperate with the system that's destroying us, we're in danger of operating out of the perpetual victim mode, always blaming someone "out there" for our problems. Much like the battered woman who finally gets out because one day she realizes that if she stays she will die, each of us must recognize when and where we're cooperating with our own oppression.

One of my friends who was brought up Catholic in the 1950s describes the effect of confession on her body. "I remember having to go to confession," she says, "beginning at age seven, searching my conscience for crimes and misdemeanors, feeling caught in the horrible dilemma of being unable to speak the unspeakable—about sexual wonderings, masturbation—who had the language for that? And were girls even capable of it? Was I the only one in this dilemma? It was suggested on a plastic card that guided the confessional process that these failings fall into the category of 'impure thoughts and deeds.' Even given this sanitized version, I could not confess to some man, semivisible behind the confessional grill, whose breath smelled of cigarettes and alcohol, the sensual dimensions of myself. Without a complete confession, however, you were not allowed to take Holy Communion, or if you did, you would be condemned to hell, with a mortal sin on your soul. (They sort of had you coming and going.) This was my first encounter with an ethical dilemma.

"And so I unconsciously and ingeniously devised a way out. When I was at the entry of adolescence, around age eleven, I began systematically to faint during mass, right before communion. I had to be carried out of church, and there on the entryway steps I remember being able to breathe, to hear the birds and feel the sun. This went on for over a year. I had no control over these fainting sessions. I was embarrassed by them and bewildered by what my body was doing—cold sweats, ringing in my ears, and the inevitable blackness closing in on me. (I have ever since felt oppressed in the confines of a church.) The intolerable and contradictory demands simply knocked me unconscious."[19]

Many women have been knocked unconscious by the conflicting demands of our culture. And many of us are waking up to it. Healing from conditions such as pelvic pain, PMS, and chronic fatigue syndrome from taking care of too many people is almost always enhanced when we realize that we are not alone in our suffering and that our problems occur in a cultural context that is often unsupportive to us. Recovery of our health and then learning to create health on a daily basis involves naming our experiences for what they are—no matter how painful—and then learning that the motor for our lives is within us, regardless of our past.

Though it is extremely helpful to have a physician or health care provider who acknowledges the mind/body connection, it is even more important that we ourselves appreciate that our bodies and their symptoms are part of our inner guidance. We can free ourselves from our overdependence on the medical system by seeing the ways in which our own beliefs and behavior perpetuate the parts of this system that do not help us create health. If we ourselves persist in thinking that our diseases and symptoms such as endometriosis, fibroids, and PMS are "just medical" and not related to the other parts of our lives, we are participating in and thus perpetuating the addictive system in medical care.

TABLE 2

The Body as a Process	Medical World View
The female body reflects nature and earth.	The female body and its processes are uncontrollable and unreliable. They require external control.
Thoughts and emotions are mediated via the immune, endocrine, and nervous systems. They are biochemical events.	Thoughts and emotions are entirely separate from the physical body.
The physical, emotional, spiritual, and psychological aspects of an individual are intimately intertwined and cannot be separated.	It is possible to separate an individual into entirely separate, unrelated compartments.
Illness is part of the inner guidance system.	Illness is a random event that just happens. There is very little a woman can do to prevent illness.
The body creates health daily. It is inherently self-healing.	The body is always vulnerable to germs, disease and decay.
Illness is best prevented by living fully according to one's inner guidance while creating health daily.	Illness prevention is not possible in this system. So-called prevention is really disease screening.
Concerned with living fully. Focuses on what is going well without denying death.	Concerned with avoiding death at all costs. Focuses only on what can go wrong.
Our true selves don't die.	Death is seen as failure and final.

On the other hand, when we learn how to tune in to the language of our bodies, we're more able to make informed decisions about medical testing and technology, which can lead to more satisfactory relationships with our health care providers. We must begin to trust ourselves and our experience as much as we trust laboratory data. One of my patients who had very infrequent periods came to see that she always got a period whenever she was "in love." She came to trust that she didn't need a lot of hormonal testing every time her period ceased for several months. Instead, she became interested in the meaning behind those periods and what emotions were associated with them. Working in partnership with such women is a true joy for me and for their other physicians as well. Both doctor and patient acknowledge our areas of expertise, our areas of ignorance, and the unknown that lies beyond.

As you read this book, remember that we all have choices—and we all have inner guidance and spiritual help available that can help us move toward optimal health, joy, and fulfillment. Recovery from the addictive system means learning to live fully from the inside out in a culture that often negates this way of being in the world. Our bodies and their symptoms are our biggest allies in this endeavor, because nothing gets our attention as quickly. Our bodies are a wonderful barometer of how well we're living in the present and taking care of ourselves.

Germaine Greer recently said in an interview about her book, *The Change,* "Nobody knows what a well woman would look like. How can you treat women if you don't know what femaleness is?" I've seen well women, and I'm becoming one myself. I'm beginning to know what wellness looks like, and it starts by embracing our bodies. Imagine yourself whole, healed, and deeply in touch with the wisdom of your female body. How do you feel? What do you know in your bones? Nothing is more exciting than knowing that our bodies and our feelings are a clear, open pathway toward our destinies.

TWO

Feminine Intelligence and a New Mode of Healing

> In the end I find I can't separate brain from body. Consciousness isn't just in the head. Nor is it a question of mind over body. If one takes into account the DNA directing the dance of the peptides, [the] body is the outward manifestation of the mind.
> —Dr. Candace Pert, former chief brain biochemist, National Institutes of Mental Health

The mind and the body are intimately linked via the immune, endocrine, and central nervous systems. Today, mind/body research is confirming what ancient healing traditions have always known: that the body and the mind are a unity. There is no disease that isn't mental and emotional as well as physical.

Energy Fields and Energy Systems

Humans are made out of energy and sustained by energy. Our bodies are ever-changing, dynamic fields of energy, not static physical structures. They are a hologram in which every part contains information about the whole. We know from quantum physics that at the subatomic level, matter and energy—which can also be called spirit—are interchangeable. The best expression of this that I have heard is that matter is the densest form of spirit and that spirit is the lightest form of matter. We can view our bodies as manifestations of spiritual energy. Our mind and daily thoughts are part of this

25

energy, and they have a well-documented effect on matter and our bodies.

Psychological and emotional factors influence our physical health greatly because our emotions and thoughts are always accompanied by biochemical reactions in our body. The mind/body continuum can be adequately understood only when we appreciate ourselves as an ever-changing energy system that is affected by, and also affects, the energy surrounding it. We don't end at our skins.

Though we cannot see this energy that makes up the bodymind and sustains us, it is nevertheless a vital part of us. It is the life-force that keeps our hearts beating and our lungs breathing even when we are asleep. Anyone who has had the experience of being with a dying person will tell you that after the moment of death, something changes. Though the physical body is still present, the person they knew is no longer there.

Energy fields interact within an individual person. They also interact between one person and another, and between one person and the world in general. These interactions, whose existence is well documented, are important for lifelong human growth and healthy development. A study at the University of Miami on premature babies, for example, found that babies who were stroked regularly gained weight 49 percent faster than did those of the same weight who weren't stroked. (Both groups of babies were fed exactly the same amount of food.) The stroked babies were longer and had larger heads and had fewer neurological problems at eight months of age than did the controls.[1] Babies who are not touched and cuddled, even though they are fed and cared for physically, are at great risk of death from the elusively diagnosed "failure to thrive."[2]

Even accidents, which we think of as "random" events, have been shown in a number of studies to be related to the emotional and psychological states (or energy fields) of the "victims." Several studies have indicated that accident-prone individuals have certain personality features that include impulsiveness, resentment, aggressiveness, unmet dependency needs, depression, sadness, loneliness, and unresolved grief. They tend to punish themselves when they feel anger toward others. So in the language of energy systems, it appears that the energy field of "accident-prone" individuals interacts with the environmental energy field in a way that increases their incidence of accidents.

Clearly, human interactions have profound effects on health. These effects can be either positive or negative, depending upon the state of mind of the people involved in those interactions. When we begin to appreciate ourselves as fields of energy with the ability to affect the quality of our own experience, we will be getting in touch with our innate ability to heal ourselves and create health every day of our lives.

Our bodies are influenced and actually structured by our beliefs. We inherit many of these beliefs from our parents and the circumstances of our upbringing. Scientific studies conducted by Dr. Leonard Sagan, a medical epidemiologist, underscore this and show that social class, education, life skills, and cohesiveness of family and community are key factors in determining life expectancy. Of all these factors, however, education has been shown to be the most important. A review of *all* the major epidemiological data on health makes clear that the major determinants of health are *not* immunization, diet, water supply, or antibiotics. In fact, the dramatic decline in death rates from infectious disease earlier in this century began long before the routine use of penicillin and antibiotics. *Hope, self-esteem, and education are the most important factors in creating health daily,* no matter what our background or the state of our health in the past.[3] Even illnesses are affected by our emotional state. Dr. Jeanne Achterberg has shown that the course of cancer can be better predicted by psychological variables such as hope than by medical measurements.[4] We always have the power within to educate ourselves more fully about what will help us heal and create health.

One of my patients told me, "I had a flash of insight on the way to your office today. When I was little, the only way I could get my mother's attention was to be sick. So I've had a lot of broken bones, then cancer, and now an abnormal Pap smear. I just realized today that I don't have to get sick to get her attention anymore!" She added that at the moment she had that insight in her car, the sun broke through the clouds, reinforcing her insight with its brilliance.

Understanding the Bodymind

The medical community is beginning to view patients as physical beings who constantly renew themselves. The body is like a river of information and energy, we are learning, and all its parts have a dynamic communication with all the other parts. Radioisotope studies have shown, for example, that red blood cells replenish themselves every twenty-eight days, while we regenerate a new liver every six months. In this continual restructuring of our physical bodies, we have daily opportunities to create health.

Though each of us is bombarded by millions of stimuli daily, our central nervous systems and sense organs function in such a way as to choose and process *only those stimuli that reinforce what we already believe about ourselves.* A Nobel Prize–winning experiment underscores the importance of this concept: Scientists raised kittens to adulthood in an environment that contained only horizontal lines on the walls of their cages and in the rooms where they were kept. Once they grew into mature cats, they were placed in a normal environment and proceeded to run into anything with vertical lines. The cats literally didn't "see" anything vertical. The opposite proved true with kittens raised within an environment of only vertical lines. Once they grew up, they bumped into everything horizontal. We can apply this insight to people, too. For instance, women who are abused as children are much more likely to be abused repeatedly as adults. They have been conditioned to being abused and have difficulty recognizing loving people and environments. As adults, our nervous systems function to reinforce what we were exposed to in our early years, unless we consciously change the effects of our early programming. The seeds of many later illnesses are sown in our childhoods, then fertilized regularly by our beliefs and thoughts that expect these experiences to be repeated.

The science of the mind/body connection, or psychoneuroimmunology (PNI), helps explain how the circumstances of our lives can affect our bodies. PNI and related research shows that the subtle electromagnetic fields around and within the body form a crucial link between the cultural wounding, which we think of as "psychological" and "emotional," and the gynecological or other problems women have, which we think of as "physical."

Many women who've survived sexual abuse, for example, divorce themselves from their bodies. Some experience themselves in their bodies only from the neck up. As one of my patients with continual menstrual spotting said, "I don't want to think about anything below my waist. I hate that part of my body. I wish that part of me would just go away." This was an important understanding for her; it indicated where she needed to take a step toward healing. Her menstrual spotting continually drew her attention back to a disowned part of her body that needed healing. An associate of mine sometimes has patients draw pictures of themselves. She told me of a patient with chronic pelvic pain who drew a self-portrait only from the waist up. My associate pointed out to this woman that maybe her pelvis, through pain, was trying to get her attention. She was leaving it out!

If the science of the mind/body connection helps explain how our emotional and psychological wounding becomes physical, it also supports our ability to heal from those conditions. All distress, all healing of distress, and all creation of health are simultaneously physical, psychological, emotional, and spiritual.

Up until fairly recently, scientists believed that information was passed linearly in the nervous system from nerve to nerve, just like electrical hard wiring. But now we know that our body organs communicate directly with the brain and vice versa, through chemical messengers known as neuropeptides. These neuropeptides pass messages between nerve cells; neuropeptide receptor molecules then receive messages that are triggered to be released by emotions and thoughts. It used to be believed that the cells' receptor sites for neuropeptides were located only in the brain and nerve tissue. But we now know they are found throughout the body. Dr. Candace Pert and other researchers have found that these brain–nervous system chemicals land on and activate receptor sites located in the body's endocrine and immune system cells, as well as in nerve cells. Not only that, body organs such as the kidney and bowel also have receptor sites for these so-called brain chemicals. These chemicals are part of the way in which thoughts and emotions affect our physical bodies directly.

Not only do our physical organs contain receptor sites for the neurochemicals of thought and emotion, our organs and immune systems *can themselves manufacture these same chemicals.* What this means is that our entire body feels and expresses emotion—all parts of us "think" and "feel." White blood cells, for instance, can produce morphinelike pain-relieving substances, and they in turn contain receptor sites for the same substances. This gives a person the capacity to modulate her own pain without medication. Though female organs have not been studied specifically, I'm certain that the uterus, ovaries, and breast tissue make the same neurochemicals of thought and emotion as the brain and the other organs. Hormones, for example, are messenger molecules for emotions and thoughts. The immune cells, too, have receptors for neuropeptides, the messenger molecules. Ovaries and probably the uterus make estrogen and progesterone—hormones that are also neurotransmitters that affect emotions and thoughts. And these organs too have receptor sites that receive messages from the brain and the immune system. It's easy, then, to understand that when we are sad, our female organs "feel" sad and their functions are affected.

Our thoughts, emotions, and brain communicate directly with our immune, nervous, and endocrine systems and with the organs of our bodies. Moreover, although these bodily systems are conventionally studied and viewed as separate, they are, in fact, aspects of the *same* system! If the uterus, the ovaries, the white blood cells, and the heart all make the same chemicals as the brain makes when it thinks, *where in the body is the mind?* The answer is, *The mind is located throughout the body.*

Our entire concept of "the mind" needs to be expanded considerably. *The mind can no longer be thought of as being confined to the brain or to the intellect; it exists in every cell of our bodies.* Every thought we think has a biochemical equivalent. Every emotion that we feel has a biochemical equivalent. One of my colleagues says, "The mind is the space between the cells." So when the part of your mind that is your uterus talks to you, through pain or excessive bleeding, are you prepared to listen to it?

When I asked a married thirty-five-year-old lawyer who had a sudden onset of bleeding between her periods what was going on in her life, she bristled. "I think this problem is medical," she said. By that, she meant that the problem was purely physical and was not related in any meaningful way to the rest of her life. I gently explained to her that I would have asked her the same question had she broken her leg, and I pointed out that all symptoms are "physical." My patient then calmed down and told me the truth: Recently she had had an extramarital affair and was feeling guilty, and she was terrified that she had acquired a sexually transmitted disease. Her irregular bleeding had started soon after her affair began. This additional history enabled me to give her better and more appropriate medical care, while she learned that she didn't have to separate herself into unrelated parts.

One of my patients went to see a biofeedback therapist about shoulder pain caused by chronic muscle tension. While she was learning to relax the muscles of her shoulder, she noticed that her muscle tension increased whenever she was thinking certain thoughts. One of these thoughts was of being spanked as a child. Another was of her husband's ill health and its possible implications for her. On the other hand, when she thought of the positive aspects of her life, her muscle tension lessened. She came to see that her fears and beliefs were encoded in her body. Through biofeedback, she learned that her muscle tissue had feelings, thoughts, and memories that were part of her body's wisdom.

The mind and the soul, which permeate our entire body, are much vaster than the intellect can possibly grasp. Our inner guidance comes to us through our feelings and body wisdom first—not through intellectual understanding. When we search for inner guidance with the intellect only—as though it existed outside of ourselves and our own deepest knowing—we get stuck in the search, and our inner guidance is effectively silenced. The intellect works best *in service* to our intuition, our inner guidance, soul, God or higher power—whichever term we choose for the spiritual energy that animates life. Once we have acknowledged that we are *more* than our intellect and that guidance is available to us from the universal mind, we have accessed our inner healing ability. As William James once said, "The power to move the world is in the subconscious mind."

Feminine Intelligence: How
Thoughts Are Embodied

Women have the capacity to know what they know, with their bodies and with their brains at the same time, in part because their brains are set up in such a way that the information in both hemispheres and in the body is highly available to them when they communicate.

In school I was taught to distrust my own thinking process because it never fit with the dualistic way in which education is set up. On a multiple-choice test, for example, I could always find a reason why almost every choice given might be correct. I could always see "the big picture," and I could see how everything was related to everything else. In going over my wrong answers, my teachers often told me, "You're reading too much into it. The correct answer is obvious." It was not always obvious to me. Now that I have learned to appreciate how intimately my thoughts, emotions, and physical body are connected, I have begun to reclaim my full intelligence. It is staggering to realize how many highly intelligent women think that they are stupid because so much of their intelligence has been undervalued. Dr. Linda Metcalf says, "Women think that their intellects are a male construct sitting inside their heads."

I have learned that like many women, I speak and think in a multimodal, spiral way using both hemispheres of my brain and the intelligence of my body all at the same time. Jean Houston describes the evolution of multimodal thinking like this: For centuries, women stood in their caves, stirring the soup with one hand, bouncing the baby on the other hip, and kicking the woolly mammoth out the door with the other foot. We have evolved having to focus on more than one task at a time—understanding innately the consequences of our actions, not just on ourselves but on our entire family unit or tribe. By having to focus on several things at once, women have, over the centuries, developed a brain structure and style of thinking that is characteristically different from most men's.

In most women, the corpus callosum, the part of the brain that connects the right and left hemispheres, is thicker than it is in most men. That is, male and female brains are "wired" differently. Men characteristically use mostly their left hemispheres to think and to communicate their thoughts; their reasoning is usually linear and solution oriented. It gets to "the point." Women, in contrast, recruit more areas of the brain when they communicate than do men. They use the right and the left sides of their brain. Because the right hemisphere has richer connections with the body than the left hemisphere, women have more access to their body wisdom when speaking and thinking than do most men.

This doesn't mean that male brains inherently lack this capacity. It's just that for centuries they haven't been encouraged to develop these capacities. For the last five thousand years, Western society has believed that a linear left-brain approach is the superior mode of communication and that a woman's more embodied way of speaking and thinking is inferior and "less evolved." The authors of the book *Brain Sex* point out, "Men, it seems, are the sex who say the first thing that comes into their heads, while women communicate by calling on a much wider repertoire. Taken all together the evidence paints a comprehensive picture of a busier and wider interchange of information in the female brain."[5] Unfortunately, instead of developing embodied thinking, we learn to reject and denigrate this capacity.

In a recent dialogue with sociolinguist Deborah Tannen, Robert Bly said, "Words are in one lobe of the brain and feelings in the other." This statement, I must emphasize, is true only for most male brains. It ignores the complexity of female brains. "So that means," Bly continued, "that women have an ability to mingle those much quicker than men can. Women have a superhighway going on there. And, as Michael Meade remarked, men have this little crooked country road, and you're lucky if a word gets over."[6]

When I'm explaining something in detail, my husband will often say to me, "Can't you say that in fewer words? Can't you get to the point?" This expresses a stereotypically male communication style. When I think or speak, I use language to express the richness of what goes on in my mind and body while I'm communicating my thoughts. I like to hang out with language and wander around in it. I often come to understand how I'm feeling by talking about it for a while, letting my thoughts arise from my whole body and whole brain before speaking them. Processing ideas verbally or writing down my thoughts helps me to know more of myself.

In contrast, my husband uses as few words as possible. He and most men want to get to the point, the product or solution, and everything has to have one, otherwise it is not worth talking about. Most men view and experience the *process* of getting to the point as tedious and worthless. (They tend to use pointers whenever they lecture, and some have a hard time giving a lecture without one. Women rarely use them unless they have selectively overdeveloped their left hemispheres.) Dr. George Keeler, a holistic medical colleague, says, "When men talk they leave out the verbs. When women talk, they leave out the nouns." Alluding to quantum physics, which teaches that particles and waves are simply different aspects of matter, Dr. Keeler observes, "Men speak particle language. Women speak wave language."

Multimodal, embodied thinking makes it possible for most women to go to the grocery store without a list and still remember everything they came to buy, plus other stuff that they suddenly remember they need. When I'm in the middle of surgery, I am also aware of what my children are doing, that we need paper towels, and that I have to pick up bread on the way home. All of this is going on in my brain at the same time. It is called *relational thinking*. My husband, on the other hand, holds and works with only one or two thoughts and tasks in his mind simultaneously. He often has to go back to the store three times to accomplish what I can do in one trip.

The differences between male and female communication styles come up repeatedly in my office. When I am explaining a woman's condition to her male partner, I often tell him, "Listen, when I talk to you about what your wife [or partner] has, I may seem to be talking in circles. I'll be going out here, out here, and over there." I motion my finger in a circle. "It may feel like a digression to you, and you may not see the relevance of all that I'm saying. But it is all related. Stay with me—I'm coming back to the main point and will tie it all together for you."

My views and other scientists' views on the differences between male and female thinking are controversial. Regardless of what we believe, however, I've come to see that to be fully healthy, women must come to appreciate the fullness of the intelligence available to them as it comes through their entire beings—body, mind, and spirit.

Beliefs Are Physical

Thoughts are just one part of our body's wisdom. A thought held long enough and repeated enough becomes a belief. The belief then becomes biology. Beliefs are energetic forces that create the physical basis for our individual lives and our health. If we don't work through our emotional distress, we set ourselves up for physical distress because of the biochemical effect that suppressed emotions have on our immune and endocrine systems. Autoimmune diseases, such as rheumatoid arthritis, multiple sclerosis, certain thyroid diseases, and lupus erythematosus, for example, are all caused in part by autoimmunity, meaning that the immune system attacks the body. Why would the immune system attack the cells of the person in whom it is functioning, unless it is getting some kind of destructive message from somewhere very deep within the body? Mental depression has been associated not only with self-destructive behaviors but with depression of immune system functioning.[7] Many women with autoimmune diseases also suffer from depression. Studies have also shown, for example, that stress and loneliness can help cause a latent (inactive) herpes virus to become active.[8] The same is true for those with Epstein-Barr virus, the virus linked with chronic fatigue syndrome. This is one reason why, even though over 90 percent of the population have been exposed to and have antibodies to Epstein-Barr virus, only a small percentage actually suffer from the disease. This information is especially relevant to women since at least 80 percent of all autoimmune disease occurs in us.[9] Even endometriosis, epilepsy, premature menopause, infertility, and chronic vaginitis have autoimmune components.

What an individual believes is heavily influenced by the culture in which she lives. Beliefs held in common perpetuate the type of society in which we live. Given our society, it is not surprising that women have so much perceived stress. In several scientific studies, "inescapable" stress has been associated with a distinct form of immunosuppression (suppression of immune system response).

Emotional shock is associated with the release of endogenous opiates (morphinelike substances) and corticosteroids (hormones from the adrenal glands), which prevent white blood cells from protecting the body from cancer and infection. People who have a sense of hopelessness or despair and who perceive their situations as being uncontrollably stressful have higher levels of corticosteroids and immune suppression than do those who attempt to cope with the stress.[10] People who are exposed to what they perceive as "inescapable" stress actually release opioidlike substances (enkephalins) that literally numb the cells of their bodies (in stress-induced analgesia),[11] rendering them incapable of destroying cancer cells and bacteria if this goes on chronically.[12] It is not *stress itself* that creates immune system problems. It is, rather, the *perception* that the stress is inescapable—that there is nothing a person can do to prevent it. This perception is associated with immune system suppression.

It is important to understand that our beliefs go much deeper than our thoughts, and we cannot simply will them away. Many beliefs are completely unconscious and are not readily available to the intellect. I know from my practice—and from my life—that most of us aren't aware of our own destructive beliefs that undermine our health. They don't come from the intellect alone, the part that thinks it's in control. They come from that other part that in the past became lodged and buried in the cell tissue.

Jean, a lovely dark-haired graphics designer, recently came for a consultation with me. She is forty-five years old and was concerned that her periods had changed over the years from a pattern of every 28 days to every 25 to 34 days. She had no spotting in between and no other symptoms. This history sounded completely normal to me, but another doctor had told her that her cycle change might represent cancer. He recommended a uterine biopsy. Because her cervical opening was too small to allow a biopsy instrument to enter, a D&C under general anesthesia was suggested. Jean decided to seek a second opinion. Her exam was normal, but she did in fact have a very small cervical opening and therefore could not have an office biopsy.

I told Jean that I thought she was a very unlikely candidate for uterine cancer and that I wouldn't recommend a D&C. If she was really worried and wanted one, I said, it could certainly be done to be sure she didn't have cancer. To help her make her decision, I asked her what her childhood experience of illness had been, since a woman's childhood experience tends to profoundly influence her beliefs around health and disease. Jean said, "I was an only child, and my mother was always sick. She constantly had bowel problems. I had to take care of her. As a result, I personally react to everything that happens in my body as though it's a catastrophe— just as my mother did."

Then I said, "If you decided to have a D&C and it turned out to be normal, would you be able to relax and stop obsessing over cancer?" She said that it wouldn't make any difference. She'd still worry. We agreed then that she had to change her belief system about her body and its vulnerability, which had been so firmly influenced by her early years.

To do this, Jean now needs to understand that her fear is not entirely accessible to her intellect. Much of it is in her body and her subconscious mind. Telling Jean, or women with similar problems, to "just relax, you're fine, it's nothing" and that "it's all in your head" is not scientifically accurate. Jean's belief is in her mind, but her mind is located throughout her body and in every organ in it.

For Jean to stop obsessing about cancer (or anything else), she will have to go through a process that every one of us must also go through to heal. To explain this process to patients, I use the first three steps of the twelve-step program, which originated with Alcoholics Anonymous. Since these twelve steps are based on spiritual truths, I've found them applicable to nearly every aspect of life about which I or my patients are seeking guidance. Step one is: "We admitted we were powerless over alcohol and that our lives had become unmanageable." Instead of the word *alcohol*, you can substitute anything that you currently are obsessing about or feel powerless over. In Jean's case, she must admit that she is powerless to change her belief and obsession about cancer with her intellect alone. She must also admit that this belief is not healthy and that it is making parts of her life unmanageable. Her belief won't go away if she beats herself up about it or tries to force herself to change it with her intellect alone.

The second step is: "We came to see that a power greater than ourselves could restore us to sanity." This power "greater than ourselves" is a part of our inner guidance and bodily wisdom. The word *sanity* means the same thing as inner peace or serenity. Acknowledging that we have access to guidance from a power greater than our own intellect is a very positive step toward actually accessing that guidance. The third step is: "We made a decision to turn our will and our lives over to the care of God *as we understood Him.*" (I automatically change the word *Him* to *inner guidance* or *divine wisdom.*) This step bypasses the intellect entirely. It is a leap of faith that acknowledges the fact that all of us have inner guidance available within us and that that guidance has the power to remove our harmful beliefs. The words *made a decision* are very important. To create health, a woman needs to make a decision to do it. Then she must be willing to stay with the process. Participating in twelve-step meetings and working the steps around a fear, a belief, or even an illness that you've found your intellect to be powerless over can be very helpful and practical.

For Jean and thousands of women like her, the knowledge that she is not alone in her fears and obsessions is itself very helpful. I've never met anyone who didn't inherit at least some health-destroying beliefs either from their families or from the culture in general. We can uncover the deep programming of our bodies and change it to support health. Many of my patients have been able to do this once they understand that although their diseases are very real and physical, these diseases are often accompanied and reinforced by unconscious beliefs. Uncovering these and healing from them is a continuous, exciting, and empowering process. It is part of the process of creating health. It requires patience and compassion.

Beliefs and memories are actually biological constructs in the body. Think of your mind as an iceberg. The conscious part—the part that thinks it's in control—is what peaks above the surface. But it amounts to only about 25 percent of the total iceberg. The so-called "subconscious" part of your mind is the much larger part— 75 percent of it lies below the surface. Our personal histories are stored throughout our bodies, in muscles, in organs, and in other tissues. This information, like the submerged portion of the iceberg, is not generally recognized by the part of the iceberg on the surface, our conscious intellect. Our cells contain our memory banks—even when the conscious mind is not aware of them and actually battles to deny them!

Once when I called a bellman to my hotel room to help me with my bags, he noticed a bottle of Chinese cough syrup near the sink. He made a face, held his stomach, and said, "I thought that was castor oil, and I remember that my mother gave it to me often as a child. I used to have stomach pains after taking it. Just looking at the bottle now gives me a stomachache!" This man had no conscious control over his body's memory of his childhood pain. His body automatically reacted to the sight of a familiar bottle that wasn't even related.

Once I was hiking with a woman who told me that two weeks before, she had gotten some sunscreen in her eye and her eye had watered all day from the irritation. Several days later, she merely smelled the same sunscreen when someone else was using it, and her eye started to water again. Her biological memory was already encoded in her eye. Her intellect had been bypassed entirely!

How Beliefs Become Physical

At any given time, our state of health reflects the sum total of our beliefs since birth. Our entire society functions under many shared and sometimes harmful beliefs. (One that I hear regularly at my office is, "Well, now that I'm thirty [or forty, or fifty], I suppose it's normal to have aches and pains.") All living things respond physically to the way they *think* reality is. Dr. Deepak Chopra, an authority on consciousness and medicine, uses the example of flies placed in a jar with a lid on top. But once the lid is "removed," they will not leave the jar except for a few brave pioneers. The rest of the flies have made a "commitment in their bodyminds" that they are trapped. In aquariums, it has been shown that if two schools of fish are separated with a glass partition for a certain amount of time, the fish will not swim into each other's space even after the partition is removed.

So it is that we can be sure the events of our childhood set the stage for our beliefs about ourselves and therefore our experience, including our health. For a woman to change or improve her reality and her state of health, she first has to change her beliefs about what is possible.

That we have the wherewithal to overcome our destructive and unconscious patterns is a truth that I see proved daily in my practice. This power has also been documented experimentally in a study of the effects of beliefs on the aging process. Dr. Ellen Langer studied a group of male volunteers over the age of seventy at a retreat center for five days. They all had to agree that they would live in the present as though it were 1959. Dr. Langer told them, "We are not asking you to 'act as if it were 1959' but to let yourself *be* just who you were in 1959." They had to dress as they had then, watch TV shows from 1959, read newspapers and magazines from that time, and talk as if 1959 were right now. They also brought pictures of themselves from that year and put them around the center. Dr. Langer then measured many of the parameters that often deteriorate with aging (but don't need to), such as physical strength, perception, cognition, taste, and hearing. The parameters reflected "biological markers" that experts in geriatric medicine often cite. Over the course of the five days, many of the chosen parameters actually improved. Serial photographs showed that the men looked about five years younger as well. Their hearing and memory improved. As they changed their mindsets about aging, their physical bodies changed as well! Dr. Langer writes, "The regular and 'irreversible' cycles of aging that we witness in the later stages of human life may be a product of certain assumptions about how one is supposed to grow old. *If we didn't feel compelled to carry out these limiting mindsets, we might have a greater chance of replacing years of decline with years of growth and purpose*" (emphasis mine).[13]

If we had the power to reverse the effects of aging, what might be possible with health! The hopefulness that these data raise cannot be overestimated. It suggests that if we can leap out of our collective cultural jars, life holds possibilities that we've not imagined before. But before we get there, we must first acknowledge the horizontal or vertical stripes that many of us keep running into. Once we *see* what has been there all along, we can create alternative routes.

Healing Versus Curing

> Freedom and fate embrace each other to form meaning; and given
> meaning, fate—with its eyes, hitherto severe, suddenly full of
> light—looks like grace itself.
>
> —Martin Buber

*T*here is a difference between healing and curing. Healing is a
natural process and is *within* the power of everyone. Curing,
which is what doctors are called upon to do, usually consists of an
external treatment, and medication or surgery is used to mask or
eliminate symptoms. *This external treatment doesn't necessarily
address the factors that contributed to the symptom in the first place.*
Healing goes deeper than curing and must always come from
within. It addresses the imbalance that underlies the symptoms.
Healing brings together the often hidden aspects of a person's life as
they relate to her illness. Healing is different from curing, though
curing and the restoration of physical function may accompany
healing. One can be healed completely and go on to die of her illness.
This is a key understanding that is often missing from treatises on
holistic medicine: Healing and death are not mutually exclusive. As a
physician, I've been trained to improve and preserve life. But sometimes we need to let go of that training and accept death as a natural
part of a process that is much bigger and more mysterious than we
realize. Patricia Reis, who works with many of our patients' dreams
and body symptoms, says, "The bigger meaning of healing is a
'wholeing,' a filling out of the missing pieces of a person's life.
Sometimes this may even mean facing death in a more fully realized
way. Certainly it is an opportunity to come more deeply and fully
into life."

Although our entire bodies are affected by our thoughts and
emotions and their various parts talk to each other, each individual's
body language is unique. *No matter what has happened in her life, a
woman has the power to change what that experience means to her
and thus change her experience, both emotionally and physically.
Therein lies her healing.* There are no simple formulae for decipher-
ing the message behind a symptom, and only the patient herself can
ultimately know what the message is about. Sometimes a woman's

body, through chronic vaginitis, asks her to leave a relationship. Sometimes headaches that occur premenstrually are a sign that she needs to give up caffeine. In other women, these symptoms may be related to something entirely different. It is up to each woman to "sit with" her symptoms in a completely receptive, nonjudgmental way so that she can begin to appreciate the unique language of her body.

We don't yet understand completely why it is that one woman who has been abandoned by her husband, for example, will seem to deteriorate emotionally, mentally, and physically, blaming this particular trauma for a lifetime of woes, while another woman with a similar background will recover fully and live a productive life. Some people can name an initially painful and traumatic circumstance as the stimulus from which major personal growth later arose. Childhood abuse, incest, loss of a parent, and other traumas are not absolutely linked in a cause-and-effect way with subsequent distress in adulthood. The effect of trauma on our physical, mental, and emotional bodies is determined largely by *how we interpret the event and give it meaning.*

Emotional factors are usually involved in common gynecological problems, along with diet, heredity, multiple sexual partners, or bad luck. I have found that most women with persistent genital warts, herpes, or ovarian cysts have experienced or are continuing to experience emotional and psychological stress or unrest. In these cases, a history of sexual abuse, abortions that haven't been resolved emotionally, or some conflict involving relationships or creativity is almost always present. These conflicts live in the body's energy field until they're resolved—they are "healing opportunities" simply waiting for our attention.

One of my OB/GYN colleagues, Dr. Maude Guerin, illustrates this beautifully by using the example of a woman named Joan who had severe endometriosis and pelvic pain. Dr. Guerin "cured" Joan with a total abdominal hysterectomy and removal of both ovaries and tubes—a standard treatment for her problem. Following surgery, however, Joan developed back pain, depression, and incapacitating hot flashes, requiring many times the regular dose of hormones. Although her pelvic pain had been "cured," in many ways she was no better off than she had been before. Instead of being "healed," she had simply traded one group of symptoms for another. The surgical removal of her uterus and ovaries had not resolved the emotional conflicts in her body's energy field that were the root cause of her problem.

Dr. Guerin discovered that Joan had been sexually abused at the age of six, had lived through the death of her sister at the age of sixteen, and had turned to workaholism to avoid her feelings. Despite these major traumas in her life, she had never been able to cry. Dr. Guerin writes, "This patient has been a wonderful teacher for me. Although I never discounted the concept that thoughts and feelings influence physical health, I had always perceived that influence to be relative. This patient taught me that consideration of the mind-body link is obligatory in the care of every patient, no matter how cut-and-dried their course seems to be.

"I certainly felt that I had cured this woman, and was proud of myself at her six week check-up. It took the two of us years to learn that although she had been 'cured' by surgery, she was not healed by it.

"Looking back on her first visit with me, which I remember vividly, and her subsequent course, there were many, many clues to a much larger picture that I was unable to see at the time. On her initial office visit, she was sitting on the examination table while still wearing her panty hose. Not only did she have trouble getting undressed for the exam, she also had a great deal of difficulty even getting her body in the examination position. Once she was there, I found that placing the speculum in her vagina was nearly impossible because of her extreme anxiety and muscle tension. Since then my patients have continued to help me see the big picture, for each of them. I know that you can 'cure' many patients without acknowledging the mind/body link, but I also know that you will 'heal' very few."[14]

One of my own patients had an abnormal Pap smear. She already knew that simply removing the abnormal cells from her cervix ("curing") would not address the underlying energy imbalance in her body that was at the root of the abnormality. She began working in her journal every morning with the intention of being receptive to what was necessary for her healing. She meditated on what this symptom was trying to teach her. After she had been engaged in this inner healing work for several weeks, she uncovered a key belief that she felt was important to her. This belief was that the abnormal cervical cells were a punishment for her sexuality. Having discovered and named this belief, she proceeded to schedule standard medical therapy so that her "healing" and her "curing" would be in partnership. On her way to the appointment to have laser treatment for this condition, she experienced a wave of forgiveness toward herself and her sexuality that moved her to tears. She even felt a shift take place in her body. When she was examined at the office, all traces of the abnormality had gone, and she didn't require the surgery. She is very grateful for the physical cure, as well as the psychological and emotional healing that took place.

In this society, when a physician acknowledges a woman's innate healing ability, she or he often seems to be saying that she *caused* her illness to begin with! But our illnesses aren't based on simple cause and effect. It is simplistic and potentially harmful to believe that we consciously and intentionally create illness or any other painful life circumstance. Our illnesses often exist to get our attention and get us back on track. Feeling that we are "to blame" for our illnesses simply reconstellates the woundings of our childhood and is exactly the opposite of healing. Feeling we are "to blame" keeps us stuck and unable to move forward in our healing. The part of us that "creates an illness" is *not* the part of us that feels the pain of the illness. It is not a conscious part of us, but it can be affected by our consciousness once we put our healing process to work.

Many physicians, however, equate taking responsibility for illness with being to blame for it. In the addictive system, we equate having responsibility with being "to blame." At the opposite extreme, other physicians feel that since their patients didn't cause their disease, they should not be overly involved in their own treatment. It is important that you have a doctor or health practitioner whose beliefs can reinforce your healing. Recent studies have shown that the expectations that physicians have about their patients' healing potential are picked up consciously and unconsciously by their patients and do affect their ability to get well.

We can begin to heal our lives at the deepest levels when we begin to value our bodies and honor their messages instead of feeling victimized by them. Trusting the wisdom of the body is a leap of faith in a culture that fails to acknowledge how intimately the mind and body are connected. By *the wisdom of the body*, I mean that we must learn to trust that the symptoms in the body are often the only way that the soul can get our attention. Covering up our symptoms with external "cures" prevents us from "healing" the parts of our lives that need attention and change.

I used to run into what I call "blame walls" when I asked my patients to participate in their own health care. Once, for example, when I explained to a woman that her fibroid (benign uterine tumor) might be related to how she was using her creativity within her relationships, she became angry and thought I was blaming her. "Do you mean I caused this?" she said. I told her that she must move beyond blame, beyond cause-and-effect thinking. To heal from her problem she needed to relate to her fibroid in a new way, seeing it not as the enemy to be "cured" but as an aspect of her own inner guidance that was trying to direct her attention toward health-enhancing changes in her life. Responding to and learning from an illness is a way to confront the addictive system in which we live our lives.

For healing to occur, we must come to see that we are not so much responsible for our illnesses as responsible to them. The healthiest people I know don't take their diseases or even their lives too personally. They spend very little time beating themselves up about their illnesses, their life circumstances, or anything else. They take their life one day at a time as it unfolds in its own way and its own time. A young woman stated this attitude beautifully when she wrote, "I take full responsibility not for getting cancer in the first place, nor for ultimately surviving it, but rather for the quality of the way I am responding to this bit of chaos thrown into my life."

The story of Martha, a close family friend, provides a most striking example of the mystery of illness and body symptoms. Though unusual in many ways, her story illustrates the range of experiences available to us when we are open to healing in whatever way it presents itself.

When Martha was in her mid-fifties, a series of painful childhood memories began to surface spontaneously. She allowed herself to feel fully how painful her childhood had been. She expressed and released these feelings through sobbing for hours over several days within the space of about a week. During this process she fully remembered the details of being taken to run-down bars by her bootlegger father. While she was at these places she had often watched him kissing women who were strangers. She recalled being left with an aunt for a few days while her mother broke her father out of jail. The aunt, who had only one eye, kept her and her younger sister in a cockroach-laden room with only crackers to eat and a single light bulb hanging from the ceiling. As Martha let herself remember those and many other things that she had "deep-sixed" fifty-five years before, she was able to cry and wail for as long as she needed to as a trusted friend sat with her. This "cleansing" went on for several days, off and on. Afterward, she said, "I realized that there was nothing of beauty in my life when I was a child. It was worse than I ever let myself remember."

Once she was able to see this part of her life for what it really was and express her emotions around it, the chronic neck and shoulder pain that she'd had for years and that had been called "degenerative changes in her spine" went away completely. It has never come back.

Last spring, Martha called me to say that she was experiencing terror of death to a degree she'd never known possible. Based on her past experience of trusting her symptoms, she decided to stay with her feelings and symptoms to see what they could teach her rather than running away from them or trying to suppress or "cure" them with drugs.

Martha is no stranger to death, having lived through the death of two of her children and her husband—two of these in the space of one year. Her fear of her own death, which she told me followed her to bed at night and confronted her in the morning, was accompanied by vague left-sided upper abdominal pains, which she at first misinterpreted as being related to taking penicillin for a dental infection. Her terror was so awful that she couldn't really talk about it for quite some time.

As her terror and the stomach pain became worse, her intuition suggested that she should drive across the country from New England to Taos, New Mexico, where one of her daughters lives. She wanted to be alone, and she felt that driving a long distance would be the right thing. I had never heard her so upset, but I was not worried. I trusted that she had something to work through and that I would hear from her afterward, when she was ready to talk to me. Several days later she called, still quite shaky. "It all started out on the prairie," she said. "For a couple hundred miles I drove, and then I felt this enormous emotional and physical pain. I was driving past the stockyards. There were all these cattle up to their bellies in their excrement. It hit me how we all live in all this crap and then gloss it over with scented toilet paper. I felt such sadness for the state of the world, for all the environmental problems. I thought of all the fear we always have. I found myself trudging across the prairie as a pioneer woman. I 'saw' thousands and thousands of women, of all races, all ages, trudging across the prairie, holding up the world through their labors. I felt the fear and the pain of all those women, the endless work. [As these images were washing over her, her stomach pain was getting worse and worse so that she had to pull her legs up to her chest. She tasted blood in her mouth, but when she spat into a tissue, nothing was there.]

"Then the flash came. I was a Viking, a male Viking. I had a huge sword. I killed a woman about to have her child. I killed them both with this sword. It was so awful to think of that. I just kept driving with tears and agony. To think that I was capable of doing such a thing! I felt such compassion for men because they were trained to do this. This pain in my stomach, the tears, the agony—this went on for about four hours. When I went over the mountain pass in the Rockies, the sun came out and I hoped it would go away. But the horror still came. It was like some horrible dream that was real, but it wasn't.

"I needed to do this alone in an environment that wasn't 'home.' All night Friday on the day I left, the pain was on the left and seemed to be leaving. But on Saturday as I continued my trip, I'd get these waves of dread in the left side of my abdomen. That's exactly where I [the Viking] put the sword.

"When I got to Taos, I had a session with Mary, a gifted intuitive. She did a reading and felt it was not necessary for me to go any farther. This vision of the pioneer women and me as a Viking killing a pregnant woman has helped me to release my fear of death.

"I know I need to put a closure on this, I need to acknowledge it and close it. Perhaps it was necessary for the female to be killed. It was the worst thing I have ever done, the thing that I have tried to hide from God and from myself. The other thing I realized is that all of mankind has done this. We have all killed and murdered. I feel as though I have just died from another lifetime. Now I'm giving birth to myself. I can never go back to what I was before, because too much has happened to me. I can't be what I was before.

"I haven't felt my full physical energy for some time. I've always been at a physical high pitch. This experience helped me in a realization of my own death. The environment, the earth, and what we've done to it is very deep in me. I think that now I have also successfully dropped my ties to my children in the sense of holding on too tightly out of fear. I can move on now."

Martha realized that a full intellectual understanding of what had just happened to her was not necessary for her healing. She did not have to interpret the vision or experience of "being a Viking" as a past life experience or anything else in order to heal. What was necessary was that she *feel* all of what was coming up from deep within her. After she acknowledged the act of murder, she felt freed of its burden and thus renewed. She also realized that she had to change the way she had been living. She needed to stop spending time with friends who contributed nothing to her life, in friendships that were based on habit, not mutual enrichment.

When Martha returned to her home a week later, she still felt some residual fear and dread from the experience and wanted to be free of it. She wrote down the whole thing, then went out into the back yard under a night sky full of stars, dug a hole, and burned her writing. She buried the ashes and stood up, and finally after weeks of dread, she felt completely released and walked back into her cabin.

About three weeks later, she was visiting her aunt and uncle in Ohio. Her Uncle Roy took her aside and said that he didn't feel that he had much longer to live and that he had something he wanted to give her. He took her into a back room, reached up on a shelf, and handed down a bronze statue. It was a Viking with a sword.

We shared our amazement at this bit of synchronicity. ("Synchronicity is God's way of remaining anonymous," says Dr. Bernie Siegel.) Martha said, "I can have this statue in my house now. It is a symbol for me of healing. I know that if I had not allowed myself to experience this memory or dream or whatever it was, I would have developed a fatal stomach condition. I am certain of this."

This story illustrates profoundly that the notion that we are "to blame" for our illnesses in any conventional sense is irrelevant and narrow. In some mysterious way, our conscious intellect is *not* in control. Another part of us—our higher power, soul, or inner wisdom—is. The concept of "the self" needs to be expanded. Studies have documented the power of prayer to heal at a distance, instantaneously. Time and space are not absolute. We are "acted upon" by forces outside of our conscious control. We can be open to learning from all of life, from our inner selves and from all that with which we are connected.

We have the body we have because it is precisely the vehicle in which we can best do what we came to do. Stevie Wonder has said that his blindness helped him feel the love that is all around him more than he would if he were sighted. Perhaps he couldn't do the creative work he's doing if he were in a "normal" body. Elisabeth Kübler-Ross points out that when our physical quadrants are sick or nonfunctioning, our spiritual and mental quadrants often expand way beyond what they would normally. She uses the example of children with leukemia who seem wise beyond their years.[15] I accept the truth of this on faith. We can't really hope to figure it out with our logical intellectual selves. There are indeed more things in heaven and earth than are dreamt of in our philosophies.

Be open to the messages and mysteries of your body and its symptoms. Be eager to listen and slow to judge. What you learn may have the capacity to save your life.

THREE

Inner Guidance

Right after Mary Lu was diagnosed with breast cancer, she called me to discuss her treatment options. I told her that part of her healing would be to learn how to trust herself to make her own decisions about her treatment after gathering information from a number of experts. She later wrote me, "I remember that I felt scared when I heard you affirm that in recovery, I would know what to do to deal with the cancer. I remember thinking that these were life-and-death choices and not on par with deciding how to spend some weekend. Then what flashed for me was that my soul has always been at stake all these years. Anne [Schaef] reminded me that I had come to my first group session with her back in 1981 concerned about my health. It was right after a diagnosis of ulcerative colitis and I was afraid I was killing myself. I do believe in the mind-body-soul connection. With decisions to make concerning my cancer treatment, *I had this sense that I would have a real chance to trust my inner guidance.* Trusting myself at such a deep level was frightening to me, but I can gratefully say now several months later that this 'stuff' really does work, that I have trusted my process a lot through this. And each time that I have guided myself to my own healing, it gives me renewed courage to continue to trust."

Our inner guidance can direct us toward that which is most life-enhancing and life-fulfilling for us. Mary Lu learned that she could find the surgeon she needed to work with and the treatment that worked best for her, even in the face of breast cancer. Not only that,

TABLE 3

External Guidance: Dominant Cultural View	Inner Guidance
Physical world is inferior to Spirit.	Spirit informs everything.
Nature is inferior to God and must be controlled.	Nature is a reflection of Divine Spirit.
Human beings are superior to the natural world.	Human beings are co-creators with spirit and nature.
Behavior is based on fear and judgment.	Behavior is based on respect for self. Respect for self results in respect for others.
Difference is suspect and must be controlled.	Difference is celebrated as a reflection of the creativity of spirit.
There's only one right way to live and to be.	There are many paths to fulfillment and joy. None are superior.
Delayed gratification. Enjoyment and fulfillment must be earned.	Live in the moment and enjoy the process of creating.
The inherent worth of an individual is arranged in a hierarchy of superior to inferior.	Life is an interdependent cooperative adventure with all beings connected holographically.
Guidance for behavior dictated by laws and institutions from external sources.	Guidance for behavior comes from connection with Inner Guidance.
There is such a thing as purely objective reality separate from consciousness.	The whole universe is a projection of consciousness.
Action and pushing against what we DON'T want is the only way to accomplish anything.	Consciousness creates all that is. Thoughts and feelings create reality.
Support and nourishment must be earned from people and institutions outside of oneself.	The individual is self-nourishing through her connection with her inner being and guidance system.
Approval from others is the basis for happiness.	Self-approval and self acceptance are the keys to happiness.

External Guidance: Dominant Cultural View (*cont.*)	Inner Guidance (*cont.*)
Humans are inherently flawed. Worth must be earned.	We are inherently worthy and precious by virtue of our existence. We have nothing to prove.
Spiritual guidance comes only from priests, ministers, or churches.	Our internal guidance and spirit are inherently loving and beneficent.
God and spirit are the ultimate judges of worth.	The universe is continually unfolding.
It is possible to control everything and everyone.	Humans are not capable of understanding everything from a strictly physical viewpoint. Mystery is part of the wonder of life.

she learned that she could even enjoy her life at the same time. She did this by *allowing herself to be led by how she was feeling in each moment of the day.* Each step of the way, she moved toward the decision that *felt best* to her. When you move toward that which is most fulfilling and life-enhancing, healing follows regardless of what your health is like in the moment.

Our inner guidance system is mediated via our thoughts, emotions, dreams, and bodily feelings. Our bodies are designed to act as receiving and transmitting stations for energy and information. Living in touch with our inner guidance involves feeling our way through life using *all* of ourselves: mind, body, emotions, and spirit. When I refer to this process in this book, I mean the various ways we listen and use our inner guidance to make conscious changes in our lives, behavior, relationships with others, and health.

Listening to Your Body and Its Needs

We can generally trust our "gut feeling" about someone or something to be accurate information. This is because the solar plexus, the place in the body where we generally feel that "gut reaction," is in fact a primitive brain. It is also a major intuitive center, the part of our body that lets us know whether we are safe and whether we are being lied to.

Each of us must develop ways to tune in to our body's needs. We can start with simple things. When you're tired, rest. When you have to go to the bathroom, go. If you feel like crying when you read a certain passage in this book, let yourself cry. If you simply can't read certain parts of the text, notice them—they may refer to subjects that are painful to you. Just make a note of your reactions. Notice your breathing as you read: Does it speed up or slow down depending upon the material you're covering? What is your heart doing? Is it racing or is it slow? Does reading about the uterus or the menstrual cycle unearth any old memories or body feelings?

I often ask women to pay attention to what their bodies feel like in the moment. In order to heal our bodies, we have to reenter them and experience them. (Right after I wrote that, I noticed that my legs were numb. I'd been sitting too long and had ignored my need for movement. After a ten-minute barefoot walk on the lawn and some deep breathing, my body felt much more alert and happy.)

We have to give our bodies credit for their innate wisdom. We also don't need to know exactly why something is happening in our bodies in order to respond to it. You don't need to know *why* your heart is racing or *why* you feel like crying. Understanding comes *after* you have allowed yourself to experience what you're feeling. Healing is an organic process that happens *in the body* as well as in the intellect. So if you are feeling "out of sorts" or "off balance," just be with that feeling, allow it to come up. After you have allowed yourself to experience it, take a moment and go back over the events of the last few hours or days. If you are feeling ill or having symptoms, reflecting on recent events may give you a clue about what preceded the symptoms.

Here's an example from my own recent experience. A few months ago, I woke up with the visual signs and hand and face numbness that are the symptoms of an impending migraine headache. I had developed classic migraines at the age of twelve, had one or sometimes two headaches approximately every month until my sophomore year in college, and then didn't get another one for twenty years. While growing up, I was a definite migraine personality, pushing myself mercilessly in school and in all my activities. I "shorted out" my body's electromagnetic system from stress on a regular basis.

So when I began to get that old, familiar, sickening feeling, I immediately used it as an opportunity to learn. I put an ice pack under my neck, lay down, kept the room quiet, and concentrated on making my hands warm. (I had learned from a biofeedback therapist that migraines can often be "aborted" by relaxing totally and warming the hands.) Gratefully, I managed to avoid getting a full-blown headache that in the past had left me in pain, nauseated for most of the day, and very weak. After about one hour, I was able to go about my activities but felt very subdued. I thought back on the previous three days.

I had been tearing around the house, trying to pick up and organize years of clutter in two days. Toward the end of the weekend, my temper had been short, I had scarcely taken time to eat or go to the bathroom, and I hadn't taken a break from the bending and cleaning for hours. I had gone to bed with a dull headache. The next morning, I woke up with the migraine symptoms. It was clear to me that my ability to put my bodily needs for rest, recreation, and nurturing aside for long periods of time was very intact. Only now my body wouldn't let me get away with it nearly as much as it used to. Hence the migraine. I took it as a warning.

The healing principle that summarizes this learning is the following: *If you don't heed the message the first time, you get hit with a bigger hammer the next time.*

The purpose of emotions, regardless of what they are, is to help us feel and participate fully in our own lives. To become aware of our inner guidance system, we must learn to trust our emotions. This isn't always so easy, because many of us have been taught to live our lives as though we were in a constant emergency situation. We think, "Oh, I'll deal with that painful emotion later. Right now I don't have time. I have to get that report out, or cook dinner," or whatever it is. This delay or denial requires our bodies to speak louder and louder to get our attention. The next time you feel moved to tears or moved to laughter, stop and experience it.

Many women have been taught to "think"—not feel—that we should be upbeat and happy all the time. Sadness or pain are natural parts of life. They are also great teachers. No one gets through life without experiencing sadness or pain. Yet our culture teaches us that there is something wrong with pain—that it must be drugged, denied, or otherwise avoided at all costs—and the costs are very high.

We are not taught that we have an innate ability to deal with pain, that our bodies know how to do this. Crying is one of the ways in which we rid our bodies of toxins. Crying allows us to move energy around our body and sometimes to rechannel it or understand it in a different way. When we don't allow ourselves to feel our emotions and instead use addictive processes such as running or tranquilizers to "get a high," we actually create hormones (enkephalins) that repress tears (and our full emotional expression).[1] Tears contain toxins that the body needs to get rid of.[2] Tears of joy and tears of sorrow have different chemical compositions and are influenced by hormones. They also serve different purposes. When we allow ourselves a full emotional release, our body, mind, and spirit feel cleansed and free. Insight about what to do in a given situation often comes *only after* we feel our emotions about it and shed tears if necessary. Interestingly, tears of joy and tears of sorrow are physiologically and chemically distinct from each other, even though sadness and joy are very much related. We cannot feel the height of our joy unless we have felt the depths of our sadness. Though joy and sadness express different emotions, both are natural parts of how our body processes and "digests" feelings.

Many illnesses are quite simply the end result of emotions that have been stuffed, unacknowledged, and unexperienced, for years. One of my patients with a long history of migraine headaches recently said, "I finally hit bottom with my headaches when my neurologist wanted to put me on lithium. I knew I didn't want to deal with the effects of that drug on my body. I started biofeedback so that I could learn to relax. I had a childhood that was so painful, I had nowhere else to go but into the pain. Now I realize that I don't have to have the pain anymore. I notice that I start to get a headache the minute I stop taking care of myself. If I don't rest or get enough sleep, or if I don't stand up for myself with my family, the headaches start. I see that all along the headaches have been trying to show me something."

Emotional Cleansing: Healing from the Past

Healing can occur in the present only when we allow ourselves to feel, express, and release emotions from the past that we have suppressed or tried to forget. I call this *emotional incision and drainage.* I've often likened this deep process to treatment of an abscess. Any surgeon knows that the treatment for an abscess is to cut it open, allowing the pus to drain. When this is done, the pain goes away almost immediately, and new healthy tissue can re-form where the abscess once was. It is the same with emotions: They too become walled off, causing pain and absorbing energy, if we do not experience and release them.

Children release emotion naturally and immediately, and each of us is born with the innate ability to do this. Yet because our culture worships emotional control, we learn early on how to suppress our emotional releases. When a woman comes to me because she is having panic attacks or crying spells, I know that some emotional material is ready to come up to be processed. To observers who haven't experienced deep process, she may appear to be "losing it," "going off the deep end," or "getting out of control." She is not "out of control," however; she is simply allowing a healing process to arise within the body. Only the intellect has lost control—it has taken a back seat to the innate wisdom of the body.

Too often, health care providers prescribe drugs in cases like this. As a result, a woman's natural healing process can get stagnated for months or years. And even if drugs are not prescribed, most people in our culture are uncomfortable with the emotions that arise when they are watching another person feel their emotions. They therefore rush to "comfort" the person who is beginning to cry or "lose it." This stops the person's emotional process and at the same time protects the "comforter" from feeling his or her feelings. The healing process stops for both of them.

On the other hand, if a woman is encouraged to stay with what she's feeling, to go into it, to make the sounds she needs to make, and to cry or yell as long as necessary, staying completely with her innermost self, she'll often discover that her body has the innate ability to heal even very painful memories and events from her past. When we are willing to be with "what is" instead of running away from it, we will often be able to work through painful experiences that have lain dormant and taken up our energy for years. Stephen Levine calls this experience "the pain that ends the pain."

When we have allowed ourselves a full emotional release, the body, mind, and spirit feel cleansed and free. Insights come up and long buried self-understanding returns. I've watched people forgive themselves and others after deep process work because they are finally at peace with painful events in their past. This can happen even after years of intellectualizing that never really healed them.

One striking example of this was the deep process of an infertility surgeon I'll call Carol. Carol had found it very painful when she was not able to help a woman become pregnant, in spite of using all of the current technology at her disposal. Though infertility is not an exact science, she took her couples' failures to conceive very personally. This made her emotional attitude toward her professional life fraught with sadness.

During a workshop I was leading, the discussion turned to the subject of "mothers," and many of the participants released a great deal of emotional material. Carol got down on a mat and allowed herself to cry and wail. During this process she kept repeating, "I don't need to create any more mommies. I don't need to create more mommies." When she was finished, she realized that she herself had never really had a mother in an emotional sense. She had been beaten repeatedly by her mother when she was a child. She had made her career choice as an infertility physician in part because of her unresolved early-childhood pain: On an unconscious level, she was trying to "create mommies" in an attempt to create the mother she emotionally needed. Following this deep insight, she was able to go back to her work refreshed and free, finally released from assuming complete responsibility for her patients' conceptions.

Dreams: A Doorway to the Unconscious

Dreams are another part of our inner guidance system. Scientific evidence shows that the amount of activity in our brain when we dream is identical to the amount when we are awake. During dreaming, our inner guidance works with our brain to lay down a map of the activities or goals that we desire or need for a healthy balanced future. Dreams also show us the beneficial and nonbeneficial directions toward which we are focusing our energy and how and where we need to make adjustments.

One of my patients who was healing from chronic pelvic pain related to me that, as she healed, she became more and more competent and powerful in her dreams. She said it was fun to go to sleep at night to see what she'd be capable of next.

Another patient, recovering from incest, said, "I recently dreamed that a little four-year-old girl was trying to tell me about someone who hurt her. I know that I am that girl—and that I need to listen to her in my dreams."

Another woman, suffering from chronic vaginitis, asked her dreams for guidance about what to do, since none of our physical treatments were helping. She came back a week later and said, "I had the dream. Everything was black, and I heard a voice say, 'When you get rid of Larry, the problem will go away.' " She eventually was able to tend to her relationship problems and her condition began to clear.

Learn to pay attention to your dreams by writing them down first thing in the morning. Plan to remember them before you go to bed at night. Keep a notebook and pen beside your bed.

Intuition and Intuitive Diagnosis

Intuition is the "direct perception of truth or fact *independent of any reasoning process.*" A very good example of intuition is when you walk into a dark room and somehow *know* that someone is in there, even when you can't see them and haven't been told they are there. We are all born with this ability, and all of us were highly intuitive as children. Most of us, however, were trained out of this way of knowing by the age of seven. The more education we get in this culture, in general, the less we trust our natural intuition. Because our society glorifies only logical, rational, left-brain thinking, we are taught to discount other forms of knowing as primitive or ignorant.

Thus, our intuitive capacity has become suspect and underutilized. Yet it is a skill that can be relearned at any time because it is a completely natural way of knowing. Although addictions keep us out of touch with *what we know and what we feel* and most of us are out of touch with our intuition much of the time, as we become more inner directed and more in touch with our inner guidance system, we automatically gain access to our intuition. Our society admits that even the geniuses among us use only about 25 percent of their brain capacity. To use intuition is simply to use more of our intelligence than we are accustomed to using.

Intuitive diagnosis is the ability to read our own (or another's) energy field. Intuitive diagnosis is centuries old and has been part of many ancient healing systems. Every traditional shaman has worked in this way, as have healers in the Wicca tradition.[3] Intuitive diagnosis can help us detect energy blockages *before* they become physical. We can act on this information and keep ourselves healthy.

How Inner Guidance Works

One of my medical student friends who has a "bad back" has noticed that her back pain always emerges when she has to do something that she doesn't want to do. (This is true in spite of the fact that she has a so-called "physical" problem that should, by itself, explain her symptoms.) Currently, she is contemplating writing a research paper. Whenever she even thinks about writing this piece and the colleagues with whom she will be involved, she gets neck pain and feels sick to her stomach. All her training has taught her that publishing this research paper is what she *should do* for her career. Yet her inner guidance, which speaks to her through her body's feelings, is telling her something quite different. She knows that she must take the radical step of choosing between her inner guidance and what society is telling her is best if she is to remain healthy.

Our bodies are designed to function best when we're doing work that feels exactly right to us. If we want to know God's will for us, all we have to do is look to our gifts and talents—that's where we will find it. Health is enhanced in women who engage in work that satisfies *them.* If a woman wants to know what her gifts and talents are, she can think back to when she was age nine to eleven, before the culture really put her into trance. What did she love to do? What did she want to be? Who did she think she was?

Another way to get in touch with our gifts and talents is to ask ourselves what we would do or be if we knew we had only six months to live. Would we stay at our current job? With our current partner?

We are meant to move toward whatever gives us fulfillment, personal growth, and freedom. We are born knowing what activities, things, thoughts, and feelings are associated with these qualities. We must learn to trust ourselves and know that we can naturally move toward that which is healing and fulfilling.

Many people have been taught that they can't have what they want and that a life full of struggle is somehow more honorable than one full of joy. We have also been taught to distrust something if it is too fulfilling or too much fun. This belief is reflected in our bodies. An eminent hypnosis researcher once noted that negative effects, like blisters, were twice as easy to induce as positive outcomes.[4] Yet when we can clearly state what we want and why, we are instantly in alignment with our inner guidance. This is because it feels good in our bodies to think about and dwell upon what we want and why. We get excited and are inspired automatically by these thoughts and feelings, which in turn keep us in touch with our inner knowing and spiritual energy. The result is enthusiasm and joy.

Our culture has too often taught us that it is selfish to have our own wants and dreams and to enjoy ourselves. Many girls, when they are in touch with their inner power, have been told, "Who do you think you are, the Queen of Sheba?" Too many of us have heard "Don't break your arm patting yourself on the back" when we have done a job we're proud of or have given ourselves credit for, something that we loved to do, just for us. All of our lives, this kind of statement has stopped us dead in our tracks. We are accused of being selfish when we've given our own lives and interests priority. We have been brought up to avoid being seen as selfish at all costs.

In general, women in our culture have a difficult time going after what they personally want and need in an atmosphere in which it is assumed that they will perform and be responsible for all of the tasks of daily living such as child-rearing, meal preparation, and general nurturing. And even if child-rearing and housekeeping are precisely what a woman wants to do the most, she may find that these activities are undervalued and underpaid. However, nothing will change in a woman's outer circumstances until she learns to value her own life and her own gifts as much as she has been taught to value and nurture the lives of others. As a friend of mine says, "If you want to be one of the chosen, all you have to do is choose yourself!"

Nearly every woman I know has been socialized to believe that putting everyone else before herself is the right thing to do. Yet we can reverse this idea and attend to ourselves. Dana Johnson, a researcher friend of mine and a registered nurse, even recovered from Lou Gehrig's disease by learning to respect all aspects of her body. After she had had the disease for some years, she began to lose control over her breathing muscles as well as the rest of her body. Her breathing difficulties made her think she was going to die. But she decided at that point that she wanted to experience unconditional love for herself at least once before dying. Describing herself as a "bowl of Jell-O in a wheelchair," she sat every day for fifteen minutes in front of a mirror and chose different parts of herself to love. She started with her hands because at that time they were the only parts of herself that she could appreciate unconditionally. Each day she went on to other body parts. Day by day, her physical body began to get better as she learned to appreciate it. She also wrote in a journal about insights she had during this process, and she came to see that since childhood she had believed that in order to be of service, acceptable to others, and worthy herself, she had to sacrifice her own needs. It took a life-threatening disease for her to learn that service through self-sacrifice is a dead end. Although feeling good about being of service simply for its own sake is health-enhancing, far too many women bake cookies, make coffee, and clean up because it's expected of them and they would feel guilty if they didn't do it. Service to others done under obligation creates exhaustion and resentment.

Knowing What We Don't Want

In addition to knowing what we *do* want, we have the capacity to know what we *don't* want. Knowing what we don't want is inborn. Every baby knows what feels good and what doesn't feel good, and up until about the age of six, a child will automatically go toward what feels good and away from what feels bad. This capacity is seen in its purest form in a two-year-old child who has just learned how to say no.

The ability to say no to what doesn't support us is an essential part of our inner guidance system. It is never too late to start saying no to those things that drain you and yes to those that replenish you.

- When a friend calls and asks for help, stop for a moment and ask yourself, "Do I really want to help right now, or would I prefer to do something else?"
- Check your body when someone asks you to do something. Are there areas of tension? Do you get a "gut reaction" of any kind? Does your body say, "Yes, this would be fun," or does it say, "No, doing this would be draining"?
- If you find yourself tired or irritable at the end of a day, ask yourself what thoughts, activities, or people drained your energy during the day.
- On the days when you are feeling wonderful, ask yourself what thoughts, activities, or people enhance your energy flow.
- Keep a journal, and begin to notice and write down everything that contributes to a positive energy flow that replenishes you. Paying attention to these things will draw more of them into your experience.

One of my patients, a social worker, originally came to see me complaining of PMS and mild anxiety attacks. In going over her history, I noticed that she never had any time to herself and that her life was overrun with taking care of others' needs while neglecting her own. I told her that she must practice noticing what activities replenished her energy and which ones drained her. Then I told her that in order to reverse her symptoms, she had to spend at least one hour each day recharging her own energetic batteries by resting or doing something she liked. She did so, and a month later all her symptoms were gone. She told me that she was learning how she drained her energy in her daily life. She said, "When I lie down or sit down to write in my journal, I can literally *feel* the energy coming back into my body. Knowing how crucial this is to my physical and emotional well-being is a revelation."

All of us receive messages from our bodies regularly about what serves our health and well-being and what doesn't. Our bodies know immediately when we are doing something or even thinking about something that doesn't support us fully. One of my friends gets diarrhea and stomach cramps when she just thinks about going to visit her parents. She was abused, both physically and emotionally throughout her entire childhood, and this abuse has continued into adulthood. Her body knows that visiting her parents will not be good for her, and it gives her symptoms as messages to stay away. When she gives herself permission to stay away, her stomach problems go away immediately.

In order to create health daily, long before illness ensues we need to pay attention to the subtle signals from our bodies about what feels good and what doesn't. Foggy thinking, dizziness, heart palpitations, acne, headaches, and back, stomach, and pelvic pain are a few of the common but subtle symptoms that often signal that it is time for us to let go of what we don't want in life. Here's an example from my own life.

Back in the 1980s, when I had two young children, I was working too many hours, and I often felt that aspects of my work weren't respected by my colleagues. My face was often broken out in large blemishes that I had never had as an adolescent or at any other time in my life until then. I tried taking vitamins, changing my diet, and using a variety of skin creams. Nothing helped—until I left my place of work. Within six months the problem cleared and has never returned.

Clearly, my face was a barometer of my well-being during those years. Through my skin condition, my body had been telling me that my work setting was not supporting me optimally. My complexion had been registering my "thin-skinned" sensitivity and my anger at not being completely accepted by my colleagues. (I hadn't completely accepted myself, either, at this point.) All of these emotions lay just below the surface, though I couldn't appreciate this at the time. Once I "faced" my innermost needs and left the situation that simply was not supporting me, my complexion improved automatically. As my life cleared up, so did my face.

Negative emotions exist to let us know that we are not facing the clearest path to what we want. When we realize that our bodies and their symptoms—feelings—are our allies, pointing out what serves our highest good and what doesn't, we become free. Whenever you feel angry or upset, have a headache or a bodily symptom, take a moment to reflect upon what the symptom is trying to say to you. When I am caught up in a downward spiral of negative feelings, I instantly know that I am out of touch with my inner guidance and that I'm giving too much attention to what I don't want. I have learned to notice when I'm feeling bad and stop for a moment. If I can catch myself at the beginning of the bad mood, I can often get my energy flowing positively again by doing the following process:

1. I acknowledge what I am feeling *without making any judgment about it.* I avoid wallowing around in the negative emotion and prolonging it, but I definitely *feel* it fully. I "stay with the feeling."

2. I acknowledge that there is a reason why I am feeling the way I am.

3. I spend twenty seconds or so identifying what is causing my energy to flow negatively. For example, yesterday I was angry because a staff member didn't get an important message to me in time for me to return a phone call promptly.

4. Having identified the source of my negative emotion, I then ask myself what I *do* want. (I have a friend do this with me if I need help clarifying my wants in a positive, nonreactive way.) What I want is usually the opposite of what I am experiencing the moment I'm feeling bad. Asking myself what I want shifts my focus back to positive thoughts and thus moves my energy toward my wants.

5. I then name what I want. Stating our wants is powerful because it defines them clearly, allowing our creative energy to flow toward them. Thus, in the example in step 3, I would say, "I want to receive my telephone messages on time so that I can respond to them promptly and efficiently." This statement reflects positive energy flowing toward what I want. Because it is a statement of pure positive energy with no negativity in it, it helps draw what I want into my experience. When I am thinking about or talking about what I want, the negative emotion often goes away by itself.

6. Finally, I affirm that I have the power within me, via my inner guidance and my power of intent, to get what I want.

Going through this process is *not* a way to deny my emotions or push them away. Rather, it helps me acknowledge them, feel them fully, and use them as guidance toward what I *do* want. I regularly sit down with a notebook and make a list of exactly what I want in a given situation. This aligns my thoughts with my inner guidance, and it feels good. Inspiration about what to do generally follows. Please note that I don't try to figure out what to *do* about a certain situation until I've gone through the entire process of looking in the direction of what I want. The reason for this is that directed thought creates vibration, which then results in inspiration. I remind myself that whenever I am reacting *against* something I don't want, I just create *more* of what isn't working and my actions are based on fixing what I don't want instead of creating what I do want. In the past, for example, my husband would often spend many hours at the hospital and wouldn't come home for dinner on time. I used to look out the window and wait for him, trying to keep the dinner warm, feeling angry at him and sorry for myself. The more I demanded that he show up on time, the more of a problem it became in our relationship. One day, I simply decided to go ahead and eat dinner myself and then get on with the evening activities and enjoy myself. I did this whenever he wasn't home when he said he would be. Eventually, he began coming home on time spontaneously, and this hasn't been a problem since.

Unfortunately, instead of using our feelings as inner guidance, we're brought up to fear, deny, or judge our negative emotions and feelings as *bad*. Most of us were taught that being able to "control" ourselves and our emotions is commendable and a mark of achievement. When John F. Kennedy was assassinated, my mother thought that Jackie Kennedy was an inspiration to the nation because she walked behind the casket with such dignity, never shedding a tear or showing any emotion—a role model for the nation. Though remaining emotionally calm and collected under pressure can be admirable, all too often this control becomes such an ingrained habit that women are out of touch with their emotions even when it would be healing and safe to acknowledge and express them. Men are even more at risk for being out of touch with their feelings than women, since they learn early on that "big boys don't cry." A friend of mine was taught that if she had to cry, she should bury her face in a pillow so that the rest of the family wouldn't have to hear it. Yet crying and making sounds are all a part of our emotional "digestive" system and a way to keep energy flowing evenly throughout our bodies.

Anne Wilson Schaef points out that the addictive system has a "nonliving" orientation. This orientation encourages us to "keep a lid on it," as in, "Don't make waves." By learning very early on that emotions are bad or shameful, we learn not to trust our inner guidance or our bodies. When we are encouraged to be out of touch with what we know and what we feel in general, we are systematically trained out of moving toward fulfillment of our innermost desires and saying no to what we don't want. Even our religions teach us to squelch our innate joy and creativity and that feeling good is a sin. As Matthew Fox points out, "Our civilization has not done a good job with the energy called delight and joy."[5] We need to know that the very essence of a life based on inner guidance is abundant delight and joy!

Every smiling, laughing three-month-old baby I've ever met reflects the true, joyous nature with which we were all born. Ashley Montagu once said that most adults are nothing more than "disintegrated children." Fortunately, our inner guidance is always available to remind us of our direction toward fulfillment. When we realign with our inner guidance and stop judging our bodies and our feelings as bad when they are offering us information, we are on the pathway to a life filled with growth and delight.

FOUR

The Female Energy System

Understanding how energy works in our female bodies can help us decipher our individual body's unique language. The location of a disease within the body—where it occurs—has psychological and emotional meaning and significance. Specific mental and emotional patterns are associated with specific body locations. Our thoughts, emotions, and behaviors are reflected or patterned simultaneously in the brain, the spinal cord, the various organs, the blood, and the lymphoid (immune) tissue, and in the electromagnetic field that surrounds and penetrates all those areas. Understanding the different dynamic patterns of energy that our bodies give rise to and operate within can help you appreciate how positive or negative energies can manifest themselves in your individual body.

The Matter/Energy Continuum

Our body's energy system is always changing, and the *potential* for healing or disease is present at all times. Precancerous cells, for example, arise regularly in our bodies. They form invasive cancers only when our own internal controls break down.[1] Mental and emotional energy goes in and out of physical form regularly, bouncing on the continuum between energy and matter, particle and wave. Quite simply, emotional and mental energy can become physical in our bodies.

When we have unresolved chronic emotional stress in a particular

67

area of our life, this stress registers in our energy field as a disturbance that can manifest in physical illness. Here is how it happens:
When we obsess about someone or something, our life-energy leaks
away from our body. When we obsess, we tie up energy—*chi, ki,
prana,* or *qi*—in a negative process that diverts it from our cells.
Vital cellular processes thereby become depleted. We leak energy in
any situation in which our anger or fear are controlling our ability
to move forward in our lives. While most doctors do not view the
onset of disease in terms of these energy leaks, it is interesting to
note that some medical research supports this observation. In one
study, for instance, cancerous cells were shown to "steal" energy (in
the form of the molecule DPN, an ATP-like molecule) from adjacent normal tissue.[2]

In any case, thinking about energy fields and energy leaks can
help us understand and begin a healing process. When we persist in
being angry with someone who has hurt us, for example, a part of
our spirit is occupied with that person and is not available to us for
healing. When a person has been severely abused, shamans believe
that part of the person's spirit may flee in order to escape the abuse.
One of the healing traditions of shamanism is called "soul retrieval,"
in which the missing "spirit" is called back. Many women who have
been sexually abused as children relate that they "left their bodies"
during the abuse. Some remember that a part of themselves actually
left and went up to the ceiling and "watched." This split-off part of
their spirit is not available to them in the present for healing.

Many times we are not conscious of these energy leaks. But if
these leaks continue without being healed, bodily distress is often
the result. Bodily symptoms can serve to bring our attention to that
area so that healing can begin. One of my menopausal patients who
came to see me with insomnia and depression told me of her sexual
abuse as a child—something she had not been consciously aware of
until a week before her visit with me. She had gone through a
painful divorce in her forties and had had a recent breakup with her
lover of seven years. She said, "I realize now that I've spent my
entire life trying *not* to remember that I was sexually abused. Now
that I know it happened, I realize why I've never had a satisfactory
relationship. I've always pushed people away. I didn't know how to
be fully present in a relationship. But I didn't know any better. I'm

grieving for my early life and the fact that it has taken me this long to remember and release the past. But finally the chronic knot in my stomach is gone. I feel free. I am so relieved." Her sleep problem and depression cleared up spontaneously as her memories of abuse arose and were released from her energy field.

How to Heal Energy Leaks

To stay or become healthy, it is useful for each of us to notice where we are "leaking" our energy. A good time to do this is when you go to bed each night. To begin the process of healing your energy leaks, simply notice who or what you are thinking about, worrying about, or obsessing about. What thoughts, emotions, events, or people keep coming into your mind? Are there any emotions or thoughts over which you are obsessing? See who you're holding resentments against. When you find these areas, you must call your spirit back. One way to do this is by using your will and your power of intent to call back the parts of you that are caught in past or present situations that don't serve your highest good. It is helpful to do this out loud. Simply state, "Spirit, come back here—I need you with me." The split-off parts of yourself are not used to this calling, but eventually they will respond to your efforts and your energy will return.

Most of the blockages in our energy systems are emotional in nature. It's helpful to think of your energy system as being like a stream of water flowing along. As long as this energy flow is healthy and you are feeling good about yourself, there's much less risk of disease. Environmental toxins, dietary fat, and excess sugar or alcohol (to name a few) usually don't manifest in disease unless other factors have already "set up" the pattern or blockage in the body's energy system in the first place.[3] Environmental or dietary risk factors can be likened to "debris" carried along in the body's energy flow. This debris stays afloat unless there is a felled tree or other blockage to the water flowing in the stream. When there is, the debris collects on the branches of the felled tree and accumulates. Over time, similar accumulations in the body's energy flow can result in physical illness. In fact, scientific research has associated a failure of the flow of information between cells with the induction of cancer in those cells. A physical barrier of any kind that blocks communication between cells is a carcinogenic influence.[4] The fat and connective tissue that form a fibroid, for example, do so only when the energy flow around and through the uterus is already blocked in some way.

Our emotions are often stuck at the childhood level, when we were not allowed to experience them fully. In this culture, which teaches us to split our adult intellectual knowledge from our emotional reality and needs, one can have a Ph.D. from Harvard but an emotional body that is only two years old. The emotions, unexpressed and unacknowledged, become energetically stuck. Emotions that are expressed and felt, on the other hand, simply flow through our energy system, leaving no residual "unfinished" business.

We do not have to wait to develop cancer or other diseases in order to get the message that we need to change our energy system and begin creating health. None of us are completely free from the fear, anger, and stress that come and go as part of normal life. When these emotions become intense enough to affect our psychological and emotional well-being on a regular basis, we are heading for physical illness unless we resolve them in a healthy way. When our daily unresolved pain, anger, and frustration rob our bodies of vital health-producing energy, it is crucial to bring healing and understanding into our daily thoughts, emotions, and actions.

Here is a crucial point: It is completely possible for a woman to go through her entire life free from physical illness, even though she was abused, beaten, or neglected as a child. Early childhood problems do not *necessarily* cause energy disturbances and physical illness. They often occur after a woman begins to develop as an individual and form her own identity and opinions *separate* from those of her family and her background. At this point she may realize that what happened to her as a child was not acceptable. However, she is realizing this from the perspective of a mature individual, not of the child she was then.

Hurts and wounds from a woman's past do *not* become potentially devastating to her, physically or emotionally, *until* she gets the idea that what happened to her in the past was *wrong,* that it shouldn't have happened, and that she was abused purposely and consciously by her family members. She has now introduced into her emotional and psychological pattern a conflicting model of how her life *should have been.* This sets the stage for the toxic effects of blame. Though a woman may have been terrified or abused as a child, this early abuse will *not* affect her or her body *unless* she starts to believe that she was *entitled* to a different life. At this point she begins to relive and reevaluate her early life-experiences from the perspective of an individual reviewing a crime scene. Energy disturbance and subsequent illness may well result at this point if she is unable to work through her emotional and psychological pain with forgiveness and understanding for herself and others.

The chemistry of conflict, or righteous indignation, requires two major energies: The first is when a woman begins to remember that she was indeed violated in some way. The second is when she interprets those events from the point of view that her family deliberately and of conscious mind chose to do that to her. This mindset, not the abuse, is what creates disease.

I've learned how to recognize the poisoning effects of "righteous indignation" in my own body. Getting stuck in this energy for a long time becomes self-destructive. The longer we stay in this mode, searching for a perpetrator to blame for what happened to us—be it men, our mothers, the government, or doctors—the more our bodies are energetically depleted.

What we now call incest, for example, was not seen as incest years ago—it was tribal sharing. Some groups in many countries still live this way. Female circumcision is routinely carried out by elder women in cultures in which it is practiced. The tribal wisdom is that the young girl will be considered "tainted goods" if she hasn't been circumcised. From our Western cultural standpoint, this is barbaric. Because consciousness of the physical, psychological, and spiritual effects of female circumcision is now growing, the entire subject is being brought out into the open, discussed, and reevaluated.

Incest and other human rights abuses have been the norm for the last five thousand years. "These did not become the crimes they are today," writes Caroline Myss, "until we began to re-evaluate our personal boundaries within our tribal settings." In my view, this collective reevaluation constitutes addictive system recovery.

Our early family life clearly has a profound influence on our character and health. A prospective study by Dr. Caroline Thomas, for example, indicates that a man's lack of closeness to his parents,

or having a father who was physically and emotionally less involved, could predict early disability and death from suicide, hypertension, coronary artery disease, and tumors.[5]

Earth's Energy

Traditional Eastern philosophies describe the profound interaction
between the Earth's energy and that of the physical human body,
and the strong connection between female energy and the Earth's
own natural pull. Understanding women's nature, with its natural
ebbs and flows, as positive and powerful gives us a chance to heal
and live in a balanced, healthy way.

According to some Eastern beliefs, women's bodies are different
from men's, in that the Earth's energy moves up through our bodies
and inward. This female energy is "drawing-in" energy or centripetal force. This centripetal female energy is irresistible. It is so powerful that if one lives in a family setting, most of the household will
want to be around the person with the most centripetal energy—
usually the mother—and will be acutely aware when she is gone.
Children will save up their complaints for their mother at the end of
the day, if she hasn't been around. My children always need to know
where I am in the house. If I walk out of a room, they call, "Mom,
where are you?" after about one minute. When they were younger,
they always had to be in the same room with me. I couldn't take a
bath alone until the oldest was about nine. In contrast, when the
children were small, my husband could have been away for much
longer before they'd notice. A woman's inward-pulling energy is at
work when she puts the baby to the breast, the penis into the vagina
(if she is heterosexual), and the egg's chemical signals to sperm
swimming toward it.

Michio Kushi, the macrobiotic teacher who first discussed and
illustrated this energy pattern for Western readers, points out that
the Earth's centripetal force coming up through the feet is present in
men as well as women, just as heaven's force, coming downward
from the sky through the head down through the body (centrifugal
force), is present in women as well. What differs is the degree to
which each energy is present. In women, in general, more "Earth's
energy moving up" or centripetal force is present. I've been told that

Navaho women wear skirts because doing so increases the body's access to this Earth energy through the circle that the skirt creates on the Earth in relationship to the body (see Figure 1).

Centripetal energy is a grounding force that affects everyone around us because women tend to be the centers of their households, taking on psychological responsibility for the well-being of other family members. Therefore, when a woman changes her life for the better, her entire family (whether or not she has children) generally benefits. She sets the tone. The well-being of the family and of society itself depends upon women becoming and remaining healthy. Part of creating health is understanding the power of female energy and its implications. The health of a woman's loved ones is directly linked to her own personal health. So we owe it to ourselves first to take the time we need to heal.

The Chakras

Centripetal "drawing-in" force is only one way to characterize female energy. We also have seven specific energy centers in our bodies known as *chakras*. Emotional-psychological patterns commonly affect women's bodies and their energy centers, the chakras. Don't be surprised if you feel some resistance to hearing this information. Don't blame yourself for events of the past that have resulted in unhealthy patterns in your present life. Simply notice them and begin the healing process. Every human being, male or female, has the same chakras, and each of them is affected by specific emotional and psychological issues. These energy centers connect our nerves, hormones, and emotions. Their locations run parallel to the body's neuroendocrine-immune system and form a link between our energy anatomy and our physical anatomy. The energy system of the human body is a holographic field that carries information for the growth, development, and reproduction of the physical body. This holographic field guides the unfolding of the genetic processes that transform the molecules of our bodies into functioning organs and tissues. Though standard Western medicine has not recognized chakras yet, Eastern cultures have long appreciated them. Caroline Myss, an internationally known medical intuitive who diagnoses illness and energy dysfunctions with whom I've

FIGURE 1: EARTH'S ENERGY GOING UPWARD
Female energy = centripetal or "drawing-in" force. Earth's energy coming upward through the feet, then spiraling around the uterus, breasts, and tonsils.

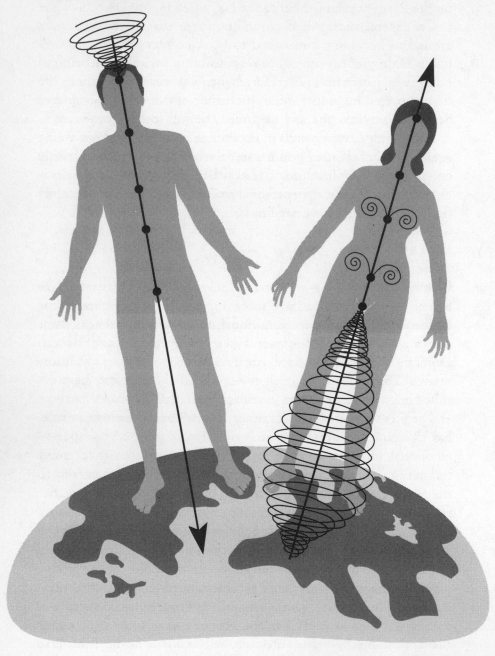

worked for over three years, has taught me the mental and emotional patterns that create either health or disease in each of our body's energy centers, the chakras. If we look at chakras as the place where energy transforms from the emotional to the physical body, we can begin to grasp how cultural wounding may have psychological and emotional consequences that set us up for subsequent gynecological, obstetrical, or other health problems. Whether you believe in chakras as literal or as metaphoric places in the body, they can help you activate mind-body connections to help you heal.

Each of the seven chakras of the human body is associated with a specific organ and emotional state. Each is also associated with a certain kind of fear and emotional insecurity. In other words, specific fears and emotions actually target specific areas of the body (see Figure 2). The location and naming of the chakras varies somewhat in different texts and different traditions, but the chakra system I use has been researched extensively by Dr. Norman Shealy, a neurosurgeon and energy medicine researcher, and Caroline Myss. Caroline Myss's intuitive ability appeared in her life rather suddenly and very unexpectedly.[6] She describes herself as a teacher whose goal is to "help people learn to think of themselves in the language of energy and to combine their awareness of energy anatomy with the care they give their physical bodies." As you learn about the chakras, listen to your own body and trust in your intuition about it and your different organs and system. Try to visualize each chakra's energy field to see if it feels healthy and whole to you or seems to need your attention and care.

Though all seven chakras are important and interlinked, I will concentrate on the ones that relate most directly to gynecological, obstetrical, and breast health. Some spiritual traditions emphasize the upper chakras as "more important" or "holier" than the "lower" or "less-than" chakras, but I want to stress that this is a typical patriarchal misunderstanding. We cannot hope to improve our health or the circumstances of our lives if we think of our body's lower centers as "less worthy" or "beneath our dignity." If humankind had collectively taken care of its lower chakra needs and viewed them as vital parts of the whole, instead of subordinating them to "higher" spiritual concerns, our planet and our individual lives would be flourishing today. Thinking that spiritual needs are more worthy than physical needs is doing a "spiritual bypass." As you work through the chakras, notice which ones you would like to spend less time on and examine why. You may want to review them until you become comfortable with them.

The Lower Female Centers: Chakras One to Four

The bottom three chakras are related to our physical life: the people, events, memories, experiences, and physical objects within our environment, past and present. All three of the lower female centers are inextricably linked and interacting. Therefore, although I address each one separately, understand that they all affect each other. (Ultimately, all seven chakras affect each other and are interactive.)

The *first chakra* area is affected by *how secure and safe we feel in the world.* The body areas that correlate with this chakra are the base of the spine, the rectum, and the hip joints. The foundation for our sense of safety usually is formed in childhood. Therefore, unresolved family and physical survival issues—like problems concerning one's house, family, sexual identity, and race—are represented in the first chakra.

The *second chakra* contains stored memories, emotions and information about *how we relate to other people.* The pelvic and reproductive organs (vulva, vagina, uterus, cervix, and ovaries) are in the second chakra. The health of this area is affected by the degree to which our relationships are based on issues of control, blame, and guilt. If we use sex, money, blame, or guilt to control the dynamics of our relationships (including our relationship with ourselves), then the organs of the second chakra will be adversely affected.

The *third chakra* is associated with a person's *self-esteem, self-confidence, and self-respect.* The foundation for a woman's sense of herself is formed by the emotions, memories, and wisdom stored in the energy fields of the first and second chakras. In order to have good self-esteem, a woman must feel secure in the world (first chakra) and have relationships based on mutual respect and support (second chakra). The gall bladder, liver, pancreas, stomach, and small bowel are the organs associated with the third chakra.

FIGURE 2: CHAKRA DIAGRAM WITH FEMALE FIGURE

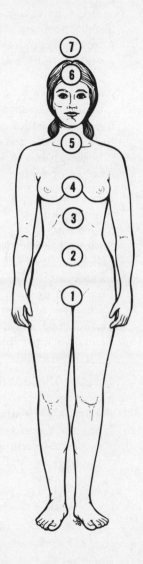

TABLE 4
ENERGY ANATOMY: MENTAL AND EMOTIONAL PATTERNS, THE
CHAKRAS, AND THE PHYSICAL BODY

Chakra	Organs	Mental, Emotional Issues	Physical Dysfunctions
7	Muscle system Nervous system Skeletal and skin	Inability to trust life Acquiring attitudes, values, ethics, and courage Issues with humanitarianism Issues with selflessness Inability to see the larger pattern in life Absence of faith	Paralysis Genetic disorders Bone cancer Bone problems Multiple sclerosis Amyotrophic lateral sclerosis (ALS)
6	Brain Eyes, ears Nose Pineal gland	Fear of self-evaluation Intuitive skills Knowledge Misuse of intellectual skill Inadequacy Fear of being open to the ideas of others Paranoia and anxiety Refusal to learn from life experiences	Brain tumors/ hemorrhage/stroke Neurological disturbances Blindness/deafness Full spinal difficulties Learning disabilities Seizures
5	Thyroid Trachea Neck vertebrae Throat Mouth Teeth and gums	Issues with personal expression Following one's dreams Using one's personal power to create in the physical world	Raspy throat Chronic sore throats Mouth ulcers Gum difficulties Temporomandibular joint problems Scoliosis Laryngitis Swollen glands Thyroid problems
4	Heart/lungs Cardiovascular Shoulders Ribs/breasts	Resentment, fear, bitterness Grief; issues with forgiveness	Congestive heart failure Myocardial infarction (heart attack)

Chakra	Organs	Mental, Emotional Issues	Physical Dysfunctions
	Diaphragm	Decrease in love of life	Mitral valve prolapse
	Esophagus	Anger/hostility/criticism	Cardiomegaly
		Demanding judgmentalness	Asthma/allergy
			Lung cancer
		Inability to give love to self or others	Bronchial pneumonia
			Upper back, shoulder
		Inability to receive love	Breast cancer
		Self-centeredness	
3	Abdomen	Inability to trust others	Arthritis
	Upper intestines	Fear, intimidation	Gastric or duodenal ulcers
	Liver, gall bladder	Lack of self-esteem, self-confidence, or self-respect	Colon/intestinal problems
	Kidney, pancreas		
	Adrenal gland		
	Spleen	Resenting care of others	Pancreatitis/diabetes
	Middle spine	Fear of assuming responsibility, or making decisions for self	Indigestion, chronic or acute
			Anorexia and bulimia
			Liver dysfunction
			Hepatitis
			Adrenal dysfunction
2	Uterus, ovaries	Blame and guilt	Ob/gyn problems
	Vagina, cervix	Problems with money, sex, and control issues with other people	Pelvic/lower back pain
	Large intestine		Sexual potency
	Lower vertebrae		Urinary problems
	Pelvis	Power/control in the physical world	
	Appendix		
	Bladder		
1	Physical body support	Safety/security in the world	Chronic low back pain
	Hip joints		Sciatica
	Base of spine	Not able to provide for life's necessities	Varicose veins
			Rectal tumors/cancer
		Not able to stand up for self	
		No place feels like home	
		Not supported by anyone	

Source: Shealy, C.N. and C.M. Myss. *The Creation of Health: Merging Traditional Medicine with Intuitive Diagnosis* (Walpole, NH: Stillpoint Publications, 1983).

All of the unresolved stresses of our early physical life related to people, events, memories, and experiences pull energy *primarily* from the three lower power centers, the first three chakras.

Lower Chakra Stresses in Women
- Any and all hostile feelings
- Resentments and feelings of rejection
- Wanting to leave a relationship but fearing the financial consequences
- Shame of one's body
- Shame about one's family background or one's husband's social status
- Guilt about the quality of one's mothering
- Being a child abuser instead of an abused child
- A history of incest or rape
- Guilt over an abortion
- Inability to conceive

These issues all have the potential to affect the organs "below the belt" because of the way in which all the lower chakras work together. Now I'll discuss the issues of each chakra in more detail.

The First Chakra: How Family Wounds Are Stored in the Body
Our first chakra health is related to our upbringing and early life. This includes our immediate and extended family, our race, social status, educational level, family legacy, and our family expectations as these were handed down through the generations. To describe the breadth of the issues involved in the first chakra, Caroline Myss uses the word *tribe*. For example, certain men learn very early on what it means to be a member of a clan. Another first chakra "inheritance" is that of many first- and second-generation immigrant families in the United States. In this tribal programming the belief is often passed on that to accomplish anything worthwhile, one must suffer and sacrifice personal happiness and pleasure. Family scars and the social and familial information that form a person's idea of reality are connected to the first chakra area.

The tribal mind is not an individual's mind. The tribal mind is primarily a survival collective brain that seeks to hold on to its own and fight for its own survival in the world. The tribal mind is concerned with *loyalty*, not love, kindness, or tenderness. What the tribe refers to as "love" is really obligation to the tribe. An example of this is a family member who says to another, "If you really loved me, you'd come to visit your family and me more often." Tribal consciousness, then, is not a high-class, highly evolved consciousness. Yet we all share it to some degree, and many women admit that as they get older, they themselves can hear that tribal mind within themselves. "I sometimes hear my mother's words coming right out of my mouth, and I can't believe it," patients often tell me.

I sometimes refer to the tribal mind as "crabs in the bucket." If you have a bunch of crabs in a bucket and one crab tries to escape over the edge, the other crabs will always pull the escapee back down with the rest of them. The same sort of thing often happens to women and their families as the women decide to break free from limiting patterns. Almost invariably, family members try to sabotage her efforts—at least initially.

Countless women have had the experience of confronting their parents about abuse or incest soon after remembering these events, only to find that their parents deny these allegations outright. The unconscious motive to preserve the tribe is the reason so many parents deny having ever violated a tribe member. At some level, their tribal memory bank has absorbed the memory very differently from the way the individual member records the same event.

First Chakra Issues That Can Set the Stage for Illness
- Unfinished business with parents
- Incest (this is a second chakra issue as well)
- Abuse or neglect in childhood
- Psychological programming from one's early years that is limiting, such as:
  - "You're stupid." "You're useless." "You're a bad girl."
  - "Only Catholics go to heaven."
  - "Your body is something to hide out of shame."
  - "Girls are meant to serve men."

- "Men always come first." (For example, in many families the men get the best cuts of meat, and the women get what is left over.)
- "Girls should not be ambitious or bright."
- "Women can't make money. They must marry it."

Most tribes or families *do not deliberately* try to poison their members—they are merely handing down what they recognize as tribal wisdom, even in the form of limiting and painful ideas. It is useful to think of yesterday's "tribe" as today's dysfunctional family.

My friend Carla recently realized, after resolving her many physical illnesses, that the seeds for these illnesses had been planted in her childhood. Her mother had repeatedly beaten her, not out of malice or lack of love but simply following her own tribal programming of how to love and prepare a daughter for life. She had told Carla that the beatings were how she showed her love. Whenever the mother saw another mother beating a child in the supermarket or elsewhere, she used to remark to Carla that obviously that mother really loved her child. Carla's mother deeply believed that life is very difficult and filled with pain and that to accomplish anything, Carla would have to suffer. Later, each time Carla reached a cherished goal, she developed a serious illness. She is now realizing that she can reach her goals joyfully by using her innate gifts and talents and her inner guidance, and that repeated illness and suffering need not be part of her experience.

The Second Chakra: Symbolic Creative Space

The second chakra is concerned with the day-to-day physical aspects of living, with the people to whom we relate, and with the quality of our relationships. The second chakra also relates to everything we own: money, relationships, and possessions. Since most of our early programming is to serve the tribe, most men and women automatically move into the roles of their second chakras in an unconscious way. They choose the partners that fulfill the needs of their second chakra. Women thus tend to marry for physical security, money, children, social status, and fear of abandonment. We then carry out our roles within these needs accordingly. We are programmed to tend to the needs of our personal tribe and often become completely controlled by the fears of the second chakra.

Second Chakra Issues: How Relationship Wounds Are Stored in the Body
- Fear of abandonment
- Financial security
- Social status
- Children
- Creativity

The uterus and ovaries are the major organs in the second chakra. This area is both literally and figuratively "creative space" out of which women can produce babies, relationships, careers, novels, insights, and other creative or artistic works. When our energy is not flowing smoothly in this area of the body, gynecological problems, such as fibroid tumors, can result.

When I think of the uterus as "potential space," I also think of what we as women are usually expected to "store" in there. A slang term for the uterus is "the bag," and as humans who have or have had a uterus, we are also the ones who carry all the stuff that others don't want to carry. Women who are married and have children often notice that their children give them (not their husband) the half-eaten food, gum wrappers, and other garbage that they no longer want to carry. We have all heard older women referred to as "old bags." When I was pregnant, nursing, and caring for small children, I felt like the "multiple bag lady."

Not only do women carry physical excess, we are also expected to carry "emotional" excess for others—usually for men, but not always. One sixty-year-old patient of mine with three grown children is living alone with her husband, who has recently retired. She tells me she is now champing at the bit to do other things in her life that she has long wanted to do, such as traveling and writing. But her husband is not enthusiastic about her endeavors. He's not sure what to do with his newly acquired freedom from work. My patient says, "But my husband still wants me to carry his anima—his moods, his enthusiasm, his fun. And when I let down and allow any of my own feelings to show, other than enthusiasm, *he* gets depressed." *Anima*, a term coined by the famous psychologist Carl Jung, is a man's inner feminine aspect that often gets projected onto the real-life women in his life when he is unwilling to feel his own emotions and work through them. What unconscious material do we store in our body centers that neither we nor anyone else really wants to carry around? When unresolved second chakra–related issues surrounding relationships, creativity, and/or a sense of security exist, the pelvic area of the body as well as the lower back can become vulnerable to disease.

A number of second chakra issues can set the stage for illness. The studies of Dr. Gloria Bachmann indicate that childhood sexual abuse is associated with eating disorders, obesity, and somatic complaints in the genitourinary system, as well as substance abuse and other self-destructive behaviors.[7] Studies by Dr. Robert Reiter and others have found that previous sexual abuse is a significant predisposing risk factor for chronic pelvic pain.[8]

Whenever I see a woman with a uterine problem such as fibroid tumors—which are present in 40 percent of American women—I ask her to meditate upon her relationships, creativity, and sense of security. What is her fibroid telling her about these areas? Fibroids, endometriosis, diseases of the ovaries, and other pelvic disorders are manifestations of "blocked energy" in the pelvis. In a misogynist culture in which 40 percent of women are sexual abuse survivors and one in three gets physically raped, it's not hard to figure out how this happens.

At the time of her annual exam, I found a small fibroid in Gina, a patient who was thirty-eight years old at the time. I asked her to meditate on "blocked energy" in her pelvis, and she later told me, "When I got home and took some time with this question, I realized that when my brother died in an accident, I was furious with him for leaving. I was twenty-five and really couldn't allow myself to feel that rage. So I just stuffed it in my pelvis. I hadn't thought about that for years." On a follow-up exam three months later, I found that her fibroid was gone. I believe that by expressing and experiencing the full impact of her anger for the first time, she changed the energy pattern in her pelvis and actually dematerialized the fibroid, transforming it from matter into energy. She told me, "I had a feeling that when I came in today, you'd say it was gone. I literally felt it let go."

I've seen other women decrease or eliminate their fibroids when they remembered and released old experiences.

Third Chakra: Self-Esteem and Personal Power

The foundation for a woman's sense of herself, her self-esteem (third chakra), is formed by her sense of security and safety in the world (first chakra) combined with the quality of her relationships (second chakra). As a result of the collective and individual histories of most women, many of us have low self-esteem. For centuries women haven't been validated or valued except in their capacity as servers and pleasers of others. Thus, as women have become individuals in their own right, their families often do not support them in becoming all of who they can be.

This is because families usually hold an unconscious "tribal" fear that their female members will abandon them to serve their own needs and live out their personal dreams without the family. We've all inherited the belief that a woman cannot develop herself fully without simultaneously sacrificing her ability to serve her family.

Besides undertaking the classic struggle to balance our personal interests and our responsibilities, women often pace our self-esteem to our mate's cycle. If a woman's partner becomes highly successful, she may become depressed because she can't keep pace with him; or she may not back her partner's new adventure into different thought or creative new territories for fear that he (or she) will leave her. On the other hand, when a mate is unsuccessful in the outside world and becomes depressed or abusive, this also affects the woman in her third (and also first and second) chakra. Conflicts such as these cause energetic dysfunction in the third chakra and can result in physical illness in the stomach (ulcers, anorexia nervosa, and bulimia), gall bladder, small intestine, liver, and pancreas (diabetes).

Archetypes and the Lower Female Centers

When a woman feels that she is forced to participate in an activity, her body, mind, and spirit are at risk for harm.[9] When she unwittingly participates in a pattern of self-abuse and abuse from others, she is acting under the influence of what in energy medicine is called the "rape" archetype.

Archetypes are psychological and emotional patterns that influence us unconsciously until we become aware of their power. Archetypes are universal ideas, images, and patterns of thought that we all share in our subconscious. Though the concept of archetypes may at first seem elusive, these unconscious patterns of thought and behavior have a very real effect on our bodies and emotions.

To help you understand the concept of archetype more clearly, I'll use an example—the "mother" archetype. A woman who is unconsciously operating under the influence of the "mother" archetype (as it currently exists in this culture) thinks obsessively about the needs of her children while forgoing her own. Even when her children are old enough to care for most of their physical needs themselves, the woman sometimes focuses her thoughts on whether they've had enough to eat, whether they are happy, and whether they are warm enough or cool enough, ignoring or suppressing her own needs to do something for them. This culturally encouraged behavior of worrying can become a damaging stereotype. Another example of an archetype is the "hero." When we see the word *hero*, we instantly think of a person who is strong, bold, and brave. A hero is one who may fearlessly rescue others and neglect his or her own safety and needs because of a compulsion to "save" someone else. If unconscious, this kind of behavior, too, can be detrimental to health.

When we are unconsciously participating in archetypal patterns of behavior, we lose touch with our deepest selves and our inner needs. When a woman is not following her own heart's desires and instead acts only to fulfill others' needs, she may be under the influence of either the "rape," the "prostitute," or the "mother" archetype, depending upon the circumstances.

The "rape" and "prostitute" archetypes are very closely related. When a woman engages in sexual activity that she doesn't really want but feels unable to do anything to prevent, she is under the influence of the "rape" archetype. The same archetype is present if she denies herself sexual pleasure because she feels that this is what her partner wants—and again feels unable to alter her situation. The "rape" archetype may occur when a woman participates in her own violation, when she participates in such things as an abortion that her mate wants but that she doesn't. A woman who resents her partner but stays in the relationship anyway for financial or other reasons is not acting from her individual strength but is under the spell of the "prostitute" archetype. Women often handle this archetype by blaming ourselves or by absorbing our own anger and rage, lest telling of these feelings results in our becoming abandoned.

A woman's second chakra organs are also put at risk when she herself becomes an aggressor or victimizer. Women participate in the "rape" archetype, for example, when they violate their children's physical and psychological boundaries. Daily enemas and rough washing of the genitalia are other common examples of women as violators. Women use emotional weaponry, while men add to that their fists. Women who victimize pay for it not only through the energy of their female organs in the second chakra but with organs in the first and third chakras as well. According to Caroline Myss, aggressive behavior can be associated with cancer in the organs of the first three chakras.

It is important for us to understand and accept that women do have the potential for aggression. When we refuse to acknowledge a problem, we simply perpetuate it. Recovering from patriarchal influences isn't about blaming men, because in our culture we're all potential victims and potential perpetrators. When I first had a reading with Caroline Myss, for example, she told me that my body registered a rape between the ages of twenty-one and twenty-nine—the years that I was in medical school and doing my residency. Though I had not been physically raped, my body's energy system had been emotionally and psychologically "raped" by my medical training—something I had not been consciously aware of at the time. Myss states that almost everyone in this culture has suffered from a psychological or emotional rape of their innermost self at least once. That is one reason why so many women who have never suffered from overt sexual abuse nonetheless have chronic pelvic pain and other second chakra problems. Many women feel stuck in jobs in which the "rape" or "prostitute" archetype is a daily reality.

When we continually see women only as victims, we do not acknowledge the damage women do to themselves and to others. If you've ever borne the brunt of female abuse or been an abuser yourself, you'll understand the significance of this point of view.

Shame and the Lower Female Centers

Another issue for many women is shame. Shame hits the lower female centers and the interior organs, including the uterus and ovaries. Shame can be a result of social programming that tells a woman she's inferior, and it can be a result of family relationships, such as unhealthy relationships with her children, or shame at her partner's social status. Shame over a rape, whether it was physical, emotional, or psychological rape, affects the vaginal area.

Research supports these energy dysfunctions. Fisher and Cleveland found that there are differences in personality between women who develop interior cancers and those who develop exterior cancers.[10] An individual's perception of whether her body is permeable and easily penetrated by external influences, either physical or emotional, is related to whether she is susceptible to cancer. Those women who perceive their bodies as permeable are subject to cancers that are located more deeply in their bodies—for example, in the ovaries or uterus. Those women who believe that their bodies are strong and protected against external influences are more prone to cancers in the external genital areas.

The Fourth Chakra

The bodily areas associated with the fourth chakra are the heart, breasts, lungs, ribs, upper back, and shoulders. The fourth chakra is symbolic of self-love and our ability to feel "unconditional love." The emotional and psychological issues associated with ill health in the fourth chakra area are an inability to give or receive love from self or others (nurturance), lack of forgiveness, grief, unresolved anger, hostility, criticism, and being judgmental.

The second and fourth chakras have a unique interrelationship. The uterus is sometimes called the "low heart," while the heart in the chest is the "high heart." It's been said that if the low heart has been closed, through rape, incest, or abuse, a woman cannot truly open her high heart. In this culture, women also tend to shut down their low hearts, or their sexuality and erotic needs, because we're taught that "nice" girls aren't sexual. We're also taught, however, that it's fine for us to be in touch with our emotions and feelings, and so we're set up for second and fourth chakra conflicts.

Energetic chakra dysfunctions often arise when a woman is confused about how to use both her loving (fourth chakra) and her creative (second chakra) energies optimally. The major conflict within women is that most of us still believe that in order to be loved, to receive love, and to guarantee that someone will need us, we must care for our loved ones' external physical needs. But such love relationships, dependent upon ties of family obligation and tribal tradition, are recognized as relationship addictions once a woman begins to individuate and become conscious of her patterns. Energy dysfunctions that arise in the second and fourth chakra areas at the same time are very common in our culture. They often result when women unconsciously participate simultaneously in both the "rape" archetype and the "mother" archetype.

Sally, a twenty-six-year-old waitress, had very early stage cervical cancer (second chakra) and multiple breast cysts (fourth chakra). When she was a girl, her father had been both emotionally and physically distant. In her early teenage years, to fill up this emptiness, she had had multiple sexual partners, boys whom she neither loved nor respected. This addictive pattern of behavior (the "rape" and "prostitute" archetypes) disrupted the energetic patterns of her second chakra area, and she suffered from very painful and frequent herpes outbreaks in her vagina. She also had genital warts.

Like Sally's distant father, Sally's mother took care of neither her own nor her daughter's physical or emotional needs. Sally never learned how to care for her own emotional needs, in that no one ever demonstrated this behavior to her. Both Sally and her mother had energetic disruptions in their fourth chakra areas related to lack of self-respect and self-nurturance. Both mother and daughter have breast problems. Sally's mother has already had breast cancer, and Sally has had two breast biopsies for benign lumps.

Neither Sally nor her mother is unique in our culture. I see women like them in my practice daily. When a woman neglects her own inner needs, when she addictively cooks, cleans, and cares for the physical needs of her family, when she works obsessively at her job, and when she provides sex on demand because of feelings of obligation or guilt, she becomes susceptible to disease in both her second and fourth chakras. Quelling her insecurities about abandonment or about being good enough, about self-esteem, uses up her emotional energy.

Supporting these energetic dysfunctions, the research of Fisher and Cleveland shows that the personality patterns of women who have disease only in the second chakra differ from those of women with disease only in the fourth chakra. An extensive literature search reveals no studies on the personality patterns of women who have malignancy in *both* the second and the fourth chakra areas.

Patients with malignant tumors in the breast (the high heart) have different personality patterns from those with cervical cancer (low heart). In one study, 50 percent of the cervical cancer patients (a second chakra disease) had physically lost their fathers due to death or desertion during their early years (a second chakra–related emotion). In contrast, in the homes of those with breast cancer (a fourth chakra disease), the father was emotionally distant (a fourth chakra–related pattern).[11] Other studies have shown that significantly more cervical cancer patients have behaviors that suggest a second chakra energy imbalance: They had married multiple times, had a high incidence of sexual activity with partners whom they neither loved nor respected, and were very concerned with body shape, and size. They also had a feeling that they had been neglected as children. In contrast, studies of the breast cancer patients suggest behavior patterns associated with fourth chakra dysfunction: They had a greater tendency to stay in a loveless marriage, had a relatively high likelihood of carrying a heavy load of responsibility for younger siblings during childhood, and had a greater chance of denying themselves medical care and physical nurturance.[12]

Caroline Myss's observations further substantiate the research above. She teaches that emotions that are of the raging variety hit below the belt. Sadness that cannot be expressed, on the other hand, is associated with disease above the belt. I will be covering this in more detail in Chapters 5 to 10.

How to Heal Lower Chakra Wounding

Lower chakra wounds *don't heal until they're witnessed.* Someone has to say, "Yes, this happened to you." Such witnessing validates the existence of the wound; then the healing process can begin. A very important part of my work with women is this witnessing process. As a physician, I represent an authority figure. When I or another person validates a woman's woundings, she can use that as a very powerful catalyst for healing. But it is even more important that the *woman herself* acknowledge her wounding and need for healing. As long as a woman is stuck in denial ("It wasn't really all that bad, he never hit me," or "My family loved me very much—my father would never have done that"), she won't be able to tell the truth to herself. Her secrets will remain locked in the cells, unavailable for witnessing and healing.

After the witnessing of her wounds, a woman must then investigate how these wounds have affected her life. This is the naming stage—the stage when she realizes that her life has indeed been adversely affected by someone or something. Denial has now left. Many women in our society are currently at this stage. The final stage required for healing and the optimal functioning of the woman's energy system involves *releasing* the power of the wound to control her life. Forgiveness is now required, for both herself and others.

Other Chakra Issues

The *fifth chakra* is related to the power of the will, communication, personal expression, and following one's dreams. This chakra is located in the throat, mouth, teeth, gums, thyroid, trachea, and vertebral bodies of the neck. Dysfunctions in this chakra include chronic sore throats, throat and mouth ulcers, gum disease, temporal-mandibular joint disease (TMJ), scoliosis, thyroid disease, cervical disc problems, swollen glands, and laryngitis. Women with fifth chakra problems often have difficulty speaking up for themselves.

The *sixth chakra,* sometimes known as the third eye, is related to personal vision, knowledge, intuitive skills, self-evaluation, and introspection. This chakra is located between the eyes, near the ears, nose, brain, and pineal gland. Dysfunctions associated with this chakra are vision problems, brain tumors, blood clots (blood clot formation is related to stopping the flow of intuitive information), neurological disorders, blindness, deafness, full spinal difficulties, seizures, and learning disabilities.

The *seventh chakra* is related to seeing the larger purpose in our lives. It's also related to our attitudes, faith, values, ethics, courage, and humanitarianism. This chakra is located near the crown of the head. The physical framework of the body is the skeleton. Skeletal system problems resulting from seventh chakra issues involve the framework around which you build your life—the metaphysical skeleton. Dysfunctions in this chakra can result in paralysis, bone cancer and other skeletal problems, and muscular system and nervous system diseases, such as multiple sclerosis and Lou Gehrig's disease.

Understanding energy anatomy holds the key to true healing, rather than just masking our symptoms, because it offers a comprehensive and holistic view of how each of us co-creates health or disease. Much of the material in this chapter may have been new to you. Take your time, and let it sink in in its own way and in its own time.

Our body heals best when we're living in the present. When we're truly present, we can heal almost anything. But most people tie up most of their energy in woundings from their past, while the rest of it is consumed by worrying about the future. You cannot heal anything unless a significant amount of your energy and spirit is available in the present moment. Dr. Lewis Thomas once said that he had come to believe that cancer was the physical metaphor for the extreme need to grow. Healthy growth involves getting as many parts of yourself as possible available in the present moment—*the now,* the only place that healing can happen. Rarely is a person always present right now, today. Living in the now is a skill that is developed through introspection, meditation, and "living in process."

Please pay attention to how you are feeling. Remember that many illnesses begin as blocked emotions. What do you remember? Is there anything you need to know or do now about the information you've just read? Chapter 15, "Steps for Healing," is designed to help you with this process.

PART TWO

The Anatomy of Women's Wisdom

FIVE

The Menstrual Cycle

How might it have been different for you if, on your first
menstrual day, your mother had given you a bouquet of flowers
and taken you to lunch, and then the two of you had gone to meet
your father at the jeweler, where your ears were pierced, and your
father bought you your first pair of earrings, and then you went
with a few of your friends and your mother's friends to get your
first lip coloring; and then you went,
    for the very first time,
        to the Women's lodge,
            to learn
                the wisdom of women?
How might your life be different?
                                        —Judith Duerk, *Circle of Stones*

We can reclaim the wisdom of the menstrual cycle by tuning
into our cyclic nature and celebrating it as a source of our
female power. The ebb and flow of dreams, creativity, and hormones associated with different parts of the cycle offer us a profound opportunity to deepen our connection with our inner
knowing. This is a gradual process for most women, one that
involves unearthing our personal history and then, day by day,
thinking differently about our cycles and living with them in a new
way.

TABLE 5
THE ANATOMY OF WOMEN'S WISDOM

Body Organ or Process	Encoded Wisdom	Energy Dysfunction	Physical Manifestation
MENSTRUAL CYCLE	Creative cycles and attunement with unconscious lunar information	Refusal to embrace cycles of darkness and light Not allowing shadow side to be seen and worked through	Lack of periods Heavy periods Irregular periods PMS
UTERUS	Creative center in relationship to self	Bondage to the emotions of others Unable to birth most creative self	Fibroids
OVARIES	Creative power in external world	Addiction to external authority or approval Inability to move forward secondary to financial, physical, or emotional abandonment	Ovarian cysts Ovarian cancer
BREASTS	Giving and receiving nurturance	Imbalance between giving and receiving	Breast cysts, pain Breast cancer
PREGNANCY	All creative processes and fertility	Insufficient energy to create and maintain new life Inability to trust the process of giving birth	Infertility Miscarriage Dysfunctional labor

Body Organ or Process	Encoded Wisdom	Energy Dysfunction	Physical Manifestation
CERVIX/VAGINA VULVA	Discretion about intimacy	Sexual relationships that don't enhance one's well-being Guilt about sexual pleasure	Herpes Warts Abnormal Pap smears Cervical cancer
MENOPAUSE	Passage into the wisdom years Reseeding the community	Unfinished business from past that is unaddressed Fear of process of aging	Incapacitating hot flashes Melancholia Depression Palpitations

Our Cyclical Nature

The menstrual cycle is the most basic, earthy cycle we have. Our blood is our connection to the archetypal feminine. The macrocosmic cycles of nature, such as the ebb and flow of the tides and the changes of the seasons, are reflected on a smaller scale in the menstrual cycle of the individual female body. The monthly ripening of an egg and subsequent release of menstrual blood or pregnancy mirrors the process of creation as it occurs not only in nature, unconsciously, but in human endeavor. In many cultures, the menstrual cycle has been viewed as sacred.

The cycle of ovulation is ruled by the moon. Studies have shown that peak conception rates and probably ovulation appear to occur at the full moon or the day before. During the new moon, ovulation and conception rates are decreased overall, and an increased number of women start their menstrual bleeding. Scientific research has documented that the moon rules the flow of fluids (ocean tides as well as individual body fluids) and affects the unconscious mind and dreams.[1] The timing of the menstrual cycle, the fertility cycle, and labor also follows the moon-dominated tides of the ocean. Environmental cues such as light, the moon, and the tides, play a documented role in regulating women's menstrual cycles and fertility.[2] In one study of nearly two thousand women with irregular menstrual cycles, more than half of the subjects achieved regular menstrual cycles of twenty-nine days' length by sleeping with a light on near their beds during the three days around ovulation.

The menstrual cycle governs the flow not only of fluids but of information and creativity. We receive and process information differently at different times in our cycles. I like to describe menstrual cycle wisdom this way: From the onset of menstruation until ovulation, we're ripening an egg and—symbolically, at least—preparing to give birth to someone else, a role that society honors. Many women find that they are at their "best" from the onset of their menstrual cycle until ovulation. Their energy is outgoing and upbeat. They are filled with enthusiasm and new ideas. At midcycle, we are naturally more receptive to others and to new ideas—more "fertile." Sexual desire also peaks for many women at midcycle, and our bodies secrete hormones into the air that have been associated with sexual attractiveness to others.[3] In fact, at ovulation our bodies secrete volatile hormones into the air that can draw men to us. (Our male-dominated society values this very highly, and we internalize it as a "good" stage of our cycle.) One patient, a waitress who works in a diner where many truckers stop to eat, has reported to me that her tips are highest at midcycle, around ovulation. Another man described his wife as "very vital and electric" during this time of her cycle.

The Follicular and Luteal Phases

The menstrual cycle itself mirrors how consciousness becomes matter and how thought creates reality. On the strictly physical level, the span of time between menses and ovulation (known as the follicular phase) coincides with the growth and development of an egg. On the expanded level of ideas and creativity, this first half of the cycle is also a very good time to initiate new projects. A researcher friend of mine tells me that she has the most energy to act on ideas for new experiments during this part of her cycle. Ovulation, which occurs at midcycle, is accompanied by an abrupt rise in the neuropeptides FSH (follicle stimulating hormone) and LH (luteinizing hormone). Ovulation represents creativity at its peak, followed by evaluative and reflective time, looking back upon what is created (ovulation through menses). The FSH, LH surge that accompanies ovulation may be the biologic basis for the increased mental and emotional creative receptivity experienced at ovulation.

My researcher friend notes that during this part of her cycle, she prefers to do routine tasks that do not require much input from others or expansive thought on her part.

Our creative biological and psychological cycle parallels the phases of the moon. From ancient times, some cultures have referred to women having their menstrual periods as being on "their moon." When women live together in natural settings, their ovulations tend to occur at the time of the full moon, with menses and self-reflection at the dark of the moon. Scientific evidence suggests that biological cycles as well as dreams and emotional rhythms are keyed into the moon and tides as well as the planets. Specifically, the moon and its tides interact with the electromagnetic fields of our bodies, subsequently affecting our internal physiological processes. The moon itself has a period when it is covered with darkness, and then slowly, at the time of the new moon, it becomes visible to us again, gradually waxing to fullness. Women, too, go through a period of darkness each month, when the life-force may seem to disappear for a while (premenstrual and menstrual phase). This is natural. We need not be afraid or think we are sick if our energies and moods naturally ebb for a few days each month. Demetra

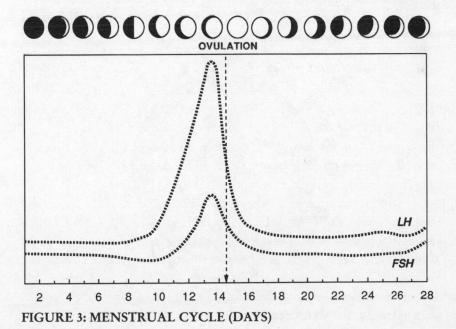

FIGURE 3: MENSTRUAL CYCLE (DAYS)

George writes that it is here, at the dark of the moon, that "life cleanses, revitalizes, and transforms itself in its evolutionary development, spiraling toward attunement with its essential nature."[4] Studies have shown that most women begin their menstrual periods during the dark of the moon (new moon) and begin bleeding between four and six A.M.—the darkest part of the day.[5]

If we do not become biologically pregnant at ovulation, we move into the second half of the cycle, the luteal phase—ovulation through the onset of menstruation. During this phase, we quite naturally retreat from outward activity to a more reflective mode. During the luteal phase we turn more inward, preparing *to develop or give birth to something that comes from deep within ourselves.* Society is not nearly as keen on this as it is on the follicular phase. Thus we judge our premenstrual energy, emotions, and inward mood as "bad and unproductive." (See Figure 4.)

Since our culture generally appreciates only what we can understand rationally, many women tend to block at every opportunity the flow of unconscious "lunar" information that comes to them premenstrually or during their menstrual cycle. Lunar information is reflective and intuitive. It comes to us in our dreams, our emotions, and our hungers. It comes under cover of darkness. When we routinely block the information that is coming to us in the second

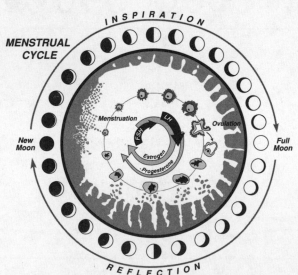

FIGURE 4: LUNAR CHART FOR MENSTRUAL CYCLE

half of our menstrual cycles, it has no choice but to come back as PMS or menopausal madness, in the same way that our other feelings and bodily symptoms, if ignored, often result in illness.[6]

The luteal phase, from ovulation until the onset of menstruation, is when women are *most in tune with their inner knowing and with what isn't working in their lives.* Studies have shown that women's dreams are more frequent and often more vivid during the premenstrual and menstrual phases of their cycles.[7] Premenstrually, the "veil between the worlds" of the seen and unseen, the conscious and the unconscious, is much thinner. We have access to parts of our often-unconscious selves that are less available to us at all other times of the month. The premenstrual phase is therefore a time when we have greater access to our magic—our ability to change things for the better. Premenstrually, we are quite naturally more "in tune" with what is most meaningful in our lives. We're more apt to cry—but our tears are always related to something that holds meaning for us. The many studies of Dr. Katerina Dalton have documented that women are more emotional premenstrually, more apt to act out their anger, and more prone to headaches and fatigue, and they may even experience exacerbations of ongoing illnesses such as arthritis. To the extent that we are out of touch with the hidden parts of ourselves, we will suffer premenstrually. Years of personal and clinical experience have taught me that the painful or uncomfortable issues that arise premenstrually are always real and must be addressed.

Women need to believe in the importance of the issues that come up premenstrually. Even though our bodies and minds may not express these issues and concerns as they would in the first part of our cycle—on our so-called "good days"—our inner wisdom is clearly asking for our attention. One woman told me, for example, that whenever she becomes premenstrual, she worries that the house, car, and investments are in her husband's name only. When she mentions this to her husband, he replies, "What's wrong? Don't you trust me?" I'd call that a premenstrual reality check that needs attention! One husband reported that in the follicular phase of his wife's cycle, she was great, was always cheery, kept the house in order, and did the cooking. But after ovulation she "let herself go" and talked about wanting to go back to college and get out of the house more. I told him that these issues that arise premenstrually should be treated seriously and asked him to consider what his wife's needs were for her full personal development. I pointed out that her difficult behavior premenstrually was her way of expressing those needs.

There is an intimate relationship between a woman's psyche and her ovarian function throughout the menstrual cycle. Before we ovulate we are outgoing and upbeat, while ovulating we are very receptive to others, and after ovulation (premenstrually) we are more inward and reflective. An astounding study done in the 1930s supports my observations. The psychoanalyst Dr. Therese Benedek studied the psychotherapy records of a group of patients, while her colleague Dr. Boris Rubenstein studied the ovarian hormonal cycles of the same women. By looking at the woman's emotional content, Dr. Benedek was able to predict where she was in her menstrual cycle with incredible accuracy. The authors wrote, "We were pleased and surprised to find an exact correspondence of the ovulative dates as independently determined by the two methods"—that is, psychoanalytic material compared with physiological findings. They found that before ovulation, when estrogen levels were at their highest, women's emotions and behavior were directed toward the outer world. During ovulation, however, women were more relaxed and content and quite receptive to being cared for and loved by others. During the postovulatory and premenstrual phase, when progesterone is at its highest, women were more likely to be focused on themselves and more involved in inward-directed activity. Interestingly, in women who had periods but did not ovulate, the authors saw similar cycles of emotions and behavior, except that around the time when ovulation should have occurred, these women missed not only ovulation but the accompanying emotions; that is, they were not relaxed, contented, or receptive to being cared for by others.[8]

Given our cultural heritage and beliefs about illness in general and the menstrual cycle in particular, it is not difficult to understand how women have come to equate their premenstrual phase not as a time for reflection and renewal but as a disease or a curse. In fact, the language that our culture uses regarding the uterus and ovaries has been experimentally shown to affect women's menstrual cycles. Under hypnosis, a woman who is given positive suggestions about her menstrual cycle will be much less apt to suffer from menstrually related symptoms.[9] On the other hand, a study by Diane Ruble found that women who were led to believe that they were premenstrual when they weren't reported experiencing more adverse physical symptoms, such as water retention, cramps, and irritability, than another group who were led to believe they were not premenstrual.[10] These studies are excellent examples of how our thoughts and beliefs have the power to affect our hormones, our biochemistry, and our subsequent experience.

Healing Through Our Cycles

Once we begin to appreciate our menstrual cycle as part of our inner guidance system, we begin to heal both hormonally and emotionally. There is no doubt that premenstrually, many women feel more inward and more connected to their personal pain and the pain of the world. Many such women are also more in touch with their own creativity and get their best ideas premenstrually, though they may not act on them until later. During the premenstrual phase, we need time to be alone, time to rest, and time away from our daily duties, but taking this time is a new idea and practice for many women. Premenstrual syndrome results when we don't honor our need to ebb and flow like the tides. This society likes action, so we often don't appreciate our need for rest and replenishment. The menstrual cycle is set up to teach us about the need for both the in-breath and the out-breath of life's processes. When we are premenstrual and feeling fragile, we need to rest and take care of ourselves for a day or two. In the Native American moon lodge, bleeding women came together for renewal and visioning and emerged afterward inspired and also inspiring to others. I think that the majority of PMS cases would disappear if every modern woman retreated from her duties for three or four days each month and had her meals brought to her by someone else.

I've personally found that simply and *unapologetically* stating my needs for a monthly slowdown to my husband is all that is needed. When I show respect for myself and the processes of my body, he shows respect as well, and my body responds with comfort and gratitude. Indeed, my experience of my own menstrual cycle began to change after I noticed that my most meaningful insights about myself, my life, and my writing came on the day or two just before my period. In my mid-thirties, I began to look forward to my periods, understanding them to be a sacred time that our culture didn't honor. When I am premenstrual, the things that make me feel teary are the things that are most important to me, things that I know tune me in to my power and my deepest truths. My increased sensitivity feels like a gift of insight. I don't become angry, though if I did, I would pay attention and not chalk it up to "my stupid hormones." I like to keep track of the phases of the moon in my daily calendar to see if I'm ovulating at the full moon, the dark of the moon, or in between. When I ovulate at the full moon and menstruate at the dark of the moon, my inner reflective time is synchronized with the moon's darkness. Getting my period at the time of the full moon results in a more intense period: I am more emotionally charged than usual, and my bleeding is often heavier than normal. I've found that sometimes simply intending to bleed at the dark of the moon tends to move my cycles in this direction, though not always. (I don't "try" to control this.) Noting my individual cycle in relationship to the moon's cycle consciously connects me with the earth and helps me to feel connected with women past and present.

Our Cultural Inheritance

The menstrual cycle and the female body were seen as sacred until five thousand years ago, when the peaceful matrilineal cultures of Old Europe were overturned.[11] The original meaning of the word *taboo* was "sacred," and women having their periods were considered sacred; now in some societies they are considered taboo. Often their dreams and visions were used to guide the tribe. Native cultures the world over have honored young women with coming-of-age ceremonies. First menstruation has meant being initiated into the "offices of womanhood" by mothers, aunts, and other initiated women.[12] Archaeological evidence from more than six thousand years ago points to the fact that the original calendars were bones with small marks on them that women used to keep track of their cycles.[13] Yet throughout much of written Western history, and even in religious codes, the menstrual cycle has been associated with shame and degradation, with women's dark, uncontrollable nature. Menstruating women were thought of as unclean. In A.D. 65, Pliny the Elder wrote:

But nothing could easily be found that is more remarkable [note the ambivalent word choice!] than the monthly flux of women. Contact with it turns new wine sour, crops touched by it become barren, seeds in gardens dry up, the fruit of trees fall off. The bright surface of mirrors in which it is merely reflected is dimmed, the edge of steel and the gleam of ivory are dulled. Hives of bees will die. Even bronze and iron are at once seized by rust and a horrible smell fills the air. To taste it drives dogs mad and affects their bite with an incurable poison.[14]

The taboo associated with the menstrual cycle has continued to this day. Generations of women have been taught that we are more physically vulnerable during our periods—that we can't swim, bathe, or wash our hair during those days. These beliefs were originally based on the Victorian theory that bathing, shampooing hair, or swimming might "back up" menstrual flow, resulting in stroke, insanity, or rapid onset of tuberculosis.[15] More recently, it has been felt that contact with water during this time would result in catching a cold. There is no scientific basis for any of these taboos, yet they have served to keep women afraid of a natural bodily process for generations.

If we are to reclaim our menstrual wisdom and honor our cyclic natures, we must at the same time acknowledge the negative attitudes that most of us have internalized concerning our menstrual cycles. We must acknowledge the pain and discomfort that many women experience monthly. Our cyclic nature has been the brunt of all kinds of jokes about being "on the rag" or having "the curse." Puberty and the first menstruation for many women have been saturated with shame and humiliation. Nothing in our society—with the exception of violence and fear—has been more effective in keeping women in their place than the degradation of the menstrual cycle.

Replacing the harmful inherited myths about our menstrual cycles with accurate information is part of women's healing. After menarche (the first menstruation), which generally occurs around the age of twelve in this society, a young woman reaches sexual maturity. A certain body composition is required for the onset of menarche. Usually the body weight must be about 17 percent fat for a young woman to start having periods. Studies have indicated that a body fat level averaging about 22 percent of body weight is necessary for sustained ovulatory cycles in most females.[16] This is one reason why anorexic young women and female dancers and athletes who are very thin don't have regular periods. Though a young woman's first cycles are usually not ovulatory, she gradually becomes fertile over the next several years, producing an egg each month from her ovaries. If the monthly egg is not fertilized at midcycle, this results in a menstrual period about fourteen days after ovulation. In the flow, the lining of the uterus (the endometrium) is shed. Each month, the lining or endometrium builds up and is shed cyclically, stimulated by a complex and amazing interaction between hormones produced by the ovaries, the pituitary gland, and the hypothalamus. (See Figure 5.) Because of the complexity of this hormonal interaction, many areas of a woman's life affect the menstrual cycle. The cycle in turn affects many areas of a woman's life.

Most girls learn about the menstrual cycle in a sterile, clinical way, without respect for their female bodies and their own sexuality. How their bodies and sexuality are linked to the menstrual cycle is rarely discussed. Very few girls are introduced to menstruation as a positive rite of passage. My mother told me the "facts of life" and explained eggs and sperm. I recall being very upset by this information. I was in the fourth grade. My sister, eleven months younger than I, had said earlier that day, "Mom, I know where babies come from, but how do they get there?" My mother took us into her bedroom and read us a book that said that girls get a menstrual period around the age of twelve, and that after they get their period they could have a baby if they had sex.

I was not happy with this information. I continued to hope that women could get pregnant by kissing rather than by the disgusting act my mother described. Why I found the whole thing so disgusting might have had something to do with my own mother's initiation into puberty. She was not concerned with the meaning of the menstrual cycle and the sacredness of the female body, though she was and is a woman who is truly wise and ahead of her time. My mother had learned that once she got her period, somehow she could no longer enjoy herself in the same way. Her favorite girlhood activities had been playing baseball and climbing trees with the boys. But once she "became a woman," she was no longer allowed to play with the boys. Years later, she told me that she begged her mother to take her to the hospital to "get her fixed" so that she

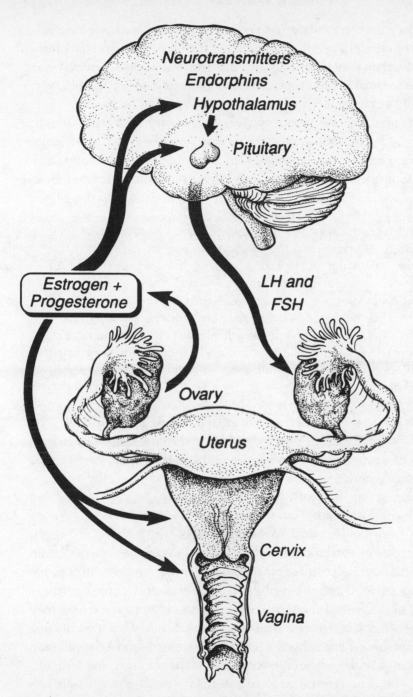

**FIGURE 5: THE FEMALE MIND/BODY CONTINUUM:
INTERACTIONS BETWEEN THE BRAIN AND THE PELVIS**

wouldn't have periods anymore and could go back to baseball. Because my mother didn't completely resolve her adolescent feelings about her menstrual cycle until she was in her sixties, I absorbed some of her unconscious feelings around menstruation, even though she presented it to me as a normal part of life.

Instead of celebrating our cyclic nature as a positive aspect of our female being, our culture teaches us that we shouldn't acknowledge our periods at all, lest we neglect the needs of our spouses and children. Consider this excerpt from a 1963 insert inside a tampon box:

WHEN YOU'RE A WIFE

Don't take advantage of your husband. That's an old rule of good marriage behavior that's just as sensible now as it ever was. Of course, you'll not try to take advantage, but sometimes ways of taking advantage aren't obvious.

You wouldn't connect it with menstruation, for instance. Yet, if you neglect the simple rules that make menstruation a normal time of month, and retire for a few days each month, as though you were ill, you're taking advantage of your husband's good nature. He married a full-time wife, not a part-time one. So you should be active, peppy, and cheerful every day.[17]

Always cheery—just like those old Doris Day movies. No wonder so many women have PMS! When I think of the indoctrination represented by that 1963 insert, in the year I got my first period, I wonder how we women have come as far as we have!

The Menstrual Cycle, Birth Control Pills, and Women's Intuition

Our intuition works differently during the various phases of our menstrual cycle. It changes again after menopause. One of my colleagues, an osteopathic physician, noticed this connection between intuition and the menstrual cycle when he referred a patient to me for a change in birth control method. She had been on the pill for a number of years, but he felt that continued use of the pill was interfering with her ability to know what her next steps in life should be. The referral note to me read: "Birth control pills are interfering with intuitive function. Suggest alternatives." I applaud this doctor for his insight.

In an age in which millions of women's bodies, due to the use of birth control pills, are more in tune with pharmaceutical companies than with the moon, it is no small task to rethink a medication that has offered so many women such highly touted advantages. After all, the pill provides women with periods that need never ruin their weekends, it often decreases menstrual cramps, and it is associated with a decreased risk of ovarian and endometrial cancer. But then, no one is sure whether it increases the risk of breast cancer, although studies have shown that it can increase the risk of cervical cancer.

Laurie, one of my colleagues in OB/GYN, was on the pill for over nine years before she changed her mind about its advantages. She had routinely "pushed" the pill as the panacea for all her patients, using her own experience as coercion. When she lectured them on why they should all be on the pill, she always ended her talk with the statement, "They'll never get my pills away from me." Only after Laurie began to see her own illnesses as physical manifestations of the diseases in her spirit was she able to reevaluate her position on the pill. The breakthrough for her happened in part because her relationship with her husband had begun to deteriorate. They were having frequent arguments around the subject of sex. "It drove me crazy," she said, "that he seemed to separate it completely from everything else that was going on in our relationship. At the same time, my own confusion about my body, my feelings of discomfort with its size and shape, my inhibitions about noise and awkwardness during sex, and mixed messages from my childhood about sex and seduction made sex something fraught with negative connotation and sometimes insurmountable obstacles."

Laurie was learning about how different parts of our bodies talk to us through symptoms as part of our inner guidance system. As she did, she realized that remaining on birth control pills might prevent her female organs from optimally communicating with her, especially in a personal crisis around her own sexuality. She began to awaken to how she had inadvertently become separated from her body by following the dictates of the culture instead of her inner guidance. This awakening was accompanied by an interest in feminism for the first time in her life. Up until then, she had considered herself highly successful and functional, which is how she seemed on the surface. Yet she had had a benign ovarian cyst, operated on several years before, and during her OB/GYN residency she had been operated on for thyroid cancer. Her emerging inner wisdom showed her that these conditions had been her body's way of trying to get her attention and let her know that something was off balance in her life. Now she was willing and eager to pay attention to what her body was saying, especially since she was healthy.

"I felt sadness," Laurie says, "that I had taken for granted, drugged away, or labeled a 'curse' all the wondrous workings of my brain, my hormones, my uterus, and my ovaries. No one ever celebrated my first period. No one had helped me connect the power of giving birth to my sexuality. I longed to recapture some of that lost magic and mystery. But it took me almost two years of pulling down the curtains of my life and dusting away the cobwebs before I felt that I could tentatively trust my body."

After these two years of personal struggle, Laurie decided to take a year off from her busy obstetrical practice in a large city. She was exhausted from the demands of three children, her practice, and now a marriage that was ending. She knew that she needed to reflect on her life and taking some new directions. She said that when she finally got around to doing it, going off the pill was "something of an act of celebration and rebellion." It was clear to her that a divorce was imminent. "Since I did not need contraception anymore," she observed, "it occurred to me that now might be the time to allow myself the luxury of my hormones. So I threw away the last dial-pack and waited. I was pretty sure that after nine years of instruction from Ortho Pharmaceutical, my ovaries would be totally confused, so I was willing to be patient. I was prepared for swelling, irritability, wild emotions, and confusion. I was not prepared for what happened."

Two weeks after stopping the pill, Laurie was sitting with a group of women and relating the events of the past two years. She noted, "Suddenly, I was in tears and I could hardly speak. I remember thinking, 'Now isn't this strange?'" It took her a while to realize that even though she did indeed feel sadness about the changes under way in her life, she had in fact told others about these changes and feelings before, while she was on the pill, without any emotional or physiological reaction whatsoever. She discovered that for her, ovulation was associated with an increased ability to feel and express her deepest emotions. She wrote, "I didn't realize for two more days that the excessive cervical mucous [a very common sign of ovulation] and the sudden opening of the emotional floodgate were signs of ovulation. Even when I did put it together, I refused to trust my body. 'Well,' I thought, 'I'll just wait two weeks and see.' Two weeks later, there she was in her red dress—my first spontaneous period in over nine years, never a more welcome sight. I felt as though I had been given a wondrous gift from a long lost friend. This body, that I had abused for so long and in so many ways, was suddenly talking to me again, giving me encouragement and reassurance. All was not lost."

In addition to finding that her emotions were now more available to her, Laurie found that she was more in touch with anger that she would have previously denied. She related that shortly after her own periods resumed, "I found my anger. My righteous, fiery, white-hot anger. Of course, my husband was the unwitting recipient of what felt like twenty years of suppressed emotion. I don't know if he deserved all of it—certainly not all at once. But as it came pouring out, I remember thinking, 'This is amazing! This is really me. My hormones. My magic!' I think now that if I had been feeling that anger as it came up all those years, I might still be married. That I would have divorced much sooner. Either way would have been better than what had happened. It was not okay that I had missed so much of myself."

Laurie knew to honor and pay attention to what was happening to her, even though some of it was painful. She later reflected, "Since then I have learned to expect to hear regularly from my hormones. They teach me where I still need to put my attention. When I am suddenly in tears, I know to pause and consider what emotional work I still have to do in that area. When anger comes, I remind myself that being able to push it down inside myself is not a gift. Anger unexpressed produces disease. It belongs outside my body."

The other thing that Laurie noticed was the connection between her menstrual cycle and her inherent sexuality. I have heard similar stories from many women. She told me, "There is this wild desire racing around in my brain for several days every month around ovulation. My friends told me about it, but this is amazing. And I thought all those years that the pill was helping my sex life by getting rid of all those messy barrier contraceptives!" She had used the diaphragm only while breast-feeding, and she realized she had blamed her lack of sexual desire on the messiness of diaphragm use. But now, she understood that her lack of desire was most likely related to breast-feeding hormones and energy drain, not the diaphragm. Many nursing mothers simply are not interested in sexual intercourse, since their energies are being quite literally "sucked away" by another very engaging human being—the new baby. Sexual desire resumes gradually as the baby gets older.

Laurie noted another change that is very common. After going off the pill, her body tended to make up for lost time, with ovulations coming more frequently for a while, then adjusting to approximately once per month. "When I first reclaimed my cycles," she wrote, "they were very short, about every three weeks. Although the thought flashed through my head briefly that it would be a pain to be bleeding one week out of every three, I realized that the thought was a conditioned one. How many forty-year-old women had complained to me about the increasing frequency of their periods and begged me to 'do something' about it. Now I realized that I had been given a gift of short cycles to 'catch up.' I loved getting to cycle more often. I got to ovulate every three weeks. I got more lessons about my body. It was like a condensed crash course in female physiology—my own. I began to celebrate getting my periods every three weeks and hoped that menopause would not come until I was sixty-five. Having given myself permission to enjoy all these new lessons, I once again learned that I was not in control—my cycles began to spread out to three and a half, then four weeks. I think it was just a test, having three-week cycles. It was to see if I really wanted this part of my body back. I do."

Laurie's story illustrates what reclaiming our menstrual wisdom and power feels like. Though "the pill" has been a boon to many women, it has also taken them out of touch with some essential parts of their female wisdom. When people are in close contact with each other, for example, one way they communicate is via hormones. Oral contraceptives, however, have been shown to eliminate part of our hormonal communication pathway, including our sexual communication with men. One study found that the volatile fatty acids in vaginal secretions known as *copulins* stimulate male sexual interest and behavior. Women on the pill, however, don't secrete them.[18] Women who live together often cycle together, in what one of my friends calls "becoming ovarian sisters." This doesn't happen to women on the pill. Studies have shown that women who have close relationships with other people have shorter and more regular cycles, whereas women who isolate themselves are more likely to have irregular cycles.[19]

Menstrual Cramps (Dysmenorrhea)

As many as 60 percent of all women suffer from menstrual cramps. A smaller percentage are unable to function for one or more days each month because of the severity of their pain. The fact that the majority of women in our culture suffer from menstrual cramps is a very clear indication that we have something wrong with our relationship to our bodies. It testifies that we have lost much of our connection to our menstrual wisdom. The psychological and gynecological literature of the 1950s was filled with studies that suggested that menstrual cramps were mainly psychological, related to being unhappy about being a woman. Caroline Myss says that cramps and PMS are classic indications that a woman is in some kind of conflict with being a woman, with her role in the tribe, and with the tribal expectations of her. Given our current society's traditional expectations for women, it's amazing that 100 percent of us don't have cramps and PMS.

Cramps are not the same as PMS, although women often suffer from both. Dysmenorrhea is divided into two types. Primary dysmenorrhea is cramps that are not secondary to another "organic" disease in the pelvis. Secondary dysmenorrhea is cramps that are caused by endometriosis or other pelvic disease. Treatments that help primary dysmenorrhea usually help secondary dysmenorrhea as well.

I had primary dysmenorrhea in my teens and up until after the birth of my first child. I sometimes had to call my mother from school and leave class because of the pain. Once during my residency I even had to leave a major surgical case because of menstrual cramps. One of my fellow residents said to me, "Gee, Chris, *you* have cramps? Must be it's not all in women's heads!" (Remember, I was "one of the guys" back then and was doing everything in my power to maintain that position. You can imagine what a blow it was to have to leave the operating room because of that dreaded female weakness, *cramps*!)

Beginning in the late 1970s, studies showed that women with cramps have high levels of the hormone prostaglandin F2 alpha (PGF2 alpha) in their menstrual blood. When this hormone is released into the bloodstream as the endometrial lining breaks down, the uterus goes into spasm, resulting in cramping pain.[20] (Menstrual cramps are not in the head after all—they're in the uterus!)

When I first got my period, I also became nearsighted and had to get glasses. I resented this—no one else in the family had glasses. I believe now that there was something I didn't want to see. My vision problem was exacerbated by reading without adequate breaks to rest my eyes. I suspect that I was conflicted about growing up in general and growing up as a girl in particular, just as my mother had been. The increased stress from puberty, together with all the dairy food I ate, increased the level of adrenaline (norepinephrine) and prostaglandin F2 alpha in my blood, resulting in bad cramps. The cramps disappeared for a while after the birth of my first child, but they came back, though much milder and not with every period, when my second daughter was about five. This time of no cramps reinforces my belief that when my life is in balance, I don't have cramps. When I become too busy or stressed out, I'll have a few hours of cramps on the first day of my period. They slow me right down and are a good reminder that I need to make some adjustments and to tune in to the wisdom of my body.

Treatment

DIET. A high-fat, high-protein diet favors the synthesis of prostaglandin F2 alpha, the hormone associated with menstrual cramps. In order to steer the body away from excess production of prostaglandin F2 alpha and into the prostaglandin E series (the ones that don't produce cramps), a woman must have enough of the essential fatty acid known as gamma linoleic acid available in her system. (See page 123.) She also requires adequate levels of vitamin C, vitamin B_6 (pyridoxine), and magnesium. Metabolically, women who have high stress levels and a poor diet are a setup for excess production of prostaglandin F2 alpha and subsequent menstrual cramps.

Other Nutritional Treatments

- Stop dairy food, especially cheese, ice cream, cottage cheese, and yogurt. (See Chapter 17.)
- Cut down on excess protein and meat. Use meat as a condiment only.
- Follow a high-complex-carbohydrate, low-fat, relatively low-protein diet. Use menus from sources listed in Chapter 17.
- Take essential fatty acids, such as flaxseed, borage, and black currant seed oil. Oil of evening primrose is also good. The usual dose is four to six 500 mg. capsules per day, in divided doses.[21]
- Take a multivitamin-mineral supplement.
- Take 100 mg. vitamin B_6 per day, in combination with B complex. B_6 has been shown to decrease the intensity and duration of menstrual cramps.[22]
- Take magnesium, as much as 100 mg. every two hours during the menstrual cycle itself, and three to four times per day during the rest of the cycle.
- Take 50 mg. vitamin E three times a day during the entire cycle. Vitamin E has also been shown to improve dysmenorrhea.[23] Vitamin E must be in the form of d-alpha tocopherol for it to have any biological effect.

MEDICATION. Nonsteroidal anti-inflammatory drugs like Advil, Nuprin, Anaprox, and Ponstel block the synthesis of prostaglandin F2 alpha, when these drugs are taken just at the onset of a period, *before* the pain starts, or as soon after as possible. Once the endometrial lining begins to shed and prostaglandin F2 alpha gets released into the bloodstream, it's much harder to interrupt the resulting uterine spasms that cause the pain.

Birth control pills, which eliminate ovulation and therefore the hormonal changes associated with cramps, work well for many women who are not interested in making lifestyle or dietary changes. Some women, however, get cramps even on oral contraceptives. The newer pills can be safely used by most women over thirty-five, as long as they do not smoke.

Energy Medicine
- Stress reduction. (See page 123.)
- Castor oil packs to the lower abdomen at least three times per week for several months, to improve immune system functioning and decrease stress and adrenaline levels. (See page 135.)
- Acupuncture, herbs, massage, homeopathy. Homeopathic remedies are best prescribed by a competent practitioner who is familiar with the field.
- Changing your view of your menstrual cycle.

Women's Stories

JANE: HEALING MENSTRUAL CRAMPS. Jane first came to see me this past winter at the age of twenty-six. She had had years of very, very painful periods, starting shortly after she started menstruating at age thirteen. She described the cramping as occurring before her actual period started and continuing after the bleeding had ended. She was worried that something might be seriously affecting her reproductive organs, such as endometriosis or an ovarian cyst.

Jane had tried birth control pills for about a month several years before, but she had stopped because she didn't like the way she felt on them. She also had tried Anaprox, a nonsteroidal anti-inflammatory medication similar to Motrin and available by prescription. It had helped her somewhat, but she was still quite incapacitated. In addition to her cramps, she complained of heavy bleeding (going through one tampon per hour on the second day), premenstrual irritability, acne, bloating, tender breasts, and vaginal itching before her period. Neither of Jane's two sisters had menstrual cramps or other gynecological problems. Jane's diet was based on dairy food, such as cottage cheese, ice cream, and yogurt, all of which she ate frequently. She said that she loved food in general, but dairy food made up the bulk of her food intake.

Jane was an elementary school teacher and was not very pleased with her work. She said that she had always wanted to move to Idaho but felt guilty about doing that because her parents didn't want her to move so far away. Her parents felt that it was very selfish of Jane to want to pursue her own interests. They felt that she should stay home near them, continue in the security of teaching, marry, and have children. Jane's childhood desire to please her parents now came in direct conflict with her own need for personal growth. She came to see that staying home and ignoring her own needs would only result in illness for herself. I pointed out that she was in a classic codependent dilemma and that she needed to come to terms with this in order to heal fully. In addition to meeting the expectations of her parents, the stress of doing work she no longer found fulfilling was weighing her down.

Jane had a completely normal pelvic exam, with no sign of a cyst, tenderness, or anything else suggestive of reproductive disease. I recommended the following course of action:

- Apply castor oil packs to the lower abdomen two times per week.
- Stop eating all dairy food and red meat.
- Take a multiple vitamin twice or three times per day.
- Begin plans to move to Idaho.
- Do some reading on codependency.

When Jane returned to my office three months later, her cramps had markedly improved. She said that she was shocked by the difference she had felt after stopping dairy food and red meat. Her bleeding had lightened considerably. She realized that her diet really had a large effect on her cramps, and she said that the castor oil packs "felt great." When she was using these, she took the time to tune in to herself and her needs, and she thought of living out her dreams instead of being stuck in old patterns that didn't serve her. She read some books on codependency and came to see that she had been trained to be a "people pleaser" since childhood. She realized that she had to learn how to please herself if she hoped to find her life satisfying. She had outgrown being the good little girl in the family.

After three months, Jane's periods were much easier and she had been able to decrease her Anaprox dose considerably, as she changed her diet and decreased her stress level. Most impressive of all, she made plans to move to Idaho and would not start the next school year in a job and a place that she didn't like. Though the prospect of moving into the unknown was frightening to her, it was also exhilarating. If she hadn't made plans to live her own life separately from her parents, I believe that her health would eventually have been at risk because of her "niceness." By using her body's wisdom, Jane healed not only her menstrual cramps but her life.

Premenstrual Syndrome (PMS)

No modern disorder points to the need to rethink our ideas about menstruation and reclaim the wisdom of our cycles more directly than the common malady known as premenstrual syndrome, or PMS. Having treated hundreds of women with PMS, I know that such a rethinking is needed to get to the root causes of PMS. Dietary change, exercise, vitamins, and progesterone therapy are all useful in treating PMS, and I initially recommend them for many women. But in persistent cases of PMS, a deeper imbalance exists that lifestyle changes alone won't help. As studies have confirmed, unresolved emotional problems may disrupt the menstrual rhythm and the normal hormonal milieu.[24]

At least 60 percent of all women suffer from PMS. It is most likely to occur in women in their thirties, though it can occur as early as adolescence and as late as the premenopausal years. PMS has been known since ancient times, but it was popularized in the 1980s by an article in *Family Circle* magazine, which articulated the monthly suffering of millions of women. The media picked up on this, and within a few months PMS became a nationally known problem and a household word.[25] It also became a hot topic with feminists, who argued that the diagnosis would be used against women. Doctors worried that it would become a "wastebasket" diagnosis that women or their families would use as an excuse when no one could figure out what was really going on. Meanwhile, scores of women finally had a name for their monthly suffering and sought medical help for it.

Interestingly, conventional OB/GYN meetings did not address the topic of PMS until *after* the *Family Circle* article came out and women began coming to doctors with their self-diagnoses. We doctors were in many cases ill-prepared for this. It had not been covered in our training. The demand created by women and the media for treatment of PMS was such that by the mid-1980s, PMS was a lecture topic at many major OB/GYN specialty meetings and research began appearing in the journals. Just as the desire for natural childbirth forced doctors to reform their patriarchal approach to obstetrical practice, women's desire to understand PMS has influenced the practice of medicine and helped move it toward a more enlightened attitude toward the female body.

Diagnosis

A wide variety of symptoms can be present with PMS. In making the diagnosis it doesn't matter what specific symptoms a woman has premenstrually. *What is important is the cyclic fashion in which they occur.* Women who chart their symptoms for three months or more often see a pattern and are able to predict when in their cycle their symptoms are likely to start. Most women will have at least three days during the month when they are entirely free from the symptoms listed here, except in very severe cases. In the second half of the menstrual cycle many underlying conditions are exacerbated, such as glaucoma, arthritis, and depression. Exacerbation of underlying conditions is not defined as PMS, though it is related to PMS. There are more than one hundred known symptoms of PMS.[26]

PMS Symptoms

abdominal bloating	fainting
abdominal cramping	fatigue
accident proneness	food binges
acne	headache
aggression	heart palpitations (heart pounding)
alcohol intolerance	hemorrhoids
anxiety	herpes
asthma	hives
back pain	insomnia (sleeplessness)
breast swelling and pain	irritability
bruising	joint swelling and pain
confusion	lethargy
coordination difficulties	migraine
	nausea
depression	rage
edema	salt craving
emotional lability	seizures
eye difficulties	sex drive changes

sinus problems	sweet cravings
sore throat	urinary difficulties
styes	withdrawal from others
suicidal thoughts	

If nothing is done to interrupt PMS, it often gets worse over time. In the early stages of PMS, women describe symptoms that arise a few days before their menstrual period and then stop abruptly when the bleeding starts. Over time the symptoms that begin premenstrually gradually begin one to two weeks before the onset of menses. Some women experience a cluster of symptoms at ovulation, followed by a symptom-free week—then a recurrence of the symptoms a week before menses. Over time, a woman may have only two or three days of the month that are symptom-free. Eventually, no discernible pattern of "good" days and "bad" days is left: She feels "PMS" virtually all the time.

Some women equate menstrual cramps and PMS, but PMS is different from menstrual cramps (dysmenorrhea). This difference is not always clearly stated in writings on PMS. Many women with PMS have completely pain-free periods. Many women with severe cramping have *no* premenstrual distress. Menstrual cramps are caused by uterine contractions and cramping that results from excess prostaglandin F2 alpha, a hormone produced as the lining of the uterus breaks down during the menstrual cycle. Some studies have shown that prostaglandin hormones are also involved in PMS symptoms. For that reason, dietary change, vitamin and mineral supplements, and antiprostaglandin medication (usually the nonsteroidal anti-inflammatory drugs like Advil) are often useful both for cramps and for PMS.[27]

Though some doctors are still looking for "the biochemical lesion" that causes PMS and hundreds of scientific papers have been published on the topic, no one has been able to find it or a "magic bullet" drug to cure it. A reductionistic approach—looking for the chemical "cause" and "cure"—simply doesn't work because the causes of PMS are multifactorial and must be approached holistically. The effects of the mind, the emotions, diet, light, exercise, relationships, heredity, and childhood traumas must all be taken into account when treating PMS.

All of the following events result in hormonal changes in the body. PMS is apt to be initiated or exacerbated by these changes unless treatment is initiated.

Events Associated with PMS Onset
- Onset of menses or the year or two before menopause
- Coming off birth control pills
- After a time of no periods (amenorrhea)
- The birth of a child or the termination of a pregnancy
- Pregnancies complicated by toxemia
- Tubal ligation, especially as done in the 1970s, in which a greater portion of the fallopian tube was destroyed by unipolar electrocautery, a method of burning the tubes that is no longer used
- Unusual trauma, such as a death in the family

A variety of nutritional factors contribute to PMS. Studies have shown that women with PMS tend to have the following nutritional and physiological characteristics.

Nutritional Characteristics of Women with PMS
- High consumption of dairy products[28]
- Excessive consumption of caffeine, in the form of soft drinks, coffee, or chocolate[29]
- Excessive consumption of refined sugar and not enough whole grains and vegetables
- A relatively high blood level of estrogen, resulting either from overproduction from dietary and body fat or from the decreased breakdown of estrogen in the liver. High estrogen levels are associated with deficiencies of the vitamin B complex, especially B_6 and B_{12}. The liver requires these vitamins to break down and inactivate estrogen.[30]
- A relatively low blood level of progesterone, the hormone that works to balance excess estrogen. This decreased level is felt to be secondary either to lack of production or to excess breakdown of this hormone in the body.[31]
- Excessive consumption of animal fat (which leads to increased levels of the hormone prostaglandin F2 and also contributes to excess estrogen/low progesterone levels in PMS[32]). Vegetarians with a low-

fat, high-fiber diet, on the other hand, are known to excrete two to three times more estrogen in their feces than nonvegetarians. They also have 50 percent less plasma blood levels of unconjugated estrogens (a type of metabolized estrogen) than women who eat meat, and as a result they have a decreased incidence of PMS.[33]

• Excessive body weight, which increases the chances of hyperestrogenism and PMS.[34] Body fat manufactures estrogen in the form of estrone (one of the estrogens).

• Low levels of vitamins C and E and selenium. As with the B vitamins, the liver also requires these substances to metabolize estrogen properly.[35]

• A deficiency of magnesium.[36] Chocolate cravings have been linked to low magnesium levels. The liver needs magnesium, along with B vitamins, to metabolize estrogen optimally.

• Inadequate exposure to natural light and a tendency toward seasonal affective disorder (SAD). Many of the symptoms associated with PMS are precisely the same as those associated with SAD. Light acts as a nutrient. It directly influences the entire neuroendocrine system through the retina, the hypothalamus, and the pineal gland. In one study, patients with PMS responded significantly to treatment with bright light. Their weight gain, depression, carbohydrate craving, social withdrawal, fatigue, and irritability were reversed with two hours of bright light treatment in the evening.[37] A similar study showed PMS improvement when bright light was used for two hours in the morning. Living under artificial light much of the time without regular exposure to natural light can not only profoundly affect the regularity of the menstrual cycle, it can create PMS. A variety of authors have studied the beneficial effects of natural light.[38]

Treatment

Many women are given symptomatic treatments for PMS that over the long run don't work. Treating a woman's bloating with diuretics, her headaches with pain-killers, and her anxiety with Valium often serves to create new side effects from the drugs themselves and ignores the underlying imbalances that led to PMS in the first place. Though psychotherapy is often prescribed for women with PMS and may provide insights about stress, it ignores the nutritional and biochemical aspects of this disorder.

Program for PMS Relief

• *A high-complex-carbohydrate, low-fat diet.* This means 35 grams of fat or less per day and 75 percent of calories from complex carbohydrates. Low levels of dietary fat and protein also favor hormonal balance. (See Chapter 17.)

• *A multivitamin-mineral supplement.* It should contain 400 to 800 mg. of magnesium and 50 mg. of most of the B complex. All women should take this daily all month long, not just premenstrually.

• *Elimination of refined sugar and refined flour products.*[39]

• *Elimination of caffeine.* As I've learned through the years, just getting off caffeine, even as little as one cup of coffee or one can of cola per day, can have a dramatic effect on PMS for some women.

• *Increased consumption of essential fatty acids—especially linoleic acid (GLA-gamma linoleic acid) for proper metabolism of hormones.* Borage oil, black currant seed oil, and evening primrose oil are good sources of essential fatty acids. Dietary sources of essential fatty acids include raw nuts and seeds, but most women prefer to use supplements, which are widely available at pharmacies and natural food stores. Generally, 500 mg. 3 to 4 times per day is prescribed, or take as directed on the bottle. Headaches may occur at high doses. The optimal metabolism of essential fatty acids in the body requires adequate levels of magnesium, Vitamin C, zinc, vitamin B_3, and B_6.

• *Stress reduction.* Women who practice meditation or other methods of deep relaxation are able to alleviate many of their PMS symptoms.[40] There are numerous types of meditation that work. Each woman should choose the type of meditation that she feels most drawn to and incorporate this discipline into her daily routine.

Meditation in the form of the Relaxation Response of Dr. Herbert Benson is practiced 15 to 20 minutes twice per day for three months. This meditation involves: (1) sitting quietly in a comfortable position with eyes closed; (2) deeply relaxing all muscles beginning with the face and progressing down to the feet; (3) breathing through the nose and becoming aware of your breath; and (4) saying the word "one" silently to yourself as you exhale. Don't worry about successfully achieving a deep level of relaxation.

• *At least twenty minutes of aerobic-type exercise three times a week.*[41] Brisk walking is all that is necessary. Such conditioning exercise decreases many premenstrual symptoms. It also increases endorphins in the blood (or naturally occurring morphinelike substances that help the body deal with depression). It is estimated that half of all depression cases can be helped through exercise alone.

• *Full-spectrum light.* Expose yourself to full-spectrum light for two hours each evening or each morning (2,500 to 10,000 lux, a measure of light intensity) from either natural light or a full-spectrum lighting source.[42] A cloudy day in northern Europe provides 10,000 lux. A sunny day near the equator provides 80,000 lux.

• *Natural progesterone therapy when indicated.* Natural progesterone, in combination with lifestyle changes, often produces profound improvement in PMS symptoms.[43] In their capacity as neurotransmitters, estrogen and progesterone clearly affect mood. Estrogen, if unopposed by progesterone, tends to irritate the nervous system. Progesterone, on the other hand, is associated with tranquillity.

I recommend natural progesterone for women who have moderate-to-severe PMS that doesn't respond to simple lifestyle changes and who often describe a Jekyll-and-Hyde personality change premenstrually. Natural progesterone also works well for women whose major premenstrual symptom is a migraine-type headache. These headaches often start with the gradual change in estrogen and progesterone levels that tends to occur in the years leading up to the menopause.

Natural progesterone is not the same thing as the synthetic progesterones (progestins) such as medroxyprogesterone acetate (Provera). There are no serious side effects with natural progesterone at the usual doses. Sometimes it might cause intermenstrual spotting or delay the period. This usually resolves itself in one to two months. Extremely high doses—much higher than I recommend—have been associated with euphoria and occasional dizziness in rare cases. Oral natural progesterone is available by prescription from your doctor. It is also available in the form of skin creams, oils, or sublingual (under-the-tongue) drops. Not all pharmacies carry it and not all physicians know where to get it. (See Resources pages 680–81.)

Synthetic progestins, on the other hand, have many known side effects, such as bloating, headache, and weight gain. Unfortunately, many women are told that synthetic progestin is the same as progesterone. But synthetic progestins can actually increase PMS symptoms because taking a synthetic progestin decreases the body's natural progesterone levels.

Women who do well on progesterone often experience a rapid change in mood that begins after ovulation and ends just as the menstrual flow starts. They describe feeling fine and then within several hours having a "black cloud" come over them.[44] When their periods start, they feel as though "a light has gone on." These women are describing a biochemical change in their bodyminds that is very real and not just "in their heads."

The relative imbalance between estrogen and progesterone associated with PMS is a dynamic, changing phenomenon that cannot be documented with current laboratory hormonal testing. A subtle imbalance between estrogen, progesterone, and other related hormones is also associated with irregular periods and emotional stress. Emotional stress increases levels of the hormone ACTH, often resulting in anovulatory cycles[45] (cycles not associated with ovulation) characterized by inadequate levels of progesterone.

Ultimately, when women are willing to look at the emotional issues behind their PMS, they are eventually able to change their internal hormonal status *without* outside hormones. In fact, most women require progesterone therapy for PMS symptoms for only six months to two years, though sometimes it takes longer. The process of healing our emotional and psychological stresses *results in biochemical changes* in our bodies. Healing emotional and psychological reality is a biochemical process.

I suggest that a woman with PMS start natural progesterone a day or two before ovulation or a day or two before she usually notices symptoms. It is important to get the progesterone into her system before she normally experiences her mood change. This will often prevent her symptoms or greatly alleviate them. Waiting until she is already symptomatic to start her progesterone treatment often doesn't work. Each woman's dose varies, so most have to experiment to find a level that works for them.

The use of the progesterone over time helps rebalance the estrogen-progesterone ratio. Using natural progesterone produces a gradual improvement of symptoms with each cycle. Many women are able to decrease their dosages over time once their symptoms have been completely relieved. It is much more effective, however, to start out with dosages that are on the high end of usual dosages and stay with these for several months.

Women's Stories

GWENDOLYN: TRANSFORMING PREMENSTRUAL RAGE. Gwendolyn was thirty-six when she first came to see me. She was tall, thin, dramatic, and articulate, with a great sense of humor, but her PMS was so bad that she routinely flew into rages and became manic. In one high-energy premenstrual manic phase, she stayed up all night painting her kitchen and then, without any rest, put in a full day of work. This was followed by several days of depression and fatigue so severe that she was unable to get out of bed. At one point her family was so concerned about this behavior that they considered removing her children from her care and called me for my advice. Her PMS and severe mood swings had begun early on in her teenage years and were often accompanied by self-destructive behavior that led her into some dangerous situations. During one of these times, she was gang raped. On another occasion, she became pregnant and later got an abortion. Because of the severity of Gwendolyn's symptoms, I initially prescribed high-dose progesterone therapy. Eventually, however, Gwendolyn healed her PMS as she addressed the imbalances in her life.

As she recovered, she told me, "In my premenstrual times, every ounce of anger, bitterness, and sense of betrayal erupted—often at such a rate that it became increasingly difficult to stay in my marriage and to continue to care for my autistic daughter and two younger children."

By the time of her first visit with me, Gwendolyn had divorced and was meditating regularly and eating a whole-foods, macrobiotic-type of diet, which was helping her to some extent. She was exercising regularly and taking the appropriate food supplements. These dietary and lifestyle practices are often enough to "cure" PMS in its mildest stages. Despite these adjustments, however, she still went through an emotional "hell" each month. She had so much unfinished emotional business in her life that her premenstrual wisdom was forcing her to look even deeper at the imbalances in her life.

By the time Gwendolyn began her progesterone treatment, many aspects of her life were totally out of control. She came to see that the emotional "crash" that she experienced premenstrually each month actually was forcing her to peel off all the layers of denial in her life. And looking back, she came to see that this process was essential for her healing. A significant factor in her healing was joining a twelve-step program known as Sex and Love Addicts Anonymous (SLA). She realized that she had a history of moving from one abusive relationship to the next, never finding the "right" man but always obsessing about whomever she was with. When her artist boyfriend expressed his need to leave the relationship, Gwendolyn was premenstrual and flew into a rage, during which she beat him physically with a vengeance that both surprised and scared her. She realized that she had a significant relationship problem and went into counseling to explore and heal her abuse issues. She learned how a sex and love addiction is often the result of childhood sexual abuse, and she began to connect an early abuse experience and the rape with her current self-destructive behavior. She began to appreciate that her premenstrual rages were those of an unhealed child and that they needed to be addressed now that she was an adult. Meanwhile, she continued to meditate, exercise, eat well, go to counseling, and attend twelve-step meetings.

Through supporting her physical body with natural progesterone, good nutrition, and the regular deep rest of meditation, Gwendolyn developed the inner strength necessary to "handle all that had to erupt and clear out of my body." During her office visits, no matter how bad she felt, I repeatedly reminded her to stay with what she was feeling, that anger and rage were okay and a natural part of the healing process. She needed to feel her anger, even pound a pillow if necessary. But instead of attacking a person with it, she needed to respect the anger as a message telling her something she needed to know. As her healing process continued, she discovered that underneath her premenstrual rage and anger, the wisdom and the truth lay waiting. By feeling her anger and staying with it, she discovered tears and a profound sense of abandonment left over from the abuses. "The feelings of abandonment are overwhelming sometimes," she told me. "But if I allow the sadness to come, in the end I come out stronger."

After nine months of progesterone therapy, Gwendolyn was able to cut way back on her dosages. "I continue on the progesterone only two days a month and only because of mild irritability," she says. "I hit an occasional emotional wall, but the difference now is that I am able to cope much better knowing where it is all coming from. I believe that when a woman has PMS, the physical, emotional, and spiritual all have to be addressed so that a human being can feel whole again—returning to the whole being—integrity, in fact."

It has been two years since Gwendolyn first began to listen to and understand her menstrual wisdom through learning to trust and transform her rage. When I recently spoke with her, she was doing better than ever. She says that if she had to describe her life in one word, it would be *empowerment*. She's taking care of old business, making amends to those she's hurt and telling the truth to those who have hurt her. She is thrilled that "the talents I was born with are flourishing: my voice, music, and art. I believe that we all have these talents. But we aren't made to feel that we have anything worthwhile." She no longer needs progesterone. She writes, "When I become angry at all, I give myself quiet space, go within, and ask myself, 'What is it that you're afraid of or what pain are you trying to escape?' I almost always get an answer that I can then work with."

PMS and Codependence

There is a strong correlation between PMS and growing up in an alcoholic family system, in which the parents or grandparents were alcoholic. The relationship between PMS and "giving your life away" to meet other people's needs—relationship addiction—is very high. In many families in which the men have a tendency to become alcoholics, the females tend to develop PMS. Children of alcoholics have a 40 percent chance of becoming alcoholic, not only because they have a genetic predisposition toward it but because they've learned that alcohol is the way to deaden their emotions. This behavior is frequently passed on to them, along with genes that predispose them to drinking. Women in alcoholic families or with alcoholic partners develop PMS as a result of cutting off their feelings. I've worked with countless women who have decided to break the chain of PMS experienced by generations of women in their families. (Hypoglycemia [low blood sugar] and a resulting tendency toward sugar craving are also very common in women from alcoholic families who have PMS. This condition tends to be much worse premenstrually and can be treated with the dietary recommendations I've already covered.)

Leslie, a forty-nine-year-old homemaker and former teacher with PMS, came to see me with severe premenstrual mood swings, sugar cravings, and fatigue. As I read through her history, I noted that her husband was an alcoholic and that she was in a teaching position that she hated. She had had an alcoholic mother and sister and had never addressed any of these family issues. During the initial visit, I counseled her about supporting her body during the menstrual cycle through nutrition and exercise, and I stressed that she wouldn't "cure" her premenstrual discomfort until she was willing to look at the messages they were sending her about her own family situation. I could tell that she wasn't ready to hear this information, and she did not return for a follow-up.

Seven years later, however, Leslie made an appointment. She told me, "When I was in to see you in 1985, you told me that I needed to check out my codependence and that my PMS and decreased energy were related to that. I left thinking, 'Dr. Northrup's a nice woman, but she doesn't know what she's talking about, and in fact I think she's crazy. How could codependence and PMS be related?' But now I realize the connection between what was happening in my life and my PMS. I finally realized that my husband has been verbally abusive for years. I am in the middle of a divorce, and I see now that I had totally 'de-selfed' myself."

Leslie told me that she had joined a twelve-step group and was picking up the pieces of her life and learning about the effects of living with verbal abuse and alcoholism for so many years. Leslie's feelings are no longer deadened. She's becoming her own person and determining what she will and will not accept about her family's behavior. She no longer has PMS most months, but when she does, she pays attention to it, slows down, and makes the necessary adjustments in her life, so that she gets her needs met.

Irregular Periods

After over fifteen years of medical practice, I continue to be amazed by how clearly menstrual cycles and bleeding are connected to the contexts of our lives. Abnormal uterine bleeding is always connected to family issues in some way. As Caroline Myss says, blood is family—always. One woman told me that she and her two sisters, who were living in different parts of the country, skipped periods in the same month when a fourth sister had a miscarriage, although they didn't realize it until they talked at their next get-together. One of my patients, age fifty-five, who had her last menstrual period at the age of fifty-two and went through a classic menopause with hot flashes and lab tests confirming "change of life," nevertheless got a completely normal period right after her mother died. When a "menopausal" woman develops "postmenopausal" bleeding, I always ask her what is going on with her and her family. She will often tell me that an emotionally significant family event preceded the bleeding.

Menstrual blood, especially when it comes at an unscheduled time, is a message. It carries wisdom of some kind. Myss points out that most bleeding problems originate from an imbalance in our system: too much emotion and not enough mental, intellectual energy to balance it. She notes that bleeding abnormalities are exacerbated when a woman internalizes confusing signals from her family or society about her own sexual pleasure and sexual needs. A woman may, for example, desire sexual pleasure but feel guilty about it or be unable to ask directly for what she desires. She may not be consciously aware of this inner conflict.

Most practicing physicians have seen the profound effect that the psyche can have on the menstrual cycle. In 1949, S. Zuckerman recognized that emotional disturbances could disorganize menstrual rhythm, accelerate uterine bleeding, and also influence the time of ovulation. Diffuse networks of nerves connecting the brain with the ovaries (called preganglionic autonomic pathways) may mediate this connection between emotions and uterine and ovarian function.[46]

What Are Regular Periods?

Before I examine the subject of menstrual period irregularity, it's necessary to explain what is normal. Women are sometimes taught that their periods are irregular if they do not occur every twenty-eight days. I consider periods *regular* when they occur roughly every twenty-four to thirty-five days. Having a period every twenty-eight days like clockwork happens for some women but not all. Thousands of women who don't fit the every-twenty-eight-day pattern are under the impression that their periods are irregular, when in fact they are completely normal.

Period regularity is determined by a complex interaction between the brain (hypothalamus, pituitary gland, and temporal lobes), the ovaries, and the uterus. Period patterns can change with changes in seasons, lighting conditions, diet, or travel, or during times of family stress. Irregular and anovulatory menstrual cycles are associated with premature bone loss. Often women can tell when they have ovulated because they have a watery discharge twelve to sixteen days from the first day of their last menstrual period. Sometimes called "fertile flow," it has an egg-white consistency. Cycles in which a woman has ovulated are also characterized by what is called premenstrual *molimina*. Molimina is a group of "symptoms" resulting from normal cyclic hormonal changes in the body. These include a slight premenstrual redistribution of body fluid often experienced as "bloating" or slightly tender breasts, slight lower abdominal cramping, and mood changes associated with being in a more reflective, less active state. Women who don't ovulate usually don't have these changes and will often get a period "out of the blue," without having any idea that one is "due." Periods in which there is no ovulation tend to be more irregular.

Excessive Buildup of the Uterine Lining (Endometrial Hyperplasia, Cystic and Adenomatous Hyperplasia)

In some women with irregular periods, a biopsy of the inside of the uterus (endometrial biopsy) reveals a condition in which the normal lining of the uterus has been replaced by an overgrowth of glandular tissue. Under the microscope, the endometrial glands look as if they are piled on top of each other and packed too closely. This overgrowth results from overstimulation of the uterine lining by estrogen without the balance of progesterone. It is known as cystic and adenomatous hyperplasia (meaning too many glands) of the endometrium.[47] (It is not to be confused with endometriosis, which will be discussed at length in Chapter 6.) Hyperplasia results when a woman's ovaries haven't ovulated regularly: Instead of a uniform thickening and then sloughing of the uterine lining (the endometrium) from the hormones associated with regular ovulation, the endometrium gets out of sync. Some parts of the lining "think" it's day 7, while others think it's day 28. This results in irregular and intermittent bleeding.

Cystic and adenomatous hyperplasia or simple endometrial hyperplasia is not considered dangerous unless abnormal cells are present in the biopsy of the uterine lining. Finding some simple endometrial hyperplasia on a biopsy is fairly normal and is not a cause for alarm if it happens only once or twice. Many women in their forties and fifties skip an ovulation every now and then as their ovaries undergo the changes leading up to menopause. When a woman's periods become irregular, she does not necessarily require a uterine biopsy, though this decision must be made on a case-by-case basis depending on her history and examination findings.

Treatment

Please note that for this and other conditions, I will be discussing the treatments that are most commonly prescribed in the United States. These treatments do not address the issues underlying symptoms. The underlying issues and what a woman can learn from them are covered in the individual stories at the end of this chapter.

Many cases of simple endometrial hyperplasia go away on their own. However, a very small percentage of women with this condition have atypical cells on their biopsies. Endometrial hyperplasia needs to be monitored and followed to be sure it is going away rather than progressing. Women with chronic anovulation over many years do have a statistically higher incidence of uterine cancer. Gynecologists are trained to treat everybody as though they were a potential cancer risk. Therefore initial conventional treatment of endometrial hyperplasia consists of giving a synthetic progestin hormone such as Provera or Aygestin for one to three months and then repeating the endometrial biopsy to make sure that the condition has cleared. I often use natural progesterone for this purpose, especially in those women who have adverse side effects from synthetic progestin. (See page 124 for the difference between synthetic and natural progesterone.) Physicians vary widely on how much of the drug they give and how long they give it. Prescribing a progestin drug is sometimes called a "medical D&C" (dilation and curettage of the uterine lining), because it causes the endometrial lining to slough off in a uniform manner all at once and helps the uterus get rid of the tissue buildup.

Some women with persistent endometrial hyperplasia do not respond to treatment with progestin or progesterone and may even require a surgical D&C in the operating room. In extremely rare instances, they may need a hysterectomy if this condition does not go away or if it progresses to produce abnormal cells.

Dysfunctional Uterine Bleeding (DUB)

Skipping periods more than just occasionally, or frequent bleeding between periods, is known as dysfunctional uterine bleeding, or DUB. These abnormal patterns are often "hypothalamic" in origin, meaning that they are related to that complex interaction between the brain, ovaries, and uterus. Severe anxiety and depression change neurotransmitter levels in the brain and can affect hypothalamic function. Dysfunctional uterine bleeding is often associated with anovulatory cycles. Though I've been trained to look for endocrine abnormalities—such as thyroid problems or pituitary problems—that can cause menstrual abnormalities, I rarely find anything wrong by using standard blood tests and a physical exam. Because DUB can also be related to high prolactin levels caused by pituitary tumors, I always order a blood test for this hormone as well. However, prolactin hormone levels that are too high, a condition known as hyperprolactinemia, is not common.

A diagnosis of DUB is made on the basis of history, blood tests that check pituitary and thyroid hormone levels, and sometimes a biopsy from inside the uterus to see if the uterine lining shows signs of anovulation or abnormal cells.

Conventional Treatment

The conventional treatment for DUB consists of giving hormones such as birth control pills to "regulate" the periods. This common treatment is now given even up until menopause in women who don't smoke. (In the past, birth control pills were not recommended for women over thirty-five, but this standard has now changed, since birth control pill hormone dosages are lower, and more recent studies have shown that they are safe in older women.) Birth control pills do result in reliable periods every month and taking them may be the first choice for women whose lives are too busy to change their circumstances. But pills don't heal anything—they simply mask the underlying issues in the body or put an imbalance "to sleep" for a while. Nevertheless, like most gynecologists, I prescribe birth control pills for many women, both for contraception and for DUB, because taking the pill is the easiest way for a woman to eliminate her symptoms without doing the work of changing aspects of her life that are contributing to the problem.

Women with DUB who are in their forties and older are statistically at greater risk for endometrial hyperplasia, and most physicians will do an endometrial biopsy before they initiate hormonal treatment. Progestin hormone (synthetic progesterone) is often the treatment of choice, both to clear up the hyperplasia if it is present and to stop the abnormal bleeding. I often use natural progesterone for the same purpose. (The dosage is 200 mg. two times per day orally, or as a vaginal or rectal suppository for thirty days or more, depending upon the patient.) If a woman is skipping periods and wants to get pregnant, the fertility drug Clomid, which tricks the brain and ovaries into producing an ovulation, will often be prescribed.[48]

A subgroup of women with DUB are overweight. They don't ovulate regularly, in part because their body fat produces too much estrogen. The estrogen overstimulates the uterine lining and can result in anovulation. These women sometimes have a condition known as polycystic ovary syndrome in which their ovaries develop a thickening outer wall, just under which many unreleased, partially stimulated eggs form cysts. On ultrasound examinations, the ovaries show up as being enlarged and having multiple small cysts in them. (Interestingly, medical intuitives report exactly the same appearance when they do readings on these women.) Polycystic ovary syndrome is also associated with too much estrogen and not enough progesterone (hyperestrogenism). Dietary change to a low-fat, high-fiber diet can help lower estrogen levels.

Unabated stress; a high-fat, low-nutrient diet; and a lack of exposure to natural light can *all* result in DUB. Many of my patients with DUB have been helped by lifestyle and dietary changes alone. Some make these changes in addition to hormonal treatment.

Alternative Treatment Program
My treatment plan often includes one or more of the following:

• A low-fat, high-fiber diet for at least two months. It should be under 35 grams of fat per day, with at least 75 percent of calories from high-complex carbohydrate, unrefined foods such as vegetables, whole grain products, and beans. (See the Appendix for healthy diet plans.)

• Multivitamin-mineral supplements and essential fatty acids that help metabolize excess estrogen and balance prostaglandin hormones. (See "Program for PMS Relief," page 123.)

• Castor oil packs to the lower abdomen, at least three times per week for sixty minutes each time. This regimen should be followed for at least three months and then can be tapered to once a week. Packs should not be used while you are bleeding heavily.

Castor oil, also known as palma Christi (the palm of Christ) has been used for healing for hundreds of years. Castor oil packs are a treatment that the medical intuitive Edgar Cayce often prescribed for many different conditions. I was introduced to them by Dr. Gladys McGarey, who has used them in her general practice of medicine for over forty years. They are made by saturating wool or cotton flannel, folded four-ply, with cold-pressed castor oil. The oil and flannel can be purchased at a health food store or directly from the company that makes them, Home Health Products (telephone: 1-800-468-7313).

The oil-saturated flannel is then placed directly on the skin of the lower abdomen and covered with a piece of plastic, such as a plastic bag. Heat, in the form of a hot water bottle or heating pad, is then applied over the pack. A blanket or towel can be placed over the heat source to keep everything in place. I prefer a nonelectric heat source and often recommend a hot water bottle known as a Fomentek bag. (See Resources for information on how to obtain one of these and for more information on castor oil packs.) The patient then reclines with this on her lower abdomen for sixty minutes. During this treatment, I ask her to pay attention to thoughts, images, and feelings that arise and make note of them in a journal. Preliminary studies on castor oil packs done at the George Washington School of Medicine indicate that they improve immune system functioning.

- *Light therapy.* Determine what the first day of your last period was as nearly as possible. (You may need to guess.) From days 14 to 17 of your cycle, sleep with a 100-watt light bulb in a common bedside-table lamp that has a shade that disperses light onto the ceiling and wall but is minimally disturbing to sleep, on the floor next to your bed. Do this for six months. In one study of two thousand women, more than 50 percent regulated their previously irregular periods to a regular cycle of 29 days by doing this.[49]

- *Natural progesterone.* This can be taken orally or transdermally. The dosage depends on the symptoms; usually it is 50 to 200 mg. orally on a daily basis, on days 14 to 28 of the cycle, for at least three months. For transdermal application, use ProGest cream, one quarter teaspoon (14 to 20 mg.) in the morning, one quarter teaspoon in the evening, on the soft areas of skin (breasts, abdomen, neck, face, inner arms). Alternate the sites with each application; apply on days 14 to 28 for at least three months. Increase or decrease the dosage depending upon rate of absorption and the severity of the symptoms.

- *Synthetic hormones.* Synthetic progestin (Amen, Aygest, Provera) can be taken, 10 to 20 mg. on days 14 to 28 of the cycle for three months, or as prescribed by your health care practitioner. Birth control pills can also be prescribed.

• *Acupuncture and herbs.* Acupuncture and herbs can help DUB and many other gynecological problems. But just as there are many emotional settings and energy dysfunctions that may set the scene for a woman's menstrual disorders, there are many appropriate and specific Oriental herbal and acupuncture treatments that may be prescribed. When a woman seeks acupuncture and Oriental herbal treatment for her menstrual disorder, she may receive one of numerous diagnoses, including (but not limited to) deficient blood of the heart, spleen, or liver; deficient *chi;* stagnant blood; and stagnant *chi.* Depending upon her history or physical symptoms, as well as her physical examination, specific acupuncture points and herbs will be selected that are appropriate for her condition. Each woman who is drawn to this approach must find an appropriately trained practitioner of oriental medicine with whom she feels safe.

• *Meditation and stress reduction.* Any modality that decreases stress can help menstrual period regulation because of the profound link between emotional or psychological stress and biochemical imbalance.

Women's Stories

DEBORAH: BREAKING FAMILY TIES. Deborah was seventeen when she left her family to go to college. She described her family as "lower middle class and not oriented to a college education." In fact, Deborah was the first person from her family ever to leave home, except to marry. Her family was not supportive of her living away from home, and they wanted her to visit every weekend.

During her first year in college, Deborah met many people who were interesting and exciting to her: A whole new world of intellectual challenge and career possibilities began opening up for her. She was happier and felt more fulfilled than at any other time in her life. Unfortunately, her mother, fearing that she would lose Deborah, began to call her on the phone every evening, telling her that she was a failure and that she would never succeed at anything if she stayed in college. She threatened to call the dean of the college and have Deborah's scholarships rescinded so that she would have no choice but to come home.

Deborah became depressed, and her periods became irregular for the first time since menarche. They came two or three times per month, or not at all for two to three months at a time. To feel better about herself, she began to run as a form of exercise. At first, this made her feel physically stronger, more independent, and more in control of her body—which seemed to be out of control for the first time in her life. But the exercise didn't help her irregular periods. In fact, it contributed to long periods of amenorrhea (no periods at all). She saw a gynecologist who told her that her pelvic exam was completely normal. The reason for her problem, he said, was, "she was fooling around with too many guys." Since she was not involved with any men at this time, she was not helped by this physician and avoided gynecologists for the next eleven years.

Deborah did, however, consult with an acupuncturist, who prescribed Chinese herbs for her in addition to acupuncture. These treatments helped regulate her periods within two months, but she soon found that she had to deal with the source of her depression that returned when she had to stop running because of an injury. (She discovered that her periods went right back to their abnormal pattern as soon as she stopped her acupuncture and herb treatments.) She came to see that her relationship with her mother was the source of her problems, and she eventually moved out of state, away from her mother's continual phone calls, to break her mother's control over her life.

When I first saw Deborah, she was recovering from addictive exercise and her relationship with her mother. She had begun psychotherapy and was exploring these issues. I recommended an intensive workshop with Anne Wilson Schaef, a whole foods diet, ProGest cream, and a calcium-magnesium supplement. Over the next six months, her periods became regular, every twenty-eight to twenty-nine days, and she was no longer depressed. She finished college and recently completed her Ph.D. She has broken the original family ties that were at the root of her problem, and her life is becoming balanced on all levels.

DONNA: DYSFUNCTIONAL FAMILY AND DYSFUNCTIONAL BLEEDINGS. Donna, a forty-two-year-old professor, came into my office with a six-month history of irregular periods—bleeding for two weeks, then nothing for six weeks, then a few days of spotting, and so on. She also had bouts of severe anxiety and depression that lasted for three weeks straight, at just about the time the irregularity started.

Donna's mother had also gone through abnormal periods and mood swings in her forties but had decided that "it is all your hormones, and you're just going to have to live with it." Donna is quite sure that her mother had had unresolved issues with her own father, since Donna remembers her grandfather as someone who was very scary to be around when she was a child.

Donna told me that she'd been having some dreams about and memories of sexual abuse by her uncles. "I've been terrified that if I tell anyone what happened or what I think happened, God will get me," she told me. "Can you force yourself to deal with this stuff any faster?" Like many women, she was under the impression that merely having the facts—who, what, where, and when—would help her deal with her discomfort and get on with her life once and for all. But that's not the way healing our lives works. We have to let healing work its way through us gently, gradually, and respectfully.

Donna's upbringing had led her to claim, "Everything in life is my fault. I keep thinking that I must be crazy and must be making this stuff up." I reassured her that in this culture women have been labeled crazy for centuries for telling the truth and that what she was going through was quite normal, given her history. She decided to do some work with an incest survivors' group to help her break through her own and her family's denial. After several months of work, she had another endometrial biopsy—to check for abnormal cells—and it was perfectly normal, as were her pituitary hormones. Her periods had gradually become more regular.

Dealing with her emotional trauma was what actually "cured" Donna's period problems. Her periods, through their irregularity, had communicated to her a bodily wisdom. Her menstrual blood turned her attention to the healing that was required in her relationship with her family, her blood line.

DARLENE: IRREGULAR PERIODS SINCE MENARCHE. I first saw Darlene, a teacher, as a patient when she was thirty years old. She was married, had no children, and had had a very long history of dysfunctional uterine bleeding since puberty. She experienced long stretches of time with no periods, followed by bleeding almost continuously for a month at a time, then spotting infrequently. Darlene had on-going anxiety issues and had panic attacks if she had to leave the house for a long period of time. Her marriage was a source of unhappiness to her rather than comfort. She was generally anxious, had trouble sleeping, and had frequent headaches.

Darlene's upbringing had been stressful. Her father and at least one grandfather were alcoholics although, she said, there was a lot of family denial around this. Her mother, her maternal grandmother, and her cousin had had lifelong problems with irregular bleeding that led to hysterectomies. Her aunt and another cousin had uterine cancer and also had hysterectomies.

Darlene originally came to my office for a fertility workup. Because of her bleeding pattern, we did an endometrial biopsy, which showed endometrial hyperplasia. For treatment of this condition, she was placed on large doses of synthetic progestin. In contrast to most women on this therapy, however, her bleeding didn't stop. A repeat biopsy after the progestin treatment again showed the abnormality of cystic and adenomatous hyperplasia. The next step would be a dilation and curettage (D&C) to be certain that she didn't have uterine cancer.

But Darlene was terrified of the procedure and begged me for an alternative. Because of her strong reaction, I compromised and recommended castor oil packs on her lower abdomen three to four times a week to help restore her immune system. I knew this would give her a chance to reflect at least three times per week on her condition and any messages it might hold for her. We agreed that if this didn't change her cells, we would go ahead with the D&C.

Two weeks later, I did another endometrial biopsy. The tissue was normal endometrium, consistent with the first phase of her menstrual cycle. Darlene was ecstatic and cried with relief. She then went on to have a completely normal period. In the ensuing months her periods were normal, too, and have remained that way. During these months she had changed her biochemistry through biofeedback, which she did for her insomnia, headaches, and intense anxiety. Realizing that her marriage had not been healthy for her, she separated from her husband, began divorce proceedings, and entered into a love affair where her sexual needs were addressed and that turned out to be deeply healing for her.

Three years later, when Darlene came in for her annual exam, she told me that she was developing a feeling of power around her menstrual cycle that was new and very exciting for her. "My breasts get bigger," she said, "I feel powerful, and I walk around like I know the secrets of the universe. I think my family has been terrified of my power for years. I can remember feeling it even when I was a little girl. Although having this power seems new, it also seems like something I've known for a long time." Darlene has reclaimed her connection to the universal feminine and her sexuality. By doing so, she has broken a cycle of irregular bleeding that was generations deep within her family—and blood ties.

Heavy Periods (Menorrhagia)

Some women bleed so heavily during their periods that they routinely bleed through one or two tampons and a pad worn at the same time. Their blood may soak through their clothing even on the second or third day of their cycles. Some are unable to leave the house during certain days of their periods because the bleeding is so heavy. One of my patients decided to have a hysterectomy after she bled through her clothes into the upholstery of her airplane seat on two different business trips to Europe.

This kind of heavy bleeding is called menorrhagia. Women with menorrhagia have periods at regular intervals, but the periods are heavy. Over time, menorrhagia may lead to anemia (a low red-blood-cell count) if a woman doesn't get enough iron in her diet or if her body can't replace the blood she loses each month. Menorrhagia can be caused by fibroids, endometriosis, or adenomyosis. Rarely, it is associated with a thyroid problem. Some women bleed heavily for no obvious reason.

Chronically heavy periods can be related to chronic stress over second chakra issues, including creativity, relationships, money, and control of others. One of my patients who sometimes had very heavy periods noted that her periods became heavy when she was upset and needed to weep. "When I bleed like that," she said, "I feel like it's the lower part of my body weeping for the losses I have suffered in my life." When she took the time to pay attention to the different problems she was having and let herself feel her disappointments and pain, her periods were normal. Another patient, who had bad cramps every month and bled profusely, began to think of the uterine pain as related to her strong need for creative space in her own life. She began to set aside one hour a day to do sculpture. Each time she did, she got in touch with the sheer joy of creating for its own sake and her pelvic pain and bleeding gradually lessened each month.

Adenomyosis, a common cause of heavy bleeding, is a condition in which the glands that normally grow in only the lining of the uterus—the endometrium—grow deeply into the walls of the uterus. (Sometimes called "internal endometriosis," adenomyosis is often present along with fibroids and/or endometriosis but not always.) This condition can result in bleeding into the uterine wall with each menstrual period, resulting in painful periods and heavy bleeding during menstrual cycles. The uterine wall becomes spongy and engorged with blood, resulting in a condition in which the normal uterine muscles can't contract normally to decrease the bleeding.

A diagnosis of adenomyosis is usually suspected from a woman's history and from a characteristic boggy-feeling uterus on pelvic examination. A definitive diagnosis can be made, however, only by magnetic resonance imaging (MRI) or by a biopsy of the uterine wall, which entails surgically removing a piece of the uterus or by removing the entire uterus.

Treatment

As for all the conditions mentioned in this section, modalities that change the electromagnetic field around the body and unblock the energy in the pelvis can have a beneficial effect on menorrhagia. Acupuncture, meditation, and massage are among these modalities.

• *Dietary change.* Whether or not a woman's bleeding is caused by adenomyosis, she may respond well to a low-fat, high-complex-carbohydrate diet that reduces excessive circulating estrogen (30 grams of fat or less, with 75 percent of calories from complex carbohydrates) followed for at least three months. Menu plans are listed in books by Dr. John McDougall, Dr. Dean Ornish, and others. (See also Chapter 17.)

Vitamin C with bioflavonoids (500 mg. per day)[50] and vitamin A[51] have also been shown to decrease menstrual blood loss. Vitamin A at doses as high as 100,000 IU per day often works well but can be given at this high level for only three months. Otherwise, there is a risk of toxicity. I also recommend a good multivitamin-mineral supplement that has adequate levels of all the vitamins, since they tend to work synergistically.

Eliminating all dairy food (even low fat) for at least three months often helps as well, for reasons that I cover in Chapter 17.

• *Medications.* Women whose menorrhagia does not respond to diet or who prefer other options can often be helped by a synthetic progestin hormone to keep the bleeding under control. My usual regimen is 5 to 10 mg. of Provera or Aygestin, taken once or twice per day during the last two weeks of each menstrual cycle. Birth control pills also can work well in many cases. Natural progesterone, either applied as a skin cream or taken orally, can also be used. The dosage depends upon the severity of the problem: For oral progesterone, 100 mg. four times per day for most severe cases, 50 mg. two times per day for milder cases, from days 14 to 28 of the cycle. For ProGest or Progestone cream, a half teaspoon twice per day on the soft areas of the skin—breasts, neck, face, abdomen, inner thighs, and inner arms; alternate the sites at each application. Following a low-fat, high-fiber diet often decreases or eliminates the need for the progestin or progesterone over time. Some women have used this treatment for months or even years as an alternative to hysterectomy.

Prostaglandin inhibitors such as ibuprofen (Advil or Motrin), naproxen sulfate (Anaprox) or mefenamic acid (Ponstel) have also helped some women decrease menstrual bleeding.[52] These are best taken one or two times per day for three to four days before the menstrual cycle is due and continuing through the days of the period that are usually the heaviest.

• *Surgery.* Endometrial ablation, in which the lining of the uterus is cauterized, is a surgical treatment for heavy bleeding in women whose menorrhagia has failed to respond to all other treatments. Several of my patients have responded very well to endometrial ablation, although for others, it hasn't worked at all. Women who opt for this procedure, which is done in the operating room under general anesthesia, must be carefully screened beforehand to make sure that their condition is likely to respond. Hysterectomy is also an option.

Healing Our Menstrual History: Preparing Our Daughters

Many women, like those about whom you've read in this chapter, have turned around their painful menstrual experiences and begun to reclaim their rightful heritage: their bodily and menstrual wisdom. As a woman does this, she passes on to the next generation a more positive body image and relationship to her body. In this way, she frees herself and others from the patriarchal degradation of the feminine, and the possibility of healing all women's cycles is greatly enhanced.

For too long, young girls have been introduced to the menstrual cycle solely in terms of sexual intercourse and the possibility of getting pregnant inadvertently. Most girls are not emotionally prepared to grasp the fullness of their female sexuality until they know about and understand the workings of their own uterus, fallopian tubes, ovaries, and cyclic menstrual nature. Reclaiming menstrual wisdom involves women envisioning a new and more positive way of thinking and talking about the menstrual experience to ourselves, our daughters, and to the men in our families. And it involves educating ourselves and others about female sexuality. Many of us have husbands who have voiced unease about their daughters' puberty. Fathers seem to hold a very old and probably unexamined sense of needing to protect their daughters from other men and boys. If this protection really worked and helped women to feel secure in their female bodies, we might feel happy about it. Realistically, however, fathers simply cannot protect their daughters effectively, and girls and women cannot and must not continue to seek out men as protectors and providers.

Many women have told me about the lack of support they felt from their own fathers when they reached menarche: "As soon as I got my period things changed between us. He never hugged or cuddled me again. Our relationship was never the same." One woman with a uterine fibroid remembered her father yelling at her across the room when she was fourteen and all dressed up to go out on a date, "You slut, you whore!" She hadn't remembered this for years. She said that it had felt as if his words went right into her body and stayed there, affecting the way she felt about herself as a woman for the next twenty years.

From birth, females are indoctrinated with the idea that our bodies are subject to the appropriating gaze of others, and to public comment and observation. We parade our little girls out for the gaze of others and often dress them up like small confections for pleasing others. One of my colleagues described how his thirteen-year-old daughter sat down at the dinner table and her older brother said, "I see we've had a visit from the breast fairy." He told this story amidst gales of laughter, but I imagine that his daughter didn't find it very amusing.

For many girls in this society, puberty has been a time of loss. When my oldest daughter was eleven and I was tucking her into bed one night, she told me that she was worried about something. She had a sore growth on her chest that was scaring her. She wanted me to check it. I did and found a small nipple budding on the left—the first sign of puberty. I told her that it was normal and that she had nothing to worry about. I congratulated her!

Later, unable to sleep, she came into my room and said, "Can we talk?" I said, "Of course," and asked what was troubling her. She burst into tears and said, "I don't want to grow up." I held her and told her that I remembered feeling the same way. I hadn't thought about it for years. But now, with her in my arms, perched on the brink of puberty, I remembered the deep sadness I had felt about growing up. I recalled never wanting to leave home and never wanting my life to change. We sat on my bed while I shared this with her and held her.

After a while, I asked her if she wanted to talk about this with her father. She said, "Yes." She asked, "Dad, were you ever sad about growing up?" He responded, "Not until the last few years." All of us laughed together at his reply. After a few more minutes of acknowledging my daughter's feelings about puberty, she thanked us and went happily off to bed. This experience was a great example for me of how our emotions, when we respect and express them, quite naturally move through the body and are released.

My daughter has not brought this issue up since, but I know she will if she feels the need for support. Her sadness had been a challenge in how we can help our daughters come of age with joy and respect. I appreciate now that at some deep, inarticulate level, she knows that moving from the innocence of girlhood to puberty is not an entirely happy prospect in a culture in which the female body is a commodity. As we work together to create new rites of passage for women, we must acknowledge that moving forward also means letting go and grieving over what we are losing.

Clearly, we cannot take our daughters into a space where we have never been. We cannot provide healing for them in areas in which we're still deeply wounded ourselves. If we still carry generations of shame about the processes of our female bodies, we cannot hope to pass on to our daughters a sense of love for their own bodies. We need new ways of thinking about this whole area. Each of us must create new ceremonies and new rites of passage for our own daughters. But before we can hope to do this effectively, we must own our own experiences, however unsupportive and painful, and work through them.

How might we think differently about our cycles? How might we celebrate our bleeding time, our time of power, our time of connection to the global female being? Tamara Slayton has made redeeming the menstrual cycle her life's work. She founded the Menstrual Health Foundation and the New Cycle company. In addition to educational services, her company makes a Coming of Age Doll kit to help mothers and daughters (or fathers and daughters, or any other combination of supporters) make a doll together to celebrate the girl's menarche, choosing fabric, beads, and any other adornments together.

Tamara conducts workshops with adolescent girls, in which pink wax is given to each girl to mold a model of a little uterus, with ovaries, eggs, and different types of cervical flow—red for blood and white for fertile, midcycle flow. The different types of flow are then charted with the monthly cycle. Little ovaries made from pink wax contain dots of green wax to show the eggs. By so combining the artistic creative process, the use of hands and mind at the same time, with information about the menstrual cycle, we can reclaim the link between our physical cycle and our creativity. Can you feel how different this is from "sex education"? Girls can't possibly integrate sexuality until they understand and respect their own cycles and inner rhythms.

I delivered my niece several years ago and saved her umbilical cord by wrapping it around a cardboard toilet paper tube and setting it inside a sunny window to dry. (If it's winter, you can do this in a slow oven.) The long, thin spiral of sinew that is left is a powerful symbol of the link that this child had with her mother. I intend to present this cord to her at her own coming of age party when the time comes. Some Native American tribes braided the umbilical cord into the mane of the child's first pony for protection. Many other cultures have special uses for the cord. My daughters were fascinated by this cord and wondered why I hadn't saved theirs. I told them that at the time I had never thought of it. I now wish I had.

Today's teenage girls are "fertile time bombs" because they have no knowledge of their own cycles and use sexuality and intercourse as a rite of passage.[53] I advocate teaching all teenage girls how to make love to themselves, so that they don't feel the need for teenage boys for an outlet! When we teach our young women respect for their bodies and for their cycles, and when we heal ourselves in these areas as well, we help break the cycles of abuse that have gone on for centuries.

After reading a newspaper article on Patricia Reis's work with the Goddess and women's bodies, Marge Rosenthal remembered that she had introduced the menstrual cycle to her daughter by creating a myth. In a letter to Reis she wrote, "When my daughter was four or five and I was premenstrual and searching for something positive about cramps, grouchiness, and all the other pleasures of being a woman, I created the Goddess Menses. She came out of a spontaneous situation: Mama grouchy—a kid wondering why, and me grasping for a believable answer.

"I told her that once a month the Goddess Menses visited a woman's body, and that she was a very mysterious goddess. Sometimes she sneaked in without us knowing, and sometimes she announced herself with powerful tuggings inside our bodies. I told her that when men bleed it is always a sign of illness or injury, but that the bleeding the goddess brought was a reaffirmation of life. A cleansing of our body. I told her that the goddess's arrival is a time of celebration, a time to buy flowers or something small and special, just for us women.

"I told her the grouchiness was because I wasn't listening to my body. Had I felt the tuggings, I would have known to be extra loving to myself (and perhaps taken a couple of aspirin!). As a result of my doing this, I saw all the positive value of creating our own goddesses. I created a little goddess to make positive association with the menstrual cycle. She is a high-spirited, energetic goddess who plays tricks with our bodies, arriving early or late, quiet or stormy, tugging or rolling over us, but once her presence is acknowledged she is very happy to quietly settle down and wait—until next time.

"As I approach menopause I will miss the goddess. It will be a time of her holding on to the youth we shared and me letting go to let the next spirit enter my body. I wonder what *her* name will be?"

Creating Health Through the Menstrual Cycle

Sitting quietly, ask yourself, "What is my personal truth about the menstrual cycle? How am I feeling about this information? What messages about menstruation and hormones have I learned from my family? What information have I handed down to the younger women in my life? What do I tell myself about my menstrual period? What can it teach me?" Regardless of where you are, be gentle with yourself.

For the next three months, keep a moon journal specifically for noticing the effects of your menstrual cycle on your life. Keep track of the phases of the moon. (These are often listed in the newspaper or in an almanac.) See if you notice any correlation between your cycle and the phases of the moon. See if you crave certain foods premenstrually. What are they? Would taking a long bath feel as good as eating that hot fudge sundae?

Give yourself time to tune in to and reclaim your cyclic nature. Write a short journal entry every day. The rewards of doing this will be beyond measure. You'll feel connected to life in a whole new way, with increased respect for yourself and your magnificent hormones.

Celebrate the Goddess Menses in your own unique way.

SIX

The Uterus

The oldest oracle in Greece, sacred to the Great Mother of earth, sea, and sky, was named Delphi, from delphos, meaning "womb."
—Barbara Walker, *The Women's Encyclopedia of Myths and Secrets*

The uterus is located in the low center of the pelvis, connected to the vagina by the cervix and to the pelvic side walls by the broad and cardinal ligaments. The back portion of the bladder attaches to the lower front part of the uterus—the lower uterine segment. The fallopian tubes come off each side of the upper portion of the uterus, known as the fundus. The ovaries are located below the ends of the tubes, known as the fimbria. The fimbria look like delicate fern fronds. (See Figure 6.)

The ovaries, tubes, and uterus are all part of the female hormonal system. Each of these structures is intimately connected to the others.[1] The circulation of blood to the ovaries depends in part on an intact uterus. Following a hysterectomy, changes in the blood supply to the ovaries result in an earlier menopause in many women. The uterus itself is very sensitive to the effects of hormones. As the central organ in the pelvis, the uterus and its attachments to the pelvic side walls, the cardinal ligaments, are important, but underrated, components of the entire pelvic anatomy.

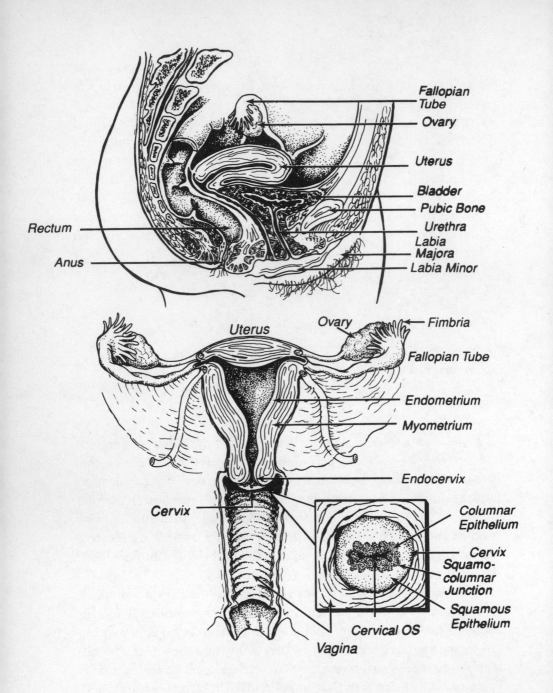

FIGURE 6: UTERUS, OVARIES, AND CERVIX WITH ANATOMIC LABELS

Our Cultural Inheritance

The uterus has hardly been studied separate from its role in child-bearing, a fact that reflects this society's baseline cultural biases.[2] The uterus is seen as someone else's potential home and is valued when it can potentially play that role. After the uterus's childbearing function has been completed or when a woman chooses not to have a child, "modern" medicine considers the uterus to have no inherent value. The ovaries are usually viewed in much the same way because medical science believes that hormonal replacement from artificial sources can perform their functions as well as or even better than a woman's own ovaries. Women are taught to view themselves in pretty much the same way—valuable as a function in being someone's mother or mate, with no inherent value of their own.

When I was in my residency training, one of our oncology fellows (a doctor doing specialty training in gynecological cancer) taught us, "There's no room in the tomb for the womb." Another slogan from my training was: "The uterus is for growing babies or for growing cancer." Occasionally, during my training, when one of our staff physician teachers removed a uterus that looked perfectly normal, we'd jokingly call the diagnosis CPU, a medicalized acronym for "chronic persistent uterus." These attitudes pervade conventional medicine.

The possibility that the uterus might have any function other than childbearing or tumor production has not been adequately addressed in conventional OB/GYN training. Even today, if a woman has a reproductive illness but wants to keep her uterus even though she has no interest in childbearing, her medical team too often views her as overly emotional or sentimental, a bit superstitious, and not well educated about that organ. The general patriarchal tone of this medical training is that if such a woman were more sophisticated, she would know that the uterus is useless to her except for childbearing.

Recently, I did a fibroid removal from the uterus of a forty-eight-year-old woman who didn't want a hysterectomy. The chief resident who assisted me said, "Why don't you just do a hysterectomy? They can have my uterus anytime they want. Now that I've had my children, it's only good for growing cancer." I told her she'd been brainwashed.

The following quote from a paper on hysterectomy sums up the attitude that pervaded the 1950s and still lives on, albeit to a lesser extent, today. "Hysterectomy is justified in women near the end of their reproductive period, in whom the uterus no longer serves a useful function . . . and . . . when reproduction is no longer desirable, the uterus can be dispensed with, for, although it contributes little or nothing, the aging organ is subject to degeneration and serious disease." This paper, written by a Dr. M. E. Davis, dismissed the possibility of any adverse reaction to hysterectomy by noting that "the complete removal of the uterus at delivery [of a baby] does not interfere with normal sex life; it actually improves it. . . . The roomy vagina, combined with the freedom from fear of conception, results in ideal marital life."[3] In fact, the uterus does seem to play a role in hormonal regulation, and its removal is not advisable unless absolutely necessary.

This undervaluing of the uterus by doctors and the public alike contributes to the fact that hysterectomy is one of the number-one elective surgeries in the United States. The current incidence of hysterectomy approaches 60 percent by the time women reach sixty-five years of age.[4] Since our thoughts and beliefs affect our bodies, these negative messages about the uterus that we internalize over a lifetime cause a large number of problems that women experience in this area.

Energy Anatomy

Though there are distinct differences between the energies of the ovaries and those of the uterus, many women have problems in both at the same time. For example, many women whose ovaries are affected by endometriosis also have fibroid tumors in the uterus. It is helpful, therefore, to discuss in general the overall nature of the emotional and psychological energy patterns that create health and disease in the pelvic organs, before we discuss these areas separately.

The *internal* pelvic organs (ovaries, tubes, and uterus) are related to second chakra issues. Their health depends upon a woman feeling able, competent, or powerful to create financial and emotional abundance and stability, and to express her creativity fully. She must be able to feel good about herself and about her relationships with other people in her life. Relationships that she finds stressful and limiting, on the other hand, adversely affect her internal pelvic organs. Thus, if a woman stays in an unhealthy relationship because she feels she cannot support herself economically or emotionally, her internal pelvic organs may be at increased risk for disease.

Disease is not created until a woman is frustrated in effecting changes that she needs to make in her life. The likelihood and severity of disease is related to how well the various areas of her life are functioning. A supportive marriage and family life, for example, can partially compensate for a stressful job. A classic psychological pattern associated with physical problems in the pelvis is that of a woman who wants to break free from limiting behaviors in her relationships (with her husband or her job, for example) but who cannot confront her *own* fears about the independence that making that change would bring. Though she may perceive that *others* are limiting her ability to break free, her major conflict is actually within herself around her *own* fears. One of my patients developed a fibroid tumor of the uterus and an ovarian cyst when she was forty. I asked her if her need for creativity was being met, and she told me that she very much wanted to leave her job and begin a florist business. She'd been interested in flowers since childhood, but her parents had always discouraged her interest since they considered it "frivolous." She had dutifully gone along with their suggestion that she learn typing and secretarial skills instead. She eventually became an executive secretary in an accounting firm. Though this work was not satisfying to her, she stayed at her job because she had a steady income and good "benefits," and was afraid of the risks of striking out on her own. As her fortieth birthday approached, she felt the need to pursue her childhood passion and had recurrent dreams about fields of flowers that she couldn't get to because they were fenced in by barbed wire. She came to see that through her ovarian cyst and fibroid uterus, her body's "birthing" center was trying to tell her something.

Another issue that affects a woman's pelvic organs is competition among her various needs. When her innermost needs for companionship and emotional support are in competition with her outer needs for success, autonomy, and tribal approval, this situation may manifest in her inner pelvic organs, the ovaries and the uterus. Our culture teaches us that we can't be both emotionally fulfilled and financially successful, and that our needs for them both are mutually exclusive; that as women, we can't have it all. Women are not usually taught to be competent in handling economic and financial assets because the patriarchal system depends on women being dependent. Since having money and status protects us and makes us feel safe, women have been taught that to find security they have to marry, and men have been taught that they have to provide women with money and social status. Success, in the addictive system, permits us to control others. These beliefs and the controlling behavior that results from them are a setup for pelvic problems.

The uterus is related energetically to a woman's innermost sense of self and her inner world. It is symbolic of her dreams and the selves to which she would like to give birth. Its state of health reflects her inner emotional reality and her belief in herself at the deepest level. The health of the uterus is at risk if a woman doesn't believe in herself or is excessively self-critical.

Uterine energy is slower than ovarian energy. The biological gestation time for the fetus is nine lunar months, while the biological gestation time for an egg is only one lunar month. Think of the uterus as the soil, either symbolic or biological, in which the creative seeds from the ovaries grow over time.

Ovarian energy is more dynamic and quickly changing than that of the uterus. In the reproductive years, healthy ovaries create new seeds monthly in a dynamic way. When this dynamic ovarian energy needs to get our attention, the ovaries are capable of changing very quickly. A large ovarian cyst can grow in a matter of days under the right circumstances.

Ovarian health is directly related to the quality of a woman's relationships with the people and things outside herself. (See Chapter 7.) Ovaries are at risk when women feel controlled or criticized by others or when they themselves control and criticize others.

Chronic Pelvic Pain

Pelvic pain can occur in one pelvic organ such as an ovary, in several pelvic organs, or throughout the pelvis, even if all of the pelvic organs have been removed. A certain percentage of women with chronic pelvic pain are not helped by surgery or medical treatment. In fact, thirty percent of hysterectomies done for chronic pelvic pain *fail* to relieve the pain, even when there is a diagnosable pathology such as endometriosis or fibroids. Women who have chronic pelvic pain often have complex psychological and emotional histories. Often, their pain is the result of pelvic endometriosis and is related to unfinished emotional pain in either past or current relationships with partners or with jobs, sexual abuse, emotional abuse, or rape (on any level). Emotional stress in a woman's personal or professional life that she perceives to be unresolvable is a big contributor to pelvic pain. Unresolved traumatic events from the past live in the energy system of the body, even after the pelvic organs have been removed surgically. I commonly see pelvic pain flare-ups in women who uncover incest memories, visit the place in which the incest took place, or work at jobs that control them but in which they feel they must continue to work. I tell these women that, through their pain, the body is asking them to pay attention to it and take care of it. The body, in its wisdom, wants to bring their attention back to the physical site of their emotional pain so that they can begin the healing process.

In many cases of chronic pelvic pain, no "physical" cause can be found and therefore the medical profession does not take it seriously. But chronic pelvic pain that comes from unresolved emotional pain from the past is *real*—it is not just "in the head." Pain is patterned or stored physically and chemically in our nervous, immune, and endocrine systems; it is in the bodymind. It cannot simply be cut out surgically.

Candace was thirty-nine years old when she first came to see me for chronic pelvic pain. She looked ethereal and delicate and worked in a school. In her teenage years she had been fascinated with ballet and had danced for a while, but she later gave it up when she moved out of state. She told me that she did not like her school work but didn't have the resources to change anything in her life. She wanted a garden, she said, but she was unable to have one because she lived in an apartment. She described her childhood as difficult but told me that she had already dealt with those issues and that they were not relevant to her current problem. Her father had been a strict disciplinarian, with high standards of perfection to which her mother had always tried to live up. Candace complained of nearly constant burning pelvic pain and suffered from chronic fatigue syndrome. Though she had tried very strict whole food diets, exercise, and a variety of holistic treatments ranging from acupuncture to polarity therapy, nothing had helped her.

Candace had a completely normal pelvic exam, and I was unable to discover tenderness or pain. But because her pain had been getting progressively worse, I scheduled her for a laparoscopy to see if she had pelvic endometriosis, an infection, or some other condition. (A laparoscopy is a procedure done under general anesthesia in which a telescopic instrument is placed in the pelvis to look at the organs directly.) It showed her pelvic organs as completely normal. Because she had already made so many lifestyle changes with no improvement, and because she told me that she had already dealt with her childhood issues, I suggested that she consult with Caroline Myss.

Myss later said, "This woman's entire system below the waist registers as if it's on fire. The pain levels are excruciating. She is one thought-form away from developing a malignancy." She said that Candace's problems dated back to a childhood, in which she had been criticized repeatedly. "Between the ages of one and seven," Caroline said, "we usually develop our link with the Earth through our relationship with our parents. But this woman has never bonded with actual physical life. As a response to her pain, she has created a fantasy world in her mind as an escape. Though she thinks she has dealt with her early history, what she means is that she can talk about it. But that doesn't count for anything."

All the energy from Candace's past was still in her body. She had not allowed herself to feel it or release it. I discovered that her apartment was set up as a refuge against the world and that she was always alone. Myss said, "Her energy is revealing that she has sent her spirit on to live in a fantasy world, a Harlequin romance, while avoiding everything and everyone who is earthy and real." As a consequence of this, Candace's bodily wisdom kept crying out for attention to its earlier wounding, even as Candace kept sending her spirit out of her body. Myss told me that Candace had almost no energy available in her system for healing because of this. "You must tell her," said Caroline, "that she must get back here, or her body will quickly manifest a way for her to leave."

When I went over this reading with Candace, she was able to appreciate parts of it but certainly not all of it. Like many women, Candace had been out of touch with her emotions for years. If it had felt safe to feel as a child, she wouldn't have needed to send her spirit into a fantasy world. The information in Myss's reading could not help Candace heal until she internalized its truth and felt it in her body. After her reading and her surgery, Candace practiced calling her spirit back. I asked her to make a list of all the reasons she wanted to live. I encouraged her to find a way to have a garden. She has taken some steps forward in her life. She now has a garden, and her pain has lessened somewhat. She has lived in a fantasy world for so long, however, that reentering real life and healing fully will require time, commitment, and the willingness to do so. She has not developed cancer.

Candace's case illustrates that healing from chronic pelvic pain often involves healing our lives at the deepest levels. Healing modalities that affect the function of the neuroendocrine and immune systems—such as massage, acupuncture, counseling, and dietary change—are all helpful, but ultimately the psychological and emotional data banks from our past must be purged and healed, and our spirit must be called back into the present moment. This can only be done when we acknowledge and have faith in our own inner wisdom and our connection to a power that is greater than our present circumstances.

Endometriosis

Endometriosis is a mysterious but increasingly common condition. The tissue that forms the lining of the uterus, the endometrial lining, normally grows inside the uterine cavity (and is responsible for monthly menstrual cycles). In endometriosis, for some reason, this tissue grows in other areas of the pelvis and sometimes even outside the pelvis entirely. (There are documented cases of endometriosis in the lining of the lungs and even in the brain.) The most common site for endometriosis is in the pelvic organs, on the pelvic side walls (which surround the internal organs in the pelvic cavity), and sometimes on the bowel.

Endometriosis is sometimes associated with infertility and pelvic pain, though not always. Since fibroids and endometriosis are often present in the same individuals at the same time, everything I say about fibroids often applies to endometriosis as well. Like fibroids, endometriosis is related to diet and blocked pelvic energy.

Endometriosis is the illness of competition.[5] It comes about when a woman's emotional needs are competing with her functioning in the outside world. When a woman feels that her innermost emotional needs are in direct conflict with what the world is demanding of her, endometriosis is one of the ways in which her body tries to draw her attention to the problem. Women are now part of the traditionally male world of competition and business. Many women do not get emotional support in their homes or personal lives. Others have abandoned the notion that they even have emotional requirements. A great many of the women I've seen who have endometriosis drive themselves relentlessly in the outer world, rarely resting, rarely tuning in to their innermost needs and deepest desires. It makes perfect sense that so many women would have this disease at this time in our history. One Jungian analyst has referred to endometriosis as "a blood sacrifice to the Goddess." It is our bodies trying not to let us forget our feminine nature, our need for self-nurturance, and our connection with other women.

Historically, endometriosis was called the "career woman's disease." Women who delayed childbearing were felt to be at greatest risk for it. In the recent past, many women with endometriosis were told that if they'd stay home and have babies, they would be okay. This is a controversial assertion, besides an offensive one, since some recent studies show that there is no difference in the incidence of endometriosis in women who have been pregnant and those who have not. Dr. David Redwine, an internationally known endometriosis expert, concludes that pregnancy offers no protection against endometriosis. What would protect against the disease would be business and personal environments that don't require a mental-emotional split. This revolution will be slow to come, so in the meantime each woman can work toward healing herself starting by understanding and listening to her body and its messages.

Symptoms

Endometriosis is classically associated with pelvic pain, abnormal menstrual cycles, and infertility. These symptoms vary a great deal from woman to woman. Some women with advanced endometriosis have never had any symptoms at all and don't even know that they have the disease until their doctor diagnoses it. Others, with only minimal endometriosis, may nonetheless have debilitating pelvic pain and cramps almost continuously. Most women are somewhere in between these two extremes. The most common area for endometriosis to occur is behind the uterus in the area between the uterus and rectum, known as the cul-de-sac of Douglas. Endometriosis in this area can cause painful intercourse, rectal pressure, and pain with bowel movements, especially before a period.

Diagnosis

Endometriosis of the pelvic cavity can be diagnosed definitively only via laparoscopy, though I often suspect it in women whose symptoms are consistent with endometriosis, such as a history of pelvic pain and intermenstrual spotting. In a few rare cases, it can be seen during a pelvic exam if endometrial lesions are present on the cervix, vagina, or vulva. Unfortunately, studies show that the average woman with endometriosis goes to about five doctors before the diagnosis is made because many other medical conditions, such as irritable bowel syndrome, mimic endometriosis.

Some authorities believe that you can find endometriosis in anyone if you look hard enough.[6] I agree with this. I've found endometriosis in a surprising number of completely asymptomatic women at the time of laparoscopic tubal ligation. Neither they nor I would have suspected it.

What I'd like to know is the incidence of endometriosis in women who have no problems. I believe that all women probably have embryonic cells in their pelvic cavities that could grow into endometrial tissue. But if all of us have the potential for endometriosis, why do some women develop symptoms while others do not? Since the medical authorities cannot tell us, the answers lie within the individual woman. It is up to her to decipher what her symptoms are trying to tell her.

Common Concerns

WHY DO SO MANY WOMEN HAVE ENDOMETRIOSIS? When I was in training, we didn't see nearly as much endometriosis as we're seeing now. There are a number of reasons for the perceived increase in the disease. First, with the advent of laparoscopy, we are diagnosing it more frequently. The patient is in and out of the hospital on the same day. The ease of looking into the pelvis without doing major surgery results in laparoscopy being offered to patients who have pelvic pain rather routinely.

Another factor in the apparent increase in incidence of endometriosis is that women today are delaying childbearing and having more menstrual cycles than in the past. When they do have children, they are having fewer of them. Since endometriosis is a hormone-dependent disorder, when the body has relatively high circulating estrogen levels without a break for pregnancy and nursing, this would favor its manifestation.

IS ENDOMETRIOSIS HEREDITARY? Endometriosis often runs in families, so there is some hereditary link. I've seen patients whose sisters and mothers all had it. Having a sister with endometriosis does not guarantee that you'll have it too, especially if you live your lives in different ways. The genetic potential for endometriosis does not have to manifest unless your environment and health habits promote it. The standard high-fat American diets and their effects contribute to endometriosis and are associated with families who have endometriosis. In my clinical experience, intake of dairy food is especially associated with exacerbated pain of endometriosis.

WILL ENDOMETRIOSIS INTERFERE WITH MY FERTILITY? Many endometriosis patients are fertile women whose main problem is pain. Endometriosis does not cause infertility, but it is felt to be a major contributing factor. Currently, 40 to 50 percent of women who have a laparoscopy to determine the cause of their problems with infertility are found to have endometriosis.[7] Many women with endometriosis have the massive pelvic scarring usually associated with infertility. Dr. David Redwine says, "Studying the disease among predominantly infertile women only serves to confuse the issue."[8] Whatever is causing the endometriosis symptoms may also be responsible for the infertility, but one doesn't cause the other.[9]

SO WHAT CAUSES ENDOMETRIOSIS? Medical theories about endometriosis abound, but no one really knows what it is and why so many women seem to have it now. The classic theory is that endometriosis results from retrograde menstruation, or menstruating backward, so that some of the menstrual blood and tissue that lines the uterus goes back up the fallopian tubes, then implants in the pelvic tissue and begins to grow.[10] Since retrograde menstruation probably occurs in every menstruating woman at some point, this doesn't explain why some women get the disease and others don't. Another theory is that pelvic tissues spontaneously convert to endometrial tissue, possibly due to irritation or hormonal activity.

It is not clear exactly what causes the pain associated with endometriosis. It is known that endometriosis is stimulated in part by the hormones of the menstrual cycle and that the pain is worse at ovulation and during the premenstrual and menstrual times of the cycle. Since endometrial lesions are the same as the tissue inside the uterus, it is understandable that when a woman bleeds with her menstrual cycle, her endometriosis implants bleed microscopically inside her body too. Some experts feel that the endometrial lesions secrete some kind of chemical that results in bleeding from surrounding capillaries in the peritoneum (the Saran Wrap–like lining of the pelvic cavity and pelvic organs where endometriosis is found). Over time, this monthly bleeding into the pelvic cavity is believed to be the cause of painful cysts and adhesions that tend to flare up under the right circumstances.

The theory that makes the most sense to me is that endometriosis is a congenital condition and is present at birth.[11] According to this theory, endometriosis arises from embryonic female genital tissue that never made it to the inside of the uterus during development.

This helps explain why endometriosis can run in families and why some girls have severe pelvic pain from endometriosis *as soon as* they start their periods. Yet in this theory all females have the capacity to develop endometriosis if embryonic cells in their pelvis get stimulated by the right set of circumstances.

Though most gynecologists have been taught that endometriosis is a progressive disease that gets worse over time, some studies, including Dr. Redwine's, show that endometriosis doesn't spread and won't recur if all of it is removed surgically. There are indications that the disease is static, that it does not spread, and does not get worse over time, though its appearance changes over time.

When performing laparoscopies to diagnose the cause of pelvic pain, many gynecologists miss the diagnosis of endometriosis in its early stages because they were taught to look only for the characteristic black "powder burn" (gunpowder) lesions. In fact, endometrial lesions come in a range of colors: clear, white, yellow, blue, and red. Many of these early lesions are very subtle and difficult to see without the proper equipment.[12]

The color of endometrial lesions may be related to blood leaking from nearby capillaries. Over time, the lesions progress from clear to black depending upon the amount of scarring present. The older the woman with endometriosis, the greater her chances of having "classic" endometriosis with black "powder burn" lesions and "chocolate" cysts of the ovaries. (Endometriosis in the ovaries can result in large ovarian cysts filled with old blood. When these are operated on, the contents of the cysts look just like chocolate syrup.)

The Neuroendocrine-Immune Connection

The intimate interactions between our thoughts, emotions, and immunity hold the key to interpreting the message that endometriosis has for the individual woman. Studies on the immune systems of women with symptomatic endometriosis show that these women often have antibodies against their own tissue, called autoantibodies. This means that at some deep level, the mind of their pelvis is rejecting aspects of itself.

The autoantibodies interfere with various processes of human reproduction, including sperm function, fertilization, and normal progression of pregnancy. Their presence may explain the association between infertility and endometriosis in those women who have both problems at the same time. Endometriosis has been clearly associated with decreased female egg fertilization, decreased success rates for in vitro fertilization ("test tube" fertilization), and increased miscarriages. The clinical experience of therapist Niravi Payne with women with infertility and endometriosis shows clearly that at an unconscious level, these women may have an ambivalence about becoming pregnant. Their minds may desire it, while their hearts aren't sure. The presence of these abnormal autoantibodies in patients with endometriosis holds the key to understanding many characteristics of the disease that scientists have been unable to explain when they have looked at it as a structural problem only, as if it were a tumor to be removed.[13]

Making antibodies against the body's own tissue is characteristic of other autoimmune diseases that stymie conventional medical science and that cannot be "cured" in the conventional sense. The immune system is highly sensitive, and our survival depends upon its ability to recognize and distinguish self from non-self. What can possibly be going on when the immune system carries out self-destruct orders? We can use the evidence that the immune system carries out the messages from our minds to help ourselves heal.

Treatment

Women with symptomatic endometriosis do best with a comprehensive treatment program that fully supports their immune systems while they remain open to finding out what they need to change about their lives. My patients have healed endometriosis symptoms through a variety of treatments. Most important, many of them have come to a greater understanding of what they need to learn for true healing, not just to mask their physical symptoms.

HORMONES. The most common treatment for endometriosis, once diagnosed, is hormonal therapy, in the form of birth control pills, synthetic progestin, danocrine sulfate, or most recently, the GnRH agonists (gonadotropin releasing hormones), such as Synarel and Lupron. These drugs act on the pituitary gland to make a woman temporarily menopausal, thereby allowing the endometriosis to regress by stopping its cyclic hormonal stimulation.

All of these hormonal therapies change the amount of estrogen and other hormones in the system, so that endometriosis is not activated. When hormone levels are decreased, symptoms often disappear and the disease itself becomes inactive. Danazol and the GnRH agonists are also used to decrease the amount of endometriosis prior to surgery—in some cases, so that surgical removal is easier. The problem with these approaches is that they don't really cure the disease; they simply shut down the hormonal stimulation of it for a while. In addition, some women do not tolerate well the side effects of these treatments. Danocrine sulfate (Danazol) is expensive—it costs about a dollar a dose—and it can have masculinizing side effects, such as hair growth and voice deepening. Most women gain some weight while they are on it. GnRH agonist therapy results in hot flashes, thinning of the vaginal tissue, and bone loss. Yet other women badly need these hormonal treatments as a respite from pain, even though the pain often recurs once the drug is discontinued.

I recently saw a patient who had been on Synarel (a GnRH agonist) all summer. "It was so wonderful to go camping, water skiing, and hang gliding and not have to worry about the pain," she told me. "I felt just wonderful. I know I can't stay on it forever, but I sure felt great." She had been off it for two weeks when I saw her, and her pain was beginning to recur. As we talked about her options, she said that when she was having the pain before she went on the drug, she would often get complete pain relief from a massage. She was surprised by that, but she felt that massage was too expensive ($30 to $45, depending on the therapist) and that dietary change was too difficult due to her schedule. Yet Synarel costs $300 per month.[14] Once she thought it all through, she decided to try to change her schedule to eat better, and she is now willing to try a few nondrug approaches for a trial period of three months. After that, if she has no relief, she knows that surgery is an option.

Even though the menopausal symptoms associated with GnRH agonists appear to be reversible once the drug is stopped, this type of therapy inherently makes me nervous. I prescribe it only in select cases, when the patient has a lifestyle that isn't amenable to alternatives. Usually, this means a very stressful job, long work hours, a lot of travel, almost no time to herself, and lack of desire or ability to change her career. Using drugs in this type of situation makes it easier for the woman to continue activities that may nonetheless be harming her at some level. I worry about her using the medication, but I also trust her process, knowing that she will learn something from whatever option she chooses. I also trust that what brought her to me has also opened her to learning about her body. She knows that she can come back to try some other things when and if it feels appropriate.

Based on the clinical experience of Dr. John Lee, an expert on the clinical uses of natural progesterone, I have recently begun using natural progesterone for some of my patients with endometriosis (see Chapter 5). Natural progesterone helps counteract endometriosis by decreasing the effects of estrogen on the endometrial lesions. Natural progesterone is free from side effects and is very well tolerated. I recommend one two-ounce jar of ProGest cream per month, applied daily to soft areas of the skin, such as the face, neck, and abdomen, alternating the sites. Use it on days ten to twenty-eight of each cycle, approximately. Natural progesterone capsules taken orally are another choice; the usual dosage is 50 to 200 mg. per day, taken on days ten to twenty-eight of each cycle.

SURGERY. Many women with severe endometriosis, having tried hormones and pain medication for years, often end up at very young ages with complete hysterectomies, including removal of their ovaries. Though this is often the women's choice at the time, many of them later learned that there were alternatives to this aggressive surgical approach.

More conservative surgery that removes only the endometriosis and preserves the pelvic organs can be very helpful. More and more gynecologists are skilled at this pelviscopic surgery and have learned how to remove endometriosis without missing any lesions. If any endometriosis is left behind after this conservative surgery, the pain is likely to recur. Pelviscopic surgery, done correctly, has a pain recurrence rate of only about ten percent. In these women, the pain is frequently associated not with endometriosis but with fibroids, adhesions, or adenomyosis (see Chapter 5). A woman who intends to undergo surgery for endometrial pain must go to someone who is skilled in this form of treatment.

ENERGY MEDICINE. Anything that improves immune system functioning and increases the flow of energy in the body is apt to help endometriosis. Ask yourself the following questions and answer them honestly:

- What are your emotional needs?
- What would you like to see happen in your job or your life that would nourish you fully?
- Are you caught up in competition of any sort in your life? Are you willing to make changes?
- Are you getting enough rest?
- Do you believe that you have the power to change the conditions of your life?

Apply a castor oil pack to your lower abdomen at least three times per week for one hour each time. (See the Appendix for instructions.) Pay attention to all thoughts, images, and feelings that arise. Consider a course of acupuncture with Chinese herbs. (See Chapter 5.) Get a total body massage at least once every other week for two months. What did you notice after the massage?

DIETARY CHANGE. Endometriosis is an estrogen-sensitive disease; excessive fat intake stimulates excess estrogen production in the body, which stimulates endometriosis. Thus, endometriosis symptoms often disappear completely or lessen dramatically when women follow a low-fat, high-fiber diet free of all dairy products (even low-fat dairy products). If you wish to try this, eliminate all dairy for at least one month.

One of my patients had had endometriosis for many years. She had unsuccessfully used danocrine sulfate and surgical treatments. But after she eliminated dairy products from her diet, she became free of endometriosis symptoms and has remained so for ten years. Recently, she conceived her first child without difficulty, even though another doctor told her that she probably wouldn't be able to get pregnant.

Take a good multivitamin-mineral supplement that is rich in the B complex and magnesium (about 50 mg. of each of the B vitamins and 400 to 800 mg. of magnesium).

Women's Stories

DORIS: LEARNING FROM ENDOMETRIOSIS. Doris was forty-one when she first came to see me. She was a highly successful professional who spent lots of time traveling and working but had little time for herself and her personal, emotional needs. She had heavy periods that got worse at night and sometimes would soak through the sheets. She complained of fluid retention, bloating, and severe menstrual cramps. Her uterus was enlarged to ten-to-twelve-week-pregnancy size from fibroids. She had a history of infertility, several miscarriages, and an abortion. A laparoscopy by another physician had confirmed the presence of endometriosis as well as fibroids, and he felt that these were associated with her miscarriages. Her gynecologist had suggested a hysterectomy because he said that her periods would continue to be difficult and that she would eventually end up with the surgery anyway. She was not happy with this diagnosis, however, and came to see me about her alternatives.

When I first saw her, she had a great deal of tenderness behind her uterus, which is very common in women with endometriosis. I asked her questions about her lifestyle, diet, previous miscarriages, abortion, exercise, and stress levels. I agreed that surgery was not something we needed to consider right then and suggested several alternative treatments. Among them were eliminating dairy products from her diet, applying castor oil packs to her lower abdomen, taking vitamin supplements, and reading about perfectionism, addiction, and whole foods. From what Doris had told me about herself, I felt that she needed to heal her feelings about her miscarriages and her abortion. She decided to follow my suggestions. To unlock her feelings about her fertility, she decided to write letters to the unborn potential beings who had been in her body. As she wrote me later, "Obviously they were still there in some form in my mind and had taken form as fibroids and maybe endometriosis in my body. The most incredible experience occurred after I wrote the letters. I had been remembering my dreams with great regularity through visualization techniques. One night in a dream, I was fully aware of my body, and I dreamed that thousands of white doves were flying out of my uterus. An unbelievable feeling of lightness came over me, and I awoke crying with joy."

Three months after Doris's dream experience, I examined her and found that many of her fibroids were gone and so was all of her uterine tenderness. The fibroids seemed to have solidified into a smooth mass that was definitely smaller than it had been at the time of her earlier examination. Doris has found that when she takes care of herself and follows her diet, gets exercise, and does some things just for herself, she feels fine and has no pelvic symptoms of any kind. Though her fibroids have not disappeared entirely, they haven't grown for years. She now has no tenderness on examination, a testimony to the fact that her endometriosis is very inactive.

Doris used the wisdom of her body to heal some very painful experiences about which she had not allowed herself to grieve. She was willing to risk completely changing the way she saw herself in the world, a change that often needs to be made if women are to heal at the deepest level. This often involves examining with microscopic honesty how we really feel about being female. It also may involve cutting way back on our worldly activities and creating a healthful balance between our inner and outer selves.

Fibroid Tumors

Fibroids are benign tumors of the uterus. They grow in various locations on and within the uterine wall itself or in the uterine cavity. (See Figure 7.) Standard medical practice to gauge the size of a fibroid is to compare the uterine size of a fibroid with the size of the uterus if it contained a fetus of that size. Thus, a woman will be told that she has a fourteen-week-size fibroid, if her uterus is as big as it would be if she were fourteen weeks pregnant. Fibroids are made from hard, white, gristly tissue that has a whorllike pattern. They are present in 20 to 50 percent of all women. One of my patients, who watched her fibroid removal via a mirror, later said,

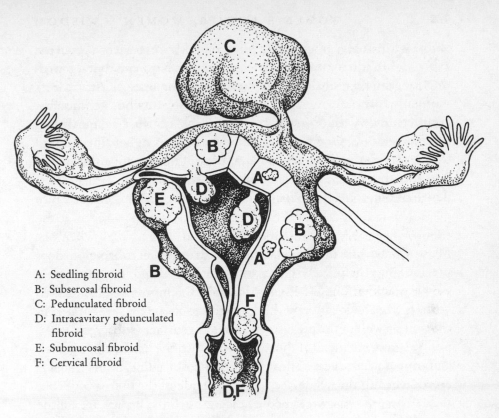

A: Seedling fibroid
B: Subserosal fibroid
C: Pedunculated fibroid
D: Intracavitary pedunculated
   fibroid
E: Submucosal fibroid
F: Cervical fibroid

FIGURE 7: FIBROID DIAGRAM

"The appearance of the fibroid surprised me. I expected it to be messy looking. A fibroid looks like a piece of high density polyethylene plastic, the stuff cutting boards are made of."

Fibroids are responsible for as many as 33 percent of all gynecological hospital admissions, and they are the number-one reason for hysterectomy in this country.[15] They are three to nine times more common in black women than Caucasian. Many women with fibroids are unaware that they have them until they are discovered during a routine pelvic examination. No one knows, from a conventional medical standpoint, what causes fibroids.

Caroline Myss teaches that fibroid tumors represent our creativity that was never birthed, including "fantasy" images of ourselves that have never seen the light of day and creative secrets of our other "selves." Fibroids also result when we are flowing life energy into dead ends, such as jobs or relationships that we have outgrown. I ask women with fibroids to meditate on their relationships with other people and how they express their creativity. Fibroids are often associated with conflicts about creativity, reproduction, and relationships.[16] In our rapidly changing culture, where women's roles are in rapid flux, it is quite obvious to me that conflicts about childrearing are a cultural, not just an individual phenomenon. One of my patients, after looking at her fibroid, said that it was easy to see a fibroid as a form of hard, implacable anger. The fact that so many women have these growths is perhaps evidence of our collective blocked creative energy in this culture.

Symptoms

Most women do not have symptoms from their fibroids. These uterine growths usually come to a woman's attention on routine pelvic examination. Whether a fibroid is symptomatic has to do with its size and location within the uterus. Those that are located in the muscle wall of the uterus just under the surface (subserosal) may not be symptomatic. But those growing into the uterine lining itself (submucosal) often cause heavy or irregular bleeding. Some fibroids are attached to the inside or even the outside of the uterus by a thin stalk. These are known as pedunculated fibroids. If they are on the outside of the uterus, they are sometimes confused with ovarian tumors. I've had two patients who "delivered" pedunculated six-centimeter fibroids through the cervical opening. I simply removed these fibroids by suturing and then severing the stalk. Neither of these women had any further problems.

Women who have both fibroids and endometriosis may experience menstrual cramps, pelvic pain, or both. Most fibroids can be treated conservatively by letting them be and having an examination every six months or so to monitor their growth.

BLEEDING.   Some women with fibroids have extremely heavy periods, resulting in anemia, fatigue, and even an inability to leave the house during the heaviest days. If the fibroids are growing quickly, if a woman's hormones are in flux (which is common around the time of the menopause), or if she's been under a great deal of stress, she can even develop hemorrhaging from uterine fibroids. Some women grow so accustomed to their large monthly blood loss that they don't even realize how a "normal" flow would feel.

Fibroid tumors can cause a lot of bleeding because the uterus is endowed with a very rich blood supply. If the fibroid is submucosal, located just under the uterine lining, the body has an especially difficult time with the usual mechanism that stops menstrual flow. Menstrual flow is stopped, in part, by muscular contraction of the uterus. Fibroids may interfere with this mechanism. An endometrial biopsy (taking a sample of tissue from inside the uterus) or sometimes a D&C is necessary in cases of abnormal bleeding to be certain that the bleeding is caused by fibroids and not cancer. This is especially true for those women who have bleeding at irregular intervals throughout the month.

FIBROID DEGENERATION. A fibroid may start to degenerate, following its rapid growth. This can happen, for instance, during a particularly stressful or emotionally demanding time, during pregnancy, or during the year or so before menopause. Fibroid degeneration can occur when the fibroid outgrows its blood supply. When this happens, the center of the fibroid is deprived of oxygen from the blood, and the nerves deep inside this tissue register a lack of oxygen as pain, in the same way that frostbitten toes do. The pain can be a nuisance but is not life-threatening. The degeneration in the center of the fibroid often causes some shrinkage in fibroid size, and on occasion a fibroid degenerates completely and disappears. Whether the fibroid shrinks or disappears, the pain usually goes away after a week or so as the nerves adjust.

PELVIC PRESSURE AND URINARY FREQUENCY. Sometimes the position of a fibroid causes symptoms because the fibroid pushes into another organ, such as the rectum or the bladder. Pressure or a sense of fullness in the rectum, lower back, or abdomen may result. If the fibroid is in the front of the uterus and relatively low, the pressure on the bladder can decrease the bladder's ability to hold urine, resulting in urinary frequency, or having to void in frequent small amounts. These symptoms are annoying but are not harmful to the body in general. I've never seen an organ contiguous to a benign fibroid that was harmed by the fibroid. An occasional very large fibroid can partially block the ureter (the tube going from the kidney to the bladder) when a woman is lying down. Neither urologists nor gynecologists know for certain whether this situation can eventually cause kidney problems. Most women with fibroids large enough to cause ureteral pressure prefer surgery. Several of my patients, however, are doing very well without surgery, and their kidneys are fine. One of these women, who has had a very large fibroid uterus for at least ten years, and whose ureter has occasionally shown some dilatation from fibroids, has just started to go through menopause. Her fibroids are shrinking rapidly now.

Common Concerns

WHAT IF I HAVE A FIBROID? When I feel fibroids on a patient for the first time, I usually get a pelvic ultrasound to measure them and to check out the status of the ovaries. Sometimes it's impossible on a pelvic exam to tell the difference between an ovarian growth and a fibroid on the uterus.

CAN FIBROIDS BE CANCEROUS? Fibroids are almost never cancerous (less than one in a thousand turn into uterine sarcomas, a very rare type of cancer of the uterine muscle. The only way to tell for sure, however, is to take them out and look at them under the microscope.) Since the mortality rate for hysterectomy itself is one in a thousand, the risk of surgery is actually greater than the risk of the fibroid being malignant.

The most common problem with fibroids is their tendency to grow and to cause bleeding. But as with many women I've worked with, if the underlying energy patterns, life questions, conflicts, and emotional issues associated with the fibroids are addressed and changed, the fibroids usually do not grow or cause problems.

ARE FIBROIDS GENETIC? Fibroids can run in families. One of my fibroid patients told me that every female in her family for three generations had fibroids. She is planning to be the first woman in her tribe to get to menopause with her uterus intact. She has changed her diet and now is completely free from symptoms.

Just as in a strong family history of alcoholism, in a strong family history of fibroids the individual woman is "up against" a family belief system, from which it is very difficult to break free. I once read an article about familial ovarian cancer entitled "My Mother, My Cells," in which the author articulated her difficulty with "inheriting" a tendency toward a disease that terrified her and over which she felt she had no control.

In this country, we tend to think of a genetic predisposition as an inevitable "sentence" that we *will* get the disease. However, environmental factors play a huge role in whether a disease ever gets expressed. For example, some individuals with the gene for cystic fibrosis show virtually no signs of the disease and live well into their fifties. Some women with very strong family histories of breast cancer never get the disease.

Women who have strong family histories of fibroids, ovarian cysts, or endometriosis have developed these conditions themselves but have healed from them. One patient summarized a necessary part of this healing when she said, "I've finally realized that I am not my mother. I don't have to live out her life in my body." In families in which there is genetic disease, we should study those members who *don't* get the disease. Most likely they are the individuals who broke the family mold, the ones who did not live out family expectations on a cellular or other level.

WILL MY FIBROIDS INTERFERE WITH PREGNANCY? During pregnancy, hormone levels are very high and preexisting fibroids can grow rapidly. If they begin to degenerate, fibroids can sometimes cause uterine contractions that can result in premature delivery. This doesn't happen with all fibroids, however. I've seen women with large fourteen-week-size fibroids get pregnant, carry to term, and go through normal labor and delivery without *any* problem.

One twenty-nine-year-old woman came to me already twelve weeks pregnant with a large fibroid in the posterior portion of her uterus. The pregnancy had been unplanned, but she was thrilled about it. Her doctor had told her to have an abortion and then have the fibroid removed before conceiving again. He told her that the fibroid would probably cause the early delivery of a baby who would be so premature that it wouldn't live. She was very upset about her dilemma and needed a physician who was willing to go along with the pregnancy, knowing that there might be a problem *while being open to the possibility* that all could go well. Her pregnancy proceeded normally, going to full term without pain, bleeding, or premature labor. She delivered a seven-pound, three-ounce girl after an eight-hour labor. Her fibroid had shrunk to eight weeks' size, by the time of her six-week postpartum checkup.

Fibroids can result in miscarriage or even infertility, particularly if they've distorted the uterine cavity enough. Whether there are problems seems to depend on the location of the fibroid within the uterus and how close it is to the developing baby and placenta. An ultrasound or hysterosalpingogram (an X-ray study in which dye is injected into the uterus and tubes) can give you some idea of fibroid location before pregnancy, as can an MRI (Magnetic Resonance Imaging).

Some pregnant women have fibroids that start degenerating. They end up in the hospital to be watched closely while they rest in bed on pain medication. Generally, fibroids don't hurt the developing baby unless they cause so much uterine irritability that the uterus starts contracting and premature labor results. There are no guarantees against developing problems with fibroids during pregnancy because the entire uterus grows, including the fibroid wall. The farther away from the uterine cavity the fibroid is located, the less likely that a woman will have problems. Some doctors are willing to take a wait-and-see attitude about fibroids and pregnancy, suggesting that a woman try to get pregnant and see what happens. Others will suggest that she have the fibroids removed before attempting pregnancy.

WILL THE FIBROIDS GROW? WILL THEY GO AWAY? Many women with fibroids are told that hysterectomy should be performed when their fibroids are relatively small so that a more risky and complicated hysterectomy in the future, should the fibroids grow, will not be necessary. Studies have shown that there is little or no justification for this.[17] Fibroids do grow sometimes but not always. They tend to grow quite briskly during the years just before menopause, when hormonal levels fluctuate widely, then shrink dramatically after menopause. One of my perimenopausal or "almost menopausal" patients, age forty-nine, whom I've followed for more than ten years, can easily feel her fibroids through her abdominal wall by pressing down with her fingers. She says that her fibroids grow up to her belly button just before her period and shrink down to just above her pubic bone within three days after her period is over! Fibroids often change size during each menstrual cycle, reaching their peak during ovulation and just before the menstrual period begins. They can also grow during periods of stress. Fibroids can be followed by a physician or other qualified health care provider with an exam every six months or so. There's no reason to rush into surgery, unless you have repeated episodes of severe bleeding that cannot be controlled with hormonal treatments or other measures.

Sometimes fibroids go away completely. I recently met a religious woman who had been scheduled for hysterectomy because of fibroids. She prayed about them daily. Six weeks later, when she went back to her doctor, the fibroids were gone and she didn't require the surgery.

One of my patients, a forty-three-year-old musician and sound healer named Persis, first came to see me with a fibroid the size of a four-to-five-month pregnancy. After two years of a strict diet, reflective inner work, massages, and therapeutic sound,[18] her very large fibroid uterus returned almost back to normal. I rarely see fibroids shrink as much as hers did. This shrinkage was not because of menopause. She is still having normal periods. Here is her story.

"In the summer of 1988, I was diagnosed with endometriosis and a grapefruit-size fibroid tumor. The preceding years had been filled with increasingly excruciating pain that left me almost blacking out while driving. I had gotten used to being in pain for two weeks, then recovering from the exhaustion in the next two weeks, and had become terrified of getting my period.

"The doctor I was seeing at the time told me about all the alternatives for correcting the problem. His favorite was hysterectomy—'At your age you don't need it anyway,' he said. Then there was hormone therapy to stop the periods for one to two years: 'Your voice will drop, and you will lose your sexual desire.' And the last offer he made was that I could continue with the pain and bleeding until menopause.

"Since I wanted to keep my body whole, didn't particularly like the idea of giving up my womanhood to hormone therapy, and couldn't tolerate the pain, I looked for other treatment. I made a commitment to my life. I accepted the responsibility for taking care of myself. I accepted the loving help of others. I began a very strict regimen of macrobiotic diet, sitz baths, exercise, and meditation. Looking back, I don't know how I fit all that into my busy life. I do know that I am a changed person.

"I also began gently to search out the reasons behind my 'woman's troubles.' I accepted my codependent nature and began opening up to the pain of my childhood and young adulthood. The pain in my belly was a culmination of a lifetime of pains. I knew just cutting it out wouldn't 'fix' all the other pains in my life.

"I now have little pain and feel extraordinarily well. I am and always will be in process throughout my life. Through meditation and sound healing on myself, I have renewed my inner faith. I accept my life and my ability to heal myself as well as to help others heal. As I do for others, I do for myself."

IF I HAVE SURGERY, WILL THE FIBROIDS GROW BACK? The answer to this question must be individualized. In general, a woman who is within five years of menopause when she has her fibroids removed is not likely to have them grow back, because her estrogen levels will be decreasing naturally. Sometimes there are many tiny fibroids in the uterine wall. It can be difficult to remove all of them at the time of surgery. If the underlying energy pattern, emotional issues, or hormonal levels associated with the fibroids haven't changed, these so-called "seedling" fibroids can start to grow. Women who change their diets dramatically decrease the likelihood that the fibroids will return. Most of my patients' fibroids do not grow back or worsen. I believe that this is because the type of woman who comes to me is ready to do the hard work of really looking at the message behind the problem. I recommend dietary change, bodywork, and other alternative methods, even for those women who choose surgery as their treatment. Surgery alone will not change the fundamental pattern in their bodies that encouraged the fibroids to grow. It is vital to listen to what our bodies are trying to teach us.

Treatment

At no point do I make dictatorial treatment recommendations about what any one of my patients should do with her uterus. There is no right and wrong. Instead, I offer them ways to think about their uterus, ovaries, and body, so that when they need to make a decision about hormones, drugs, or surgery, they'll know what their personal truth is regarding those organs. More treatments for fibroids are now available than ever before. Once a woman has gathered the facts about treatment choices, she can tune into her own inner guidance to decide what treatment choice is the best for her.

For many women, just knowing that they have a choice in the matter is a huge relief. Some women interpret surgery, for example, as further abuse, when they have not freely chosen to undergo it. Incest survivors sometimes tell me that the very thought of an invasive procedure in their body, particularly of a gynecological nature, feels just like rape. Obviously, alternative modes of treatment should be tried in these cases, rather than allow the abuse cycle to once again be ignited.

The following cases illustrate different treatment approaches to problems in the uterus. These cases show that there is no one right way to treat uterine problems. Each of these women needed help for fairly straightforward and common symptoms, and each chose a different treatment. Only one woman wanted a hysterectomy. Each woman was able to arrange treatment that respected her individual choice. Medical technology, when consciously used in an individualized treatment, can be a major aid in healing women's lives. To claim that hysterectomy is always the wrong or inferior choice is as dualistic and harmful as claiming that all natural remedies are quackery. I do not address the specific psychological and emotional issues connected with "blocked energy in the pelvis" for any of these cases. Not all women are open or ready to explore their deep issues, and I respect their choice to wait for the right time.

CONSERVATIVE: WATCH AND WAIT. If a woman's fibroids aren't causing her any problems, I recommend a pelvic exam every six months to a year, depending upon her situation. I also order a sonogram (ultrasound) initially to be sure that I'm dealing with a fibroid and not an ovarian cyst or tumor. Sonograms can be ordered to measure fibroid size and check ovaries. Conservative treatment is sometimes called "benign neglect" or the "tincture of time." Sometimes it's the best therapy.

HYSTERECTOMY.   Hysterectomy is probably the option most commonly offered to American women who have fibroids. This option is often chosen in the following situations: When a woman has been bleeding for months or even years, is anemic from the blood loss, has an abdomen that looks pregnant, can't leave home for fear of bleeding through her clothes, and has urinary frequency from a fibroid pushing on her bladder.

A hysterectomy can improve the quality of a woman's life, and I do perform them. If a woman has surgery for which she isn't really ready, without adequately exploring the alternatives, however, the results can be devastating. Over the years, I've come to see that women who give their options a great deal of consideration before deciding on surgery are much happier with the outcome. (On how to prepare for surgery and the recovery process, see Chapter 16.) Unfortunately, there's often a tendency in medicine to create a crisis situation and rush in. Sometimes a woman who has had a single frightening episode of bleeding with a fibroid will be told to have a hysterectomy as soon as possible. Because of her fear and the sense of being pushed by her doctor or family, she will often go along, when she could have waited. The women who often regret their decisions later, I believe, are the ones who did not feel that they had any choice except surgery, usually hysterectomy. Before embarking upon any course of treatment, a woman should allow herself the time to gather all necessary information and weigh all her options.

Fran, a teacher with one daughter, came to see me when she was forty-two. Over the previous six months, she had developed bleeding between periods, increasing cramps, and some pain during intercourse. When I examined her, I found that she had a fibroid the size of a large grapefruit (about 11 centimeters in diameter). I had known Fran for many years before this, and I had delivered her daughter. She traveled to many different schools during the course of her teaching day and had always found it difficult to maintain a healthy diet. She was significantly overweight and married to a man who hated his job and was somewhat depressed. Given her life situation, her treatment choice was hysterectomy with preservation of her ovaries. She knew that although I could remove the fibroid and leave the uterus intact, this would not guarantee that she'd be rid of her cramps and irregular bleeding.

Fran wasn't interested in taking the time to pursue alternative treatment modes; nor was she interested in learning about what her fibroids might be saying to her. The idea of being free from periods, cramps, and the fear of pregnancy was very appealing to her. She had her surgery without complications and returned to her normal routine within one month. She has never had second thoughts or regrets. Fran is a good example of a woman who knew she had options and who was very clear about her choice.

Before I do a hysterectomy or any other surgery, I always point out that the removal of the organ may change the woman's experience of her body. Much more research needs to be done about the effects of hysterectomy on women's physical, emotional, and psychological health and body image.

• *Sexual Response.* In studies conducted in the United Kingdom, 33 to 46 percent of women report a decreased sexual response after a hysterectomy-oophorectomy (removal of the uterus and the ovaries).[19] Most establishment doctors regard this decreased sexual response as psychogenic, or "all in her head." The psychogenic theory is based on the patriarchal assumption that a woman's ovaries, cervix, and uterus have little connection with her libido and are not essential to her sexual gratification. Such patriarchal thinking likes to divorce the body from the mind and feels that the brain is the source of our primary inclinations, thoughts, and feelings. Since this thinking denigrates the female body and our organs, it is not surprising that it views the libido as primarily psychic in origin. As most women know, the mind and the body are a unity. Quite simply, if a woman feels positively connected to her sexual organs, then their removal will affect her sex life.

We now know that there is a physiological basis for decreased sexual response in *some* women following hysterectomy-oophorectomy. (A percentage of women actually report *increased* sexual response after hysterectomy.) Researchers know that the androgenic hormone loss associated with the removal of the ovaries is a factor in loss of libido following surgery.

Even if the ovaries are left intact, some women experience orgasm differently after hysterectomy, probably because the cervix and uterus act as a trigger-point for orgasm. These women feel the deep, rhythmic contractions of the uterus as a very satisfying part of orgasm. Once the uterus is gone, they sometimes experience the loss as a change, an actual decrease in orgasmic depth. Women who experience orgasm mainly through clitoral stimulation may not have this same experience.

On the other hand, for women who have experienced pain with intercourse for years or who have had pelvic pain from uterine or ovarian problems, a hysterectomy can greatly enhance the quality of their sexual experience and the overall quality of their life.

• *Menopause.* If the uterus is removed and the ovaries remain, the blood supply to the ovaries will be altered. This may result in an earlier menopause. In one study this occurred in about 50 percent of the sample.[20] (Many women report hot flashes for several months following hysterectomy, even when the ovaries are left in place. The same thing can happen after removal of an ovary alone, with no other surgery. It sometimes takes a while for an ovary to "recover" function post-op or for one ovary to take over the function of two.) There is some evidence that women who have had hysterectomies have an earlier onset of osteoporosis than other women, even when the ovaries are left in.

• *Urinary Problems.* Women who have had hysterectomies are more likely to develop urinary stress incontinence later in life. The reason for this is that the nerves innervating the bladder are very close to the uterus. Some of the nerve fibers may be damaged during hysterectomy.[21]

• *Heart Disease.* Some studies have shown an adverse cardiovascular effect from ovarian removal prior to a woman's natural menopause (average age of menopause is fifty-two). Since the ovaries continue to contribute hormones even after menopause, it is possible that there are adverse effects from ovarian removal even after menopause.[22]

MYOMECTOMY (SURGICAL REMOVAL OF FIBROIDS). Myomectomy is a surgical procedure in which the fibroid tumors are
removed, but the uterus is repaired and left in place. Advances in
surgical techniques over the past ten years have made this a very nice
option for women who want to keep their pelvic organs intact or
have children.

Many of my patients elect to have myomectomies even after they
eliminate all of their symptoms with dietary changes. The presence
of the fibroid may still cause an enlarged abdomen that affects how
they look and feel about themselves.

Gloria was forty-five when she first came to see me. She had had
two children, and her husband had had a vasectomy. Gloria had a
large fibroid uterus that was pressing on her bladder, causing
urinary frequency that kept her up at night. Her periods were
regular, and she had no pain. Her gynecologist had recommended a
hysterectomy, but this choice felt entirely too drastic to her. Instead,
she opted for a myomectomy. Her gynecologist wouldn't do this
procedure "because of her age," an ageist attitude on his part. Like
many conventionally trained gynecologists, this one felt that
Gloria's uterus was useless since she was over forty and didn't want
more children. The myomectomy that Gloria ultimately had
completely relieved her urinary symptoms, and she now sleeps
through the night. She is very glad to have kept her uterus.

When the position or size of a fibroid makes childbearing an
issue, myomectomy is a good choice. Before they undergo
myomectomy, many women are told that once they are in surgery
the surgeon may find it necessary to turn the procedure into a
hysterectomy. I have not seen a case in which this was necessary,
even though I do deal with a healthy patient population and work
with other skilled gynecological surgeons. When I see patients from
out of state who require that the surgery preserve the uterus and
ovaries, I often refer them to doctors who have specialty training in
infertility surgery. This type of surgery focuses on repairing the
pelvis, not on removing organs. The surgeons who are best at this
are those who are highly trained and skilled, who love to do surgery
and get a great deal of satisfaction from fixing and repairing pelvic
organs.

HORMONE THERAPY: SYNTHETIC PROGESTIN OR NATURAL PROGESTERONE. To women whose primary symptom is bleeding, I often offer synthetic progestin hormone or natural progesterone as a treatment, to keep the lining of the uterus from building up too much. In many cases this therapy works very well to control bleeding and is much more benign than major abdominal surgery. Progesterone or progestin is an option for women who are unable to change their diets or whose symptoms weren't alleviated by dietary changes. Some women become depressed while they are on synthetic progestin; others feel bloated or premenstrual or get headaches. The way I prescribe this hormone varies with the patient. Since each woman's life situation is different, her medical treatment needs to be individualized.

GNRH AGONISTS. GnRH agonists (gonadotropin releasing hormones) such as Lupron and Synarel are synthetic hormones that cause the pituitary gland to shut down the function of the ovaries. After about one month on these drugs, a woman's body becomes artificially menopausal. Her estrogen levels fall very low, and her periods cease. The cyclic stimulation of her fibroid tissue ceases, and in most cases the fibroids shrink in size. GnRH agonists are currently being used in select cases to shrink fibroids before surgery or to shrink them enough so that surgery is not necessary. Some physicians use these drugs to keep a woman's fibroids asymptomatic until she reaches menopausal age, at which point the fibroids naturally shrink. In this way, she can avoid surgery. It takes about three months to get the maximum effect from these drugs, but not everyone gets the same result because not all fibroids are created equal.[23]

As I mentioned earlier, GnRH agonists are very expensive—about $300 per month—and they are not recommended for use longer than six months. Once use of the drug is stopped, the fibroids grow back quite rapidly unless a woman became naturally menopausal during the time she was on the drug.

Many of my patients are understandably hesitant to use such synthetic hormones because they are relatively new. Too many of them remember that diethylstilbestrol (DES) was enthusiastically used several decades ago to prevent miscarriage. The drug was subsequently linked to certain rare vaginal cancers and other genital tract abnormalities in some of the female (and even male) offspring of the women who used it. The drug companies that manufacture synthetic hormones have heavily infiltrated the OB/GYN establishment with lectures and information about this form of treatment. I do occasionally recommend GnRH treatment but with caution and only in selected women.

ENDOMETRIAL ABLATION VIA HYSTEROSCOPY OR HYSTER-OSCOPY AND ENDOMETRIAL ABLATION. Christine had heavy periods for years—she had to use two super tampons at a time, as well as a pad. Sometimes these needed to be changed every half hour during day two of her period, making it very difficult for her to travel or even leave the house to grocery shop. The minimal dietary changes she made had not worked. Further testing revealed that she had multiple, very small fibroids in the uterine wall.

Christine very much wanted to avoid hysterectomy, so we tried synthetic progestin therapy for the last two weeks of each month for three months.[24] Even though this treatment almost always decreases bleeding, it didn't work in her case. A D&C also failed to alleviate her bleeding. I referred her to a physician who performs a procedure called endometrial ablation using a hysteroscope. Hysteroscopy is a surgical technique in which the lining of the uterus can be visualized and operated on by passing a scope into the cervix from the vagina. Submucosal fibroids can sometimes be removed this way by surgeons skilled in this technique. This procedure, done under anesthesia in the operating room, cauterizes and obliterates the endometrial lining—the part of the uterus that bleeds every month. When it works, menstrual periods cease or become very light. For Christine, the procedure worked beautifully. Instead of recuperating for a month from the removal of her uterus, she went into the hospital the day of her surgery and left the next. Though this type of surgery isn't appropriate for everyone, it is a great option for some. It cannot be done in some cases depending upon the position of the fibroids.[25]

AFTER MENOPAUSE: NATURE'S HORMONAL TREATMENT. Fibroids often shrink dramatically once a woman reaches menopause
(usually between fifty and fifty-two). Women with fibroids
frequently experience symptoms only when they are in their mid-
to late-forties, the age when hysterectomy is most often performed.
If a woman prefers it, hysterectomy can be avoided by keeping the
fibroids manageable until they naturally shrink during menopause.
This can be accomplished by a combination of dietary change,
castor oil packs, progestin therapy, and stress reduction.

Bea, a single teacher with no children, first came to see me in 1984
with a fibroid uterus and a history of heavy bleeding for twelve to
eighteen hours each menstrual cycle. Because of anemia from the
blood loss, she was taking iron. Her fibroid was submucosal, the
type that impinges on the endometrial lining and is often associated
with heavy bleeding. She had started a macrobiotic healing diet but
continued to bleed rather heavily each month. She took iron,
maintaining a blood count that was slightly but not seriously low.
When I first saw her, her uterus had been twelve-to-fourteen-week
size. Within six months it was down to an eight-to-ten-week size,
which I attributed to her diet. Several months after starting the diet,
she began weekly shiatsu massage treatments. She feels that the
shiatsu was more beneficial than the diet.[26] Over the next eight
years, depending on how well she was following her diet, Bea's
uterine size varied from ten-week to twenty-week size, which
occurred just before menopause. I repeatedly reminded Bea that
myomectomy and hysterectomy were options she could choose at
any time, but she was simply not comfortable about having surgery.
During the three to four years just prior to her menopause, a time
when estrogen levels swing up and down in an irregular fashion,
Bea required progestin therapy to control her heavy bleeding.
Occasionally, her bleeding was so heavy that it frightened her
family. Despite that, she avoided surgery and gradually entered
menopause. She now finds that the fibroid is shrinking quite
rapidly—from twenty-week size down to fourteen-week size in
only one week! Throughout the decade that I followed Bea, she
stayed with her dietary approach and remained firm in her decision
to avoid surgery.[27] She is now moving into menopause and grieving
the loss of her periods.

After menopause, any hormone replacement therapy may theoretically cause a woman's fibroids to grow again, but the low levels of hormones used in such therapy generally do not cause problems.

DIETARY CHANGE. Dietary change is the mainstay of my treatment approach for women interested in alternatives to drugs and surgery. Since the uterus (like fibroids and endometriosis) is estrogen-sensitive, anything that changes circulating estrogen levels can affect it. There is ample evidence that a diet high in fat and low in fiber can increase circulating estrogens. The standard American diet is precisely the diet that puts a woman at risk for fibroid tumors (as well as endometriosis and breast cancer).

A woman who changes from a high-fat, high-protein diet (rich in ice cream, red meat, and cheese) to the low-fat, high-fiber, mostly vegetarian diet will often experience decreased bleeding, bloating, and even a decrease in the size of her fibroids. Many women are eager to try this approach first, knowing that they can have surgery later if the regimen does not work out.

The same low-fat, high-complex-carbohydrate diet that I mention throughout this book can halt the growth of fibroids and in some cases, result in their disappearance.

If a woman is willing to make changes in her diet and lifestyle, I usually suggest a three-month trial of a low-fat, high-complex-carbohydrate diet that eliminates dairy food, red meat, chicken, and refined sugar. A diet used to treat fibroids must be quite strict for a while, to decrease circulating estrogens. The lipotropic factors methionine, choline, and inositol (1000 mg. of each per day) are available as dietary supplements; when these are used along with the vitamin B complex, excess estrogen levels can be lowered and symptoms alleviated. I advocate a multivitamin-mineral that contains at least 600 mg. of magnesium.

The vast majority of women who treat their fibroids through diet get rid of their pain and heavy bleeding within three to six months of following this diet. A low-fat, high-fiber diet "puts the fibroid to sleep" but doesn't "cure" the problem. The energy blockages in the pelvis must also be worked with and released. In fact, I've seen women on very strict low-fat macrobiotic diets whose fibroids have actually grown. These women usually had unresolved childhood issues, such as incest, or were married to abusive partners.

FREEING BLOCKED ENERGY. These therapies can be very healing when done by a person who is well trained and gifted.

Acupuncture, acupressure, polarity therapy, or massage often work very well for fibroid symptoms, though the fibroids don't always shrink with these therapies.

I have had very little experience with homeopathic medicine, but its practitioners have reported that fibroids shrink and symptoms can be alleviated with the right homeopathic remedy. Homeopathic medicine is a type of natural medicine that was very popular at the turn of the century and that is now gaining widespread acceptance.

The Chinese acupuncture literature indicates that it often takes a hundred or more daily treatments to eliminate large fibroids. Daily treatments require a major commitment from both the patient and the practitioner. (See explanation of acupuncture in Chapter 5.)

Almost every community in the United States and abroad has holistically oriented practitioners, although often they are not integrated with the orthodox medical community, which views them still with skepticism and rarely makes referrals to them.

Healing Program for Fibroids

• Low-fat, high-fiber diet—20 grams of fat or less per day; no animal protein, including chicken, fish, and dairy products; many whole grains, beans, and vegetables

• Supplements: methionine, choline, and inositol—approximately 1000 mg. of each per day; a comprehensive multivitamin-mineral combination containing the B complex

• Aerobic-type exercise for 20 minutes three times per week

• Massage, tai chi, meditation, acupuncture—to increase energy flow in the pelvis

• Castor oil packs to lower abdomen three times per week at minimum; attention given to thoughts, images, and feelings that arise during the treatment

• Journal: Write down everything that you'd like to create in your life. See how much enthusiasm and energy you can muster simply by imagining what it would be like to let your creative talents or secret selves manifest fully. Note where you have any blocks to this process. They will usually be identifiable as "yes, but" statements, such as "Yes, I'd love to sew beautiful clothing regularly, but there's no way I can get the time." You will soon be able to identify the limiting beliefs that are blocking your creativity.

- Go through the steps in Chapter 15 of this book.

Try this program for at least one month, then make adjustments as necessary. Each woman's needs are different, and you must therefore individualize this program. See what you can learn about your body and its responses to this new regimen. Listen to your body's messages.

Women's Stories

Fibroids, like other disorders, don't just come out of nowhere and land on your uterus. When you become willing to be in relationship with your uterus by letting its messages speak to you, you have taken the first steps toward healing, instead of just masking or eliminating symptoms. After you get in touch with the messages from your uterus, you can choose a treatment that works best for you, whether it's surgery or brown rice or both.

Many women can chart the onset of their fibroids to the onset of verbal abuse from their mates, job stress, or other problems in their relationships with the outside world. Inner work is often very useful for finding new ways to deal with these hurtful or limiting situations.

SHIRLEY: FIBROIDS AND CREATIVITY. Shirley, a nurse in her midforties, had been experiencing irregular periods and heavy menstrual flow when she was diagnosed with a small fibroid at the time of her annual exam. Shirley had been in treatment for an eating disorder and codependency a year before this. When I diagnosed her fibroids, she was in the midst of a career change, trying to decide whether to leave a stifling but lucrative management job.

I suggested she go on a low-fat, high-fiber diet and use castor oil packs. I also asked her to think about what she really wanted to do, what she would find truly satisfying. As she thought about it, she realized that her creativity had been stifled at work. She asked her body what it was telling her and to reveal it to her in dreams or meditations. Several months later, she told me, "I learned to surround myself with healing energy and love through the use of castor oil packs, meditation, and therapy."

She used Reiki treatments, a type of energy treatment similar to therapeutic touch, involving healing with the hands. Two weeks after her office visit with me, she reported, "I had a vision of the masseuse lifting a bowling-ball-shaped apparition from my abdomen. She had me draw it, and I drew what looked like a burr that you would find on your socks in the woods. It had exactly forty-five spikes on it. [Shirley was forty-five years old.] My apparition, the burr, represented me and how I cling to things in an unhealthy way. It symbolized clinging to work and people through whom I try to find fulfillment. From my dreams and meditations, I learned that my uterine growth was a physical manifestation of my own stifled creativity that could never be expressed fully through depending upon others. Through my emotional and physical healing process, my fibroid reduced in size, and I was led to a more creative, satisfying job in direct patient care." Her follow-up exam three months later showed that her uterus was much smaller, and I could find no fibroid.

MARSHA: UNSUPPORTIVE RELATIONSHIPS. Marsha, a massage therapist from out of state, first came to see me in 1986, when she was forty-one years old, to get a second opinion about her fibroids. Though her uterus was only moderately enlarged, to the size of a twelve-week pregnancy, and she was having no symptoms, she had been told that she should have a hysterectomy. Her mother had also had fibroids and had had a hysterectomy. Marsha wanted to avoid surgery. Marsha had mistreated herself for years by overeating and getting involved in harmful relationships with abusive men. She had had three abortions and no children. When she came for her first visit, she had already started a macrobiotic diet to keep her fibroids from growing.

Since everything else was normal on ultrasound testing, I affirmed Marsha's choice to treat her fibroids with dietary changes and suggested that she visit her gynecologist back home every six months. Given her insight into her own patterns of behavior, I felt she should work with alternatives to surgery. She followed the treatment plan in her home area.

Four years later, she returned to see me. Around this time, she had had several episodes of very heavy bleeding, and her gynecologist had strongly suggested surgery. Marsha, who was in the twelve-step program Sex and Love Addicts Anonymous, told me that she had just gotten out of a very unhealthy, addictive four-year relationship. She was still completely consumed by the relationship, even though both of them had agreed that it was over. She told me that she had begun to appreciate that "all the anger I've felt toward my old boyfriend has been a way to avoid doing my work on myself, my emotions, and my past." Now she began to take responsibility for her life and her situation and to get on with self-healing. Through her recovery work, she was finding that every relationship she'd ever been in since her childhood, with an alcoholic father, had been dysfunctional. She admitted that she was very good at creating drama in her life to fill the void of deadened feelings within herself and to compensate for her lack of connection with her own body.

Marsha was just starting to realize the profound connection between her relationships and her sense of self, and how they manifested in her body. She knew that not all the aspects of her fibroid were related specifically to food, but yet she used food to cover up her emotions. Her recovery, one day at a time, has gradually put her in touch with her inner wisdom. When I saw her for a check-up in 1992, her fibroid size was stable and she was having regular periods. She has entered a stage of healing that is sometimes necessary for many women, though not all: She is needing to withdraw from men for a time and be mostly with women. Each time I see her, she is more centered, more positive, and stronger. She realizes that her fibroids were a signal, calling her back to herself and her own life.

LOUISE: CHILDREN AND LOSS. Louise is a woman who is willing to assume partnership in her health care and who is not afraid to express her views. A producer for a radio station, she came to see me for a second surgical opinion regarding her fibroid uterus. Her fibroid had developed shortly after her second daughter had decided to leave home for boarding school. After her visit to me, Louise wrote the following letter to her gynecologist, who had suggested a hysterectomy.

Dear Dr. _____

On your recommendation I went for a second opinion for hysterectomy because of my uterine fibroids. Let me tell the story behind my process, in hopes that you can incorporate a broader, less conventional approach to other women who present with fibroids in the future.

First I was struck by how powerless I felt by your recommendation for surgery. Suddenly, I began to think of myself as sick, diseased. But my heart was telling me, "No, there's nothing the matter with you!" So I followed my heart's voice. I got my hands on everything I could read about fibroids, especially books and articles presenting alternatives to surgery.[28] I have learned how many unnecessary hysterectomies are performed each year in this country, and I learned of the significant, often long-term post-operative problems.

Even the small amount of research on the function of the uterus, especially postmenopausally, suggests that it is integral to overall good health. Chemical hormones cannot substitute for the magnificent functioning of the female organs.

So I became determined to keep my uterus—and not just for physical reasons. You didn't ask me anything about my feelings, about my family or lifestyle, or about how a hysterectomy might affect all that.

My two beautiful daughters have both left home within a year's time. My nineteen-year-old is in her second year of college, and my fifteen-year-old has gone away to private school in Vermont, at *her* insistence. Though I am supportive of them, at the same time it is a major life adjustment for a mother to have them both leave home so close in time. My children are gone, the offspring of my uterus, and then you tell me I should have my uterus removed as well. No, thank you. I'll hold on to it for the time being and, I expect, always. If I had a life-threatening disease of the uterus, I might feel differently.

All of this may sound bizarre to you, but I firmly believe that we contribute to illness in our bodies. The flip side is that we can contribute to healing our bodies as well. I urge you to take a little

extra time with your patients to hear their full story. If I had not
questioned what you were telling me, I might have been one of those
unnecessary hysterectomies. It would have been a convenience, perhaps, to be rid of the heavy periods, but it would have been at such a
cost—in dollars, lost work, and long-term hormone replacement
therapy, and in long-term psychological damage.

Please give your patients all the options, and the time to consider
them.

Sincerely,
Louise T.

Louise's gynecologist is not unusual. We doctors are not trained
to listen to our patients' feelings about what their diseases mean to
them. Dr. Larry Dossey, in his book *Meaning and Medicine,* tells
the story of Frank, a patient with chest pain whom he admitted to
the coronary intensive care unit. Frank was able to change his heart
rate at will by thinking about what his chest pain *meant* to him. He
told Dr. Dossey that if he let the pain mean a heart attack, he
immediately got anxious thinking about his damaged heart, clogged
vessels, the loss of his job, and the possibility of another heart
attack. But if he let the chest pain mean just a muscle ache or
indigestion, he felt relieved and his heart rate came down. Dossey
discovered that Frank's heart monitor acted as a "meaning meter."
The same is true for fibroids.

When I saw Louise seven months after her initial visit to me, she
had taken a job in another state, at a radio station where her work
was truly appreciated. She had realized the degree of loss associated
with her daughter's leaving home and had taken the time to grieve
that. While she was interviewing in the new city, she had realized
that her relationship with her husband had been unfulfilling for
years—that they had really stayed together only for the children.
She saw it clearly and began plans for a divorce, which was accomplished mutually. She then met a new lover, something she never
dreamed would happen and hadn't been seeking. This relationship
proved very sensual and meaningful to her. She had changed her diet
significantly and stopped eating dairy food. When I examined her,
the fibroid was almost completely gone. She had basically changed
her entire first and second chakra energy.

PAULA: FIBROIDS AND ABORTION. I occasionally see women whose fibroids appear to be related to an abortion or abortions. When I say "related" I don't mean "caused by." Abortion, in study after study, has *not* been associated with adverse physical effects on the body. The problems that women have after abortion, if any, are related to the *meaning* of abortion in their lives, and in the society in which they live.

Paula came to see me for an annual exam in 1987 at the age of thirty-six. She had had three abortions when she was in her teens and her twenties and had no children. I do not know the circumstances of her abortions except that she was matter-of-fact about them. She developed fibroids in her early thirties and had suffered from pelvic pain for at least five years. When I saw her, she was feeling well and healthy and felt that her well-being was related to the following story: "I was having increasing problems with bleeding between my periods and pelvic pain. Not happy with the prospect of surgery or hormones, I went to a Native American healer. He told me that I had to release the spirits of the beings who had been with me before my abortions. He performed a releasing ritual with me in which I literally saw and felt white wings flying out of my lower pelvis and away. I cried for hours with grief and relief. After that my periods went back to normal, and I've never had a day of pain since."

Paula's story is a dramatic example of the power of emotional release for healing. Though I could still feel an enlarged fibroid uterus of about eight-week size in her, this was not a problem that required more than regular check-ups. She told me that it was a relief to be able to tell her story to a doctor, since she was certain that most doctors would laugh at her and think she was nuts. That, of course, is why doctors rarely hear these stories of wonder and healing from their patients. The stories are common, and yet they are kept secret because they are too often discounted or patronized by medical professionals.

True healing, not just curing our body or soothing our mental anxiety, involves transformation of our energy field and consciousness. In the women I've just described, the healing came in part because each woman created meaning from her fibroid, menstrual problem, or other symptom. Scientists can argue all they like about whether what I'm suggesting is possible, but getting caught up in this argument for me would be participating in the addictive system. It's infinitely more desirable to get on with healing.

SEVEN

The Ovaries

... she sings from the knowing of *los ovarios*, a knowing from
deep within the body, deep within the mind, deep within the soul.
—Clarissa Pinkola Estes

From an energy medicine standpoint, ovaries are the female
equivalent of male testicles. They can be thought of as "female
balls" because they represent exactly the same thing in the world.
When a man goes out into the world to perform acts of difficulty or
courage that require manipulating the external world of things or
people, he's said to "have balls." For a female, going out into the
world, particularly a male-oriented world, also "takes balls," but she
must use her ovarian energy. She should not try to imitate a man,
because her ovaries and their energy field can be adversely affected
by her relationship with the outside world. To maintain health, she
needs to understand how to use her "balls" in a life-enhancing way.

Our ovarian wisdom represents our deepest creativity, that
which waits to be born from within us, that which can be born only
through us, our unique creative potential—especially as it relates to
what we create in the world outside of ourselves. Biologically, when
a woman ovulates, the egg attracts the sperm to it by sending out a
signal to the sperm. The egg simply waits for the sperm to arrive; it
does not go actively seeking sperm. The resulting biological creation, a baby, has its own life and consciousness connected to, but
also separate from that of its mother. Although its growth and

development are influenced profoundly by the mother, they are at the same time separate from her. She cannot use her will to force her baby to develop faster; nor can she use her will to determine when her child will be born. And once the child is born, she must acknowledge that her creation has and always will have a life and personality of its own, even though it was created from her own flesh and blood.

Similarly, all of the creations that come from deep within us, from our ovarian wisdom—whether they be babies, books, or works of art—have a life of their own that we have a responsibility to initiate and allow but ultimately not to control. Just so, our deepest creativity cannot be forced. It must be allowed the time and space to grow and develop in tune with its own internal rhythm. Like biological mothers, we as women must be open to the uniqueness of our creations and their own energies and impulses, without trying to force them into predetermined forms. Our ability to *yield* to our creativity, to acknowledge that we cannot control it with our intellects, is the key to understanding ovarian power. We must *allow* this power to come through us.

Society tries to control creativity through the imposition of deadlines (note the connotation of this word—sometimes the time factor literally kills our creativity), quotas, and productivity ratings. One of my colleagues, who has always maintained very healthy ovaries, used to do scientific research as a research assistant in laboratories. Whenever she entered a new lab, the lab director would always tell her exactly what he wanted her to produce. Once, for example, he wanted her to manufacture an artificial cell called a liposome. Whenever she tried to create this cell model by running the experimental design according to his predetermined directions, using her will and intellect to try to force and control the setup, the attempt failed and the artificial cell was nonfunctional. She felt miserable. She would then look beyond the lab director's specific demand and ask herself, "What do I want to know in this situation? How can I find out more about an aspect of life by doing this experiment? What can this teach me about cells in general?" At these times she connected with the broadest possibilities inherent in the experiment. Invariably, in the liposome experiment and in others, she would design an experiment that yielded far more information than had been originally expected of her. The end result was never exactly what the lab director had asked for, but it was usually far more valuable and enriching. In the liposome experiment, my colleague ended up creating not only an artificial cell model but an experimental design that could potentially be used to produce a vaccine against a serious disease. A by-product of this was that the lab director was always thrilled with her results and eventually learned to allow her to design her own experiments without interference. Her scientific work was brilliant. By remaining true to her deepest creative wisdom, her end results benefited everyone concerned. This is women's creativity at its finest. We can do this in our own lives and jobs by always considering how one task is connected to others and by remembering our interconnections and how one act can give birth to or build bridges to others.

Anatomy

Ovaries are the small, oblong, pearl-colored organs that lie just below the fallopian tubes on each side of the uterus. Ovaries produce eggs. A woman has the greatest number of eggs in her ovaries that she'll ever have—about 20 million—when she is a twenty-week fetus inside her mother. From that moment on, she starts losing eggs. Our biological time clock for reproduction begins ticking before we are even born!

Ovaries produce eggs about once a month, from about age fourteen or fifteen onward—sometimes earlier, sometimes later. After a girl's first period, it takes two or three years for ovulation to get going regularly—just as at menopause, it takes a number of years for ovulation to cease altogether. Because ovulation always produces a small cyst in the ovary, it's very common for ovaries to have small cystic areas in them that are either the result of newly developing eggs or ovulations that have already occurred. As the egg begins to develop each month, a nourishing fluid-filled area forms around it, so that it is encapsulated or walled off from the rest of the ovary. This fluid-filled area, known as a cyst, is physiologically and completely normal, a fact that many women don't appreciate. At ovulation, when the egg is released and picked up by the fallopian tube, the cyst actually bursts as part of the ovulatory process, and the surrounding fluid, known as the liquor folliculi, is released into the pelvic cavity along with the egg.

After ovulation, in the space where the egg used to be, a second small cystic area known as the corpus luteum develops and begins to secrete progesterone. The corpus luteum eventually gets resorbed by the ovary. Frequently the process of egg development begins and a small cyst forms, but ovulation doesn't occur in that particular site. In this case, a small cyst will be left in that area of the ovary for a while. Because of this monthly process of egg development and cyst formation, it is perfectly normal for a woman to have small fluid-filled ovarian cysts at almost any time throughout her reproductive life. In fact, ovaries almost always have small cysts in them.

Whenever a woman gets a pelvic ultrasound for chronic pelvic pain, a fibroid, or any other reason, her ovaries are also scanned and these cysts show. Small one-to-three-centimeter cysts are almost always normal, because producing small physiological cysts that come and go is part of what normal ovaries do. They gestate little eggs, little cysts—or in energy medicine terms, young ideas ripe with potential.

Ovaries also produce hormones—including estrogen, progesterone, and androgens—throughout the life-cycle, though the amounts they produce change (not necessarily declining), depending upon a woman's age. Androgen, the hormone type associated with libido, was thought in the past to be produced almost entirely by the adrenals, which are the endocrine glands located at the top of the kidneys. In the last two decades, however, various studies have established that both premenopausal and postmenopausal ovaries produce a significant quantity of androgens, perhaps as much as 50 percent of the body's entire supply.[1]

It has been commonly thought that ovaries become essentially nonfunctional after a woman stops having periods, but the role of the ovary in the second half of life is now being reevaluated. Some studies suggest that the ovary should not be surgically removed because it maintains its ability to produce steroid hormones for several decades after menopause.[2] Parts of the ovaries do start to decrease in size when a woman is in her thirties and they do lose mass more rapidly after age forty-five on average, but they are *not* the inert fibrous tissue masses they've been thought to be.

As women age, only part of our ovaries regresses, the part known as the *theca*. The theca is the outermost covering of the ovary where the eggs grow and develop and where physiological cysts form. In midlife the theca regresses, but the innermost part of the ovary, known as the inner stroma, becomes quite active for the first time in our lives.[3] In other words, as one function is winding down, another one is starting up. This process deserves much more study than it has heretofore received. In the second half of life, women's ovaries still produce significant amounts of a hormone known as andros-teinedione, a type of androgen. This substance is often converted to estrone (a type of estrogen) in our body fat deposits. Studies have shown that our ovaries can produce progesterone and estradiol even after menopause. These hormones are significant in preventing osteoporosis.[4]

Up until fairly recently, menopause has been studied mostly as a "deficiency disease." Because of this cultural attitude toward menopause, scientists have studied this natural process only to find what is lacking. If we were to design studies of postmenopausal women in which the ovary was viewed as active and useful, we would probably find out more and more about the ovary's role in maintaining normal balance in our bodies as time goes on. Our ovaries should be appreciated as dynamic organs that are part of our body's wisdom throughout life, not as something useless or potentially harmful to us when we are over forty!

Some ancient traditions have supported this view. In Taoist cultures the ovaries are thought to contain large amounts of the life-force that constantly produces sexual energy. Special "ovarian breathing" exercises can be learned to release the life-force energy that the ovaries produce and "store" it to revitalize other organs of the body, while the person achieves a higher state of consciousness. Ovarian sexual energy is thus transformed into *chi* (life-force energy) and *shen* (sheer spiritual energy).[5] Learning ovarian breathing and other Taoist meditation techniques takes time and discipline, but simply knowing that ovaries have a special energy and function besides producing the next generation of people can be emotionally healing in itself.

When a woman does not heed her innermost creative wisdom because of her fears or insecurities about the world outside herself, ovarian problems can arise. They may arise in situations in which she perceives herself as being controlled or criticized by forces outside herself. Financial or physical threats in the outer world affect the ovaries, particularly if a woman believes that she has no way to alleviate the threats. Thus, a woman who is abandoned by her mate or feels stressed on the job may develop ovarian problems if she feels that she has no means of escape from her situation and that the "outer" world is preventing her from changing. Just as life stresses may cause uterine problems, they may also cause ovarian problems. Uterine and ovarian problems are often intimately related, but there are also differences. The primary energy involved in uterine problems is a woman's perception in her innermost self that she can't or shouldn't or doesn't deserve to free herself from a limiting situation or create solutions that can support her. The uterus is very intimately linked with the third chakra and self-esteem. Uterine problems result when a woman's personal and emotional insecurities keep her from expressing her creativity fully. In these cases, she believes that she herself lacks the inner resources to do so; in other words, "she" is doing it to herself.

Ovarian problems, on the other hand, result from a woman's perception that people and circumstances outside of herself are preventing her from being creative. "They" are doing it to her. An additional energy affects only the ovaries and not the uterus—the energy of vengeance and resentment, or the desire to get even. The second chakra area is the part of the body where we traditionally wear weapons, such as guns, knives, and wallets. When a woman uses her emotional weaponry to indulge in being highly critical or wanting to get even, it is her ovaries that are at risk, not her uterus.

Benign ovarian growths differ from cancer only in the degree of emotional energy involved. Cancer in a woman's ovarian area is also related to an extreme need for male authority or approval, as she gives her own emotional needs last priority. A woman at risk for ovarian cancer may feel that she doesn't have enough power, financial or otherwise, to move or to change even an abusive situation. In contrast to cervical cancer, which may incubate for years, ovarian cancer usually develops rather quickly due to a precipitating psychosocial trauma, such as a mate announcing that he or she is leaving.[6]

A friend of mine developed an ovarian cyst when she began to realize that her job was not good for her and that her relationship with her husband was not mutually supportive. During the same time period, her husband began having an affair. Dealing with her cyst helped her to realize that there were real problems in her day-to-day life that she had to deal with. Her body was concretizing her emotional dissatisfactions and, in its wisdom, drawing her attention to her need to care for herself.

One of my patients, Beverly, had a long history of endometriosis, and her right ovary had been removed because of a benign growth four years before I met her. When she first came to see me, she was complaining of intermittent pain associated with her left ovary. She was worried that she might have to have this ovary removed as well, but she did not want to do this. She was only thirty-two and didn't want to be on artificial hormones to replace her body's own supply. She was ready to work toward the deepest levels of inner healing. On ultrasound, her remaining ovary had some small cysts in it, consistent with endometriosis of the ovary. Medical intuitive Caroline Myss did a diagnosis that revealed that Beverly had a lifelong history of truncating her own creative needs in order to meet the demands of her family, who lived close by. She also hated her high-powered executive job that took up about seventy hours of her time per week.

Caroline told Beverly that she would not get well until she allowed herself at least one hour a day of creative time just for her. During this time, she was to release all expectations of productivity. She should simply allow her creativity to flow in whatever way it needed to. Beverly had always enjoyed working with fabric and was accomplished at needlecraft. She began to sit each day and create small, very magical-appearing dolls that, she said, "seemed to have a life of their own." She told me that the dolls themselves dictated to her how they would look and what they would wear. When she first brought a few into my office, I was enchanted by them and purchased two for my daughters for Christmas. As she allowed herself this creative time, her pelvic pain eventually disappeared. It returned intermittently when she got caught up in the demands of the external world at the expense of her own creative work. Her ovary, through its persistent voice, became a personal barometer for her of how well she was allowing her innate creativity to flow. She has begun to change her entire approach to life. The dolls that are being birthed through her continue to evolve and change as well.

Ovarian Cysts

Women are meant to express our creative natures throughout our lives. Our creations will change and evolve as we ourselves grow and develop. Our ovaries, too, are always changing, forming, and reabsorbing those small physiological cysts. As long as we express the creative flow deep within us, our ovaries remain normal. When our creative energy is blocked in some way, abnormally large cysts may occur and persist. Such energy blockages that create ovarian cysts may result from stress. Such stress is not necessarily negative; for example, a woman may have a job that she loves but may sometimes simply neglect her need for rest. A cyst may be the result.

The left side of the body represents the female artistic reflective side, while the right side is the more analytic male side. Each woman will have to decide for herself what this means, but most of the ovarian cysts I see are on the left side—symbolic I feel, of the wounded feminine in this culture. Many women try to imitate male ways of being in the world that don't always fit their inner needs. When I had my first energy diagnosis with Caroline Myss, she told me that if I had stayed in my former medical group, I would have developed a nonphysiological ovarian cyst within the next year that probably would have required surgery. It had already been forming in my body's energy field.

In premenopausal women in general, cysts that are less than four centimeters in diameter are considered normal. An ovarian cyst is called a *functional cyst* when it arises as part of the ovulation process. A cyst larger than four centimeters may be watched for a few months to see if it goes away. An abnormal cyst may contain fluid, blood, and cellular debris under the surface covering of the ovary or within the body of the ovary itself.

Symptomatic Functional Ovarian Cysts
FOLLICULAR CYSTS. Many ovarian cysts that grow bigger than four centimeters and persist after two or three menstrual cycles are actually functional. Such cysts form when the follicle, the

physiological cyst in which the egg develops, fails to grow and discharge the egg in the normal way. When this happens, the ovarian follicle may continue to grow beyond the time when ovulation should have taken place. It sometimes grows as big as seven or eight centimeters in diameter and can be painful. These cysts are described on ultrasound as "unilocular" and thin-walled, meaning that they consist of just a single fluid collection contained within a thin membrane. They usually go away on their own, but some persist and require surgery. Although some physicians prescribe birth control pills to stop the ovulation process and allow the cyst to regress, the newer low-dose-estrogen birth control pills do not contain enough hormone to shut down the ovary and influence the cyst.

LUTEAL CYSTS. Another type of functional cyst is known as the corpus luteum. A corpus luteum or luteal cyst forms when the mature egg is discharged from its follicle at ovulation. This process is sometimes accompanied by a small amount of bleeding into the ovulation site on the capsule of the ovary—and sometimes into the pelvic cavity as well—at the time when the egg erupts from the ovary.

Some ovarian cysts are completely asymptomatic, while others cause pain. The pain can be sharp and knifelike if, for example, the cyst bursts and spills its contents into the pelvic cavity. Or the pain can be dull and aching if the condition is more chronic, as in many cases of endometriosis of the ovary. A small pain sometimes accompanies ovulation, caused by the release of blood into the pelvic cavity. It is known as *Mittelschmerz* (middle pain). Bleeding into a cyst cavity or the pelvic cavity often causes pain because it stretches the ovarian capsule (the tissue on the surface of the ovary). This pain can last from a few minutes to a few days. If the bleeding continues into the cyst wall for longer than a few hours, the corpus luteum becomes known as a corpus hemorrhagicum, which simply means "a body that bleeds." Bleeding from a corpus hemorrhagicum can last for several hours or even days and sometimes mimics an ectopic (tubal) pregnancy. It may be accompanied by vaginal bleeding. Hemorrhagic cysts usually go away on their own, but they can cause several days of pain. Very occasionally, the bleeding doesn't stop and surgical intervention, usually through the laparoscope, becomes necessary. Most often, this procedure stops the bleeding and removal of the ovary isn't necessary.

Most functional ovarian cysts are diagnosed by a pelvic examination, followed by an ultrasound evaluation. Both ovaries are examined and compared to be sure that it is an ovarian cyst and not something else, such as a fibroid, that is being felt.

Neither type of functional ovarian cyst—follicular or luteal—leads to cancer. Some women have symptoms from them repeatedly, while others have them only once in a lifetime. The important point to keep in mind is that these cysts can arise in only a matter of hours or days because our bodies are able to produce ovarian cysts rapidly. They can also go away rapidly.

BENIGN NEOPLASTIC CYSTS. Because ovaries contain cells that are capable of growing into complete human beings, they also contain cells that are capable of growing into a wide variety of cysts and growths, reflecting our enormous creative potential. When our creative expression is frustrated, this creative energy calls our attention to it through our body and physically manifests itself in the ovary rather than moving through us smoothly into the outer world. Conventional medical training teaches that the cause of ovarian cysts is not known unless they are of the "functional" variety and related to ovulation.

Benign, nonfunctional ovarian cysts occur when those cells of the ovary that are not associated with ovulation begin reproducing. The term *neoplastic* is often used in discussing these and other growths, both benign and malignant. *Neoplasia* simply means "new growth."

OTHER CYSTS. Besides follicular, luteal, hemorrhagic, and benign neoplastic cysts, some ovarian cysts are solid in character and don't go away after two or three menstrual cycles. This kind of cyst is assumed to be an ovarian growth arising from something other than ovulation. They require further investigation and treatment via surgery, because until a doctor has surgically removed tissue and examined it under the microscope, it is not certain whether the cyst is benign. I've occasionally had patients with ovarian cysts that were present on pelvic exam and visible with ultrasound for many years but that did not change in any way or cause any symptoms. These women know that they are taking a risk, in the conventional sense, by not having surgery. Some are willing to take that risk and live with their ovaries untouched and undiagnosed for years. Though this approach is not advocated by my training and I always offer a surgical approach as the conventional standard of care, I also respect the decisions of well-informed adults to avoid surgery.

Polycystic Ovaries (PCO)

Many women have a condition known as polycystic ovaries. So-called "polycystic ovaries" are a sign of hormonal malfunction. PCO is a complex disorder because it is so affected by a woman's emotions, thoughts, diet, and personal history.

Currently PCO is not considered a disease, although doctors used to call it "polycystic ovarian disease." It is, rather, the end result of a complex series of subtle hormonal interactions. A few cases are genetic and therefore run in families, but most cases have no known genetic link. Conventional medicine cannot explain why or how PCO occurs.

The major problems associated with polycystic ovaries are the following: The woman's ovaries do not produce eggs, and her body produces too many hormones known as androgens. Androgens occur naturally in both men and women, but in women with PCO they are present at higher levels than normal. Chronically high levels of androgens prevent normal cyclic egg development in the ovary, blocking the growth and development of eggs before they reach full maturity. When a woman's normal hormonal cycle is blocked by chronic androgen overproduction, neither she nor her ovaries will experience the natural cyclic changes associated with normal ovarian function. Her hormonal levels remain static. Thus, a woman's ovaries contain many small cysts from under-developed eggs. On ultrasound, the ovaries look enlarged, with multiple small cysts just below the entire surface of the ovaries (hence the name polycystic ovaries). Chronically high androgen levels also create a tendency toward obesity, diabetes, heart disease, and hirsutism (excess facial hair).

The Mind/Body Connection in Amenorrhea

Whenever a woman has a problem with something as complex as the ovulation process, we know that there may be a problem with the regulatory mechanism of the menstrual cycle in the brain. The hypothalamus is affected by emotional and psychological factors such as stress and repressed pain from the past, which can cause menstrual cycle dysfunction. Because most causes of amenorrhea are "hypothalamic" in nature, which means they are somehow associated with alterations in the fine tuning of brain neuropeptide levels that are poorly understood, it is possible that the hypothalamus may have something to do with PCO. In women with PCO, the cyclic release of hypothalamic hormones from the brain is changed from what it is in normal ovulatory women. It is not known whether this change is the result of the ovarian problem or the cause of it. Although the relationship of stress to women with PCO has not been studied, the stresses that have been associated with "functional amenorrhea" can give us a clue to how a woman's emotions and personal history may affect her menstrual cycle and ovarian function. These clues may well apply to those women with PCO, as well, so you should refer to the menstrual cycle discussion in Chapter 5.

Stresses that have been found to suppress ovarian and menstrual cycle functioning include negative feelings about being female. I have found that when a woman has grown up being told that women are inferior, on some level, she wants no part of being or becoming a woman. In some women, these negative feelings may work in the body to cause it to stop ovulating and become more "androgynous."[7]

Studies have shown that women who don't ovulate are often tense, anxious, more dependent, and less productive mentally compared to ovulatory women. They may also have suppressed rage at their mothers. Some feel guilt and fear about their need for parental care and protection and also fear losing this protection. As they grow up, this can manifest as amenorrhea—an attempt to "halt" becoming fully mature women.[8]

Treatment of PCO

Since standard medicine doesn't know the cause of most cases of PCO, treatment is aimed at quelling the symptoms only. Therefore, most women are currently placed on birth control pills or progestin hormones to create cyclic menstrual periods. These treatments do not address lack of ovulation or the hormonal status of the brain. Birth control pills or progestin (such as Provera) also prevent excess hormonal stimulation of the uterine lining. These agents, therefore, decrease the risk of uterine cancer, which may result from years of build-up of the uterine lining if a woman doesn't have her period. Though birth control pills do prevent some of the risks and symptoms associated with PCO, they only partially mask the problem and never address the baseline cause.

In the past, women with PCO often underwent surgery to remove a part of each ovary, known as a "wedge resection." This sometimes resulted in a lowering of hormone levels (by decreasing the amount of ovary, the amount of hormone it produces is also decreased) and in some cases, cyclic function was restored. In others, however, the surgery resulted in scarring and adhesions. It is no longer done.

In those women who desire pregnancy, ovulation can sometimes be induced with drugs. The most common one is clomiphene citrate (Clomid).

A woman with PCO can help restore cyclic ovulatory function through the following:

• Look carefully at any negative childhood messages you may have internalized about being a fertile woman. Commit to bringing these messages to consciousness so that they no longer control your body and your ovaries. Example: One of my patients who had been diagnosed with PCO three years before I first saw her realized that she had internalized feeling bad about herself as a woman because of being raped by her father. She unconsciously blamed her mother for not protecting her and so saw women as powerless. When she became aware of these messages, got off birth control pills (for PCO), and began to celebrate her female nature, her periods and her ovulations re-established themselves in about six months. (She also needed to hear from me that PCO did not need to be a life-long chronic condition for her.)

• Re-establish cyclic emotional flow. Allow yourself a full range of emotional responses to the events in your life. Try recording these in a journal to discover the natural rhythm of your emotions and moods. Are they related to the seasons, the time of day, and other cycles? Keep track of the phases of the moon on a calendar. It is well known that the menstrual cycle is affected by the cylic waxing and waning of the moon. If you live near the ocean, keep track of the tides. As already mentioned, simply paying attention to environmental cues including the light, the moon, and the tides may regulate a woman's menstrual cycle and fertility.[9]

• Re-establish cyclic ovulatory flow through connection with light and nature. Get out in natural light as much as possible. Natural light affects the hypothalamus and pituitary gland and affects ovulation. Sleep with the light on for 3 days each month. (See Chapter 5.) It might even be helpful to purchase a source of full-spectrum light and have it in your home—especially during the fall and winter months. (See Resources for sources.)

• Nourish your body fully via a low-fat, whole foods, mostly vegetarian diet. This helps decrease cholesterol levels, weight, risk of diabetes, and coronary artery disease. Such a light diet also can increase a woman's attunement to her spiritual, intuitive side. This helps re-establish emotional flow, can often help normalize a woman's hormonal levels and alleviate PCO.

Women's Stories

The following stories illustrate how several of my patients have used their ovarian cysts to change and improve their lives. These stories show women waking up to the messages their bodies were sending them and then changing their lives. The message to all of us is particularly clear: to pay attention to the ways in which we unconsciously participate in the addictive system and allow ourselves to be swayed by outside authorities rather than following our inner guidance.

GAIL: CRYSTALLIZED OVERDRIVE. Gail has been a friend of mine for years. In 1989 she first consulted me about a persistent ovarian cyst, and eventually, when she was in her late thirties it required surgery. Here is her story.

"In 1984, during a routine gynecological exam, a woman doctor found a large ovarian cyst on my left side. This sleek doctor in New York's SoHo district announced to me that this was dangerous and that I should have surgery to remove it as quickly as possible. I should then expect to be completely laid up for about four to six weeks, she said. She, of course, would be glad to perform the surgery. All of this transpired in about fifteen minutes. •

"I was terrified, completely blown away. At the time I didn't know enough about myself to know why I was so scared by this information. As was my pattern in those days, I covered the terror by increasing my activity and going into high gear. This was supremely easy for me to do in 1984, as I was directing a massive global peace initiative that had me traveling to several different continents a month. Besides covering my feelings by going into action, I had a strong intuitive sense that this ovarian cyst was neither as urgent nor as serious as this doctor seemed to think. I did not have the surgery.

"Several years went past, and I didn't really think about the cyst too much. I was in warrior overdrive, changing the world and lots of people's lives while ignoring my own. Though much of this activity was positive and deeply meaningful to me, I was out of balance in my life.

"In late 1987 my father died. Though he was well into his eighties and had led a full life, I had no idea the impact this would have on me. I experienced a kind of spiritual crisis. Through what I consider pure grace, a friend recommended a therapist who might help me. My journey with this wonderful man changed my life. With consummate skill and rare gentleness, he empowered me to recognize and heal much about myself that I had been afraid to look at. A pattern that was enormously important to my healing was my understanding that I had betrayed my feminine/mother and sided with my masculine/father. For much of my life this had resulted in my absolute allegiance to doing over being, thinking over feeling, and the outer world over the inner world. For me, this was a deeply personal betrayal, as well as a symbol of the collective societal betrayal of the feminine that has so profoundly wounded our culture.

"I began to experience my ovarian cyst as a physical manifestation of the warrior/masculine part of my personality that caused me to be so driven all the time. I called it 'crystallized overdrive.' I had betrayed my deep feminine side to such a degree that this warrior cyst was literally taking up much of the room in the feminine creative center of my body. It had grown to the size of a large grapefruit.

"Though I began to have more spiritual and emotional clarity about my cyst, I still struggled with how to deal with it on the physical level. I never felt it—I had absolutely no pain. Rather, it had a kind of looming presence, reminding me that something in me was out of balance."

In the fall of 1991 Gail came to see me. Her most recent ultrasounds showed that the cyst was beginning to grow again and that the inside was changing, becoming more solid and dense. When a cyst becomes more solid, it means that its fluid parts are being replaced by more cells and growth within it. It was becoming more substantial. I felt that she had watched it long enough and that these changes signified the potential for the cells to become precancerous. (If an individual does not heed the body's wisdom that is announced by a bodily growth, the growth often needs to speak louder and more clearly. Thus, it may grow more quickly and become symptomatic. Nonphysiological ovarian cysts have the capacity to become large very quickly, depending upon the circumstances.) Gail was also starting to get some pressure on her bladder. I suggested surgery since I felt that the persistent and now-changing cyst was a drain on her energy. As we have seen, unhealthy tissue literally "drains" the molecules needed for cellular metabolism from adjacent healthy tissue. (See Chapter 4.)

A consultation with Caroline Myss confirmed my suspicions. She said that the cyst was now "waking up" and becoming active. It had the capacity to undergo rapid growth under the "right" circumstances. She felt that it should come out within three months. She confirmed that the growth had developed because of Gail's conflict between her personal inner needs and the demands of her outer world. Myss also said that the energy difference between Gail and her husband was at its most extreme ever; Gail felt drawn toward the quiet, reflective archetypal feminine, just as her husband (her partner in work as well as marriage) was reaching his peak in recognition and activity in the outer world. This was recognition in which Gail could share if she wished. She felt acutely the competition between this "drawing inward energy from the core of her being" and the demands of success in the outer world, for which she had worked for years. If she didn't participate in this worldly success, the culture would judge that she was now "throwing it all away." Despite this conflict between her inner and outer worlds, Gail's deep ovarian wisdom was drawing her more inward than ever before in her life. This is a classic example of the type of competition in energy and body language that hits women in their ovaries.

Gail agreed to have the surgery, performed by me, whom she trusted. As part of her preparation, she worked with a spiritual studies group. The process included a kind of guided meditation in which she experienced her surgery in archetypal images, her warrior/masculine aspect standing behind her hospital bed protecting her emerging mystic/feminine aspect. As she remembered it, "The warrior reached to stroke gently the mystic's forehead. At the conclusion of the surgery my mystic held the cyst and handed it to the warrior. The warrior took the cyst and bowed deeply to the mystic. This was a profound image for me. I knew at that moment that through this surgery something very old, at my very essence, would come into balance.

"In partnership with this mythic changing of the guard, another friend led me through a meditation several days before my surgery. I had a dialogue with my cyst. I visualized it as being like the inside of a gold ball. I told it I was ready to release its 'crystallized overdrive.' I was ready to balance my outer warrior side and my inner reflective mystical side. I truly yearned for this as a healing for me.

"During this second meditation, I gave Chris [Northrup] permission to cut open my body and remove the cyst. I meditated about the removal of the cyst. I experienced vast space in my body, the turquoise color of the Caribbean Sea healing and cleansing me. Into that infinite turquoise, the female lineage of my family appeared—a long line of sister, mother, grandmother, and on and on back. They acknowledged me for reclaiming my feminine self for myself and for them."

With these healing images instilled in her mind and heart, Gail created a medicine pouch of items of significance to her. It included some crystals that had been given to her, some special stones from a beach she loved, pictures of her mother and grandmother, and some childhood toys. She packed her bag and left for Maine, to have her surgery at the hospital where I do surgery. As she later said, "My husband and two of my dearest friends were with me before and after my surgery. Their presence created a calm, loving, and joyful center from which my surgery/initiation could unfold.

"The surgery went smoothly and gracefully. Chris removed the benign cyst that had replaced my left ovary. She reported to me that I had a gorgeous and healthy uterus and right tube and ovary. When she showed my dear friends the cyst she had removed, one of my friends said that it looked like the bulging red muscles in the neck of a runner who is overexerting. Overdrive itself.

"I felt only a small amount of pain from the surgery and only mild effects from the anesthesia. I left the hospital after two days with an enormously positive feeling about my adventure there. My body then began the miraculous process of healing itself.

"I am enjoying my time of healing retreat. It's too soon to understand all of what has changed and transpired in me. What I do know is that I have faced one of my scariest dragons, and for that I am a fuller, richer person. I know that I can ask for support when I am afraid, and I know that I am loved and cared for by many dear ones. I know that I have shifted and balanced an ancient partnership within myself where the warrior waltzes with the mystic."

In many cases of large complex ovarian cysts like Gail's, the healthy ovarian tissue is replaced almost entirely by that of the cyst, and there is almost no way to distinguish healthy from unhealthy tissue. Therefore, the entire ovary requires removal.[10] Gail continues to do well, however. The very way in which she approached her cyst, her hospitalization, and her post-op care are good examples of allowing more feminine, intuitive, nurturing energy into her life, part of the lesson she learned from her left ovary.

MARY JANE: MARRIED TO THE JOB. Mary Jane is a molecular biologist who has spent her entire career working in male-dominated institutions. When she was in high school, she wanted to take physics and advanced mathematics, but her father, a physics professor, told her that she should take typing instead, because it would be much more useful to her. Like many men of his generation, he felt that his daughter would only get married and have children and that higher education would be wasted on her. Ironically, Mary Jane eventually went on to get an advanced degree in science, and she published many more research papers than her father. Though she was once married and divorced and has one child, her marriage was unsatisfying to her almost from the beginning. She then became married to her job.

Mary Jane had been a patient of mine for a few years, always traveling from out of state to my office in Maine for her annual exam. At one of these exams, I felt a seven-centimeter left ovarian cyst, which was confirmed by ultrasound. Because she was very open to working with the symptoms in her body in a conscious way, I told her that this manifestation was there to teach her something about second chakra issues, specifically her relationships and her creativity. I told her to talk with her ovary and see what it was telling her. My plan was to reevaluate her in three months or less.

An energy diagnosis by Caroline Myss revealed that the cyst was filled with anger, the anger of violation. It also had "cancer energy." This isn't the same as physical cancer but is moving toward it, and Caroline felt the cyst would have to be removed soon. Although there was no cancer now, the angry energy in the cyst was very strong.

After Myss's intuitive reading, Mary Jane started a dialogue with her ovary. As she discovered, "I found that it was filled with anger, a sense of abandonment, and also jealousy. But there was love there as well. Though I had felt this love, on occasion, I couldn't express it. I had needed a place to put all of this—it went into my ovary."

Mary Jane took a leave of absence from work. She had decided to have the surgery because of Myss's warning. I affirmed her decision and told her that she should not look at surgery as a giving-up on her self-healing capabilities. Surgery can be a very healing choice, and it would allow her to move forward quickly with healing her life on all levels. Mary Jane's personal healing issues would mean working to heal her relationship with her father and her work.

Mary Jane had her surgery and all went well. The cyst was benign. During her immediate postoperative period, she went through a process of deep grieving and let go of the unattainable vision of the relationship with her father that she had always wanted but could not have. She realized that her longing for paternal approval that never came had set up a lifelong pattern of unsatisfactory relationships with men that also affected her work and work relationships. She realized that she had to release her father from her expectations and demands. She realized that she had used her research as a method to win the approval of her peers, not simply for the joy of scientific discovery. Four weeks later, at the time of her check-up, she was doing beautifully—grateful to her ovary for showing her a truth about her life that was not obvious to her intellect. Mary Jane used her ovarian growth as a transformational journey that reconnected her body's wisdom and joy in her life's work.

CONNY: TRUNCATED CREATIVITY AND NEED FOR OUTER APPROVAL. Conny was thirty-eight when she developed a six-centimeter benign left ovarian cyst. It was removed surgically, leaving some normal left ovarian tissue behind. During the time she was developing this cyst, she had been trying to decide whether to have a child. At the time of her surgery we had discussed how she could best maximize her cyst experience for change and growth. She knew that her job was stifling her. She very much wanted to pursue making pottery and was, in fact, very good at it—she was always able to sell what she had time to make. But her job had great "benefits." I told her to check out whether it was worthwhile to kill herself for her "benefits."

A year after her surgery, Conny was back in my office, reexperiencing the pain in her left side that had been there when she had had the ovarian cyst. This time there was no cyst, but the pain was the same. She found that as soon as she arrived at work, the pain started and was getting worse. Her body was speaking loudly to her this time. She had already had one surgery. The conditions leading to the cyst in the first place—the energy pattern in her body—hadn't really changed.

Conny understood her dilemma intellectually, and she knew that something had to change. But somewhere deep inside, whenever she thought about leaving work to pursue her creative instincts, she heard her father's voice in her head saying, "You're a fool to leave your job security. Making art is not a job. That's a hobby. That's what you do when you've finished your work." She'd been carrying this belief from her father since childhood. Her job represented his approval in her life. She thus allowed forces outside herself to control her inherent creativity. Meanwhile she was denying the anger and rage associated with this situation.

I asked Conny to consider what she would do if she were given six months to live. She gave it a great deal of thought. Finally, exhausted, depressed, and in pain, she took a three-month leave of absence from work with the blessings of her company in order to sort out her priorities. The pain went away almost immediately, her energy returned, and her artistic side began blossoming. Her challenge was to balance her creative needs with her job.

When she first returned to work after her leave, her company put her in a different location, one in which she didn't have to deal directly with the public. Instead, she worked behind the scenes processing paperwork and invoices. This change fit her needs only temporarily. It was not satisfying work, and she was still allowing many aspects of her life to be controlled by her need for approval from her parents and her bosses. Within three months of a completely normal pelvic exam, she developed a very large precancerous tumor of the left ovary. It was growing so fast that she noticed a bulge in her abdominal wall that hadn't been there the week before. At surgery, the tumor was found to be a "borderline tumor"—halfway between benign and malignant. The tumor growth at the time of surgery appeared confined to the left ovary only, and after consultation with a gynecological oncologist, only the left ovary was removed—leaving Conny with a normal uterus and a normal right ovary.

However, she now knew at a deep cellular level that her creativity was desperate for expression and that her body would not settle for anything less than her complete yielding to her innermost wisdom.

She quit her job and spends as much time as she can making pots. She plans to return to school to study holistic medicine. When I last saw her, the veil of depression that had surrounded her for the previous three years had lifted. She is blossoming into the fullness of her creative self. Her relationship with her parents has never been better. She is making peace with the fact that they may never understand her creative needs, but that doesn't mean she can't have a relationship with them. She also learned that she cannot hold them responsible for the years when she chose to curtail her creativity. She regards her ovarian message as a "kick in the pants" that she really needed. She is grateful.

Ovarian Cancer

Many American gynecologists are trained to remove the ovaries after the age of forty if a woman has pelvic surgery of any kind. The reason for this is to prevent ovarian cancer. Yet ovarian cancer affects only one in eighty women in the United States. This means that scores of women throughout the country are having normal organs removed to "prevent" a condition that will actually affect very few of them. Thousands will be deprived of the essential benefits that these hormone-producing organs provide. In fact, premature removal of the ovaries is associated with increased risk for osteoporosis and heart disease, as well as a host of menopausal symptoms, including decreased skin thickness, which results in a more aged appearance and possible increased susceptibility to bruising and injury.[11]

Medicine in this culture, however, focuses on ovarian removal for its potential cancer prevention benefits and downplays any adverse factors possibly associated with it. Removal of the ovaries to prevent ovarian cancer is based on the assumptions that (1) "prophylactic" removal of the ovaries during hysterectomy is associated with lower incidence of ovarian cancer, and (2) a woman's own hormones can be easily replaced with hormone medication. But studies have shown that assumption 1 is not always true.[12] In the absence of ovarian disease, the ovaries are best left in place. Synthetic hormones cannot match the complex mix of androgens, progesterone, and estrogen that the normal ovary produces. When actual drug-taking behavior of patients is considered, given their lapses in taking medication and other erratic factors that impede a drug's absorption and performance, retaining the ovaries results in longer survival.[13]

We need another approach, so that thousands of women's ovaries are not sacrificed to save one or two from getting ovarian cancer. Understanding ovarian wisdom and energy holds the key to this approach. Ovarian cancer may result from the energy of unexpressed rage or resentment, encoded in the second chakra area of the body. A woman may not be consciously aware of this encoding. But this energy may be present in a woman whose mate or boss is always angry with her and who may be otherwise abusive. A woman can be in an abusive partnership with her work, and it may affect the ovaries in the same way. A woman who stays in this type of relationship because of her fear of physical, emotional, or financial abandonment does not believe in her own inner ability to change her circumstances. She is out of touch with her innate power, and sometimes her body will try to get her attention via the ovaries, especially if she feels resentment or anger or blames others for her circumstances. (Remember that the uterus has a more passive energy than the ovaries.)

Though other choices may be available to her, such a woman consciously believes that she is being *forced against her will* to stay in the relationship. She is being controlled unconsciously by the pattern of behavior I discussed in Chapter 4 as the "rape" archetype. If the woman stays in an abusive relationship in which she is continually violated either emotionally or physically, she is, in energy terms, being raped. Neither she nor her abusive partner or abusive work situation recognizes her inherent dignity and inner creative power, and so her dignity too is raped. Such a woman often feels paralyzed by her rage—an energy that, if it were recognized and expressed, could help her create change. Another part of her paralysis is the belief that her job, husband, or other external source has control *over* her. Finally, her emotional wound may not have been validated or witnessed on some level and in some way. Yet in most abusive situations in which women feel powerless, a husband, boss, or other external authority rarely assumes any responsibility for their part in the continued abuse—they too are unable to validate the wounding. To deal with this, women in these situations often blame themselves or absorb their own anger and rage deep within themselves. They are often afraid that if they were to let their feelings be known, they would be abandoned. Such women can begin to listen to their bodies' wisdom, and their inner guidance systems can help them create the changes needed in their lives.

The Golden Handcuff Syndrome

Ovarian cancer is linked epidemiologically with high socio-economic status. Women of higher socioeconomic status often suffer from the "golden handcuff" syndrome—that is, a situation in which a woman is unhappy with her marriage and even despises her husband or job, yet that same husband or job provides her with the financial wherewithal to take expensive vacations, live in a beautiful home, and belong to a fancy country club. Fearing that she would lose all these "benefits" if she left her situation, the woman stays— meanwhile stuffing her emotions into her body and feeling miserable and trapped on some level.

I've seen several women with ovarian cancer whose husbands have accompanied them into my office. The energy of criticism coming from these men has been palpable. I recall feeling suddenly vulnerable, guarded, and defensive in their presence. Though they said nothing, I was sure that they were silently criticizing everything about me and my office. One man shook my hand at the end of the visit without looking at me! When this man and his wife left, I said to my nurse, "How could any woman live with that energy day in and day out? I felt battered simply being in his presence."

There is such a wide variety of types of ovarian cancer that a full discussion of them all is beyond the scope of this book. Basically, ovarian cancer occurs when some kind of ovarian cells begin to grow abnormal tissue. Ovarian cancer can grow very rapidly. Almost every gynecologist I know has had the experience of seeing a woman with a normal pelvic exam who three to six months later had a pelvis full of ovarian cancer that had spread rapidly and widely.

Possible Contributors

Conventional medicine doesn't know what causes ovarian cancer, though epidemiologically it's linked to a high-fat diet and consumption of dairy food. These environmental factors can clog the system, once the energy blockages in the second chakra are already present, and swing the body's cells into disease. Studies have shown that ovarian cancer patients consumed 7 percent more animal fat in the form of butter, whole milk, and red meat than do healthy controls and eat more yogurt, cottage cheese, and ice cream.[14] The higher the socioeconomic status and the richer the food, the higher the rate of ovarian cancer.

Ovarian cancer incidence is known to be highest in those countries with the highest consumption of dairy food (Sweden, Denmark, and Switzerland)[15] and lowest in those countries with low dairy intake (Japan, Hong Kong, and Singapore). Galactose, a sugar produced during the digestion of dairy products, has been associated with ovarian cancer. Cottage cheese and yogurt appear to be the *worst* culprits in the production of this ovarian toxin because in these foods the dairy sugars are "predigested" into galactose as the end product. The body doesn't even need to accomplish this step. Meanwhile, women who are lactose intolerant and therefore cannot tolerate dairy products are at a lower risk for ovarian cancer.

Several studies have linked the most common types of ovarian cancer, known as epithelial cancer, with the use of talcum powder applied either to the external genitalia or to sanitary pads. The talc can migrate into the pelvic cavity via the cervix and vagina, and then out the fallopian tubes.[16] Talc, and possibly other substances, might act as an irritant to the covering of the ovary and thus be a risk factor for ovarian cancer. It has been shown experimentally, for example, that carbon particles applied to the vulvar area can migrate into the pelvic cavity via the pelvic organs in a rather short period of time.[17] Other factors linked to ovarian cancer:

- A variety of toxins, which poison the oocytes (the eggs of the ovary). This may increase a woman's risk of having ovarian cancer.
- Radiation, mumps virus, polycystic hydrocarbons (which are present in cigarette smoke, caffeine, and tannic acid).
- Drugs such as birth control pills that decrease gonadotropin levels. These may block the effect of oocyte toxins on the ovary.[18] This may be why oral contraceptives are associated with decreased ovarian cancer risk.
- Fertility drugs such as Clomid and Pergonal, which increase gonadotropin levels.

Several studies have demonstrated a significant reduction in ovarian cancer risk of up to 37 percent following either tubal ligation or hysterectomy.[19] The explanation for this might be, in part, because after either of these procedures, the passageway from the external genital organs to the inner pelvic cavity is permanently blocked.

What these data suggest is that women who are concerned about ovarian cancer would do well to avoid dairy food consumption, especially yogurt and cottage cheese, after the age of thirty-five, when gonadotropin levels normally tend to rise. Since there are so many other health problems besides ovarian cancer that are associated with dairy food and dietary fat, it is prudent for some women to consider changing their diets *now*. The data do *not* suggest that all women over forty should go on oral contraceptives, since these too have side effects and risks.

Diagnosis

One of the biggest problems with diagnosing ovarian cancer in the early stages is that there are very few symptoms. Vague abdominal complaints such as indigestion are often cited. Unfortunately, a number of other problems can cause such pains too.

OVARIAN CANCER SCREENING. Ovarian cancer is most often diagnosed in the late stages, but by then it is not considered curable. We *still* do not have any well-tested screening methods to diagnose ovarian cancer in the early stages, let alone prevent it. Hundreds of women are now asking for sonogram screening and the blood test known as Ca-125, which checks for tumor antigens—proteins that are shed from the surface of cancer cells. Unfortunately, neither test can give a guaranteed yes-or-no answer to the question: Do I have ovarian cancer?[20] That is the current irony of the situation with ovarian cancer screening.

A high Ca-125 reading in an otherwise normal woman creates a great deal of anxiety and fear. Yet a high reading in itself doesn't necessarily mean ovarian cancer. Endometriosis, fibroids, liver disease, and other unknown factors can also give high readings. No one can guarantee that everything is all right until laparoscopic surgery is performed and the pelvis is explored. This requires general anesthesia. If the laparoscopy fails to show the source of the elevated Ca-125, the woman will still be left with anxiety and fear about where the abnormality is coming from.

At the same time, if a woman's Ca-125 level is normal, it doesn't guarantee that she *doesn't* have ovarian cancer. A percentage of women with ovarian cancer have false negative Ca-125 results. In women who've had their ovaries removed, 10 percent can go on to develop a form of cancer that originates in the peritoneal lining of the pelvis. Although this type of cancer does not originate in the ovary itself, it looks and acts just like ovarian cancer!

Ovarian cancer, a very real dilemma for women and their doctors, requires an entirely different diagnostic approach from the one we have used for the last forty years. As one of our medical center's gyn oncologists (gynecological cancer specialists) recently stated at a conference, "Everything seems to succeed initially, but nothing works long term. Wake me up when it's over." The interface between the immune system, the emotions, nutrition, and genetics in ovarian cancer deserves further exploration in new and creative ways.

Familial Ovarian Cancer

A woman who has a sister, mother, first maternal cousin, maternal aunt, or other first-degree female relative with ovarian cancer has a higher than average risk of getting the disease herself. Familial ovarian cancer was brought to general public awareness by the Gilda Radner story.[21] Some women who have a very strong family history of ovarian cancer (20 to 30 percent chance of getting the disease) opt for prophylactic oophorectomy. Prophylactic removal of the ovaries after childbearing is over is often recommended for these women. Yet even in women who have family histories of ovarian cancer, prophylactic ovarian removal does not necessarily prevent the disease. Even after prophylactic removal, ovarian cancer or cancers indistinguishable from it can still occur from cells in the lining of the pelvic cavity.[22]

I've noticed that women who have seen a close friend die of ovarian cancer are more inclined to have their ovaries removed because of fear. Though this might be unscientific, I find that most of our lives' major decisions are based on our emotional realities and not on statistics.

Whenever a disease runs in families, we need to realize that we're not dealing solely with a simple matter of genetics. Attitudes also run in families. It would be very interesting to study only those females, in families with a history of ovarian cancer, who did *not* get the disease. Most likely, these would be the women who have broken the family mold and left their tribe, on both an energetic level and a physical level.

Oophorectomy During Other Pelvic Surgery

When a woman chooses to have a hysterectomy, to remove a fibroid uterus or undergo surgery for any other benign condition, she must also decide whether to remove the ovaries too. I ask each individual woman before surgery how high her fear level of ovarian cancer is, and I ask her to check out how she feels about her ovaries. I tell her that we can't always discern the condition of the ovaries until we're in the operating room. If we find that there's a problem at that time, I say, they may need to be removed.

If the patient decides to preserve the ovaries, she still knows that she will defer to my judgment during surgery if the ovaries look abnormal. My patients know that I tend to be "ovary friendly." Occasionally, I work with a woman who wants to be awake during surgery so that we can discuss this decision at the time. That's fine with me. I refuse to make a decision for a patient about what she should do with her ovaries. There are many factors, conscious and unconscious, that come into play when each of us makes major decisions about our bodies.

As you might imagine, most of my patients choose to keep their ovaries during hysterectomy because they—like me—value their female organs. Though my training led me to believe that ovaries should be removed as early as age thirty-five, I'm past that age now, and I value my ovaries as parts of my body that will continue to function and support me as long as I live. I know that they are part of my inner guidance system and that they will let me know if adjustments are required for their health.

Most gynecologists train in large university centers that, because of their specialty nature, treat more women with ovarian cancer in a week than the average practicing gynecologist sees in a decade. Thus, gynecologists tend to see more ovarian cancer in their training years than they ever see again. This creates a biased attitude against the ovaries. An ovarian cancer death is difficult to watch and difficult to treat. It can be associated with pain, recurrent bowel obstruction, huge amounts of fluid collecting in the abdomen, and a variety of other extremely uncomfortable sequelae. A doctor who has seen someone die of ovarian cancer is apt to be prejudiced in his or her relationship to ovaries from that point on, even though the vast majority of women will *not* get ovarian cancer.

One of the hospitals in which I work is the major referral center for our state. The gyn oncologists there see a lot of ovarian cancer. One of our pathologists said recently, "I'm scared to death of ovarian cancer. I'm having my wife have her ovaries removed when she's forty, and I even think she should have her breasts removed prophylactically." He was not completely serious about this recommendation, but this physician spends his days doing autopsies on women from all over the Northeast who have died of breast and ovarian cancer. He sees the devastation of these diseases as a daily part of his work. He cuts into huge tumors and receives surgical specimens in which a woman's uterus, tubes, ovaries, and even vaginas, bladders, and rectums, have been replaced by tumor. He sees the devastation of breast tumors that have eroded into the chest wall. It is little wonder that he feels the way he does, and it is no wonder that routine ovarian removal is advocated so strongly!

Conventional Treatment

There has been no appreciable reduction in mortality rates from ovarian cancer in the last forty years. It is a difficult disease to treat. Conventional treatment is surgical, sometimes followed by chemotherapy and radiation, depending upon how far it has spread. The diagnosis itself is usually made definitively at the time of surgery for some kind of pelvic growth. Without looking into the abdomen and taking a biopsy, there is no way to tell whether an ovarian growth is benign or malignant.

If an ovarian growth is malignant, treatment usually consists of removing the ovaries, tubes, uterus, omentum (the apron of fat covering the bowel), and any tumor that has spread into the pelvis. There are a few exceptions to this that are beyond the scope of this book. In the very early stages, surgery can be curative.

Women's Stories

One of my patients who died of ovarian cancer healed her life and her emotional issues more in her last month of life than in all her prior years. She had gone through extensive surgery and had also followed a dietary approach to her problem. She had done all the "right" things. But still her tumors grew. A physical cure was not part of her healing, though her healing came in the course of her search for a physical cure.

A doctor friend of mine who was working with her for her pain took her through a process of meditation during deep relaxation in which he asked her body to tell him what was feeding her tumors. She replied, "Fear and sadness." He then asked her to remember and reexperience a time when she did not have this fear and sadness. She went back to a time when she was a twelve-week fetus in her mother's uterus. Her mother had tried to abort her with a red and white pill. In her final days she was able to bring this information to consciousness and share it with her mother, who herself was in need of healing around this incident from many years before. My patient died in her mother's arms, free of pain, and finally free from a lifelong burden.

Caring for Your Uterus and Ovaries, or Pelvic Space

• Know that the inherent creativity symbolized by your ovaries is always present for you, regardless of whether they are still physically present in your body.

• Is there a creative endeavor that makes time stand still for you? Is there some activity or process in which you can immerse yourself and forget to eat? What is it?

• Make time each day to do something of creative value that has meaning for you. Let it come through you.

• Do any of your past creations have a life of their own? Can you celebrate being the woman who gave birth to them and then let them go? Are you still hanging on and trying to control anything you've created?

• Your creative power is sorely needed in the outer world now. This power can serve you and others very well when you access it fully and don't try to control or force it. Acknowledge your ovarian power—your female balls.

EIGHT

Reclaiming the Erotic

When I speak of the erotic, I speak of it as an assertion of the lifeforce of women; of that creative energy empowered, the knowledge and use of which we are now reclaiming in our language, our history, our dancing, our loving, our work, our lives.
—Audre Lorde

We Are Sexual Beings

Our culture associates sexuality with genitalia, even though the expression of sexuality involves much more than that. Humans are the only primates whose sexual desire and functioning are not necessarily related to the reproductive cycle. Women's sexuality is involved in giving and receiving sexual pleasure, as well as reproduction. In fact, the clitoris is the only human organ whose sole function is to generate sexual pleasure. Women's experience of sexuality is not determined by our genitalia; nor is it limited to the external genitalia, any more than male sexuality is defined solely by the penis.

Sexuality is an organic, normal, physical, and emotional function of human life. Women's vaginas have a cyclic sexual response of lubrication about every fifteen minutes throughout the sleep cycle, while men get erections. During sexual arousal the female clitoris is engorged with blood and becomes very sensitive, the vagina elongates, and the innermost third of the vagina balloons out, lifting the uterus and cervix. If intercourse occurs after full female sexual response, this changed shape in the vagina helps bring sperm to the cervix, facilitating conception.

Some women experience pain during intercourse if penetration occurs before their arousal has been sufficient to lift and move the uterus and cervix out of the way. In these cases, the ovaries may be hit during repeated thrusting, resulting in pain. This generally doesn't occur when a couple allows enough time for full female sexual arousal prior to actual intercourse.

During sexual arousal, the vagina produces lubrication from a number of sources. The glands (Bartholin's and Skene's glands) at the junction of the vulva and the vaginal opening (the introitus) secrete fluid. The walls of the vagina itself produce a fluid known as a transudate during sexual stimulation. Some women experience a gush of fluid from their vaginas during orgasm, called female ejaculate. The female ejaculate is actually made up of different fluids from different parts of the urogenital system, including a female "prostatic" gland.[1] In tantric yoga, an ancient Eastern practice that combines sexuality and spirituality, this fluid is called the *amrita*, or divine nectar.[2] A number of my patients mistake this female ejaculation for loss of urine at the time of orgasm, but this fluid is not urine, even though it does come in part through the urethra. This fluid release, which may amount to a cupful or more at a time and may occur more than once during lovemaking, is a normal component of female sexual response. Knowing its true nature is very reassuring for women.

Caroline and Charles Muir, experts on tantric sexuality, say that this nectar is often produced once an area deep inside the vagina, known as the "sacred spot,"[3] is activated (usually through gentle and compassionate lovemaking), though direct stimulation of this spot is not always necessary for production. Release of the *amrita* may occur even without an orgasm, such as when a woman "loses it" during laughter, joy, or love. In such a case, the woman is not "losing it"—she is actually *becoming* the energy of joy or love and, far from losing anything, is *gaining* the essence of these ecstatic feelings.[4] Though every woman has the potential for experiencing this outpouring of her divine nectar, she can do so only by learning to surrender herself to deep happiness—which may or may not be sexual.

The Muirs teach that the "sacred spot," deep inside the vagina and well hidden, is often the place where women store all their personal hurts and pain about sexuality. For many women, arousal of this spot for the first few times is often associated with pain or unpleasant memories. A woman and her partner who understand this will proceed slowly with their lovemaking and persevere, and the pain will begin to heal on all levels. Healing in this way can awaken a woman to joy that she has never before known.

Elizabeth, a forty-seven-year-old accountant who is beginning to go through menopause, recently came in for a check-up. "Over Thanksgiving vacation, I met a wonderful man through a mutual friend," she said. "We were immediately attracted to each other and began a relationship. When he made love to me for the first time, it was such a beautiful thing. But at one point, when he was stimulating me deep in my vagina, I had a flashback to my sexual abuse. I began to shake and to cry. I couldn't seem to help it, and I was worried that he'd think he'd done something wrong. But he just held me and told me that everything was all right and that he was there for me. Now when we make love, I still sometimes find myself getting upset, but it doesn't last nearly as long and I feel safer each time. My pleasure also increases. I had no idea that being with a man could be this wonderful. He was gentle and caring and took his time. I am so grateful."

Regardless of where a woman begins to reclaim and explore her sexuality, it's helpful to know that female sexuality, by its very nature, is a total sensory experience involving the whole body (not just the genitals). A woman's sexuality may include actual genital contact with someone, or it may not. She does *not* need a partner or a significant one-to-one relationship to be in touch with her sexuality. She may not even require orgasm or physical touching. Each woman's bodily wisdom dictates what is right for her sexually. In today's society the prevalence of sex and relationship addiction, the lack of self-esteem, and the fear of abandonment all seem to impede women's ability to listen to their body's wisdom and messages. Sometimes what a woman desires sexually may be far removed from what our culture considers normal for women—it may even mimic what is considered culturally normal for a man.

The functioning of our sexual organs and our sexual response is determined in large part by our cultural conditioning concerning sexuality. To understand female sexual response and the workings of the organs involved in it, we must also understand women's cultural inheritance. In this society, sexuality is closely linked with body image and self-esteem. There's a saying, "Men and women will never be equal until a woman can be bald and have a pot belly and still be considered good-looking." Women are brought up to feel that they deserve sexual pleasure only if they look a certain way or weigh a certain amount. Not only that, women are taught that female sexuality and procreation are two distinct things—though one may lead to the other. There is reason to believe that in ancient prepatriarchal times, women knew how to control their fertility naturally and understood the importance of sexual pleasure as a natural part of human experience. Many couples who follow natural family planning as a method of birth control become acutely attuned to each other's fertility and sexual cycles. Not only does this method afford them the means to plan or avoid conception when they desire, they often find that their intimacy and pleasure increases as well.

The culture also believes in the "big bang" theory of heterosexual pleasure, which holds that the thrusting of the penis into the vagina is the most pleasurable part of sexuality. Though this is true for some women, it is not true for others. It's only one aspect of sexuality and pleasure, and women who do not enjoy it need not feel abnormal in any way. For many women, penis-in-vagina intercourse—the kind that we're taught is the "real" thing—is not particularly satisfying. Therefore, many women "fake" orgasm to make their male partners feel that they are "good" lovers.

In her 1980 survey of 486 women, Nora Hayden found the following:

- 310 said they faked orgasm every time they had intercourse.
- 124 said they faked orgasm most of the time they had intercourse.
- 52 said they faked orgasm some of the time they had intercourse.[5]

Obviously, the big bang doesn't work for many women. Recent

research demonstrates that clitoral, vaginal, and uterine stimulation, or a combination of these, leads to orgasm.[6] Many women reach orgasm through means other than intercourse.

It is not uncommon for *frequency of intercourse* to be the sole measure by which the quality of a sexual relationship is judged— especially in medical circles.[7] It is clear, however, that many other factors determine actual relationship quality besides the number of times per week that a couple has intercourse.

Nor is the quality of a person's sex life determined by the number of sexual partners he or she has or has had. An unhealthy, potentially destructive sex life is one in which a woman bases her sexual relationships on working out her emotional needs using another person's body. Some women medicate their fears of loneliness and abandonment by having sex with people they do not love or respect, using sex addictively. Women in these unhealthy sexual relationships often had childhoods associated with sexual abuse, either subtle or blatant.

The cultural imperative that judges a woman's worth by her attachment to a man and by her sexual attractiveness to men—all men—runs very deep. Far too many women have internalized the culturally sanctioned sexual habits and needs of men as their own, when in fact male sexuality and sexual needs are probably more different and varied than we've all been led to believe.[8] Even in lesbian relationships, a woman's partner or whom she is sleeping with can be used to define a woman's worth. One of my lesbian friends told me that because of her engineering degree, she is considered a "good catch" and "good income potential." In the lesbian community in her western city, she says, there is a phrase, "You are who you sleep with."

Clearly many women believe that it is their duty to fulfill their partner's sexual desires and frequently ignore their own erotic needs. They may engage in sexual behavior from which they receive very little more than an unwanted pregnancy and/or various diseases. In November 1991, when the news came out that Magic Johnson had AIDS, an article in *Time* magazine pointed out, "Sex and sports have almost become synonymous." The article reported that "Wilt Chamberlain boasts having slept with 20,000 women—an average of 1.4 per day—for 40 years." It quoted another basketball player: "After I arrived in L.A. in 1979, I did my best to accommodate as many women as I could—most of them through unprotected sex."[9]

In wondering what kind of woman would have a one-night stand with a man—even one who is famous—the article informed us that "for women, many of whom don't have meaningful work, the only way to identify themselves is to say whom they have slept with."[10] In their own eyes, these women weren't *nobody* any longer: They had had sex with a sports star. Even though this man didn't care for them at all or even remember them, they had achieved some perverse kind of status by letting their bodies be used in this way.

Men may exert a very strong influence over women's contraceptive practices and childbearing choices. A Planned Parenthood project in Chicago in the late 1970s aimed at educating men about birth control and teaching them to take responsibility for their sexual behavior. This project surveyed over one thousand men ages fifteen to nineteen.

- The men were asked whether they agreed with the statement: "It's okay to tell a girl you love her so that you can have sex with her." Seven out of ten agreed that it was okay.
- The men were asked to agree or disagree with the statement: "A guy should use birth control whenever possible." Eight out of ten disagreed and said that the guy should not use it.
- The men were asked to agree or disagree with the statement: "If I got a girl pregnant, I would want her to have an abortion." Nearly nine out of ten said no, they would not want her to have an abortion, because it is wrong.

In other words, in this study it was morally acceptable for a man to lie to a girl to obtain sex and to be irresponsible about contraception, but it was immoral for her to have an abortion.[11]

Many women are so invested in their sexual relationship at the expense of themselves that they repeatedly put themselves at risk for pregnancy or sexually transmitted diseases rather than jeopardize the relationship. A teenage girl wrote a letter to Ann Landers in which she complained that all her boyfriend wanted to do was have sex. He barely even talked to her anymore, and they no longer did much of anything together except have sex. She was afraid to say anything to him, however, for fear of losing him!

I lectured at a local private high school several years ago on prochoice issues. Afterward, several young men came up to me and told me that the girls they were having sex with didn't even ask them to use condoms—in fact, they had even told these boys, "It's okay—you don't have to use anything." These girls (they were upper-middle-class, mostly white students at a private school) perceived discussing contraception with their boyfriends as putting their social worth at stake. Women have been socialized for centuries to put their physical bodies at risk in order to sustain interpersonal relationships that really don't support them or their well-being.

Women who have experienced rape and incest have even greater trouble than nonabused women in establishing fulfilling sexual relationships that are free of abusive elements and victimized behavior. Many of these women have never had a sexual encounter that was supportive and pleasurable.

Patricia Reis, a therapist who worked at our office for a number of years, counseled one of my patients, Jane, for several years concerning her chronic vaginitis. Reis learned that Jane's husband liked oral sex a great deal and rented numerous pornographic movies to try to stimulate her to perform oral sex. Jane had been raped as a teenager. During the rape she had had to perform oral sex on her assailant. She recalls that the odor and the trauma of the event were so bad that the thought of oral sex had disgusted her ever since. Fortunately for her, after two years of therapy she was finally able to tell her husband firmly that oral sex was not something she could cooperate with willingly at that point. She had felt used by him sexually for years and needed to distance herself from this kind of sex for a while and reestablish comfort with her own sexual desires before she would be ready to consider the possibility of lovingly providing oral sex.

Whenever people use sex to diminish, control, or harm others, it does not contribute to the health of either participant. Women who were brought up in the 1950s or even the 1980s know well the controlling attitudes and negative effects of certain religions on female sexuality. As I write this, the newspaper headlines are full of stories about priests who have routinely sexually abused children for years. The tenets of the Roman Catholic and other Christian churches degrade sexuality—a normal human function—and subordinate it to reproduction. The consequences of such repression are seen in the problems women have in expressing their sexuality as well as in the sexual deviancy of some church representatives.

Most Western religions seldom perceive female sexuality and motherhood as component parts of the same whole.[12] Christian churches have, for instance, a very long history of separating motherhood and sexuality, resulting in a virgin/whore split in our psyches that has caused much distress for many women. Barbara Walker, who has researched this history and its purpose extensively, writes, "The impossible virgin mother was everyman's longed-for resolution of Oedipal conflicts: pure maternity, never distracted from her devotion by sexual desires. . . . Theologians severed the two halves of the pagan Goddess whose femininity combined abundant sexuality *and* maternity. One half was labeled harlot and temptress, the other a mother devoid of human or female needs. Churchmen often still present the doctrine of the virgin birth as 'ennobling' to women, since they view women's natural sexuality as reprehensible and in need of control." Elizabeth Cady Stanton, one of the most famous early feminists, wrote the following at the end of the nineteenth century: "I think the doctrine of the Virgin birth as something higher, sweeter, nobler than ordinary motherhood, is a slur on all the natural motherhood of the world. . . . Out of this doctrine, and that which is akin to it, have sprung all the monasteries and nuns of the world, which have disgraced and distorted and demoralized manhood and womanhood for a thousand years. I place beside this false, monkish, unnatural claim . . . my mother, who was as holy in her motherhood as was Mary herself."[13]

Finding Our True Sexuality

Our task as women is to distinguish our own personal truth about our sexuality from the distortions that we've inherited from the culture. Our first step in defining our sexuality from the inside out is to consider ourselves as sex *subjects* rather than sex *objects*. What makes up your sexuality? Which of your ideas have you inherited from society and absorbed into your psyche and which are your own? When we reclaim our own sexuality, we find that it doesn't look anything like what the culture has led us to believe. How many women, for example, are really ready for physical lovemaking at the end of a day of work, just before they go to sleep? I've seen countless women in my practice who feel that something must be wrong with them because they don't want to have sex at night. I rarely do. For me, afternoons are much better. (I'll admit, it can take some planning.)

Frankly, nothing kills the libido faster than a day of work, then coming home to do housework, then cleaning up after dinner and doing the other attendant family tasks. For most women, their desire to make love is directly related to the quality of their connection with their partner. Ideas are sexy for women and men alike because sex is a form of nonverbal communication—good communication and good sex are directly linked. And you can't do it well or be fully engaged in it, mind and body—and you probably shouldn't—when you are exhausted.

Everything a woman's partner said or didn't say during the day affects her desire to be sexual with that person. For both men and women, attentiveness and tenderness *are part* of lovemaking, whether or not intercourse happens. So many women have asked me, "Why can't I kiss or hug my partner without it always having to lead to the bedroom?" Tragically, too many men have learned to separate sexual functioning from the other aspects of the relationship. Too many take a caress or a hug as a signal that it's time to have sex. I'd like to see the concept of "making love" extended way beyond simply genital contact.

Both men and women should make love and have sexual contact with each other when it feels right to them and not because of the need to please, to be liked, or to have power over someone. The original meaning of the word *virgin* had nothing to do with sexuality. It referred instead to a woman who was whole and complete unto herself, belonging to no man.[14] Many people would do well to reestablish their virginity. Fortunately, celibacy and virginity are being endorsed and increasingly practiced by a lot of young people now.

If a woman believes that it is her duty as a wife to have sex with her husband even when she's tired or doesn't want to, simply

234

complying with his needs while ignoring her own, she is not creating health in her life or following her own inner guidance. Some women watch and enjoy the occasional "dirty" movie and learn about sex that way; they feel that this is part of their sexual freedom. Other women who enjoy sex fully find that watching "porno" movies diminishes their sexual desire completely. They feel degraded by the way in which sex is portrayed there. One of my lesbian patients, who was in a new relationship and had always enjoyed a healthy and robust sex life, was asked by her new lover to make love while watching a pornographic movie. My patient was open to trying this new experience, but she found that her body was revolted both by the movie and by the entire evening's activities. There is no wrong or right in such a situation. A woman will need to let her body decide.

Women's Sexuality and Nature

For many women, myself included, sexuality is profoundly connected to nature. One of my friends recalls that when she went out the door of her church one Sunday morning last spring, the warm, earthy smell of a newly plowed field nearby awakened her senses. She recalled the combination of the smell and the sunshine as very erotic.[15] This makes sense—the brain pathways for the sense of smell are very close to those associated with arousal and sexuality. Another woman, a lesbian, says that she always thinks of the Grand Canyon when she's making love. A third describes swimming with dolphins as the most erotic experience of her life.[16] Sunbathing is also associated with sexual arousal for many men and women. In ancient Greece, men used to run on the beach naked to expose their testicles to the sun. Modern studies have shown that this increases their testosterone level. It is likely that in women sunlight increases the level of androgen, the testosterone-like hormone associated with sexual desire.

The ocean and waves are erotic images for many people. Before patriarchal societies became dominant, fertility, sexuality, and nature were celebrated together as aspects of the same energy and the same phenomena. The pagan festival of Beltane in the spring celebrated human sexuality and the earth's fertility at the same time.

(This festival is beautifully described in the book *The Mists of Avalon* by Marion Zimmer Bradley.) Most of the Christian holidays were originally Earth-based festivals, celebrating the cycles of Earth's fertility. To women who live in cities or other places where their contact with the natural world is minimal, the subtle erotic forces connected with the earth are not perceptible. Barraged by artificial light and noise for much of the day, they are prevented from tuning in to the smells, rhythms, and feeling of the natural Earth.

Ancient Taoist practices, still taught today, view sexual energy as life-energy. When it is consciously directed during meditation, this energy can help rebuild organs within the body. Sexual energy is one of our most powerful energies for creating health. By using sexual energy consciously, whether we are in a relationship or not, we can tap into a true source of youth and vitality. Using certain techniques combined with loving and conscious intent, we can learn to direct orgasm upward through the body so that every organ benefits from this rejuvenating experience, not just the genitals.[17]

Although it takes time to learn these techniques, every woman's health can benefit from developing a strong pubococcygeous (PC) muscle, the major muscle of contraction during female orgasm. Women who have healthy, strong pelvic muscles are less prone to vaginal problems and urinary stress incontinence, and they tend to have more fulfilling sexual functioning. To find out where your PC muscle is, simply stop the flow of urine voluntarily next time you go to the bathroom. The muscle that you must contract in order to do this is the PC muscle. Another way to find it is to put two fingers in your vagina and open them slightly. Now squeeze your PC muscle enough to close your fingers. Notice that although the abdominal and anal sphincter muscles may contract at the same time, it is the PC muscle that stops the flow of urine and closes off the vagina as well.

You must learn to tell the difference between the PC muscle and the others. Kegel's exercises were developed by a Dr. Kegel as a way to strengthen the pelvic floor and alleviate urinary stress incontinence. When done properly, Kegel-type exercises are 90 percent effective in alleviating mild urinary stress incontinence. But to do them properly, women must learn how to contract the PC muscle itself. Many women fail to strengthen their PC muscle when they do Kegel's exercises because they contract only the abdominal muscles and not the PC muscle. Notice that to engage the PC muscle, you must contract the band of muscles that circle the vagina. To strengthen this muscle, practice contracting it regularly. Here's how: Stop your flow of urination two to three times every time you urinate. As the muscle strengthens, you will be able to distinguish it from the other muscles that also contract when you do this. Three times per day, contract your PC muscle and hold for a count of three. Gradually work up to holding for a count of ten, doing five to ten total repetitions of ten counts. You will definitely notice a difference within one month.

Weighted vaginal cones, known as Femina cones,[18] can be inserted into the vagina and held there as a way to strengthen the pelvic floor muscles. These cones are an updated version of the obsidian eggs with graduated weights that have been used in Taoist practice for centuries.[19] The main muscle required to hold a cone in the vagina is the PC muscle. When a woman uses the cone, she doesn't have to think consciously about holding the "right" muscle. Her body does it automatically for as long as she has the cone in her vagina. I have recommended the use of these cones as a very effective pelvic floor exercise for over two years. My patients and I have been very pleased with the results.

The human experiences that cause us the greatest ecstasy and the greatest pain are sex, love, and religion. One reason that they cause so much pain is that we have not culturally allowed ourselves to fully experience the natural joy and pleasure available to us from them. It is natural for humans to seek out joy and pleasure. Given the nature of our society, however, it is little wonder that we've been taught to search for their intensity through drugs or even addictive sexual practices.

Sexual energy, or eros, is life-force that permeates all of creation and is part of the joyfulness of life creation. It is exactly the opposite of thanatos—the force leading to death. For too long, our culture has dwelt on thanatos, without a balance from eros. It has taught us to fear, denigrate, and suppress our own eroticism, when we should be allowing its natural expression to live fully and healthfully.

It is important to understand that the human capacity for ecstasy is a normal part of who we are and that the ecstatic sensual experi-

ence can be a spiritual one. We can experience the uplifting ecstatic
energy through art, through intense feelings of love, and during the
act of creating from deep within ourselves. Even during mystical
experiences, such as those we feel in religious worship or meditation, we partake of an ecstatic energy that can be erotic in nature.
Only by recognizing that ecstasy and spirituality are part of human
nature can we generate ways to provide experiences of ecstasy and
connection with one another that are nondestructive and nonaddic-
tive. We must feed our souls as well as our bodies.

Women's Stories

Once we have named the societal inheritance that no longer serves
us, we must let go of thoughts and behavior that are not in our best
interest. For many women, this is a lifelong process. The following
is the story of a patient who discovered that her sexuality had been
influenced adversely even in her mother's womb.

ELAINE: OLD MEMORIES LOCKED INSIDE. Elaine first came to see
me when she was in her early thirties. She had a very long history of
pelvic pain, particularly in the vaginal area. For her entire adult life
she'd had painful intercourse (dyspareunia). Several treatments that
she had undergone to remove the painful areas of tissue in the vagina
had been unsuccessful.

Standard medical care, a macrobiotic diet, and the practice of
yoga improved Elaine's health a great deal but provided her with
little relief from the pain. She divorced her husband simply because
they didn't get along. After a few years she found herself in a new
relationship, but she would have urinary tract infections and
outbreaks of herpes when the relationship became sexual. She came
in to my office very upset, saying, "I don't know what's happening.
And if I don't know what's happening to me, I can't fix it. I don't
even know what to eat. Am I too acid or too alkaline? Have I had
too much juice? When am I going to have a healthy sex life? When
will I feel normal in this area?" And on and on her intellect went,
circling, circling, obsessing, and obsessing.

I asked Elaine to stay with the despair she was feeling and not
instantly jump to the what-should-I-do-to-fix-it mode. She had
already been on medication for the urinary tract infection and the

herpes; over the next few weeks, she let herself feel the depth of her despair completely. Then she remembered being *in utero* when her mother was pregnant with her. (No technique, meditation, or therapy was required for her body to give her this information. It arose spontaneously, as it often does when a woman is ready to hear it.) She remembered the feeling of her father's penis against the amniotic sac. She felt clearly and viscerally her mother's disgust and "just get this over with" indifference. Elaine told me, "I feel as though I inherited my mother's sexual revulsion before I was born."

Within a few days of this memory and allowing herself to experience the accompanying emotions, Elaine's pelvic pain and vaginal pain with intercourse gradually lessened for months. Both of us were encouraged. Unfortunately, however, she is not yet pain free. Though she uncovered a very significant body memory concerning her sexuality, she has yet to change and heal the sexual memories and programming so deeply encoded in her body. Each person's timing for this process is different. For some, years of releasing and change are necessary. For others, the process is shorter. Each woman must learn to respect her body's healing process and timing.

Only when we are in touch with our sexuality on our own terms can we hope to share it with someone else in a meaningful relationship. A wise woman once said to me, "If you can't give *yourself* the tenderness, the love, and the caresses that you want another to provide for you, you'll never find them anywhere else." This statement is so true. I have seen it happen many times with my own patients—as soon as a woman learns to provide these things to herself and for herself, her personal life and her relationships almost invariably improve.[20]

KAREN: HEALER IN CELIBACY. Karen was thirty-five when she first came to see me, with a history of having difficulty reaching orgasm. Her pelvic exam was completely normal. While she was a child and teenager, her father, a very successful businessman, had rarely been home. Like so many women, Karen grew up without the affirmative physical presence of a loving father. She told me that she had come to associate the notion of a "loving relationship from a man" with "emotional and physical distance." She had found herself in several consecutive relationships with men who traveled a great deal and often canceled dates with her at the last minute. Each time this happened, she felt emotionally abandoned and angry that she could never count on them. Finally she went to a "Living in Process" intensive with a trainee of Anne Wilson Schaef's and began to name and confront her own part in attracting addictive relationships.

"Looking back," Karen said later, "it's no wonder that I was never able to experience any sexual pleasure when I made love. A part of me always held back—not able to surrender to the experience. Though I had sex, I faked liking it and only did it to please my partner at the time. Opening myself up to the possibility of feeling real love and passion would mean having to feel the same things that I had felt as a little girl—disappointment, vulnerability, and a sense of abandonment from the first male relationship in my life. I wasn't conscious of any of this, of course. But after hitting the despair I felt about my continual bad relationships, I knew I needed help. At the intensive, I went through several deep processes in which I felt what it was that I had been running from all of my life—the pain and despair of my childhood. Now I am in recovery, going to twelve-step meetings, and I've recently started a friendly, nonsexual relationship with a man who lives nearby and rarely travels. Initially, I wasn't attracted to him. In fact, I found him boring. He never 'hooked' me in the same way as the others had, and so I don't feel the same fascination and obsession for him as I have for others.

"As I live my life one day at a time and pay attention to receiving the small sensual gifts of life, I know that my relationship with myself is healing and that a loving relationship with a man is a possibility. But first I need a loving and sensual relationship with myself. I've decided that a period of celibacy is in order for me now. I feel more alive than I have in years. Every day I notice how good the breeze feels on my face and how loving the warmth of the sun feels on my skin. I go to the beach and watch the waves every chance I get. I pay attention to sunsets and how beautiful the moon looks in the sky. I chart my menstrual cycles and notice that I feel increased sexual desire at ovulation. I am free now to feel it but not to act on it. It is simply part of how I am reclaiming my own bodily, sensual wisdom."

Rethinking Sexuality: Concluding Thoughts

• As women, we need to consider becoming "virgin" again by being true to our deepest selves. We must do and be what is true for us—not to please someone else but because it is our truth.

• We need to acknowledge that we all have access to the life-force—the erotic, ecstatic energy of our being. It is part of being human.

• We need to imagine what our sexuality would be like if we thought of it as holy and sacred, a gift from the same source that created the ocean, the waves, and the stars.

• We, each of us, need to try to reconnect with our sexuality simply as the expression of this creative life-force.

• We need to learn how to experience and then direct our sexual energy (with or without actually having sex) for our greatest possible pleasure and good. Secondarily, we need to imagine how we can use it to benefit other people in our lives as well.

• We need to think about new attitudes toward being sexual. Ask yourself how your emotional and mental health, apart from your physical health, would improve if you were to change your thoughts and actions.

NINE

Vulva, Vagina, and Cervix

"This . . . is dedicated with tenderness and respect to the blameless vulva." *Possessing the Secret of Joy* by Alice Walker, from which this quotation comes, names and bears witness to the extreme suffering of tens of millions of women around the world whose external genitalia have been cut off and who have otherwise been mutilated in girlhood because of the dictates of their patriarchal cultures. This practice still goes on, even in some areas of the United States.

A culture more hospitable to women could appreciate the lower entrance to the female body as simply part of the normal functions of birthing, bleeding, sexuality, and elimination. It is through this area of the body, after all, that every human being must pass to be born on Earth. As the gateway to life, the vagina, vulva, and cervix should be celebrated, not mutilated.

But Western culture considers the vagina "dirty" and defiles it by this attitude. Every function associated with this area of the body— birthing, bleeding, and elimination—is *highly* charged emotionally and psychologically here. Since childhood, most of us have picked up the idea that this part of our body is different from other parts: It is taboo, dirty, and unworthy. Over the years, many patients of all ages and backgrounds have asked me during their pelvic exams, "How can you do this job? It's so disgusting." The most common reason that women douche, moreover, is their mistaken belief, handed down from mother to daughter, that this area of the body is offensive and requires special cleaning. Even though douching is not necessary and may even be harmful, about one-third of all women do it regularly.[1] The promotion and sale of feminine hygiene deodorants and deodorant-impregnated tampons and sanitary pads give women the impression that the vagina in its natural state is unacceptable, that it must be sanitized and deodorized.

Our Cultural Inheritance

The very word *vagina* comes from the Latin *vaina,* meaning the "sheath for a sword"—or the sheath for a penis.[2] Once again, women's bodies are defined only in reference to men. In prehistoric egalitarian societies, vulvas and pubic triangles were frequently drawn or inscribed on cave walls to symbolize a sacred place, a gateway to life. Unfortunately, our own culture distorts language about the vulva and vagina and has inflicted unconscious negative symbols on how we think about this area.

The vagina has long been a source of anxiety for men in male-dominated societies. *Vagina dentata*—the toothed vagina—is a common male fear. Popularized by Freud, it dates back centuries. Scholar Barbara Walker writes that "the *vagina dentata* is the classic symbol of men's fear of sex, expressing the unconscious belief that a woman may eat or castrate her partner through intercourse."[3] Both men and women associate this area of the body with mouth symbolism: The anatomical names of the vulvar parts—*labia majora,* the outer or major lips, and *labia minora,* the minor or inner lips— reflect this conception.

Given our collective history, it is little wonder that the entry points to the female body are associated with problems for so many women. Problems in the vulva, vagina, and cervix are primarily associated with a woman's feelings of violation in her one-on-one relationship with another individual or in her job. A woman who has been in a sexually active love relationship and is rejected may perceive her rejection as a violation, and vulvar or vaginal problems can result. Incest memories, confusion about sexual identity, and guilt feelings about sexuality can also result in repeated episodes of vaginitis.

A woman who has a health problem in the vagina, vulva, or cervix may be involved in a situation in which she is being used sexually without her complete conscious cooperation and consent. Or she may be feeling forced to do something against her consent or to act in a sexual way about which her emotions are divided. In such a situation her body is likely to respond with problems that we associate with sexual violation. These physical problems can appear if, for instance, she is using sex to obtain financial, physical, or emotional security or to manipulate another person, rather than to bring mutual pleasure. Feelings of being used or raped are associated with chronic vaginitis, chronic vulvar pain, recurrent warts, herpes, cervical cancer, and associated abnormal Pap smears (cervical dysplasia).

Chronic vulvar problems such as pain and itching are associated with stress from anxiety and irritation related to being controlled either by a partner or by a situation that in energy terms is equivalent to a partner. An example would be a woman who feels so "married" to a job that totally controls her that, unconsciously, she is not free to experience her life on her own terms. Medical intuitive Caroline Myss suggests that we might think of this external control as a modern-day "chastity belt." A woman's mate may control her either by forcing her to have sex or by withholding sexual activity that she desires.

Ruth came to see me with a history of recurrent vaginitis that did not respond to the usual treatments, such as antifungal creams and antibiotics. Her husband wanted sex every night, and she believed that filling his sexual needs was part of her "job." She did love him, but she was often too tired to make love in the evening. Nevertheless, she forced herself to do it, even as her unconscious resentment grew. Like many women with this problem, Ruth equated having a lot of sex with having a "satisfactory" sex life. At first she denied to me that her sex life had any problems.

The sexual imperative of our culture—that desirable women serve men sexually—is largely what gets women "into trouble" in the first place—in other words, into sexual situations that don't serve their needs and that are in fact harmful. Many women are conflicted between needing to be loved and needing sexual pleasure on the one hand, and wanting to say no to intercourse on the other. Gynecological problems in the vulva, vagina, and cervix are often related to a woman's inability to say no to entry into this area of her body when she wants to but doesn't believe she "should." These problems are quite literally related to allowing herself to "get screwed." One of my patients developed chronic vaginitis, for example, when her college (illegally) refused to award her credit for courses that she had completed. At first, she decided that she had no choice but to accept their mistreatment because she didn't want to "make waves." Despite many external remedies for vulvovaginitis, however, she did not get better until she appealed her college's decision about her credits and then refused to back down. She was eventually awarded the credits due her, and her vaginitis cleared up.

Besides frustration and anger, another emotion that generally tends to affect our health adversely is guilt. When our guilt is centered on our sexuality, it can become associated with problems specific to our entry points. The sexual revolution of the 1960s and 1970s broke down some of our culture's puritanical views about sexuality, but a sexually repressed culture cannot be healed just by taking off its clothes. Now it is even more important for women to be clear about their sexuality and their choice of sexual partners. It is especially important that women consciously use their freedom to understand what their bodies really want and not be led by the blandishments of partners who equate freedom with irresponsible behavior.

Scientific research supports the premise that certain emotional factors are associated with chronic vaginal or cervical problems, including cervical cancer.[4] One study showed that, compared with women with other types of cancer, women with cervical cancer are more likely to have poor sexual adjustment, lower incidence of orgasm during sexual intercourse, and a dislike of sexual intercourse amounting to an actual aversion. They make poorer marital adjustments, as evidenced by the increased incidence of divorce, desertion, or separation.[5] Another study was done on women who had severely abnormal Pap smears that required further evaluation to assess whether the women had progressed to actual cervical cancer. The authors found that they could predict which women had progressed to cervical cancer based on the women's responses to their questions about recent stressful life events. If a husband or boy-friend had been unfaithful, was drinking, or was running around, for example, a woman with cervical cancer would always say something like, "I should have left him, but I couldn't because of the kids" or "I thought he needed me." When responding to the same situation in their own lives, the women without cervical cancer would say, "I can't trust him—he wants more than he gives." In this same study, if a family member got a major illness or died, the women with cervical cancer would say, "I should have worked harder and taken better care of him [or her]." The noncervical cancer patients, on the other hand, were more realistic about the limits of their responsibility to others and about their ability to change the natural course of events.[6]

Most women with chronic vaginal and vulvar problems have had them for years. These problems are usually associated with unexpressed complaints about a situation in their lives that have been accumulating for years. Clinically, it is well known that treating women with chronic vulvar problems is often unsuccessful if the psychological and emotional aspects of the problem are ignored. Unfortunately, many such women have been to scores of doctors, looking in vain for the physical cure for their problem.

In energy terms, a woman sets the stage in her body for chronic vulvar problems when she *lacks the courage to change* the negative aspects of an unhealthy relationship. If she stays in a relationship with someone she doesn't respect or even like because she is afraid to leave—for whatever reason, be it fears about financial or physical insecurity, about being single, or about her own dependence—she is participating in a "prostitute" archetype. If she continues to have sex with someone whom she doesn't respect or love, she is participating in an energy pattern that is associated with chronic vaginal, cervical, or vulvar problems that are documented "prostitute" diseases.

The vulva and the vagina form the outermost points of entry into the female genital system. The cervix and its opening, known as the cervical os (*os* is an anatomical word for "entrance" or "mouth") forms the entryway into the uterus and inner pelvic organs—the tubes and ovaries. (See Figure 6, page 150.)

Anatomy

The vulva comprises the labia majora (outer lips) and labia minora (inner lips). The pubic hair on the vulva forms a protective barrier to the more delicate tissues of the vagina and the cervix. The vulvar skin contains apocrine sweat glands, identical to those under the arms. Apocrine sweat glands differ from regular sweat glands in that their secretions are triggered by emotional situations, not just by physical exertion. The vulva "sweats" more than any other part of the body.

The outer entrance from the vulva to the vagina is known as the *introitus.* The vagina constitutes a passageway to the cervix, which is actually the lowermost part of the uterus (sometimes called the uterine cervix). The cervix protrudes into the uppermost part of the vagina and is covered by the same type of cells as the vaginal lining.

The Pap smear, a screening test for abnormal cervical cells, is taken from the opening in the center of the cervix, where the squamous cell covering (squamous refers to a flattened type of epithelial cell that covers mucous membranes of the body, e.g., inside of vulva, vagina, and mouth) of the outer cervix meets the inside of the cervical canal. This area is known as the *squamocolumnar junction* (SCJ), a very dynamic junction in which endocervical gland cells constantly change through a process known as *squamous metaplasia.* In the SCJ the glands are constantly changing, in part because of the acid environment of the vagina. As a result, the normal mucous secretions from the endocervix sometimes get trapped, causing mucous-filled cysts in the cervix (Nabothian cysts). These feel like little bumps on the cervix and can sometimes grow to one or two centimeters in diameter. Though many women who feel these bumps think they have an abnormality, they are completely normal and don't require treatment.

In some women and most teenagers the SCJ is located way out on the outer part of the cervix, with the inner, redder-appearing cells of the endocervix extending outward onto the cervix. In the past many physicians have confused this normal anatomy with pathology, referring to this normally red glandular area out on the cervix as "cervical erosion" or "chronic cervicitis." Many women have had normal cervical tissue cauterized because of this misunderstanding.

At this time in our history, chronic vaginitis, sexually transmitted diseases such as venereal warts and herpes, and abnormal Pap smears (also considered a sexually transmitted disorder) are virtually epidemic. These disorders can affect the vulva, vagina, and cervix all at the same time. Though these disorders are often blamed on certain viruses that are present in these areas at the same time, *countless women who do not develop symptoms also have these same viruses present in their bodies.*

Gynecologists work right in the middle of women's most secret and painful issues. To be healers, they must recognize that a woman's sexual vulnerability often hovers around her gynecological exam. When a woman is diagnosed with a sexually transmitted disease or has an abnormal Pap smear, all her fears, beliefs, and misconceptions about her sexuality and body may well come up. It's vital for healers to be sensitive to these emotions and try to help their patients articulate their distress and grief, as well as their questions. If you as a patient do not think that your feelings about an exam or diagnosis are being treated with concern, tell your practitioner that your feelings are important to you and that you've learned to respect them as a necessary key to eventually understanding yourself better. Ask her or him for help and compassion during the pelvic exam. Though strong emotions may occur during a pelvic exam, don't expect your practitioner or yourself to know exactly why at the moment they first arise. Simply stay with what you are feeling with the intent to heal the situation. Then relax and allow the healing to come, by turning the situation over to your inner guidance. Eventually when you are ready, you will get the insight you need about the situation.

When I do a pelvic exam, I usually give the woman the option of having the back of the exam table pushed up so that she can watch me the entire time. I carefully explain what I will be doing and why, and I ask her permission before I proceed with each step. I offer her a chance to watch the exam in a mirror if she would like. I move slowly, and I tell her where I will be touching her first. I use the smallest speculum that is adequate. (I keep the speculums on a heating pad so that they are always warm.)

I often teach patients who are nervous about pelvic exams how to relax their pelvic muscles so that the speculum goes in more easily. I first help them identify the PC muscle that contracts the vagina, then have them contract it as hard as they can; then I have them release the contraction. When the contraction is released, they experience the relaxation that will help with the exam. I repeat this exercise several times until they can appreciate the difference between muscle tension and relaxation. When the woman is extremely frightened, I tell her that she can stop me anytime she wants to. This way, she knows that she is in control of the exam. In some cases, both the patient and I decide not to proceed with a pelvic exam on a particular visit, if she is feeling too vulnerable or afraid. We simply talk over her fears, and I offer information and support. When she feels ready, she returns for the exam. I reassure my patient that many women feel uncomfortable about pelvic exams, even if they are not afraid they have a disease, and that she is not alone in her fear or discomfort.

Human Papilloma Virus (HPV)

Human papilloma virus (HPV) is a very common virus that can cause venereal warts and is associated with abnormal Pap smears, or cervical dysplasia. At least 50 percent of the normal adult population and 40 percent of children are estimated to show evidence of HPV infection.[7] The vast majority of women who have been exposed to HPV do not develop any warts or cervical dysplasia. But in others HPV is associated with cervical cancer.

Controversy abounds in the OB/GYN literature as to whether HPV actually *causes* cervical dysplasia or whether the virus and the dysplasia are just in the same place at the same time—that is, in the abnormal cervical tissue. The DNA of HPV (the genetic material of the virus used for identification) has been found in virtually all abnormal Pap smears and cervical cancer cells. However, the majority of women who have been exposed to HPV do *not* get cervical dysplasia. HPV is only a cofactor in cervical dysplasia and so cannot be considered a single cause of it.

It has recently been found that some strains of HPV are more virulent than others.[8] These strains are more commonly implicated in cervical cancer and other severe Pap smear abnormalities. But efforts to determine which women have the most virulent strains of

HPV in order to prevent cervical abnormalities have not proved very effective. That's because even the so-called benign viral strains are sometimes implicated in the growth of abnormal cervical, vaginal, or vulvar tissue. In other cases, the more virulent strains cause no abnormality at all. We don't really know, in a conventional sense, who will develop abnormalities from the virus and who won't, unless we look at the factors that can contribute to decreased immunity. Abnormalities start to grow and cause damage only when the immune system has already been weakened in that area of the body and is unable to maintain the health of the tissue. One study showed that chronic stress and specific attitudes about sex change the blood flow to cervical tissue and affect its secretions. This suggests a link between stress and the subsequent development of disease in this area of the body.[9] Suppression of the immune system from chronic emotional or other stress can lead to changes in immunity that allow increased virus production in the first place. The link between abnormal Pap smears and deficient immune system functioning is well known: Women who have organ transplants and are on drugs that suppress the immune system (such as prednisone) have a much greater chance than normal of developing abnormal Pap smears. They also frequently have recurrent wart and herpes outbreaks. (Emotional reaction to the diagnosis of venereal warts can be similar to that of herpes. If you have concerns about either condition, please read through both sections.)

If our bodies are a hologram in which each part contains the whole (see discussion of this on pp. 25–26), then the HPV virus and the abnormal cells associated with the virus are two interrelated aspects of a greater whole that is not as yet entirely understood. For a variety of reasons, depressed immunity makes it much more likely that any HPV present on the cervix or in the vagina will attack already weakened cells. I think of the HPV virus as an opportunist at the scene, like buzzards around a dying calf. The virus doesn't "cause" cancer any more than the buzzards caused the calf to get sick. But once the calf is sick and dying, the buzzards start to hover. Since most women who have the HPV virus *don't* go on to develop abnormal Pap smears or cervical cancer, most viral activity and infections are halted by good immune functioning.

Symptoms

Classically, women with HPV have painless warty growths (condylomata acuminata) on the outside of the vulva that are painless but can be seen and felt. These can grow and multiply during pregnancy, when the hormones associated with pregnancy stimulate their growth. They often disappear on their own following delivery, when the hormones once again change. Warts can vary in appearance, from plaquelike growths to pointy, spiky lesions. Some women have only a few, while others have many all over the vulva. The virus can also cause warty growths on the tongue, the lips, and in the throat, though these sites are rare. Sometimes a woman has no obvious warts on the vulva but has them in the vagina or on the cervix. She may not be aware of these.

HPV infection is sometimes associated with chronic vulvar pain, chronic vaginitis, and chronic inflammation of the cervix (cervicitis). A vaginal discharge is usually not present, though it can be. Because some women have HPV infection in association with vaginal infections from yeast or the bacteria known as Gardnerella (see page 276), it is not always possible to tell exactly what virus or bacteria is causing what symptom. Unless a woman has actual warty growths on her vulva or has chronic vulvar or vaginal irritation associated with HPV, she won't know that she has it.

Diagnosis

Warty growths on the vulva, vagina, or cervix and abnormal cells on a Pap smear or cervical biopsy are usually associated with HPV. If these appearances are a first occurrence, a biopsy is taken and sent to the lab to confirm the diagnosis. Sometimes HPV is diagnosed by a colposcopy or cervigram, a screening test in which a photograph of the cervix is made after applying dilute acetic acid (vinegar) to the tissue. When vinegar is applied to the vulva, cervix, or vagina, and HPV is present in the tissue, the tissue often turns white. (This tissue is then called acetowhite epithelium, or white skin cells.) Biopsies of the white area often reveal HPV.

Common Concerns About HPV

WHY DO SO MANY WOMEN HAVE IT? HPV has probably always been present in the human genitals. You can certainly find it on old slides of Pap smears from twenty years ago. Back then, HPV simply wasn't recognized or studied as much as it is today. Several factors have contributed to its more frequent diagnosis now. One is the advent of colposcopy, a diagnostic technique developed in the 1970s to evaluate abnormal Pap smears. A colposcopy is an examination of the cervix and vagina through a magnifying lens. It may include biopsies of the vagina or cervix if any abnormal areas show up on exam. (See pp. 261–64 for more details.) As more cervical biopsy specimens were read and cervical abnormalities came to be diagnosed in their earlier stages, pathologists began to recognize the cellular changes associated with HPV more frequently.

The sexual revolution and multiple sexual partners have increased the number of women who have been exposed to the virus. Condoms don't prevent the transmission of HPV because the largest reservoir of the virus in the male is in the scrotum, and transmission is by physical contact. Even if a woman is monogamous, she can be exposed to warts depending upon the number of sexual partners that her partner has had. Factors implicated in HPV leading to abnormal growths include a depressed immune system from suboptimal nutrition, emotionally unhealthy relationships, excess alcohol, and cigarette smoking. Therefore, it's not simply the viruses from our past sexual partners that we bring to our current sexual partners. We also bring our current state of emotional health, which in part determines whether those viruses will become active.

HOW DID I GET THIS? WHO GAVE IT TO ME? This is one of the big questions for most women with the whole issue of HPV infections. The truth is that HPV, like the herpes virus, can be dormant for years! That means theoretically that a virus a woman "caught" in 1967 may not express itself in any visible way until 1992. This also means that whoever "gave" it to her may not have known that he or she had it. I've seen monogamous couples in whom one partner has warts or herpes but the other does not, despite twenty or more years of sexual relations without condoms.

In a culture that believes in "cause and effect," HPV and herpes infections are mind-numbing. These little viruses and their complex interactions with our immune systems dash our illusion of control. Some people are "asymptomatic shedders"—that is, they shed the virus potentially to others without ever knowing that they have it—so no one can be 100 percent sure that they won't give it to another person once they've got it, if they even know.

What this means for women is the following: To the degree that a woman has guilt or self-loathing about her sexuality, she will worry or obsess about herpes and HPV infections to some degree. Countless women, most of them from strict male-dominated religious backgrounds, have gone into massive shame attacks when I made the diagnosis of herpes or warts. Somewhere inside, they believe that people who get herpes or HPV have done something wrong. I have seen many other women with these conditions become paralyzed with guilt and feel they will be tainted forever. They are terrified that they will pass on the germ to someone else. Because they already feel themselves to be unworthy, the herpes or HPV diagnosis pushes their self-esteem even lower. Thus begins a vicious cycle in the body that continues to depress the immune system and that can potentially result in continual outbreaks. Media stories linking HPV and herpes with cervical cancer make their state of mind even worse. Shame combined with fear is a very deadly combination for the immune system. (Later in this chapter, I will give some recommendations for dealing emotionally and mentally with these conditions and for boosting your immune system.)

WILL HPV INTERFERE WITH PREGNANCY? Vulvar warts are often stimulated to grow by the hormones associated with pregnancy. In rare instances, a woman's warts will cause bleeding at the time of delivery, especially if an episiotomy is made through an area of the vulva that is affected by warts. In general, though, warts do not interfere with pregnancy. They often disappear without treatment once a woman has delivered. A woman with HPV can theoretically transmit it to her baby at delivery. Some babies can theoretically get vocal cord papillomas from HPV, which can be treated with surgery. This is very rare, however, and is not a reason to do a cesarean section in a woman with HPV. I have never seen a case of it. The immune system of the baby protects it almost every time.

Treatment

Once a woman has HPV, she has it forever, so treatment is aimed at removing the visible warts and making sure that she isn't growing any of the abnormal or precancerous cells that are sometimes associated with the warts. Once the bulk of a wart is removed, the immune system can deal with and remove the remainder more easily.

It is controversial as to whether it's important for males to get treated for warts. Many doctors downplay the male role in HPV and don't know how to diagnose warts properly. Therefore many men don't know that they have them.[10] The female cervix, as opposed to male penile or scrotal skin, is a unique environment and appears to be more susceptible to viral-associated abnormalities.

LASER TREATMENT. Laser treatment, very popular for warts several years ago, has not lived up to the medical profession's initial expectations. If a physician is highly skilled in the use of laser, it can be a good way to remove persistent warts, but a few studies have even shown that once warts have been "lasered" off the cervix or even the vulva, they come back faster after laser treatment than after other treatments. Perhaps this is because laser vaporizes tissue and spreads the wart virus even further into the surrounding areas. HPV on the mucous membranes of the vagina and cervix can be compared with the virus in the respiratory tract that causes a cold. We would never think of using a laser to denude the surfaces of the trachea and bronchial tree of the cold virus. But using laser to remove warts from the genital tract is really no different—we know that ultimately we can't eradicate the wart virus, any more than we can eradicate the common cold virus. Since there are many different strains of wart virus, as of cold virus, making a vaccine is impractical. I have not been impressed with the effectiveness of this modality over the long term and prefer other treatments.

PODOPHYLLIN. Podophyllin is a chemical resin derived from the May apple. It interferes with cell division and therefore stops genital warts from growing. It can be effective in some people, but it is for use with external warts only, because it can get into surrounding tissues and have toxic effects on tissues whose cell division is normal. Podophyllin is used only on the wart itself and must be washed off within several hours.

Podofilox (Condylox) is a topical 0.5 percent antiviral treatment that a woman can apply herself to external warts after an initial treatment from her health care provider. This convenient treatment may decrease the number of office visits she must make for recurrent warts. This medication is related to podophyllin and is available by prescription.[11]

ACIDS. At our office we use trichloroacetic acid (TCA) to treat warts on the cervix, vagina, and vulva. This acid is very effective but doesn't "cure" the warts—it just burns away the visible ones. This acid must be applied in minute amounts and only to the warty areas themselves because it causes painful burns to healthy tissue. (It also can burn through clothing.) Even on warty areas, it can cause immediate stinging, followed later by ulceration of the skin. If the acid gets on any area other than the wart (and it often does), it takes from one to two weeks for the skin to heal. It also takes about that long for the ulceration of the wart to slough off. The treatment may need to be done more than once.

CRYOCAUTERY. Warts can be frozen with a cryocautery device in the office. Freezing a wart causes it to disappear over a one-to-two-week period. I have found this treatment to be time-consuming and often painful for the patient. I don't use it.

ELECTROCAUTERY. Removal of very large collections of warts is possible using electrocautery. In this treatment the wart is burned off by a heated electrical device. This procedure is usually done under anesthesia in the operating room. We only resort to it when all other methods haven't worked.

LEEP. A relatively new technology, Loop Electrode Excision Procedure (LEEP), also called Large Loop Excision of Transformation Zone (LLETZ), is used to remove warts and wart-affected tissue on the vulva, cervix, and vagina. It removes warts by electrocautery, using an electrically charged wire loop. It is also used to treat cervical dysplasia. We use this technology in our office for treating cervical dysplasias in some cases, but we have not used it to remove benign warty growths. I am very pleased with this technology, however, and I feel that it can be a good treatment.

I've seen all manner of treatments "work" for warts. Warts on the hands, for instance, are known to come off after a variety of treatments ranging from applying cold potato to hypnosis.[12] We just don't know the physical mechanism that is mediated by the immune system that makes warts go away, even after thousands of years of observing that warts *are* responsive to suggestion and folk remedies.

Even though removal of warts doesn't really "cure" anything, it does help the body fight HPV. One reason for this is that treatment reduces the amount of virus that the warty growth sheds. Another reason is that the immune system is enhanced by the feeling that we're "doing something." We live in a very active culture, and Americans want to get things done. When we treat a wart and get rid of it, the patient at some level feels that it's been "taken care of." The immune system gets the message and continues to "take care of it."

NUTRITIONAL APPROACH. At our center, we enhance wart-removal treatment with dietary change, supplements, and education about immune system functioning. Persistent warts are an indicator of immune system depression—that is their message to the body. We tell our patients that the "expression" of the warts is dependent to some degree on how well they take care of themselves. Studies have shown that foods high in antioxidants—such as vitamin C, folic acid, vitamin A, vitamin E, beta carotene, and selenium (or supplements containing these)—help heal and prevent cervical dysplasia.[13] Because of the connection between HPV, cervical dysplasia, and cervical cancer, we recommend that a woman with HPV take a good daily multivitamin containing those supplements and/or a whole-food diet.

ENERGY MEDICINE. Spending time outdoors and doing activity you love will enhance immune system functioning. Of course, none of us has complete control over whether we catch a virus or whether we express it once we have it. Especially in persistent cases of warts or herpes, however, tuning in to oneself with love, forgiveness, good food, and a good multivitamin can work wonders to keep the warts or herpes from showing up again.

Herpes

Herpes is a kind of virus that can cause small, very painful ulcers on the vulva, in the vagina, or on the cervix. Herpes viruses can also cause cold sores. Herpes viruses are divided into several types. Type 1, the kind that causes cold sores, tends to live "above the belt" but can occasionally cause genital infections as well. Type 2 tends to live "below the belt" and is the most common herpes virus associated with genital herpes. Type 2 can occasionally live "above the belt," too, and cause oral infections. Once a person has herpes, he or she has it for life. A herpes virus that is dormant (or latent) resides in the infected tissue around the lips (either genital or oral) or in the spinal nerves.

Symptoms

As with HPV, many women who have been exposed to herpes never get sores and therefore have no reason to suspect that they have the virus. In fact, in one study of women at high risk for sexually transmitted diseases, 47 percent had evidence of the virus on testing, though only one-half of these had ever had any symptoms.[14] When the virus becomes active, however, it causes very characteristic small ulcers on the genital organs. The first episode of herpes outbreak that a person has (known as a primary herpes infection) can be extremely painful, resulting in a fever, systemic illness, swollen lymph nodes in the groin, genital pain, and even an inability to urinate secondary to pain and herpes infection in the bladder or urethra. After a primary herpes outbreak, a person will almost never have symptoms this severe again since the body produces antibodies to the herpes in his or her system.

Subsequent outbreaks are known as secondary herpes. These

usually start with a sensation of tingling in the affected area, prior to the outbreak of an actual sore. Some women will feel pain down their legs as well, because the herpes virus lives in the spinal portion of the nerves that innervate both the genitals and the inner thighs. Emotional factors such as depression, anxiety, or hostility may allow increased production of the herpes virus and subsequent chronic vaginal irritation.[15]

However, herpes tends to "burn itself out" after a number of years. That means that a person may get outbreaks frequently for a year or two, but they usually don't continue. One of my patients had only one outbreak. At the time of this outbreak she had found out her husband was having an affair. She eventually divorced him, is now in another relationship, and has *never* had a recurrence. Her immune system has kept the herpes virus inactive, even though her lifestyle includes behaviors that are often associated with immune system depression, like heavy smoking and the stress of constant dieting. In this woman's case, her immune system in the genital area is keeping her herpes in remission—further evidence that the immunity of our entry points is enhanced when our one-on-one relationships are going well.

Diagnosis

The best way to know if you have herpes is to see an experienced health care practitioner at the time of the actual outbreak. Though herpes ulcers have a characteristic appearance, sometimes chronic yeast infections can produce ulcerated areas of the vulva that look like herpes. Diagnosis is confirmed by taking a culture from an active herpetic sore. Even then, these cultures are often negative because the herpes virus is sometimes difficult to grow in cell culture. A blood test can also be done to see if a woman has antibodies to the herpes virus, but the majority of people already have antibodies to the herpes virus because herpes is so common.

Common Concerns

WHERE DID I GET HERPES? CAN I GIVE IT TO SOMEONE ELSE? The answer to this question is the same as for HPV: The virus can be dormant for years, so a person who has a primary outbreak may have "caught" it twenty or more years ago! I've seen first-time genital herpes outbreaks in eighty-five-year-old women who've been celibate and widowed for twenty years. Women can spread the virus to other areas of their own bodies through what's called *autoinoculation,* by directly touching a herpes sore and then other body parts. That's why it's best to carefully avoid contact with an active herpes sore.

People with herpes cold sores can spread the virus to the genital area through oral sex. Theoretically, anyone who has ever had a cold sore can develop genital herpes sores. Although the oral herpes virus (Type 1) and the genital herpes virus (Type 2) are different and generally grow best either in the oral cavity or in the genital tract respectively, they can sometimes cross-inoculate. Thus, an oral herpes virus sometimes grows in the genital area and vice versa. There is no guarantee that these viruses will stay put.

I have seen monogamous couples in which one member had herpes outbreaks while the other never got it, even though they did not use condoms during their many years of sexual relations. But it is generally recommended that people with herpes do use condoms to cut the risk of infecting someone else.

WILL HERPES INTERFERE WITH PREGNANCY? A great deal of fear and misinformation still abounds about herpes in pregnancy. Herpes does *not* cause problems in pregnancy before delivery, unless the woman's first exposure to it is during the pregnancy itself and the virus reaches high enough levels in the blood (known as viremia). It is very rare for a mother to transmit a herpes infection to the baby during the pregnancy.

The worry for most women is whether they'll need a cesarean section because of an active herpes sore on the vulva, vagina, or cervix at the time of delivery. Delivery by C-section to prevent possible exposure of the baby to the virus from the mother is not uncommon, even though the number of babies with documented herpes infection from their mothers is very, very low. C-section is often done, however, because the few babies who do contract herpes can develop life-threatening infections.

Worrying for an entire pregnancy about having an active herpes sore at the time of labor may, in my view, actually increase the chances of an outbreak. There are some very positive steps to take to prevent this. (See "Treatment.")

Treatment

MEDICATIONS. Acyclovir (Zovirax) is the most widely available antiherpes drug on the market at this time. It comes in both pill and ointment form, and some people have taken it long-term (for two to three years). When taken orally, this antiviral medication works like any antibiotic in the system. Within twenty-four hours of taking the pills, the virus is inactivated. The topical ointment for actual outbreaks takes a bit longer to work. Acyclovir is available only by prescription and is particularly effective in primary (first-time) infections.

Though I prescribe acyclovir to women who want it, I'm concerned that chronic use of it may result in resistant viral strains that will be even stronger and harder to treat than the current ones. This has happened with other disease-causing organisms over the forty years that doctors have been prescribing antibiotics and antivirals. Routinely giving antibiotics when they were not indicated and failing to look at other ways to support the immune system's own ability to fight germs have resulted in our current battle against "superbug" strains of tuberculosis, pneumonia, and staphylococcus. For that reason, I prefer an approach that bolsters a woman's inherent ability to keep the virus under control.

NUTRITIONAL TREATMENT: GARLIC. Garlic is a highly effective remedy for herpes recurrence, and it has no known side effects. It also works for cold sores. Garlic has been shown to have a number of antiviral, antibacterial, and antifungal properties.[16] For women with recurrent herpes, my center recommends the following: When the familiar "tingling" sensation starts, signaling that an outbreak is about to occur, take twelve capsules of deodorized garlic (available in health food stores) immediately to prevent an outbreak.[17] Then take three capsules every four hours while you are awake for the next three days. In almost every case, the herpes outbreak will be prevented. Take the deodorized variety of garlic, to prevent the bad breath that is the only detractor to garlic's use.

For women with a history of herpes who are planning a pregnancy or who are already pregnant, I recommend they take two garlic capsules every day. This can be increased to six to eight capsules per day if they are under more stress than usual. In my clinical experience, women who do this and who increase their garlic capsules under times of stress, don't get herpes outbreaks.

NUTRITIONAL TREATMENT: MELALEUCA OIL. Melaleuca oil, from the Australian tea tree, can be applied directly to the tingling area just prior to a herpes outbreak, either using a Q-tip or your finger. In most cases, this topical treatment will prevent an outbreak.[18]

DIETARY SUPPLEMENTS. Some people take vitamin C or bioflavonoids, while others apply zinc sulfate ointment, vitamin E ointment, or lithium succinate ointment to prevent or treat herpes outbreaks. Still other people use the amino acid lysine to prevent outbreaks. I would recommend these only if garlic and melaleuca fail to prevent an outbreak.

Use of Supplements
- Vitamin C, zinc, and bioflavonoids: 200 mg. of vitamin C and bioflavonoids; 100 mg. of zinc. Each of these is taken three times a day with meals, at the onset of discomfort.
- Lithium, zinc, or vitamin E ointments: These are applied within forty-eight hours of the onset of a herpes sore and are continued four times a day until the sore disappears.[19]
- Lysine/arginine ratio: Some women have very good success in preventing herpes outbreaks by taking the amino acid lysine as a food supplement. Lysine is taken at 400 mg. three times per day. At the same time, the amino acid arginine is restricted in the diet, to maximize the lysine/arginine ratio. This suppresses symptoms and decreases the rate of recurrence. Good foods for increasing dietary lysine are potatoes, brewer's yeast, fish, beans, and eggs. Foods high in arginine which should be avoided are chocolate, peanuts, and

other nuts. If lysine therapy is used, cholesterol levels should be followed, as this therapy may stimulate the liver to manufacture cholesterol.[20]

Cervicitis

True cervicitis is an inflammation of the cervix caused by the same infectious agents that cause vaginitis, such as trichomonas or yeast. Cervicitis and vaginitis are usually present at the same time, and treatment for them is the same. (See "Vaginitis," page 275.)

In some women, the mucus-secreting cells of the endocervix sometimes extend out onto the outer cervix (the exocervix). This is a normal anatomical variation and is not true cervicitis. Though these women sometimes experience a bit more vaginal discharge than usual, this only rarely requires treatment. In cases in which the discharge is truly a problem, cryocautery (freezing) of the cervix or LEEP cautery can be done. (See pages 254 and 255.)

Cervical Dysplasia (Abnormal Pap Smears)

Cervical dysplasia is the name given to cellular abnormalities that arise in the endocervical canal or on the cervix itself: *dysplasia* simply means "abnormal." A Pap smear shows when the cells of the cervix are abnormal, and the cells are classified according to nationally agreed-upon standards. The terminology used to classify these abnormalities is cervical intraepithelial neoplasia (CIN), which means abnormal cells in the epithelial layer of cells covering the cervix; or squamous intraepithelial lesions (SIL), which means abnormal cells in the squamous layer covering the cervix, vagina, or vulva. SIL is replacing the term CIN in some medical centers. The pathologist who reads the Pap smear ranks these cells numerically, according to the degree of the cellular change. Thus, CIN 1 or SIL 1 is considered mild, while CIN 3 or 4 or SIL 3 or 4 is severe.

Whenever I have to tell a woman that her Pap smear is abnormal, I know that her intellect will immediately jump to the worst-case scenario: *"Oh, no. I have cancer!"* Prompt investigation of the abnormal Pap smear generally results in her being reassured. Most abnormal Pap smears *do not* mean cervical cancer, though a certain percentage of dysplasias will go on to become cervical cancer if they are not diagnosed and treated. Some CIN abnormalities, particularly the mild ones, will go away by themselves. This is probably because the majority of mild dysplasias are actually HPV infections that are self-limiting. Self-limiting infections are those that the body's immune system takes care of on its own.

Cervical dysplasias can result when a woman is conflicted about wanting to be all things to all people, such as the woman who is a mother, works full time, and is worried that she does neither of these jobs well enough. Nonprofessional women experience the same thing—the treadmill dysfunction. Feeling as though we're on a treadmill certainly doesn't enhance our immune system functioning. A poor diet, environmental pollution, low self-esteem, and a bit of religious shame can set the scene for cervical dysplasias.

Scientific studies have shown that there are emotional differences between women whose cervical dysplasia progresses and those whose dysplasia remains mild or goes away. Women whose dysplasia became more severe were those who were passive and pessimistic in stressful situations; they avoided and somatically acted out their anxiety. For instance, they tended to get physical symptoms such as migraine headache, backache, and other disorders. Women whose dysplasias remained mild, on the other hand, were those who dealt with stress in a more optimistic and active fashion, effecting change in their lives by seeking creative solutions to their problems.[21]

Symptoms

Cervical dysplasias are not usually associated with symptoms, though some women who have had abnormal Pap smears have told me that they knew something was wrong because they felt a "burning" sensation in the cervical area. (Cervical cancer can be asymptomatic as well, but its symptoms usually include bleeding between periods, pelvic pain, foul discharge, and/or bleeding after intercourse.)

Diagnosis

THE PAP SMEAR. Cervical abnormalities are diagnosed initially by a Pap smear. The Pap smear (named after Dr. George Papanicolaou) was developed in the 1920s and during the late 1930s was refined and applied as a screening test to help prevent cervical cancer by identifying and treating abnormal cervical cells in their earliest stages. A Pap smear is made by taking a sample of cells from the transformation zone in the squamocolumnar junction (SCJ) of the cervix, up inside the cervical opening. At our office, like most practitioners in our area, we use a soft brush called a cytobrush to facilitate getting a good sample. The cells are then "fixed" onto a slide by spraying them or covering them with a cell-preserving chemical. A person trained in reading cellular abnormalities under a microscope then reads them. As a result of this test, there has been a 70 percent decline in the death rate from cervical cancer.

The Pap smear is not perfect; cervical cancer is not yet eradicated. About seven thousand women still die from this condition annually—and not all of them failed to get a regular Pap smear. At our hospital laboratory the false negative rate for Pap smears is about 13 percent, which means that 13 percent of the women whose Pap smears showed no abnormality actually had an abnormality on their cervix that the Pap smear screening didn't pick up. This is mainly caused by what's known as a sampling error—the technique used to get the cells for the Pap smear didn't pick up any of the abnormal cells on the cervix.[22]

Abnormalities from the upper genital tract, the endometrium, the fallopian tubes, and occasionally the ovaries sometimes show up on Pap smears, but only rarely. The Pap smear screens for cervical abnormalities *only*. Many women don't understand this limitation in their health care practitioner's ability to diagnose.

CERVIGRAPHY. At our center we partially correct for the sampling error by offering a test called a cervigram. A cervigram is a photograph of the cervix taken at the same time the Pap smear is taken. We offer the test (which isn't always covered by insurance) to any woman who has had an abnormal Pap smear or who desires extra reassurance. A negative Pap smear and a negative cervigram give the patient a 90 percent assurance that her cervix is normal.[23] The problem with cervigraphy is that it's so sensitive that sometimes women are told they have abnormalities that on further study turn out to be benign.

The American College of Obstetrics and Gynecology recommends yearly Pap smear screening for most women starting at the age of eighteen. I personally recommend an annual Pap smear for teenagers only if they're sexually active. The American Cancer Society recommendations are for yearly screening between ages eighteen and thirty-five, then every five years until age sixty. Regular Pap smears are also recommended for women who have had a hysterectomy, because the tissue of the innermost vagina, the area where the cervix was before the hysterectomy, is susceptible to the same abnormalities as the cervix. No one knows exactly which screening interval is best for all women.

COLPOSCOPY.   Once a woman has an abnormal Pap smear or cervigram, the next step is to further delineate the extent of the problem by a test known as colposcopy. In this test the cervix is observed through a magnification lens, to check the blood vessel and tissue patterns. Biopsies are taken from the areas that appear abnormal, and these are sent to the lab. Special attention is paid to the SCJ, making sure that this entire region is seen. Sometimes the abnormal cervical cells extend up into the endocervix, where they cannot be seen or tested. In these cases, a cone biopsy (a biopsy of the internal cervix in the shape of a cone) or a LEEP procedure (see page 255) is recommended to further test the tissue in the endocervix. (This procedure is not only diagnostic; it is often curative.)

A Common Concern

HOW DID I GET IT?   No one knows precisely why one woman develops cervical dysplasia and another doesn't. Like HPV, cervical dysplasia is related to the immune system functioning. In one study, women who were on immunosuppressive drugs for kidney transplants had a seven times greater chance of an abnormal Pap smear than did a control group of nonimmunosuppressed patients. Smoking is a definite risk factor for cervical abnormalities leading to cervical cancer. Women with cervical abnormalities have been found to have lower levels of antioxidants and folic acid in their blood. There is a known link between birth control pills and certain kinds of cervical dysplasias.[24] This may be in part because the pill decreases nutrients such as the B vitamins. (See "Human Papilloma Virus" in this chapter.)

Treatment

Women need to know that some studies have found that up to 50 percent of mild cervical abnormalities return to normal without treatment. A smaller percentage of the more severe abnormalities also regress. But sometimes they get worse rather quickly. Since no one knows whose "lesions" are going to go away and whose are going to grow rapidly, I recommend treatment to every woman with a cervical abnormality.

The treatment goal for cervical dysplasia is to eradicate all the abnormal tissue. Standard gynecological medicine has excellent tools to treat both cervical dysplasia and early cervical cancer. The cure rate by standard methods is over 90 percent.

Methods to destroy abnormal cervical tissue include laser, cryocautery, trichloroacetic acid, and LEEP. We are now using LEEP in the center as a method to diagnose and treat some cases of SIL that in the past required cone biopsy under anesthesia in the hospital. Some practitioners use laser in the same way.

Regular follow-up with a Pap smear every three months for one year, and every six months thereafter, is necessary to be sure that the abnormality doesn't return. After several years of normal six-month Pap smears, some of my patients are tested yearly. This decision is made on an individual basis. As one of my colleagues says, "No one ever died from close follow-up." Women who have had cervical dysplasia are likely to "get into trouble" if the disease progresses, which is why more frequent screening seems appropriate.

NUTRITIONAL APPROACH. Numerous studies have linked low levels of vitamins A and B complex with cervical dysplasia. Oral contraceptives can increase a woman's chances of getting an abnormal Pap smear, though the data supporting this are not well known by gynecologists; the pill lowers B vitamin levels in the blood. In women whose diets are already low in nutrients, the pill can set up a slight deficiency state. Even high doses of folic acid have been used to reverse cervical dysplasias in women who developed them while on the pill. That's why, whenever I prescribe the pill, I also recommend a good multivitamin rich in B complex and containing folic acid.

Women's Stories

When a woman is willing to look at the stress points in her life, then combines this inner work with standard medical techniques, she is almost guaranteed a successful outcome. Three women's stories of their reactions to their bodies' messages of cervical cancer and their struggles to understand and deal with their emotional issues follow.

SYLVIA: A WAKE-UP CALL. Sylvia was thirty-nine when she first came to see me. Two years earlier, she had been diagnosed with the beginning stages of cervical cancer and underwent a cone biopsy treatment. She had had normal Pap smears for two years, but a follow-up smear came back with the rating CIN 2. Following that diagnosis, as she was going out of the room, the nurse had remarked, "Too bad this is going to keep recurring every two years."

Sylvia later said that that remark finally galvanized her into action. She had always intended to get around to stopping cigarettes, alcohol, and caffeine, but this time she realized that it was a matter of life or death and that she had to clean up her act. She also said, "I realized, too, that it was time to stop hating my mother. I was a typical 'bad' girl until about a year ago. I then began doing healing visualizations and meditating. I realized through my healing work that I came from a family in which many generations of women have hated themselves. My sister-in-law died of lung cancer from smoking four packs per day, and at her funeral my mother was more abusive to me than I can ever remember. About two days after that, I was diagnosed with cervical cancer. I'm grateful, because I feel like I'm alive now and I hardly was before." Sylvia also told me that her sisters had all had hysterectomies and that one had had a breast removed for breast cancer. She said, "My mother has had her uterus removed, and she is a woman who is filled with self-loathing. Now suddenly I'm realizing that all of these women in my family just hate themselves and have done so for years."

Sylvia decided to break this pattern. To do so, she improved her diet, stopped smoking, and began to keep a journal in which she recorded any insights that arose about beliefs that no longer served her. She began to treat herself with more respect on every level. Her Pap smears have all remained normal since the CIN 2 was excised.

FAITH: HEALING CERVICAL AND VULVAR DYSPLASIAS. Faith, a woman in her early thirties, first came to see me in 1989. She was a nurse and was taking art classes. She had been diagnosed the year before with CIN 1 of the cervix, VIN 1 of the vulva (vulvar intraepithelial neoplasia), and VAIN 1 (vaginal intraepithelial neoplasia). All of these abnormalities were felt to be secondary to HPV infection and had been treated with laser a year before. Now the same abnormalities had returned. Faith's doctor had recommended laser treatment again, but she was reluctant to proceed. It had been quite painful, and there were no guarantees of success.

By the time Faith came to see me, she had already made some dietary improvements that she was enjoying. I explained to her the viral nature of her HPV infection and the subsequent cellular abnormalities, and I told her that she could improve her immune system by further improving her diet and by using the healing practices of her choice. I also recommended that she take dietary supplements for a while. She understood the importance of careful follow-up.

Then I didn't hear from her again until three years later, when she came in for a consultation. She told me that within six months of her dietary changes and meditation practice, all her HPV abnormalities had gone away. Her doctor couldn't believe it. Her Pap smears had remained normal. But now she was contemplating entering a sexual relationship once again, and she was worried about the HPV. Would it flare up again? She had already done a great deal of inner work around her sexuality through reading and going to twelve-step groups, particularly Sex and Love Addicts Anonymous. She realized that she had had sex in the past when she didn't want it and had participated in it almost automatically, as a way to stave off her fears of abandonment. She had been brought up in a religion that made her feel guilty about her sexuality. Her brothers had been taught by her parents not to get anyone pregnant, while she had been taught that she wasn't supposed to be sexual at all—or at least, not until marriage. Having gone through a period of celibacy, she felt that she was once again ready to explore her sexuality with another person. At the time I saw her, she had developed a supportive and loving relationship with a man that did not yet include sex.

Faith and her potential lover had both had HIV tests that were negative. I suggested that he be checked for HPV, simply to see if it was active—though both of us agreed that we couldn't be sure this would help anything. I asked her to consider whether the relationship would be a source of nourishment and joy for her. She is in the midst of deciding and doesn't plan to proceed until she and her inner guidance are in complete agreement about it.

BARBARA: WHEN SURGERY FAILED. Barbara was thirty-nine when I first saw her. Her story illustrates beautifully the connection between her past, her social situation, her body's "entry points," and her subsequent healing of them all.

The first time I saw Barbara, she was blond, petite, perfectly dressed, and had a smile on her face that looked permanently glued in place—a mask to cover what was going on underneath. Though she loved her work as a teacher, her body was giving her a lot of signals. Her mother had died at sixty-three of ovarian cancer. Her maternal grandmother had had the same disease. Over the previous nine years, she herself had had over fifteen different surgeries for early stage cancer, first of the cervix and later of the vagina.

She said of her earlier history, "As time passed, subsequent doctors' reports continued to show precancerous cells. Biopsy after biopsy led to one surgery and then another. Laser treatments proved ineffective. Finally a total hysterectomy, with removal of the ovaries, was done nine years after the first signs of abnormal cells appeared. I was advised not to worry. There was still some normal tissue. I was grateful."

Barbara's hysterectomy was done when she was thirty-six, three years before she came to Women to Women. At her first visit, we took a Pap smear of her vagina,[25] which once again came back abnormal. It was read as "mild dysplasia with koilocytotic changes (refers to specific changes in the nucleus of the cell usually associated with active HPV viral infection)." Koilocytotic change is a type of cellular feature typically seen with HPV or wart virus. She underwent a colposcopy and biopsies, which confirmed that she still had the abnormal cells in her vagina. Treatment consisted of removing the abnormal cells.

Because of the recurrent nature of Barbara's problem, we knew that there was nowhere for her to go but inward—to explore, if possible, why her body kept giving her the same message. We wanted to work with her to bolster her immune system and stop the process of disease that was resulting in more and more pieces of her vagina being surgically removed, frozen, or cauterized. All the treatments that she'd had so far—surgery, laser, cautery, and various medications—had failed to "cure" her problem.

As we took a deeper history, we found that Barbara's husband had been an alcoholic for the first fifteen years of their marriage. Much later, she found out that he had been having a series of affairs for years. As she put it, "He'd be holding my hand in the morning, and that of another woman in the afternoon. All the lies he told me were finally confirmed a few nights prior to when I asked him to leave, truths I had known in my heart. One affair after another, moments with prostitutes, encounters in large cities. He had previously denied this and more. The truth left me empty and alone." When she originally came to the center, Barbara had started to see a therapist and was in the process of piecing together her family history.

Barbara gradually began to put her life back together. She said, "I embarked on a journey that would eventually lead me to believe that I could make it on my own. Asking my husband to leave was the first well-thought-out decision I had made on my own. I was fully cognizant of the impact it would have on my life, and I had the courage to initiate and pursue a life outside the marriage. I missed the closeness and the union one feels in marriage. I missed that special person next to me and the knowledge that he would come home. He was my rock. He defined me. He owned me. He abused me. He left me. It hurt, and the pain has lightened, yet it will never fully go away." (This series of revelations on Barbara's part nicely illustrates the lifting of denial. As Anne Wilson Schaef once remarked, "It's hard to lose what you never had.")

Barbara kept a journal and told me that its pages revealed a frightened woman—a child, in many ways. She said that she feared tomorrow and that staying positive felt unnatural and uncomfortable to her. Aloneness and learning to live alone seemed insurmountable to her. Her one real joy was caring for her daughter, then eleven, and watching her grow.

Barbara started to do creative visualizations of her tissues as strong and healthy while Marcelle Pick, R.N.C., one of the founders of our center, did therapeutic touch treatments with her to help her move the "stuck" energy in her pelvis.[26] This modality has helped her learn how to relax and become less stressed. She told us that up until that time she had never thought about her sexuality, her breasts, or her vagina as free of disease, clear, healthy, and pink. "My body parts had always been dirty and not a part of me. They did not exist," she said.

She describes her therapeutic touch sessions as follows: "Therapeutic touch began as I sat in the chair. I was asked to put my hands on my knees and to think about warm water and a clean healthy body. Trust this woman, I kept saying. Trust! For the first time—ever—my body felt free of anxiety. A true sense of peace prevailed, a high that was truly unexplainable. Empowered. They want me to become empowered. I should change my diet and continue to vision my life as it could be. Trust, I kept saying. This may work. This *will* work."

Barbara attended a conference with Dr. Bernie Siegel and Louise Hay and went through a guided imagery experience that focused on the highlights of her life. She said that during this experience, pictures and pain surfaced that caused a knot in her stomach that she thought would never go away. She also did some releasing rituals to try to let go of her past. One of these was to bury her wedding ring in a creek that flowed away from her home. She said the affirmation "I'm open to receive myself." She continued working with this theme repeatedly, returning to it over and over.

Despite all of this work, another Pap smear returned as abnormal six months after her first treatment. This time Barbara was treated with a chemotherapy cream called 5 FU for ten weeks. (This treatment is reserved for very resistant cases.) She decided at this point to work with her dreams and try to listen more deeply to her cells.

Around this time Barbara's father died, and another part of her past began to surface. A mentally ill woman had lived with Barbara's family ever since Barbara was born. Barbara noted that this woman, Kerry, had great power and controlled the entire family through manipulation. Barbara wondered if Kerry had been having a lesbian relationship with her mother all these years. Was that why Kerry had always come first in the eyes of Barbara's mother—first over her husband and children?

Barbara writes, "My dreams eventually revealed the horror that I had denied. Kerry had sexually abused me as a child. My anger at this was profound. She had violated me, and how I hated her for what she had done! She often told me that I was dirty. I can still feel her hands on my body. And then she would place me in the tub and tell me to wash all the dirt away. She made me scrub my vagina until it was raw. I felt ashamed and feared the loss of those who loved me.

"I'll never know where my parents were and why they did not protect me from the witch that had bound me for so many years. She can no longer hurt me. She is old now and suffering from the pain of her own cancer, a cancer that has bound her for many years now in a home. The family's codependency has been altered. My work with the twelve-step programs has confirmed my thoughts that we all must separate and become individuals and learn to live alone.

"I struggle to forgive her for taking my mother and father from me. She also took my freedom, my dignity, my sexuality. These attributes are returning, and I've begun to love myself. The shame has lessened and the guilt is dwindling. I have begun to recognize other Kerry figures in my life. I am drawn to them; I fear them; I now avoid them.

"In my search for peace and contentment, I continue to take three steps forward and two steps back in all phases of my being. I refuse to give up the fight. I have fulfilled my promise to see my daughter through college and to present her with a model that strives to validate her while validating others and their efforts."

Barbara is making peace with her losses—her loss of her mother and father, and her loss of her relationship with a brother who is alcoholic. She says that she is grieving the "loss of the dream that someone special will come into my life and rescue me from my aloneness." She is angry that it has taken her so long to realize that no one can save anyone, she says.

"Now I know that no one can get under my skin and do for me what I must do for myself. I have let my daughter go. I have released her from being my social support and comfort. The aloneness is a new reality that I no longer deny. I will look to embrace special times with others and special times with myself. For I now see myself as a person who does not have to change. I like me. I like the warm, loving woman who peeks her head out occasionally. I will work on showing her off more. I have some wonderful qualities that can be offered to the universe. I'll be there if you'll be there."

Barbara's body is now healthy. Her six-month check-ups and Pap smears have all been normal. Now when she comes into the office, I see a vibrant, beautiful woman whose entire being radiates health. When she smiles, her smile comes right from her center. Her mask is gone. She is a healed woman.

The entry points of our bodies have been defiled and denied as part of us for too long. Though we often have much pain stored there, we can commit to listening to these forgotten parts of our bodies and reclaim them as sacred and worthy—as worthy as our minds, our hearts, and our dreams.

Cervical Cancer

I've seen several women who had the beginning stages of cancer on their Pap smears—microinvasive cervical cancer, confirmed by cone biopsy—who refuse hysterectomy, the recommended treatment. Though conventional thinking would never condone their choice of treatment, these women have gone on to live free of cancer for years.

Women's Stories

CONSTANCE, J.D. (JURIS DOCTOR): MICROINVASIVE CERVICAL CANCER. "Cancer I can cope with; it is men that perplex me," says Constance, who was diagnosed with cervical cancer. "I interpreted my cervical cancer as a signal to reassess my life. Although I meditated daily, did some exercise, and was generally aware about nutrition, I found my emotional life was out of control. In short, 'my woman,' a part of me that's very deep inside, was enraged at sexual rejection by my partner. He did not send me a clear message, he didn't just say, 'Let's be friends instead of lovers,' but instead gave me a mixed bag of approach and avoidance.

"Our relationship was of several years' standing. We had chosen to have a child together after my firstborn was in a fatal auto accident at age four. We had a daughter, but our relationship was not what I wanted or needed. My disappointment and rage ran deep and manifested themselves in the cells of my cervix.

"When I heard the results of my Pap smear and colposcopy, I stopped to reassess while I waited for my cone biopsy surgery to tell me how deeply the cancer had invaded and whether more surgery or other treatment would be necessary. I realized that the essence of my problem was a pattern of victimization by men, manifested in my body.

"In my immediate situation, the sexual rejection of me by my child's father, alternating with sweet nurturing and occasional lovemaking a few times per year, left me angry. This behavior paralleled how most men in my life had alternated nurturing with mistreatment. My past shows a pattern of classic codependency. My father had suddenly died when I was in first grade. He had been a warm, jovial man who loved children in general and me in particular. My brother, seven years my senior, had alternately accepted and rejected me as a sister. My mother's boyfriend and ersatz father figure had sexually abused me as a teenager, and my mother refused to believe me when I told her about it. My first husband, in spite of two degrees from Harvard University, physically and emotionally abused me and gambled compulsively. My second husband was an active alcoholic and was emotionally and verbally abusive.

"In the month between my abnormal Pap smear and the cone biopsy surgery, I became proactive regarding my health. I reached out to women friends and invited them to participate in my visualization of health. I scheduled extra visits with my spiritual teacher. I let go of my rage and desire to be intimate with my daughter's father. I repeatedly fed my unconscious and my soul with this little song/mantra:

> *My anger's gone.*
> *Forgiveness is on*
> *I don't want '_____.'*
> *I don't need him either.*
> *I am free, free, free to be me.*
> *My woman's healed*
> *By a fine blue light.*

"This song/mantra came to me spontaneously as I went deeply into my healing process. My goal was to stop wallowing in my martyrdom and my anger. This goal was only intellectual at first. I chanted and sang my song to get the information into my cells. A mantra is very portable. I had read about other people healing on a 'soul' level, and I realized that I had to do this too. This would involve releasing my pain and letting in forgiveness.

"My song/mantra symbolized forgiveness for me. The biggest piece of my healing was forgiveness 'from the gut,' not just intellectually. This process was a slow wearing-away and letting-go that took several months.

"Once the cone surgery was completed, my surgeon said she personally called the pathologist to discuss my biopsy because the results showed such marginal abnormality—or at least, less than expected. Her interpretation was that I had sought medical intervention earlier than is the rule. My interpretation is that because I had let go of my rage, my woman had begun to heal.

"Choosing to be proactive regarding my cancer meant choosing to follow the path of rediscovering my authentic self, which I had started to lose after the death of my father. Instead of a knee-jerk yes to others' requests, I am learning to say no and to say, 'I need some time to think things over. I'll get back to you.' Now I'm much more respectful and considerate of myself. I am cultivating a love relationship with my inner self."

Constance's Pap smears and exams have remained normal for more than five years.

Vaginal Infection (Vaginitis)

Almost all women normally have some kind of vaginal discharge. A yellowish or whitish stain on a woman's underwear at the end of a day, particularly if she has been wearing pantyhose or pants, is almost inevitable. Many women don't know this and often think that they have some kind of infection, but it is quite normal and does not require a visit to a gynecologist. Vaginal discharges of some kind can begin the year before a girl gets her first period. Her gradually increasing estrogen levels stimulate the estrogen-sensitive cells of the vagina and cervix, resulting in an increased production of cervical mucus and increasing the cell turnover time in the vagina.

A normal vaginal discharge comprises vaginal and cervical cells mixed with cervical mucus. When I look through the microscope at a smear on the slide, I see mostly normal vaginal squamous cells. Normal cell turnover of the lining of the vagina can increase when a woman is under stress, so that she will have an increased amount of discharge. But this discharge, too, will comprise normal cells.

Vaginal discharges differ at different times in the menstrual cycle. Many women notice an increase during the days surrounding ovulation, and some feel that they have "wet" themselves. Ovulatory flow, or fertile flow, sometimes resembles egg white. Some women have premenstrual spotting of brown old blood. This in itself is not an abnormality.

Just about every woman, however, is susceptible to a vaginal infection at some point in her life. Both the vagina and the vulva are often involved in these infections. Hence, when I use the term *vaginitis*, understand that the more inclusive term would be *vulvovaginitis*.

Common organisms that produce infection under the right circumstances are chlamydia, Gardnerella, trichomonas, and yeast. The key concept here is "the right circumstances." The vagina, which normally maintains an acidic pH, is colonized by many different types of bacteria. Yeast and Gardnerella, for example, live in the vagina normally.[27] When a woman is healthy, these bacteria do not cause problems. Only when something in this area becomes imbalanced are these organisms associated with infection.

Almost every type of bacteria that can cause a vaginal infection when conditions are *out of balance* can also be found in women who have *no symptoms*. For instance, some women have trichomonas protozoans, a well-known sexually transmitted cause of vaginitis, present in their vaginas for years with *no* symptoms whatsoever. Others are incapacitated by the itching and burning the protozoans can cause.

Symptoms

Most vaginal infections make their presence known by a burning or itching sensation, sometimes accompanied by a change or increase in vaginal discharge.

Common Causes

Anything that disrupts the pH balance or bacterial balance of the normal vagina can result in an infection.

REPEATED INTERCOURSE OVER A SHORT PERIOD OF TIME. Semen is a buffered alkaline fluid, with a pH of about 9. One episode of intercourse can increase the pH of the vagina for eight hours. When vaginal pH is higher than normal for long periods of time, the bacterial balance can be lost. Those bacteria that are normally present only in small numbers can begin to grow and "cause" infectionlike symptoms. If a woman makes love with ejaculation of semen into the vagina three times in a twenty-four-hour period, her vagina will not return to its normal pH for that entire twenty-four-hour period. For some women, this is a setup for infection, particularly women who are in long-distance relationships and whose sex lives are sporadic and limited to increased activity over a few days. (To prevent problems, you can douche within a few hours of intercourse with Summer's Eve Medicated Douche, which contains potassium iodide and lowers vaginal pH. Or use a vinegar douche—one tablespoon per quart of warm water.)

CHRONIC VULVAR DAMPNESS. The vulva sweats more than any other place in the body, especially when a woman is emotionally stressed. Thus, wearing restrictive, nonabsorbent, synthetic clothing close to the skin in the vulvar area can be a setup for chafing and subsequent infection. This is especially true if a woman exercises in this type of clothing. Riding a bike or a horse or using a rowing machine in such clothing can cause vulvar irritation.

CHEMICAL IRRITANTS. Some women develop vulvar irritation through chemical irritants found in perfumed, scented, softened, and colored toilet paper; bubble baths; and sanitary tampons and pads that contain deodorants. All women should avoid using pads and tampons that contain deodorants. These tampons can result in the production of vaginal ulcers, and the pads can cause vulvar irritation. No tampon should ever be left in more than eight to twelve hours at a time. Other irritants can include chemicals in swimming pools and hot tubs, scented douches, and vulvar deodorants.

STRESS. Some women respond to increased stress with a yeast infection. Many yeast infections occur premenstrually, and they often clear up spontaneously once the period starts.

ANTIBIOTICS. After the introduction of broad-spectrum antibiotics in the 1940s and 1950s, the incidence of yeast vaginitis has actually increased—dramatically. Many women can date the onset of their vaginitis to their teen years, when they took antibiotics such as tetracycline to treat acne. Unfortunately, every time we take an antibiotic, we disrupt the natural vaginal and bowel bacteria environment, and a yeast infection, either full-blown or chronic, can result. In the last decade, while the percentage of women over the age of eighteen has increased by only 13 percent, the number of antifungal prescriptions for women has increased by 53 percent.[28]

DIET. Many books have now been written on the connection between repeated courses of antibiotics, a refined food diet, and excessive yeast growth in the vagina and the bowel. Eating a lot of food made with refined sugar and flour can favor the overgrowth of vaginal yeast. Dairy products, particularly milk and ice cream, can also contribute to yeast vaginitis because of their high lactose (milk sugar) content, which favors the overgrowth of yeast in the bowel and vagina. One of my patients developed recurrent yeast infections when she drank an instant-breakfast-type drink every morning. The high sugar content of this so-called "healthy" meal substitute threw off her body's ability to fight excess yeast growth.

Many conventionally trained physicians don't look at repeated antibiotics courses and poor diet as factors in chronic vaginitis. I've worked with women who have seen ten or more doctors for their vaginitis and who have had every conventional culture and biopsy without results. Once these women begin to support their bodies' natural healing abilities through emotional work, dietary improvement, and supplements, their vaginitis problems have often gone away.

Diagnosis

The vast majority of common vaginal infections can be diagnosed by looking at a sample of the vaginal secretion under a microscope and testing it for pH. Some infections, like chlamydia and herpes, require that a culture be sent to a laboratory for further testing.

Women with chronic vaginitis are suspected to have a condition known as intestinal dysbiosis, or an imbalance of bacteria in the bowel that is often accompanied by an overgrowth of yeast. Women with this condition often reintroduce yeast back into their vaginas, even after repeated treatment for yeast. This is because yeast in the bowel reinfects the nearby vagina.[29] When intestinal dysbiosis is suspected, our center sends a special stool culture to a laboratory that specializes in proper diagnosis of intestinal dysbiosis.

Evidence also suggests that some women have chronic yeast infection even after treatment because they are continually reinfected by their sexual partners.[30] In these cases, treatment of the partner is helpful.

Treatment

OVER-THE-COUNTER PREPARATIONS. Many women can treat an occasional episode of vaginal burning or itching with one of the over-the-counter preparations that are now widely available. Yeast-Gard is a homeopathic remedy that is well tolerated. The Melaleuca Company makes an excellent preparation known as Nature's Cleanse that works well for uncomplicated vaginal infections caused by an overgrowth of normal bacteria or yeast. Resistant cases of bacterial vaginitis can be treated with vaginal antibiotic creams available by prescription: Cleocin (clindamycin) vaginal cream or MetroGel (metronidazole) vaginal cream.

A trichomonas infection can be treated with the oral antibiotic metronidazole or Flagyl, available by prescription. The side effects from this treatment are nausea and an adverse reaction to alcohol drunk during the treatment period. If a woman has trichomonas and has a male sexual partner, both partners must be treated. Otherwise, he will reinfect her. The male has no symptoms but carries the trichomonas in his genital tract.

If you've tried an over-the-counter preparation for a week or so with no improvement of your symptoms, see a health care practitioner to be certain that you're not missing something. Once a diagnosis of a vaginal infection is made, the practitioner can prescribe the proper treatment.

PREVENTING RECURRENCE. Avoiding the chemical irritants involved in vulvovaginal infections can be very helpful for susceptible women. Women with a history of repeated infections may choose to avoid using tampons for six months.

DOUCHING. I don't recommend douching except for specific symptoms that you are treating or after repeated intercourse to prevent infection. Especially with commercial preparations, douching simply disrupts the normal bacterial flora of the vagina and may actually increase the risk of infection.

For women with recurrent yeast infections, I recommend a high-fiber diet, in which all sugar and refined carbohydrates are eliminated, all cookies, cakes, juices, soft drinks, and the like. I also suggest avoiding all antibiotics. Some women have recurrent vaginitis because of an overgrowth of yeast and an imbalance of bacteria in their intestines. This condition is sometimes called systemic candidiasis or intestinal dysbiosis.

To eliminate yeast in a woman's intestinal tract and rebalance her intestinal flora, our center uses a variety of supplements, such as superdophilus and bifido factor, both intestinal biocultures. These are often available in health food stores. We also recommend that she decrease stress and enhance her immune system functioning. (See Resources for an example of a low-yeast diet we suggest for this condition.)

Psychological and Emotional Aspects

Some women with chronic vaginal infections fail to respond to any treatment. Some, too, are not open to trying any but the most conventional treatments, convinced that "there's a reason for this that you doctors are simply not finding—so do more tests." These situations present a very difficult dilemma for both the patient and the health care practitioner.

For a true "cure" of the problem, the emotional aspects of chronic vaginitis and vulvovaginitis must be looked at and worked through.[31] This is *not* to say that the problem is just in these women's heads. What might have begun "in the head" becomes physical. Studies have shown that many women with these infections have antibodies that work against their own immune and reproductive cells.[32] A gifted medical intuitive once did a reading on one of our patients who had a chronic vaginal condition. The intuitive said, "She's got Doberman pinschers in there. You go near there, and you'll lose a limb." As it turned out, this woman had experienced incest as a child. She came to see that one of the decisions she had made in her early teens was that no one was ever going to get near her vagina again. Because she had not made this decision with her intellect, on a conscious level, it was manifested through her body.

Chronic vaginitis is a socially acceptable way for a woman to say no to sex. For some women, saying "No, I'm not interested in having sex with you tonight or the rest of this week" is not acceptable, given the mate they have chosen and the home in which they grew up. If they believe that sex is one of their duties, regardless of whether they derive pleasure from it, no matter how unconscious this belief may be, chronic vaginitis may well represent an "out" for them.

Another common problem associated with chronic vaginal and vulvar infections is infidelity of the woman's partner. Even when a woman doesn't intellectually "know" that her husband is having an affair, her *body* may well be aware of it. I've seen several women in whom chronic vaginitis began at about the same time their mate started an affair. Of course, we might explain by saying that the husband was bringing something home to his wife in the form of germs, and that does happen. But in most of these women, I've been unable to find a physical cause for the vaginitis.

In a woman who has been in a monogamous relationship for years, a sudden onset of primary herpes, fever, or general illness, or genital sores, warts, or other obvious infections can be classic indicators of infidelity. For reasons already discussed, however, this is not always the case and is almost impossible to "prove." Women have also come in to our center with vaginal problems exacerbated by guilt over affairs that *they* were having.

It's not uncommon for a spouse to lie if he or she is confronted about having an affair. Several of my patients, especially premenstrually, have had dreams that their husbands were lying to them. After years of questioning their own sanity, they've found out that the dreams had been correct—they had in fact been lied to for years. And guess what? A woman's body knows it, often long before her intellect accepts the information.

Women's Stories

JOYCE: VAGINITIS AS A MESSAGE. Joyce was fifty-three when she first came to see me. For almost twenty years she had had chronic vaginal infections that always returned after treatment. When I met her, she was bitter and angry over her recent divorce. Her husband of many years, a wealthy and charming alcoholic, had left her for one of her own friends. She felt abandoned and cast aside, even though further questioning revealed that her relationship with her husband hadn't been satisfying for a long time. His drinking and workaholism had been constant problems, and her sex life had been complicated by painful intercourse and frequent infections for almost twenty years.

Joyce's physical exam on this first visit was basically normal, though her vaginal tissues were thin and tender. As long as she wasn't having intercourse, she didn't have any vaginal infections or other discomforts, and no treatment was necessary. Over the next several years, I saw Joyce for her annual exams. Each year she was a little less bitter about her ex-husband and was slowly able to see how much better she felt without him. She then remarried. When she moved in with her new husband, she had a dream in which their house was part hospital and part school. This dream was very meaningful for her because it symbolized this new marriage as one in which both healing and learning would take place. She felt cared for for the first time in her life. She realized that she had never experienced true intimacy before her marriage to this new man.

Her sex life with her new husband was wonderful, she reported. In fact, she had never dreamed that it could be so good. She has never had another vaginal infection, and her vaginal tissues are normal and healthy in every way. She has come to see that for years her body, through chronic vaginitis, was sending her a message about her prior relationship, before her intellect "got it." It is entirely possible to heal chronic vaginitis once the stage is set for healing.

KATHERINE: THE BODY'S WISDOM. Katherine came in for her annual visit, complaining that she had had several recurrent vaginal infections in the previous two months. But by the time of her visit, these infections had started to go away by themselves and she was already virtually free of the symptoms. She had recently ended a relationship that she'd been in for only two months. She said, "When he said to me, 'I want to keep you all to myself and keep you away from the world,' I knew I had to get out of there." After leaving this man, Katherine thought she would feel better—but instead she found herself bingeing on food a great deal.

As we talked, I suggested she look back over her life since her last visit a year earlier. She said that she had gotten out of a ten-year relationship with a drug addict and was in a group working on incest issues. When I asked her if she'd listened to Pia Mellody's tape on love addiction, something I'd suggested the year before, she replied, "I don't even dare to." We both laughed, and I reminded her how much progress she had made. As we were discussing the fact that the body gives us signals long before the intellect is willing to hear them, she said, "You know, I developed endometriosis in the second month of my relationship with that drug addict, and I knew at that time that it was probably caused by the stress of the relationship. But I didn't let my intuition speak to me."

Looking back, she was able to appreciate her body's wisdom, both in her long-term relationship and in the one she had just ended. I suggested to her that her vaginal symptoms—now going away— might have been telling her something.

Sexually Transmitted Diseases

For a sexually active person, there is no one-hundred-percent-guaranteed way to avoid exposure to sexually transmitted diseases (STDs), any more than there is to HPV and herpes. Despite this, exposure in itself does not make developing a sexually transmitted disease inevitable. Even with repeated exposure to HIV, the AIDS virus, some people have not gotten the disease.[33] A woman's biggest defense against sexually transmitted disorders is self-respect, self-esteem, a functional immune system (which is often associated with self-love), and commonsense measures, such as the use of condoms and the exercise of discrimination in choosing her sex partners.

You have only two choices when dealing with these diseases:

1. Gear up your illusion of control, become paralyzed by fear, make a vow of celibacy, and don't touch anyone—including yourself—down there. Sterilize everything in sight. (This doesn't work—the world is crawling with germs, and so are we all.)

2. Practice safe sex as best you can until you've made a monogamous commitment, eat well, take a good multivitamin-mineral supplement, and accept yourself for who you are and what your natural talents are. Expand your understanding of what sexuality is and how your views of it affect you.

I believe that the only way we can get out of the STD dilemma is to learn to cherish our bodies. We have to learn to be discriminating about what we put into them, and to think about and work with sexuality as a form of communication based on mutual respect and commitment, not as a way to "hold on to a man" or fill an inner emptiness and be comforted. I understand that internalized oppression leads many women to carry unwanted pregnancies and put themselves at risk for sexually transmitted disease, but I also know that women must awaken from the effects of that oppression and learn how to control their fertility and sexuality on their own terms. The reality of AIDS and other STDs may help women change the age-old, gender-imbalanced relationship between sex and power and really take control of their own bodies and health.

A Word About AIDS

I am no expert on AIDS, and I'm not involved in treating women who have it. I *am* often asked questions about it, and I frequently send women for testing. Though it is a much more serious disease, AIDS is related to herpes and warts in that one of the modes of transmission is sexual contact. Because people can have the HIV virus for years before it shows up, there are potentially *no* safe sex partners until we have been monogamous with someone for at least six months and both have negative HIV tests. (Even a negative HIV test is not a 100 percent guarantee, because you can have the virus when the test is taken but not yet have the antibody in the blood that is the basis for the HIV test.) The concept of the asymptomatic shedder that I mentioned in reference to the herpes virus essentially applies, in my opinion, to almost *all* infectious diseases, especially the sexually transmitted ones.

I believe that the AIDS epidemic is a consequence of a large-scale breakdown in human immunity, resulting from such factors as the pollution of the air and water, soil depletion, poor nutrition, and generations of sexual repression. AIDS has been called a metaphor for the breakdown of planetary immunity as a result of excessive dumping of toxins into the earth's—and thus our own—lymphatic systems.[34] Long-term AIDS survivors and those who have reversed their HIV status to negative all have the same things in common:

They have chosen to transform their lives and their immune systems through the healing power of nature and love.[35]

At the 1992 annual meeting of the American Holistic Medical Association in Washington, D.C., a panel of long-term AIDS survivors and their doctor said that despite what *The New York Times* and the Centers for Disease Control would have us believe, AIDS is not necessarily fatal. Dr. Laurence Badgeley, an expert on natural therapies for AIDS, said that many people are HIV positive and are perfectly well—*until they find out.* When they're told that they are HIV positive and that the disease is inevitably fatal, they almost immediately get sick.

In some cases the information itself, not the HIV virus, is what causes immune system depression. Obviously, the HIV virus does do damage, but its effects can be alleviated greatly through a program that includes dietary change, supplements, social support, and spiritual attunement.[36]

Breasts

I like mine—both of them. And they don't match.
—Debbie, receptionist, Women to Women

Our Cultural Inheritance

In a culture in which women and men alike are brought up on Barbie dolls, Miss America pageants, and *Playboy* images, breasts are a very charged part of our anatomy, both physically and metaphorically. Dr. Norm Shealy once remarked, "Freud had it all wrong. I've never seen a woman with penis envy, but I sure have seen a lot of men with breast envy." On some level, I believe, many people when they were children didn't get nearly the ideal amount of contact with their mothers' breasts; too many of us have been nurtured not by maternal breasts but by cold, plastic nipples and chemical formula made by multinational corporations. No wonder our society is so hung up on the female breast! No wonder the stage gets set so early for distress in this area of the female body!

Our cultural ideal is of a woman with a matched set of erect eighteen-year-old breasts. This causes all those women who don't match this ideal (the vast majority) to feel that something is wrong with them. I wish that every woman could have an opportunity to know how truly diverse breast sizes and shapes are, could see how much they vary among women. They would then realize how skewed our perceptions normally are about our breasts. We'd have a chance to begin loving the breasts we have, instead of comparing them with an impossible ideal.

Undeniably, an occasional woman has a size discrepancy or other abnormality between her breasts that is striking and a source of great psychological pain to her. Others have breasts that are so large, they cause back pain. Plastic surgery can correct such problems and can be a blessing. But most cosmetic breast surgery is undertaken because women feel they don't look as good as the models in magazines or as good as their lovers want them to look, or because our breast-obsessed culture so favors large breasts. This size concern is medicalized in plastic surgery jargon, which writes the indication for breast augmentation as *chronic bilateral micromastia*. That simply means "two small breasts that have been there for a while."

Women often feel that their breasts exist for the pleasure and benefit of someone other than themselves. I've heard former colleagues of mine discourage women from breast-feeding because it would "ruin their breasts." Many husbands forbid their wives to breast-feed because of their jealousy of the baby! Clearly, the current flap over breast implants is a symptom of a much deeper, culturally supported discontent. (I discuss implants later in this chapter.)

Breasts are the physical metaphor for giving and receiving. In ancient times they symbolized nature's abundance and nurturing qualities. That the breasts are symbols of nurturing was demonstrated well by the case of a woman whom I saw in the early 1980s. Jennifer, four years past menopause, had been referred to me with two very large cysts in her right breast that had manifested almost overnight. (They were five and seven centimeters in diameter.) When I asked her if anything was going on in her life in the area of nurturing others, she told me that her last child was leaving home for college and that a beloved cat, a pet for fifteen years, had recently died. Jennifer was grieving the loss both of her daughter and of her beloved pet. The night before the cysts appeared, she dreamed that she was nursing her baby daughter—the same child who was now about to leave home. When I aspirated the fluid from the cysts, I found that they were filled with milk! Jennifer's body had manifested the fluid of maternal nurturing in response to the change in her own nurturing role.

Our culture has skewed the nurturing metaphor in order that

women will give themselves away to others, without nurturing themselves. Women give and give and give until the well runs dry. If men and women generally went around without shirts, people would see that the major wound for women is the mastectomy scar. In contrast, the major scar for men would be the coronary artery bypass scar down the center of their chests—because men need to learn how to open their hearts.

Much breast cancer is related to our need to be self-contained and self-nurturing. According to Caroline Myss, "The major emotion behind breast lumps and breast cancer is hurt, sorrow, and unfinished emotional business generally related to nurturance." Breasts are located in the fourth chakra energetic center near the heart. Emotions such as regret and the classic "broken heart" are energetically stored in this center of the body. Guilt over not being able to forgive oneself or forgive others blocks the breasts' energy. (The other organs in the fourth chakra are also susceptible to this energy pattern.)

As far back as the 1800s, the medical literature has noted associations between breast cancer and loneliness, sorrow, and even rage and anger.[1] Women with breast cancer frequently have a tendency toward self-sacrifice, inhibited sexuality, an inability to see themselves as supported by others, an inability to discharge anger or hostility, a tendency to hide anger and hostility behind a facade of pleasantness, and an unresolved hostile conflict with their mothers. There is evidence that women with breast cancer who perceive themselves as having high-quality emotional support from a husband or other source have an enhanced immune response.[2] In one study, breast cancer patients were more likely than women without breast cancer to be committed to maintaining an external appearance of a nice or good person. They were also more likely to suppress or internalize their feelings, particularly anger.[3] It is not the emotion itself that causes the problem—it is the inability to express the emotion and then release it. In fact, one study found that the suppression of anger over many years is correlated with adverse changes in the immune system.[4] Given our society's tendency to suppress, ignore, or denigrate women and their anger, it is easy to see why so many women have breast problems. A nurse practitioner once told me that several months before her death, one of her friends with breast cancer had the following insight: "I finally realize that I didn't have to die of cancer in order to rest."

Anatomy

The female breast is designed to provide optimal nourishment for babies and to provide sexual pleasure for the woman herself. The breasts are glandular organs that are very sensitive to hormonal changes in the body; they undergo cyclic changes in synchrony with the menstrual cycle. They are very intimately connected with the female genital system. Nipple stimulation increases prolactin secretion from the pituitary gland. This hormone also affects the uterus and can cause contractions. Breast tissue extends up into the armpit (axilla), in what is known as the tail of Spence. Lymph nodes that drain the breast tissue are also located in the armpits. After a woman has had a baby and her milk comes in, she may develop striking swellings under her arms from engorgement of the breast tissue in that area. Breasts come in all sizes and shapes, as do nipples. Most women have one breast that is slightly smaller than the other.

Breast Self-Exams

Breast self-exams are best done just after the menstrual period is over, when hormonal stimulation of breast tissue is least apparent. At the Women to Women Center we always ask women if they perform monthly breast exams. But few women do them as directed—even nurses and those who should "know better."

Why do so few women examine their breasts regularly? Some women feel that their breasts are lumpy and scary and are designed for someone else's pleasure or judgment anyway. Most women who think their breasts are lumpy don't understand the breasts' normal glandular anatomy. Although the vast majority of the women I see have completely normal breasts, many feel that something is wrong with their breasts. The diagram of normal breast anatomy indicates that what we sometimes feel as tiny "lumps" or "BBs" are simply normal glands. Occasionally, one of these ducts or glands will swell and feel like a hard pea. Generally they go away by themselves over time, but it is always recommended that a woman tell her doctor about them and go in for an exam to be sure. Statistically, women find the vast majority of breast abnormalities themselves.

No matter how much intellectual information a woman has, however, doing a thorough self-exam in a clinical and systematic way may bring up all her fears about her breasts. Why search meticulously each month for something that you don't want to find, in an organ whose texture you don't understand? When it comes to our female anatomy, we're always ready to believe that something is *wrong*.

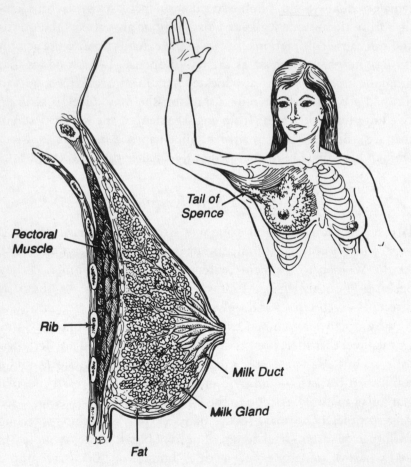

FIGURE 8: BREAST ANATOMY

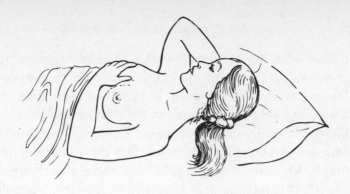

FIGURE 9: BREAST EXAM

Transforming the Breast Self-Exam

A good time to change how you think about and do your breast exams is right after you've had a normal exam with your health care practitioner and you know that everything is currently normal. When I am examining a woman's breasts, I tell her what I am feeling there and I will often have her repeat the exam, so that her fingers, too, will begin to know what "normal" feels like. From then on, whenever she touches her breasts, I ask her to do so *not necessarily to find suspicious lumps* but to send energies of caring and respect to this area of her body.

Approach your breasts with respect. If you are currently afraid of your breasts and find them "too lumpy," start changing your attitude toward them by paying special attention to them during your daily bath or shower. When you wash this area of your body, pay attention to how the skin feels under your fingers. Imagine that you have healing power in your hands (which you actually do). As you wash your breasts and under your arms, do so in the spirit of blessing this area of your body. As you do so, you will be learning the basic contours and feel of your own breasts. Do this daily as part of your bathing until you have reclaimed some respect for your breasts as an important part of your anatomy.

Once you are completely comfortable with this exercise, proceed with learning how your breast tissue feels when you use deeper pressure. You might approach this step in a spirit of curiosity, the same way that you might examine your own hand or the sole of your foot. Your breasts are a vital part of your woman's wisdom, and you want to learn to listen to them. Lie on your back with one

291

hand behind your head. This will flatten your breast tissue against your chest wall and make it easier for you to feel and appreciate your breast tissue as it lies on top of the underlying muscles and ribs. With your right hand, using the flat part of your fingers, not your fingertips, explore your left breast. Fingertips are so sensitive that they pick up all the little ductules. You may find this frightening until you know what is normal for you, so use your fingertips to explore your breast tissue only after you have become completely comfortable with your breast anatomy and trust yourself. Repeat the exercise, using your left hand to explore your right breast. It is initially helpful to divide your breast into four quadrants and examine each one separately. Then move up to your armpit and back to your nipple so that you can feel the differences in the different breast areas. Breast tissue tends to be the densest in the upper, outer quadrants of the breasts. Eventually you will be able to feel the difference between this area and others and to know that these differences are all normal for you.

The main thing I'd like women to learn is that they can get to know their breasts by understanding their anatomy, feeling their breasts (both from within and without), and looking at them. Women need to learn that their breasts are a normal part of the body and that they deserve as much or more loving attention than their hair or complexion. If a woman approaches her breasts in this way, to get to know them and *not* just to find lumps, she'll be surrounding them with a much more positive energy field than the usual energy engendered by the breast self-exam, in which you "examine to find what you don't want to find." Examining your breasts in a spirit of fear simply increases the fear and is the opposite of what you need to create healthy breast tissue. One of my patients who has had a lumpectomy for breast cancer embodies this healthy way of examining her breasts. She feels her breasts regularly and knows their anatomy well. And every morning, before she gets up, she says to them, "Girls, you're safe with me!"

Benign Breast Symptoms: Breast Pain, Lumps, Cysts, and Nipple Discharge

Breast Pain (Cystic Mastalgia)

The most common reason my patients seek medical consultation is breast lumps or cysts. Though most of them are benign, these must be closely monitored to make sure that they are not cancerous. (Nipple discharge is a less common symptom but can still be cause for concern.)

Approximately half of all women who go to doctors go because they have some kind of pain in their breasts. Cyclic mastalgia, or breast pain that comes and goes depending on the menstrual cycle, is usually caused by excess hormonal stimulation of the breast from hyperestrogenism, excessive caffeine intake, or even chronic stress. It is *not* a risk factor for breast cancer.

Dr. Mary Ellen Fenn, one of my colleagues, once remarked, "Have you noticed that men *never* complain about pain in their testicles, but that women are always complaining about pain in their breasts and even their ovaries? Do you suppose it's because men know that if they complained, someone would want to cut into them? Or is it because in our culture, these organs in men are not as much at risk?" If women learned how their inner guidance is advising them through breast symptoms to give more time and energy to themselves, they might begin to appreciate their breasts in a different way.

"Fibrocystic Breast Disease"

Currently about 70 percent of women have been told by a health care provider that they have "fibrocystic breast disease." In the past decade a few studies seemed to indicate that women with so-called fibrocystic breast disease had a two-to-three-times higher incidence of breast cancer. A panic ensued, and women were told conflicting stories by different doctors. When the National Cancer Association Consensus Committee investigated the issue in 1985, it discovered that 70 to 80 percent of what is called fibrocystic breast disease is actually normal changes in breast anatomy and is *not* associated with an increase in breast cancer. Yet many women still believe it is.

Breasts are composed of fat and connective tissue. Over time, the ratio of connective tissue to fat changes. It is therefore normal for some areas of the breast to be denser on exam than others—breast tissue is not homogeneous. One area may be denser than another simply because there's more connective tissue in that area than in another. Most women normally undergo what pathologists call fibrocystic changes in their breasts, so the chance of finding them on a biopsy is very high. Unfortunately, because the term has been used to describe just about any breast thickening, tenderness, or symptoms of any kind, women whose breast tissue is merely dense with connective tissue are sometimes given the diagnosis of fibrocystic breast disease, as are those who simply have variations in tissue density throughout their breasts, all of which are variations of normal.

Like the term *cervical erosion,* which simply pathologizes a normal change in the cervix, *fibrocystic breast disease* is basically not a disease, in the opinion of many. I think the term should be discarded. Misinformation about fibrocystic disease, the constant media exploitation of women's breasts, and our culture's ambivalence toward breasts set up a psychological dynamic that is loaded with potential harm for many women. Not only are they made to feel that their breasts are too small, too large, or the wrong shape, now they are told by someone whom they trust that their breasts have a disease!

Nipple Discharge

Nipple discharge most often happens after nipple stimulation, usually from lovemaking. It is not dangerous. After a woman nurses a baby, it may take a year or more for milk discharge to disappear completely. In cases of persistent nipple discharge that are not associated with nipple stimulation—the discharge can be anything from milky to greenish clear fluid—a blood test to measure the hormone prolactin should be drawn to be certain that the woman doesn't have a rare pituitary tumor known as a pituitary microadenoma. A bloody discharge should always be investigated to be certain there's no cancer. Sometimes, however, this very rare condition is caused by benign growths in the ductal tissue of the nipple.

Breast Cysts

Breasts are very sensitive to hormonal changes, and nonmalignant lumps or thickenings often go away over time. But it is a standard medical recommendation that you tell your health care practitioner immediately about any lump you find. When I find a lump on examining a woman, I want to know whether it is a cyst. Breast cysts, which are fluid-filled, are diagnosed by placing a needle in them under local anesthetic and aspirating the fluid contents. Sometimes a physician cannot tell a solid lump from a cyst on exam, so ultrasound is sometimes needed to make the distinction. If the lump is a cyst, its contents, usually yellow or greenish-brown fluid, can sometimes be aspirated. Though many experts feel that cyst fluid can be discarded because it is rarely helpful to analyze it, I routinely send the fluid to the cytology lab to have it checked for cancer cells.[5] In most cases, the cyst will disappear following aspiration, and no further treatment is required unless the fluid contains abnormal cells.

If the lump is *not* clearly a cyst, I very often refer the patient to an excellent general surgeon for a second opinion, including a mammogram, to be read by the radiologist *and* the surgeon. I feel strongly that women should get the best medical opinions possible about their situation before they embark on any treatment for a breast problem. In women younger than thirty-five (with some exceptions), a breast mass can be watched for several menstrual cycles to see if it goes away.

Treatment for Benign Breast Symptoms

Assuming that your breast exam and mammogram, if you have had one, are normal, here's my approach to treating breast pain, benign lumps, and other symptomatic changes. Studies have shown that the breast, like the menstrual cycle and the uterus, is stimulated by conditions that result in hyperestrogenism, or too much estrogen in the system. Not only does chronic hormonal overstimulation of breast tissue result in pain, it may even be a risk factor for breast cancer. There are many ways in which women can alter their diets to counteract this overstimulation.

For breast pain, the following treatments have been shown to work in a great number of women. Experiment with them, and pick the ones that you're most likely to stick with.

STOP ALL CAFFEINE. Studies have repeatedly shown that some women—not all—are helped by this.[6] For optimum benefit, stop not only caffeine but all methylxanthine-containing compounds, including all cola, root beer, chocolate, and even decaffeinated coffee. You may want to stop all of these for a time, then add a little back into your intake and see what happens. For some women, the caffeine restriction makes a huge difference in their breast pain. I've had patients who had breast pain before their periods if they ate as much as one chocolate candy during their menstrual cycle. Others aren't affected at all.

TAKE GAMMA LINOLEIC ACID. Supplement your diet with a source of gamma linoleic acid, such as oil of evening primrose, borage oil, flaxseed oil, or black currant seed oil (500 mg. taken four times per day). Some studies have shown that women do very well on this supplement.[7] You can also obtain gamma linoleic acid by taking one tablespoon of ground-up flaxseeds daily. Add them uncooked to soups, salads, cereals, or any grain dish just before you eat it. (You can buy flaxseeds at health food stores and grind them up in a small coffee or nut grinder.)

IMPROVE DIET. Follow a high-complex-carbohydrate, high-fiber, low-fat diet that contains no dairy food. Generally after two or three months, you can restore low-fat dairy foods and see if they make a difference.

TAKE NUTRITIONAL SUPPLEMENTS. Take a good multivitamin supplement containing high levels of vitamin E, or add vitamin E (400 to 600 IU per day) to your regimen. Studies have shown that many women with breast pain are helped by the antioxidant vitamins E and A and selenium.[8] R. S. London's studies showed that vitamin E actually decreased serum pituitary hormone levels (LH and FSH) in women treated with it for breast pain.

Note: All the studies done on the various supplements that help breast pain studied a particular supplement individually. I believe that since all of these factors work together, it's best to use them synergistically.

USE AN IODINE SUPPLEMENT. When a woman isn't helped by any of the other treatments, I prescribe an iodine supplement. It appears to change the way estrogen binds to breast tissue. In our center we use an iodine formula especially made for us by a research chemist. Others use SSKI (1 to 10 drops per day; SSKI 1 drop = 30 mg.).[9] Sea vegetables are another good source of iodine.

APPLY CASTOR OIL PACKS. Castor oil packs applied to the breasts three times per week for one hour, over two or three months, often eliminate breast pain, particularly if there is inflammation of breast tissue. Maintenance of once per week thereafter is recommended.

Discovering the Messages Behind the Symptoms

Sometimes a woman's breast pain persists until she addresses a deeper cultural wounding. One of my patients got over her breast pain only after she remembered that at the age of five she had been playing in a barn and some boys forced her to pose nude for them. She remembered that her chest was a large focus of this activity. After her breasts grew at puberty, her emotional and psychological discomfort at this kind of attention became chronic and eventually manifested as physical pain.

A forty-seven-year-old woman told me that when her daughter turned thirteen and became quite independent from her, she became acutely conscious of her breasts for a while. She said that they ached at times, as though they were longing to nourish or cradle a baby. She hadn't given birth to her daughter, she had adopted her. She said, "Heading into menopause, I remembered that I never beheld her infant face, nor did she drink from my breast. I experienced an intense desire to hold a baby for as long as I needed to. Several months later, a thickening in my left breast was found during my routine annual exam. It was near my heart. I knew what it was about. I needed to deal with renewed feelings about my infertility and its losses. I felt intense sadness over not giving birth to this wonderful child of mine. Now for the first time, my body was letting me know that it too was sorry." Two months after she had this realization, her breast thickening was gone at her follow-up exam. Sometimes the body heals simply when you give yourself permission to listen to its messages.

Any persistent mass requires a biopsy for definitive diagnosis. Most breast biopsies are done on an outpatient basis under local anesthesia by a general surgeon. A frozen section of the tissue done in the pathology department of the laboratory to which we send tissue specimens can often tell the pathologist who examines the tissue whether cancer is present during the biopsy procedure itself. Sometimes, however, the diagnosis must wait for several days until the pathologist can perform further diagnostic tests on the breast tissue.

One of the most unpleasant experiences a woman can have is living with the uncertainty about whether a breast lump is cancerous. Therefore, if I have any doubts about a breast mass, or if a woman herself is inclined toward further testing, I often refer her to a general surgeon whose skills I trust so that she will have the advantage of another set of trained hands examining her. A breast biopsy, though common, can leave dents and scars in the breast tissue. Though it is often necessary, it is not something to be entered into without a thorough understanding of its consequences and without considering whether it is really necessary.

Mammograms

A mammogram is an X-ray study of the breasts used to diagnose breast cancer in its earliest stages before it can be felt on clinical exam. Mammograms are currently recommended for all women starting at ages thirty-five to forty as a baseline and at regular intervals thereafter. Controversy exists over how often women with no family history of breast cancer who are in their forties should have mammograms. Several groups, such as the American Cancer Society and the American College of Obstetricians and Gynecologists, have agreed that mammograms should be obtained every two years between the ages of forty and fifty and yearly thereafter. These recommendations are based on general consensus only. Some women might do better with yearly mammograms, some every three years. You and your health care provider need to discuss how often you should have a mammogram.

Mammograms aren't a cure-all for all breast cancers—they miss 10 to 15 percent of all cancers. They're the best test we have at this time, however, for early detection. If something is called "probably benign" on a mammogram, the odds of it being cancer are less than 2 percent, according to the radiologists at our medical center. The rate of false positive mammograms (saying that there's something abnormal when there isn't) is 6 to 10 percent.

Mammogram reports sometimes seem punitive and confusing to women. Here are a few examples:

A routine mammogram in a thirty-eight-year-old woman who had completely normal breasts was reported this way: "The breasts are extremely dense and poorly suited to mammography." From reading this, one would think that breasts were created *for* mammography and that this woman's breasts were to blame! Having breasts that are dense to an X-ray beam is *not* an abnormality—it is a variation of normal.

A forty-five-year-old woman who also had completely normal breasts went in for a routine screening mammogram. She had benign calcifications of a small amount of her breast tissue, which is quite common and no cause for alarm. Her mammogram report, though normal, was written in extremely convoluted and frightening language: "Trabecular derangement and mazoplasia cystica with adenosis bilaterally. Some prominence of the suspensory ligaments. No evidence for superdensities, skin thickening, or unifocal hypervasularity. Scattered acinar, punctate, singular calcifications in both breasts, the largest 1.5 mm. They are quite discrete and do not have the same appearance as microcalcifications associated with malignancy."

Both these mammogram reports quoted above were brought into the center from outside hospitals by the patients themselves. Every radiologist reads a mammogram a bit differently. Reading them is an art, practiced by imperfect human beings—it's not an exact science. Women are led to believe, however, that a normal mammogram reading is a kind of guarantee that everything is all right. They don't understand the limitations of the test. Thousands of women with benign breast findings are put through an incredible amount of fear each year due to mammogram readings. Some, of course, do get diagnosed with early stages of breast cancer as a result of the test. Many physicians believe that diagnosis in the early stages is the best strategy for saving lives, though this is controversial. Many women undergo a breast biopsy because of abnormal findings on a mammogram. Even though most biopsies are benign, a lot of women go through hell thinking they have cancer, and the experience understandably makes them fearful. Almost everyone has had a friend die of breast cancer. That's the not-so-benign fallout from the best test we currently have for picking up breast cancer early. I like to go over mammogram reports with women whenever they have any confusion about the wording that is used.

Most mammogram reports also contain a statement that reads: "A negative mammogram should not preclude biopsy of a clinically palpable lesion." This is dictated into the report for legal reasons, to put the doctor and patient on notice that there are limitations to the diagnostic capabilities of mammograms (as there are with all diagnostic tests). Breast problems are diagnosed via a combination of physical exam, mammograms, sonograms, aspiration of lumps, and surgical biopsy if necessary. When a woman knows her own breasts well, this entire process is enhanced because she trusts herself to know what is normal and what is not. I don't doubt a woman's ability to find an abnormality and I always pay attention when a woman who is tuned in to her body tells me that something is wrong. If a woman or her doctor feels a lump that hasn't been there before, a biopsy is necessary to rule out cancer, even if the mammogram is normal.

A few women in my practice have had a stable lump in a breast for many years and have decided not to have biopsies of these areas. The lumps have not changed, the women themselves know these areas of their breasts intimately, and they take full responsibility for avoiding a biopsy. On the other hand, I've seen women with breast lumps who have delayed seeing a doctor for months even when they knew the lump was there. One of my patients who was eventually diagnosed with breast cancer delayed diagnosis and treatment for two years because she was immobilized by her grief about the loss of her father several years before. She was a working woman and told me that she simply "didn't have the time or energy to seek help." This is a dangerous attitude to have toward your health. Most of my patients are well informed and come in to be examined for reassurance and diagnosis very shortly after noticing a change in their breasts that is unusual. I always ask them what is going on in their lives, especially how they are nurturing themselves or others. We then proceed with an exam and further diagnostic testing if it is warranted. Regardless of the diagnosis, the patient knows that she is being asked by her breast to look within and to tune in to her inner guidance system.

Some of the women I treat don't want mammograms and won't get them. One said to me recently, "I've seen far too many women have a mammogram that was positive who then became frozen with fear. I can't help but think that that's a threat to their health. I've watched them go downhill very rapidly." This is the same reaction that some people have to getting a diagnosis of AIDS. Fear and the feeling of helplessness are indeed very detrimental to health. This same woman said, "I'll have a mammogram as soon as I'm ready to deal with the consequences, no matter what they are. For now, I believe that I may be creating cancer daily—but I also believe that my body probably handles it."

My patient may well be correct. Mammograms may pick up very early breast abnormalities that may not go on to become actual invasive cancer. These early changes are known as carcinoma-in-situ or mammary dysplasia or atypia. Because their natural history has never been studied over a long period of time, doctors automatically assume that they are all fast-growing and potentially lethal. Since these lesions often occur in many areas of the breast, mastectomy is often recommended. Dr. H. Gilbert Welch, a general internist and senior researcher at the Department of Veterans' Affairs in White River Junction, Vermont, has researched the problems associated with the ability of technology to overdiagnose diseases such as breast cancer. He points out that in the breasts of women who died of other causes, 40 percent had microscopic precancerous changes in their breasts. These same types of lesions commonly show up on mammograms and no one knows which ones will remain dormant and which ones will actually become invasive cancer.[10]

Another woman, vibrant and healthy in her fifties, said that she doesn't want a yearly mammogram, even though that's the current recommendation for a woman of her age. She feels that yearly radiation exposure to a radiation-sensitive organ is probably not benign. As she put it, "I intend to live into my nineties. I'll be damned if I'm going to zap my breasts once every year. That adds up to over forty X-rays!"

I've heard her fear voiced by others. My job is to tell women what the American Cancer Society (ACS) recommendations for mammography are and tell them that mammograms pick up breast cancer years before a woman would ordinarily feel a breast lump. I assume that my patients are intelligent adults who are "allowed" to make up their own minds about a test, even though failure to diagnose breast cancer is the most prevalent reason for lawsuits against gynecologists. Patients who want to be partners in their own health care need to hold up their end of the bargain and take responsibility for the consequences of *not* having a mammogram if they don't want one. It's very tough for me to argue with a woman who does not want a mammogram, since I don't practice "should-ought" patriarchal medicine. I advocate following the wisdom of our intuition. A woman who is willing to live with the fact that *not* getting a mammogram may mean that an early breast cancer goes undetected is making an informed choice. As I also tell my patients, however, in the current, dualistic, lawsuit-driven medical system, *I* am responsible for their breasts and for what happens to them. That's what my malpractice insurer tells me, and that's why doctors push mammograms. I don't like the system because it erects a wall between my patients and me. So I explain the problem with my patients whenever it comes up—that way, we both know what we're up against.

I do prescribe regular mammograms, even though mammograms are not perfect and they *do* involve radiation, which is also not entirely harmless. Right now, I can't guarantee the absolute safety of a mammogram. (It appears to give the same dose of radiation as flying in an airplane from Portland to Chicago. The Earth is bombarded daily with cosmic radiation that increases the higher up in the sky one goes.) If a patient doesn't want a mammogram as often as the ACS recommends it, I can understand that. Neither I nor any other doctor can guarantee that diagnosing a breast cancer in the earliest stages will necessarily save a woman's life. Far too many women have been diagnosed early with cancer who have died within two years. Others, however, *have* lived for another forty years or more.

Doing breast self-exams and getting mammograms regularly is *not* the same as *prevention*. As one of my colleagues said of breast cancer, "We identify the risks, but we don't know what to do until they manifest as disease." Our culture uses mammograms as a fix but doesn't encourage women to change their diets, stop smoking, and learn how to be in relationships that nurture them. These are preventive changes that I believe would result in healthy breasts. But as one researcher has said, it's difficult to put together a constituency for prevention. It is treatment that gets our attention. If your sister or mother dies of breast cancer, you usually give money to programs that do research to produce better treatments; you don't start a macrobiotic restaurant in your neighborhood or school. This culture likes to act only after the horse is already out of the barn.

Breast Cancer

Currently, one in nine (some studies say one in eight) women in the United States between the ages of one and eighty-five years gets breast cancer. This does not mean that one in nine forty-five-year-old women will get it. But breast cancer is the leading cause of death among American women who are forty to fifty-five years of age.[11]

When I was in medical school, I was taught that one in twenty-five women would get breast cancer. No one is sure whether the incidence of breast cancer is actually on the increase or whether we are simply diagnosing it earlier these days, with the increase in mammography and public awareness. Regardless of statistics, however, most of us know at least one person who has had or currently has breast cancer.

For this to be the case, clearly something is out of balance. I see far too much breast cancer—it currently kills many more women than AIDS. Evidence is accumulating that certain environmental pollutants contribute to estrogenic activity and may contribute to the incidence of breast problems in the industrialized world.[12] Whether or not breast cancer is on the increase statistically, and whether or not industrial toxins and pesticides are a contributing factor, every woman has to be proactive about her breast health now. We cannot wait until further studies on environmental toxins come in or the definitive treatment for breast cancer is figured out.

I'm concerned about possible links between birth control pills and breast cancer, and between estrogen replacement and breast cancer. The breast is an estrogen-sensitive organ. Many women who have been on birth control pills or estrogen replacement have found that the medication resulted in enlarged and often tender breasts. The effect of this medication, combined with the standard American high-fat, low-fiber diet, which overstimulates breast tissue, could be a setup for breast cancer. And with one in nine women currently getting breast cancer, how would we even know if we had an epidemic of the disease? It's already far too common to wait for the medical profession or the government to do something. Women must decrease their risks *now*.

The Breast Cancer–Diet Link

Breast cancer has been associated with high levels of dietary fat and low levels of certain nutrients for many years. As far back as 1977, Wynder and Gori at the National Cancer Institute showed that countries with the highest intake of animal fat had the highest mortality rates from breast cancer.[13] Excessive estrogen (relative to progesterone) over the life-cycle appears to be associated with increased risk of breast cancer. Though no one knows exactly how the diet fat–estrogen link is actually implicated in the cause of breast cancer, research has given us some clues.

• Animal fats stimulate colonic bacteria to synthesize estrogen from dietary cholesterol, thus contributing to hyperestrogenism in the body.

• The body fat itself manufactures estrone, a type of estrogen.

• Hyperestrogenism can be modulated by a high-fiber, low-fat diet, because dietary fiber increases fecal excretion of estrogen.[14]

• Oriental women who consume a traditional diet—including the soy-based products tempeh, tofu, miso, and natto—excrete estrogen at a much higher rate than those who don't. They also have a much lower risk of breast cancer. These soy products, rich in what are known as phytoestrogens, which are substances found in some plants that have biochemical properties similar to weak estrogens, appear to be protective against breast cancer, in part because the weak estrogenic activity of certain plant foods tends to block estrogen receptors on the cells from excessive estrogen stimulation from other sources.[15]

• A compound called indole-3-carbinol (I3C), which is a plant chemical obtained from cruciferous vegetables (like cabbage, broccoli, brussels sprouts, kale, and collard greens), changes the way estrogen is metabolized. This compound "predictably alters endogenous estrogen metabolism toward increased catechol estrogen production and may thereby provide a novel dietary means for reducing cancer risk."[16]

• Women with breast cancer have been shown to have selenium levels that are lower than those of women without cancer.[17] Selenium is a trace mineral that is often lacking in refined food diets.

• Hyperestrogenism and possibly breast cancer itself may be decreased by including lactobacillus acidophilus in the diet. This helpful bacterium helps metabolize estrogen properly in the bowel.[18] It is available in capsules from health food stores; health-conscious medical practitioners can usually suggest a reliable brand. Most commercially available yogurt does not contain enough of the live bacteria to make a difference.

• The use of bioflavonoids (found in the vitamin C complex) may inhibit estrogen synthesis.[19]

• In one study of women with breast cancer, low serum retinol (a vitamin A byproduct) was associated with a decreased response to chemotherapy.[20]

• Some studies have shown a link between high sugar consumption and breast cancer.[21]

• Alcohol consumption is associated with breast cancer risk.[22] In one excellent study, this link was felt to be secondary to the fact that alcohol consumption increases hormone levels in the blood. In women age fifty and over, the type of alcohol associated with the highest risk was beer.[23] Given the fact that many women drink to medicate their emotions, women's unexpressed emotions may enhance the alcohol–breast cancer link.

• Although a preliminary study by W. Willet et al. did not show a marked decrease in breast cancer incidence when the nurses in his study decreased their dietary fat intake to 30 percent,[24] other studies have shown that in countries where the breast cancer rate is very low, dietary fat accounts for only 20 percent or less of daily caloric intake. Animal fat appears to be a bigger risk factor than fat from vegetable sources. I suspect that a larger group of women would have to make a more substantive change in both fat content and nutrient density of their diet before a study would show a decreased incidence of breast cancer.

Family History of Breast Cancer

Certain families have been identified with genetically higher chances of early onset breast cancer and sometimes ovarian cancer.[25] For women in these families, the Strang High Risk Center provides information on how to accurately determine breast cancer risk. (See Resources.) The majority of women diagnosed with breast cancer *don't* have a positive family history, but for those who do, a proactive approach is important. The first thing I tell my patients who have a positive family history—usually a mother with breast cancer—is that they are *not* their mothers and that genetics is only *one* part of whether somebody gets a disease.

Here's the story of one woman, a social worker, who has resolved her family history eloquently. "Life had been hectic for some time. Working as a social worker in a large Boston teaching hospital, I covered the oncology unit and the two ICUs [intensive care units] and had a beeper that went off nonstop. At home, I felt continuously assaulted by the noise from the street and from the huge radios that every kid on the block played. I vowed that by the age of fifty I would retire from the rat race and find someplace quiet where I could do some teaching and consulting and have a small private practice and a big garden.

"I had been working in oncology for a few years. Initially, I felt somewhat compelled to do so, knowing that it had to do with my own mother's death, at the age of forty, from breast cancer. It was something of a death-defying act. If I could learn as much as possible about cancer, it would never 'get' me. All I had to do was get past the age of forty. In my own therapy, as I approached forty, I faced the issue of 'having' to do oncology work. After some struggle, I finally decided that I did what I did because I was very good at it, and that when the time came to work in some other sphere, I could do it.

"The age of forty came and went. And the angst remained.

"In September 1990, I came to Maine for a vacation. I was having dinner with an acquaintance and we were talking about our dreams for the future. When I said that my dream was to retire to a place like this when I turned fifty, she challenged me with the question, 'Why not now?'

"My answer was that I made good money for a social worker, I had a manageable mortgage, and I was vested in the hospital pension plan. Her observation that I was being held by the 'golden hand-cuffs' irked me, because I like to think my values are elsewhere. 'Besides,' she said, 'what makes you think you'll get to fifty?' Not only did my mother die young, but every day I was working with people younger than I who were dying.

"At that moment I know that my life changed. I felt it in every cell of my body. And I *knew* there was no reason not to come to Maine. The next day I told a realtor what I wanted, and on the following morning at nine A.M. I walked into the house that I now own. That first house that I looked at was just what I had dreamed about.

"In January I moved to Maine and continued to work in Boston, never minding the commute, which was made easier by a flexible schedule. In March, Claudia, a young leukemic of whom I had become very fond, died. I had worked with Claudia and her family for four years. I dreaded her death. The morning she died, I experienced chest pains. Knowing that there was no physical problem with me, I paid attention and tried to figure out what my body was saying to me. By the end of the day, I had named that pain 'collective heartbreak.' I realized that I knew more dead people than live people and decided that I needed a weekend away to think about things. A few Sundays later, I was sitting out on the rocks in front of a big resort, looking at the ocean. My thoughts were of Claudia, of many of the others I had worked with who had died, and eventually of my mother.

"For some reason I was curious about exactly how old my mother had been when she died. Surprisingly, I had never done the arithmetic that would give me that information. Simple calculations told me that she had been forty-one years and nine months old when she died. On that very day, I was exactly forty-one years and nine months old! And I had been working on the oncology unit for five and one-half years—the same length of time she had been sick with her breast cancer. I had done it! I had survived!

"The next day I handed in my resignation. I took the summer off to think about what to do with my life. Those few months turned into a few more, and before I worked again, nine months had passed—an appropriate amount of time to be reborn.

"During that time, I had the birthday my mother never had and began to rethink my identity and priorities. Eventually, I began what has turned into a very successful psychotherapy practice. I get to teach now and then, do a bit of consulting, and have that big garden. And I know for sure that I'm my mother's daughter, yet I never have to *be* her.

"As part of my journey, I have come to believe in the strength of the body and spirit—a helper even in the most impossible situations. In the 1950s, when my mother had breast cancer, I know that there were few options for a Roman Catholic woman stuck in a bad marriage, even fewer if she had been physically disabled in childhood, as was my mother. I now believe that my mother's breast cancer was her only way out of an impossible situation, a bad marriage, a stultifying existence of guilt and self-sacrifice. I regret that her escape cost her her life."

Women's Stories

Treatment modalities for breast cancer are beyond the scope of this book and are not my specialty. I'm not particularly happy with the cure rate from the current approaches. Though the experts may disagree somewhat with the statistics, the data suggest that the overall mortality rate from breast cancer hasn't changed appreciably in forty years, despite new drugs and surgical techniques.

Yet breast cancer need not be a death sentence. Many of my patients are living proof that there is life—vibrant healthy life—after the diagnosis of breast cancer.

In my experience, dietary change, certain types of support groups, and inner reflective work are important parts of treatment, regardless of whether one has a lumpectomy, uses herbs, or undergoes mastectomy and chemotherapy. Though the vast majority of women with breast cancer choose surgery, chemotherapy, or both for treatment, I've worked with several women whose choice has involved dietary change and inner healing work only—without any aid from conventional medicine besides the initial biopsy to make the diagnosis. After several years, two of these women now have clear mammograms and no evidence of cancer anywhere. One was called at home by her surgeon at the time that she first refused treatment and was told that if she didn't have the recommended surgery she would die. She refused, and now seven years later she's cancer-free. One of these women, Mildred, was forty-three years old when her diagnosis of breast cancer was made. She was married to a university professor and lived in a midwestern college town. She had never worked outside of her home, having chosen instead to marry in her early twenties and raise three children. Shortly after she turned thirty-five, she realized that her husband had been having a series of affairs with students. For financial reasons, she chose to stay with him until their children were older. When her diagnosis of breast cancer was made, however, she left her marriage, went back to school, and got a job. She is now living happily and independently. She had a lumpectomy only. When her daughter asked her why she didn't get a mammogram and exam every six months, Mildred replied, "I know why I got breast cancer. I knew what the problem was in my life, and I got rid of it. I know I will not get it back again." She knew that she could not maintain her health and stay in a marriage with a man who was sexually unfaithful to her. After more than ten years, she hasn't had a breast cancer recurrence.

Another of my patients, Julia, was thirty-eight when she had a lumpectomy. The biopsy showed that not all the tumor had been removed during this procedure. A mastectomy and lymph node dissection were recommended because of the nature of her cancer. Instead, she chose to return to her childhood home in the South and confront her demons—a lifetime of codependence and a marriage she had outgrown. This process was accompanied by a deep emotional cleansing and a letting-go of her past ways, unhealthy behaviors, and habits. Julia also changed her diet to a healthy vegetarian one. Though she is cancer-free at this time, she knows that she must stay in touch with her innermost needs and her bodily wisdom. She recently felt "called" to move to the Southwest. Though unsure of how she would make a living, she decided to go anyway. Almost immediately she found a job at a bed and breakfast. Her circumstances there were very healing and afforded her not only room and board but a great deal of time and space alone and close to nature. Julia is extraordinarily courageous and continues to do well.

Another of my patients, Gretchen, was diagnosed with a type of breast cancer that is known to be very aggressive and fast-growing. She refused conventional treatment and instead changed her diet and left an abusive marriage. She eventually found a job in a publishing house doing work that she loves. Three years later, she has no obvious cancer. But she lives from day to day and doesn't think in terms of "being cured." She says, "The essence for me is living my life one day at a time." Gretchen believes that the lifestyle changes she made have been the major factors in her healing.

I believe that some cases of breast cancer cure themselves before we even know about them. Nevertheless, the vast majority of my patients diagnosed with breast cancer undergo some type of surgery, sometimes followed by radiation and chemotherapy. I am concerned about the practice of removing lymph nodes in the armpits of women with very small breast cancers. Though lymph node removal and analysis are part of how a surgeon determines how far the cancer has spread and are therefore used to make treatment decisions, they often leave women with swelling and pain in the arm that doesn't always resolve itself. I feel that the lymph nodes are part of the body's immune system and exist to help the body fight the cancer. However, I do not treat breast cancer, and so I must defer treatment decisions to those who do.

Caroline Myss and other healers teach that cancer is the disease of timing. It can result when most of a person's energy is tied up dealing with old hurts and resentments from the past that they can't seem to release. These old hurts need a witness—someone who validates the wounds—before healing can begin.

Our relationship to time can and does make us sick. Sonia Johnson says, "Time is not a river, we all have all the time there ever was or ever will be right now. Linear time, itself, is an addictive construct."[26] In a materialistic, addictive culture, we learn that time is money and that we should spend each minute of our lives accomplishing or producing more and more. Instead of enjoying each moment we have to live our lives fully, we are instead taught at an early age that "there is never enough time." We are always "running out of time." Far too many of us suffer from "hurry sickness." We rush around, our hearts beating faster, feeling that there is too much to do and not enough time to do it. The state of our bodies and the cells that constitute them reflect this.

Monica was forty-eight when she first came to see me. She had recently had a positive biopsy for breast cancer. Her general surgeon wanted to do a mastectomy as well as remove the lymph nodes from underneath her right arm. Monica and her partner owned a used book store and ran a service for procuring hard-to-find books. Both of them had read extensively on the topic of breast cancer. She objected to the mastectomy and after full discussion, the surgeon stated that he felt comfortable doing a lumpectomy. They had been to see an on-cologist and knew that chemotherapy was a standard recommenda-tion for her type of cancer. But they wanted to find out about other things that she could do in addition to conventional treatment.

I suggested to Monica that she could eat a vegetarian diet to lower her circulating estrogen levels and apply castor oil packs to the affected breast to enhance her immune system functioning. I stressed that these measures were not considered "cures" in a con-ventional sense and that they hadn't been studied nearly as well as surgery and chemotherapy. She understood that. I told her that it was imperative that she spend the next few months learning how to take care of herself and do things that brought her pleasure. She and her family left to consider all her options, and I planned to see them three months later, in September.

When Monica returned three months later, she looked fifteen years younger and was radiant with health. I asked her what she had done. She told me, "When I left here, I knew that I had to change my life. This summer I decided to do whatever felt wonderful and healing. So I rode my bike every day and spent long hours lying in the fields looking up at the sky and the clouds. I took summer into every cell of my body. I haven't had a summer like this one since I was a kid. It seemed to go on forever."

Monica had changed her relationship to time. She had literally "stopped the clock" and brought her cells into the present. Many of us need to take the time to "take summer into every cell of our bodies." It has been six years since Monica has had any evidence of cancer. Though she eventually decided *not* to have chemotherapy or further surgery, she has remained cancer-free.[27]

Ellen is another woman whose life seems to have blossomed and improved since her diagnosis of breast cancer. When I first saw Ellen at the age of forty-six, she was just finishing up chemotherapy for her breast cancer, and she wanted some nutritional advice to help her hair grow back faster. She was the mother of grown children and lived with her husband. Her lumpectomy and lymph node dissection had been followed by some chemotherapy to decrease her chances of a recurrence. I recommended a multivitamin-mineral program and suggested that she get started on a whole-food diet gradually. Her hair grew back quickly and beautifully—and she was happy. Within one year, though, she developed a metastasis of the cancer to her spine. She underwent "palliative radiation" for this. No one was offering her a cure now—the cancer had spread to the bone.

I talked to her about what she could do to improve her immune system functioning. It turned out that her mother-in-law lived next door, and this woman's demands for attention had been a source of irritation for Ellen for years. Her husband had a lot of unresolved guilt about his mother, and the burden of caring for her endless needs had fallen to Ellen. I told her that she needed somehow to create a boundary between herself and this woman's demands. She decided to let her husband visit his mother and take care of her needs, thus freeing her to concentrate on her healing. This worked out well. She also changed her diet and took time out every day to play the piano, something at which she is very accomplished and from which she receives a lot of enjoyment.

Ellen pulled together a program that has worked well for her. Over the next seven years she had no recurrence of her cancer, and her bone scans are now negative. Her radiation therapist even wrote, "This turn of events approaches the miraculous," on his last office note. (I love it when doctors use words like that.) When I asked Ellen for some of her thoughts about her healing, she said: "I am feeling very happy to have survived seven years since the initial cancer bout, and I believe I have overcome the odds and am cured of this dread disease. It's good to put it all in perspective. I can be more detached now that I'm away from the immediacy of my recovery. However, my family doctor advised me to 'never stop fighting' when he told me about alternative choices—not popular at the time.

"There are many reasons why my breast cancer has been arrested. The work of my surgeons, my oncologist, and my radiation therapist all come to mind. I have the utmost respect, admiration, and affection for all of them. The love and concern of my family—particularly my husband and my friends—has also helped. Another great help was the counseling I went through during that first year of surgery, chemotherapy, and radiation. The books I read were also helpful. My first was *Living Well Naturally,* by Dr. Anthony Sattilaro.[28] It was very inspirational, and I keep it close by in my kitchen to this day. I don't begin to do all the things he advises; however, I do keep up my 'Do-In' exercise daily[29] and try to keep my dietary and spiritual life in order.

"The spiritual part of me has been brought out by this and has been a great comfort. Meditation, as originally suggested by my family doctor, has led me to the study of Zen Buddhism. This, along with the practice of yoga and tai chi and nutrition, has given me a mind/body connection that brings personal faith and physical strength to aid in the healing process, along with a high level of awareness.

"On a day-to-day basis, I start out each morning with a fifteen-minute routine that involves yoga exercises, tai chi, and Zen for both physical and spiritual well-being. At night, I do the 'Do-In' exercises. I watch my weight and spend a great deal of time planning, preparing, and cooking meals that are health-supportive. I eat whole foods, little fat, very little meat, chicken and fish three times a week, and lean red meat once a week. I also eat very little dairy food and many more complex carbohydrates—vegetables, salads, fruits, whole grain breads, brown rice, and soups. I also eat very little sugar. I take vitamins and eat what is available seasonally.

"If I had to talk to other women with this illness, I would tell them to get involved with their illness. They should do everything in their power to help their body become healthy and free of cancer! Have a sense of humor about it—see the positive, good things in life, and *go for it!*

"Keep yourself looking attractive when things are rough. Plan a trip or treat for yourself after chemotherapy. Keep active, and read as many books as possible. Seek out the counsel and support of others. Have a therapeutic body massage. Keep your energy flowing. There is a lot of love out there to help you. Get second opinions!

"I play tennis twice a week and golf in nice weather. I have an herb and a flower garden, I study the piano, and I meditate and listen to tapes. (I particularly like Joan Borysenko's book *Love Is the Lesson*.[30]) I try to stay centered and avoid the stresses of modern life. The study of Zen means a great deal in my life. I am fortunate to have a very loving husband and two lovely animals to share my life, as well as three grown sons, a daughter-in-law, and grandchildren nearby to light up my life.

"As far as my relationship with the breast cancer at this time, I feel that I am in control now. A diagnosis of cancer can make you feel out of control at first. It is very negative—the ultimate fear, when Darkness comes into one's life. Now that six years have passed, however, I am feeling a positive wellness of body and mind. I am increasingly peaceful and secure. I feel energy in my body and want to enjoy life. I feel the life-force within that will help me be in touch with greater forces. I feel like a person in tune with the universe. I want to let go and also to give of myself. Cancer initially makes one feel introspective and afraid—really scared. I like to be happy and satisfied without anxiety.

"My life has improved since being diagnosed with cancer. My relationships with others are more open—there's more give and take. I'm more honest. I feel more 'in the moment,' enjoying and being a part of the moment now, not dwelling on the past or worrying about the future. Zen has helped me to deal with the good and the bad."

Though Monica and Ellen chose entirely different healing approaches, both have changed their relationship to time, and both believe that they've chosen the right path for themselves.

Cosmetic Breast Surgery

Implants: A Smokescreen for the Real Problem

Recently, the news media have highlighted the problems that some women have been having with silicone breast implants. Chronic fatigue, arthritis, immune system depression, and other problems have been linked with these implants. Though I have seen no women with these particular problems, I have seen dozens of women with implants over the years of my practice, and most of them have done well. Therefore, whenever I read a headline that says something like WOMEN ARE ENRAGED AT DOW CORNING, I ask myself, "Why is it that these enraged women were moved to get breast implants in the first place?" Jenny Jones, whose breast implant story was on the cover of *People* magazine, said candidly that at the time she had her implants, no one could have talked her out of it. Her father had made comments about her breasts for years, and she wanted to change how she looked. Her honesty was refreshing, and her story is an example of how we women cooperate in our own oppression.

The current uproar masks a deeper cultural problem: On some level women know that our concern with breast size is not healthy, but we haven't yet found out what healthy is. It doesn't take a sociologist to figure out why women would want to look like the images that have been burned into our brains since childhood by everything from *Playboy* to MTV. (My ten- and thirteen-year-old daughters have already been concerned with their body shapes and weights for several years now.) Women's bodies are cultural battlegrounds, and we have taken on the impossible task of trying to look perfect according to standards that are not based on reality.

I disagree with women who feel that women who have had plastic surgery have "sold out." If there were an easy way to move fat from the buttocks to the breasts, I might consider having an augmentation myself! I have a very small breast size—they don't make an underwire bra small enough for me. And one of my breasts is smaller than the other from having had that huge breast abscess. Overall, though, I'm quite happy with this area of my body. When I first watched a breast augmentation and saw the amount of tissue damage done when lifting the chest wall off the underlying tissue, I instinctively held my own breasts protectively. I realized that I could never elect to have this procedure done to me for cosmetic reasons as it is currently performed. For one thing, implants can decrease or eliminate nipple sensation, which is part of a woman's sexual pleasure, and the implants can become very hard and encapsulated. They can cause the formation of fibrous capsules around the implant and the inability to nurse a child. But I do not judge women who have had this procedure, any more than I would judge women who have had their nose size and shape cosmetically altered.

Breast implants and the newer breast reconstruction—using a woman's own abdominal tissue—can give women who have lost a breast to cancer a body image that approaches wholeness. This surgery can be key to a woman's healing. Dr. Sharon Webb, a plastic surgeon who specializes in breast reconstruction following breast cancer surgery, says that she often receives letters from her patients and their family members telling her how grateful they are for her work and how much the surgical breast reconstruction has contributed to their overall sense of well-being. None of us is immune to our cultural inheritance and its impact on how we approach our breasts, and we need to exercise compassion for our own and other women's choices. Each woman has to decide for herself what feels best for her body and why. Here are a few stories concerning cosmetic breast surgery and its consequences.

Janice: Family Pressure

Janice came to Women to Women ostensibly for a routine annual physical exam. She had been there on two previous occasions for diaphragm fittings. A working woman, she was slim and attractive. When I entered the exam room, she said that she had some other issues she wanted to discuss after her exam, so afterward she came into my office.

Janice told me that she had had a breast-enlargement procedure a few years before and that everything seemed fine. (My exam had confirmed that.) In my office, however, her eyes filled with tears, and she said she was afraid she would cry because she had something to ask me that she had never before asked a doctor. I suggested that she stay with her emotions because whenever we're moved in this way, we are on to something very important. She continued, "I first went to see a gynecologist when I was sixteen. I was having terrible menstrual cramps, and I wanted to see if anything was wrong with me. He wouldn't let my mother remain in the room with me when he examined me. His exam was very painful and I asked him to stop, but he wouldn't. Then when he saw my breasts, he laughed and said, 'Maybe if you marry and your husband fondles you enough, they'll grow.' " He prescribed birth control pills for her cramps, and she left the office feeling humiliated.

Janice went on to describe her early breast development. She said that at first her nipples had grown and started to stand out. It felt, she said, as if she had a walnut-size mass under each nipple. This tissue grew to about the size of an avocado pit and stopped. What she was describing was normal breast budding, with normal glandular tissue underneath the nipple. This had happened around the time she got her first period. I told her that it all sounded very normal to me. She cried again. Her breasts were naturally small, but her mother, her brother, and a sister had always referred to her as "deformed."

One day while clothes shopping with her mother, her mother commented on Janice's "deformity" and told her that if she ever wanted anything done about it, she'd be willing to pay for it. (I frequently hear stories of mothers telling their daughters that their breasts are not big enough. Sometimes they suggest that their daughters wear padded bras or stuff their bras with tissue.) Janice surprised her mother and said that she did in fact want something done. Soon after, she had an augmentation mammoplasty, or breast-enlargement procedure, with silicone implants.

I asked Janice how she felt about her breasts now. She replied that she had mixed feelings because of the circumstances under which she had had the surgery. Since she was also having acupuncture treatments and was more interested in natural healing than she had been in the past, she was afraid that she'd messed herself up by doing something so "unnatural."

My reply was to share with Janice that quite a few of my patients had elected to have their breasts enlarged and had been very happy with the procedure. The ones who were happiest were those who had given it a lot of thought beforehand and were doing it to please themselves and not anyone else. These women had good results and no complications. When someone feels positive about a decision such as this, I believe that their immune system functioning is enhanced and that the complication rate is apt to be lower. I wanted Janice to know that I didn't think that having the breast surgery had damaged her health in any unalterable way.

Most important I affirmed that she was normal, not "deformed," and that she had always been normal. She simply had small breasts, like all the women on her father's side of the family. Unfortunately, she had grown up in a family that was emotionally abusive about her body at a time when she was very vulnerable. Her visit to the gynecologist had reinforced that pathology.

Now at the age of thirty-three, Janice was finally ready to bring up this history about her body. Before she left, she said to me, "You have no idea how important it is for me to hear this stuff from a doctor." I suggested that she spend the rest of the day staying with her tears and any other emotions that came up. I asked her to express them through sound. All of the tears and all of the emotions that we stifle stay in our physical bodies as unfinished business and are waiting for us to attend to them. Janice now had the opportunity to finish a significant amount of healing. She was ready to heal on all levels her relationship with her breasts.

Sarah: Implants to Please Her Husband

Sarah was about fifty-five when I first saw her. She had raised several children and had been married for twenty-five years to an alcoholic but was now divorced. As is so often the case with people like Sarah, her father had also been an alcoholic. Fifteen years before, Sarah's husband had become impotent. He had blamed her for his condition, telling her that her body just wasn't the way it needed to be for him to be able to get an erection.

Like so many women who are in addictive relationships, Sarah believed him and took on his problem as her own. Her husband said that maybe he wouldn't be impotent if her breasts were bigger. She dutifully went to New York and had breast implants placed. She hated them from the first, and her husband's impotence remained— except that now he told her something must be wrong with her vagina. Their relationship continued to deteriorate, and his drinking worsened.

Several years later Sarah's husband left her. (He is now with a younger woman for whom we can all feel sorry.) Sarah went into codependence recovery and realized that she was *not* the cause of her husband's impotence and never had been. But now she is stuck with silicone implants that she hates. She said that when it's cold outside, her breasts don't get warm because it takes so long for the implants to warm up. She has looked into having them removed but was told that it would cost her $3,000, which insurance won't cover. (This is not always the case.) Every day she is reminded of the price she's paid with her body.

Kim: Implants to Please Herself

Kim is a vivacious woman in her late thirties. She works in the fashion industry now, but she was a teacher for years. When she was a teenager, she had had large hips and very small breasts. She was never able to buy a suit because she could never find a top and a bottom that both fit. For years she was unhappy with her figure, even though she was a multitalented woman. She exercised and followed diets to correct as much of the imbalance as she could, and she elected to have her breasts enlarged after giving it years of thought. The procedure went beautifully and has been a real healing for her because she chose this procedure under optimal circumstances: She did it for herself. She already had high self-esteem, and her expectations for the procedure were appropriate.

Beth: Caught in the Middle

Beth has been a patient of mine for years. She has had two pregnancies and nursed both children. Her husband left her after her second child was born, and she's been raising her children by herself. She's independent and strong. Several years ago, she had a breast augmentation. After childbirth and nursing, her breasts seemed to be flaccid. She couldn't find a bra to fit, and she was uncomfortable with her appearance. She had always had a very attractive body. (I realize that this concept is loaded: attractive to whom? Why? For what purpose?) In any case, though she had a very low income, she managed to get the money together to have her breasts enlarged. The outcome was excellent, and she's pleased with the results. An anthropologist might say that her "social" body was improved by this surgery. (She's currently at work on overcoming her uncanny ability to attract men who aren't supportive of her.) My plastic surgery colleagues tell me that at least in the Northeast, most women who have breast augmentation are like Beth—they have it following childbearing.

.   .   .

The patients just described had their surgery four to five years *before* the current flap over silicone implants. I have no doubt that the current adverse publicity about implants will cause as much harm to Janice and thousands like her as the silicone itself—not because of problems with the silicone (and I'm not denying that there are potential problems) but by planting seeds of fear and doubt that in and of themselves can affect the immune system.

I believe that the circumstances surrounding a woman's breast implantation—why the surgery was done—are as crucial to her freedom from side effects as any potential problems from the silicone. Kim had implants so that she would be happier with her own appearance, and she has been very happy ever since. Now everything matches, and she's content. I spoke with her recently, and she said she loves her implants and is certain she'll have no trouble with them. She's not concerned about the media hype. I believe that the same holds true, in general, for postmastectomy reconstruction patients and for those who have had implants to equalize the size of their breasts.

Silicone leaks, which occur in about 5 percent of breast implants, can and do undoubtedly set up potential problems in *some* women. But not *all* women react to the leak problem. Breast implants have been used for decades with varying degrees of success.

I learned a very big lesson from my own breast abscess, so I routinely send it a lot of positive feedback—after all, its function died for my sins. Women with silicone implants are also learning a very big lesson, though the lesson for each of them will be different.

A Healing Program for Implants

• Understand that thousands of women have *no problems* with implants. Consider the fact that you have a good chance of being one of those women.

• Forgive yourself for not knowing things that Dow Chemical didn't tell you or your doctor, and that it perhaps didn't know itself. Don't waste any of your precious energy beating yourself up.

• Talk with the surgeon who placed the implants. The plastic surgeons to whom I refer patients make information packets available for all women who've had implants.

- Make sure that your diet supports your immune system: vegetables rich in beta carotene, whole grains, and beans are excellent. A low-fat, high-fiber diet is best. I also recommend a multivitamin-mineral supplement. Consider consulting a nutritionist.

- Castor oil packs applied to the breasts once per week are an excellent immune system enhancer and are also relaxing and soothing. I believe that taking the time to use packs lets your breasts know that you care for them. This could decrease adverse effects from the implants.

- For some women, having the implants removed is the right choice. One of my patients recently had her implants removed by the surgeon who put them in nine years before. The removal was done under local anesthesia at no charge to her. She said that it was very easy, and she is happy she had them removed. "I'm at a very different place in my life than I was when I had them inserted," she says. "Even though I haven't had any trouble, I don't want to worry about any potential problems."

- Understand that only you can decide what is best for you concerning implants or any other cosmetic surgery.

Breast Surgery to Decrease Breast Size

Sharon's breasts started to develop when she was only eleven years old. By the time she was fifteen, she wore a size 38D bra. She felt embarrassed at school and was self-conscious about sports. Running was uncomfortable for her, and in the summer she developed painful rashes under her breasts from sweating. Buying clothing was difficult because her hips were slim relative to her chest. At about thirty she had a reduction mammoplasty—a breast reduction procedure. Even though she now has visible scars across each breast, she is thrilled that she had the procedure done.

Erin, a strikingly beautiful woman in her thirties, came to see me for a tubal ligation. During her physical, I noticed that she had the characteristic scars of a breast reduction procedure and asked her when she had had the surgery. She told me that she'd had it in her mid-twenties, because she had simply been tired of all the attention that she got from being both beautiful and having an ample breast size. Though her size had only been about 38C—not unusually large—she still had elected to have the procedure.

One of my friends has a jogging partner who is about a 38C as well. Men slow down their cars and make comments as she jogs by. Even twelve-year-old boys feel that they have the right to follow her on their bicycles and make comments!

These experiences are typical of women who have chosen to have their breast size reduced. Though this procedure often decreases or eliminates nipple sensation, leaves scars, and prevents a woman from nursing her babies, most of my patients who've had this surgery are very happy with the results. In general, however, I would recommend delaying this procedure until childbearing is finished, so that you can have the option of breast-feeding.

Women have had a range of experiences with cosmetic breast surgery. Plastic surgery of the breast or any other area of the body is neither right nor wrong—the demand for it merely reflects the values of the culture. The changes it effects can be very rewarding, but as Naomi Wolf so aptly points out in *The Beauty Myth*, they are not a panacea. Surgery will not heal a woman's life or her relationship with her body. The most important factor in a successful outcome, aside from a skilled surgeon, is the context in which the procedure is done and the expectations that the woman has of it.

Caring for Your Breasts

RESPECT THIS PART OF THE BODY. Our task as women is to learn, minute by minute, to respect ourselves and our bodies—whether we have small breasts or large breasts, implants or mastectomies. When we appreciate our breasts as sources of nourishment for babies and sources of pleasure for ourselves, our relationship with them is bound to improve.

When you examine your breasts each month, do so with respect and caring. Thank your breasts, chest, and heart area for being a part of your body. Ask them to forgive you if you've continually showered messages on them that they're too large, too small, too droopy, or too lumpy. Then let them know that you are committed to respecting them and accepting them as worthy parts of your body. If you still think they're ugly after a week or so, respect them anyway—as an act of courage. Eventually, your attitude will soften. Remember, thoughts and feelings have *physical* effects.

NOURISH YOURSELF WELL. Consider changing your diet to a more high-fiber, low-fat, nutrient-dense approach *now*. Critics argue that we don't have enough data yet. Although further studies are needed to absolutely lay this issue to rest, why wait?

IF YOU'VE HAD A MASTECTOMY. If you've had a mastectomy, touching your scar with respect and reverence is a help—an acknowledgment of your sacrifice. A thirty-eight-year-old midwife that I met at a conference had had a breast removed at the age of twenty-one. She said that in looking back, she realized that she had profoundly rejected her breasts early on in life because she'd been given the message since birth that she should have been a boy. She attributed her breast cancer to her chronic negativity about being female. Now, more than twenty years after her mastectomy, she has decided to discard her prosthesis. She told me that the "fake" breast created a block between her chest, her heart, and the loving energy that this part of her body needed to feel. She said that now when she gets a hug from someone, all of her chest gets in on that loving energy, too.

Breast reconstruction following mastectomy can be a blessing. If this is your truth, spend some moments regularly appreciating the work of the surgeon, combined with the healing power of your body.

A few women who desired larger breasts have told me that they were able to increase their breast size by positive affirmations and by sending love to that area of their bodies. Several studies have documented that creative visualization and self-hypnosis can increase breast size or firmness; women have used the power of their own minds to duplicate, physically, the conditions that existed in their breasts at puberty.[31] If our bodies are nothing but a field of ideas, let's make sure that those ideas represent our best interests.

ELEVEN

Our Fertility

A fertile, sexually active woman using no contraception would face
an average of fourteen births or thirty-one abortions during her
reproductive lifetime: altogether, a mind-boggling disruption in
this period of hoped-for independence and equality for women.
    —Dr. Luella Klein, former president of the American
    College of Obstetrics and Gynecology, 1984

*I*deally, prenatal life, close to the mother's heart, is bliss for the
unborn. Women need to choose to live out their pregnancies
wisely, because the way they do so affects both themselves and their
offspring. Babies remember their lives—*all parts* of their lives—and
their experiences have a potentially large effect on them.

All of us retain the imprint of our entire lives within our cells. If,
during those vulnerable first nine months, a mother is emotionally
unavailable to her baby—for whatever reason—her baby often
picks up on this. Prenatal and birth memories, and their potential
impact on the unborn, are one of many reasons why women must
learn to manage their fertility well and learn how to conceive consciously. Women must become conscious vessels.

Many women have told me that they knew their parents didn't
want them, and that they had felt it their entire lives. "I know I was
conceived during my mother's grief for a son who died nine months
before," one woman said. "I remember taking this on in utero. I
vowed to try to make it better for her. I've spent sixty-four years

trying to do that for her. It has never worked." One menopausal woman, Beverly, said that her mother visited her on her fiftieth birthday with balloons and a rose, then proceeded to tell her, "You are fifty. Your life is downhill from now on. You're not a kid anymore." She told her daughter how much she had suffered in giving birth to her, and she went on to say that when Beverly was born, she had been ugly. She sang the praises of her son, however—Beverly's brother—saying that that labor had been virtually painless and that the son had been beautiful ever since birth. Listening to her mother, Beverly felt that in a perverse way she had been given a true gift on her fiftieth birthday. Her mother had confirmed what she had always thought—that she had been rejected since birth.

An existential depression can be felt by people who have been gestated and born under circumstances in which they are not wanted. One woman described feeling ashamed for breathing the air and for taking up space—she had a sense of never belonging, that she was causing someone else pain simply by being here. She told me that she had felt this as far back as she could remember. She knew that she hadn't been wanted.

Another woman, a physician in her fifties, said that she recently had gone through an emotional healing session in which she realized that she had never felt safe in her mother's womb—that she knew she hadn't been wanted. She had been trying to compensate for this her whole life by studying, becoming a doctor, and having a series of relationships. But none of this ever fulfilled a need that had been within her since before she was born—the need to be well loved and desired as a child. As she recalled, "My mother's heartbeat, so close to my own, was *not* a comfort and reassurance to me." Though her mother is now dead, she has gone through the process of forgiving her. In tears she said to me, "Now I finally miss the mother I never had. I realize that she was doing the best she could. She never had a chance for herself."

Abortion

For many women, abortion is an area of "unfinished business," and as such it deserves a thorough discussion. If we lived in a culture that valued women's autonomy and in which men and women practiced cooperative birth control, the abortion issue would be moot. If abortion were forced on women in the United States as it is in China today, it would hold a different meaning here than it does now.[1]

Abortion deliberately ends one potential life. But *not* allowing an abortion potentially murders two lives. The bond between mother and child is the most intimate bond in human experience. In this most primary of human relationships, love, welcome, and receptivity should be present in abundance. Forcing a woman to bear and raise a child against her will is therefore an act of violence. It constricts and degrades the mother-child bond and sows the seeds of hatred rather than love. Can there be any worse entry into the universe than forcing a child to inhabit a body that is hostile to it? Life is too valuable to inhibit its full blossoming and potential by forcing a woman to bear it against her will. Since we know that the early lives of criminals and societal offenders are often filled with poverty and despair, it may even be dangerous to bring a being into the world who isn't wanted. The specter of more and more women trapped in unwanted pregnancies looms on the horizon as women's reproductive capacity is treated as political barter.

On some level, everyone knows this—even those who publicly would deny women the right to control their own fertility. During my residency in Boston, it was not uncommon for pregnant young Catholic women to be brought to me by their parents, who would say, "We don't believe in abortion, but if our daughter had this child, it could ruin her life. Can you arrange something?"

One thing I've learned over the years is that there is no such thing as "sexual freedom." I think that's why I've always been uncomfortable with the phrase "abortion on demand." Having worked in the area of women's reproduction for years, I realize that the current abortion debate is a symptom of the much deeper problem I described in earlier chapters: As long as women continue to misunderstand how to meet their erotic needs, as long as they continue to sacrifice their bodies for the sexual pleasure of men, we will get nowhere. And as long as abortion is seen solely as a "women's issue," we'll get nowhere.

I performed abortions for years, and I will always be a proponent of reproductive choice for women. But I've come to see along the way how complex the issue of abortion is, and I've learned that there are no easy answers.

Abortion is always a loaded topic because it forces each woman to face her deepest feelings about men's ability to impregnate women and women's power to either retain or reject the result of this impregnation. Abortion hits at the heart of our society's beliefs about the role of women. Is society committed to women's full participation in the economy? What is our appropriate role in the home and in society? "Abortion exemplifies political control of the personal and the physiological," writes historian Carroll Smith Rosenberg. "It thus bridges the intensely individual and the broadly political. On every level, to talk of abortion is to speak of power."[2]

I always felt as though I were sitting in the middle of a minefield when I performed abortions. Sometimes I got angry when I performed a fourth abortion on a woman who simply didn't use contraception. At other times I'd perform abortions on women who really didn't want them but felt they had no alternative.

The call for "abortion on demand" implies that women need take no responsibility for their sexual behavior or its consequences. It implies that it's fine to have intercourse with whomever we wish, whenever we wish, and without having to deal with the consequences—just as men have done for centuries. Many women who have had repeated abortions have told me that they later came to realize that their sexual acting-out with men was a form of self-abuse, stemming from their self-loathing and lack of self-esteem. "Abortion on demand" implies that having sex somehow can and should be divorced from the other aspects of our lives, such as the need to be nurtured, held, or respected. It implies that the same behavior that we find abhorrent in men—having sex with no heed for its consequences—is okay for women. Why would women want to imitate (some) men in the sexual arena? We should be resisting *any* sexual contact with men who don't also respect our souls and our innermost selves.[3] In the 1990s and beyond, women are going to have to rethink their sexual programming. But first we need to be clear on what that programming is.

When a woman chooses to have an abortion on behalf of herself and her own life, she is swimming against a five-thousand-year-old tide of conditioning, of social agendas propounded by churches and other male-dominated institutions, that say that woman's primary purpose is to have children and to serve her children and her husband. Allowing women to choose the course of their own lives goes very deeply against a very old grain.

Over the past twenty years, as the number of women going against this grain has vastly increased, the political and societal forces that want to "keep us in our places" are becoming more vocal—and more destructive. A century and a half of rhetoric designed to make women feel guilt and shame surrounding abortion should give little wonder that abortion is not an easy issue for women to talk about freely. Yet if every woman who ever had an abortion, or even one-third of them, were willing to speak out about her experience—not in shame, but with honesty about where she was then, what she learned, and where she is now—this whole issue would heal a great deal faster.

The cultural climate of any historical era can have profound effects on the overall emotional and physical well-being of that era's people. Currently, as women's power is rising, so is the antiabortion rhetoric. Though no culture has been a stranger to abortion, Smith Rosenberg's research documents that abortion becomes a political issue only when there are "significant alternations in the balance of power between women and men, and of male heads of household over their traditional dependents."[4] At just such a time, these changes are reflected in laws concerning women's right to manage their own fertility.

Healing Postabortion Traumas

The technical aspects of the various abortion procedures are very simple and don't usually cause women any physical problems, though it is always a shock to the body when the process of gestation is abruptly halted via outside intervention. All the studies done so far on the long-term health consequences of abortion, whether done by D&C or suction, have failed to show an increase in infertility or other problems. The antiprogesterone drug RU486, the newest morning-after pill, is even safer, according to preliminary studies conducted in Europe.

With decades of guilt and shame as an emotional backdrop, however, many women never adequately process the emotional aspects of abortion. Many have never even told another person that they had one. Not infrequently, a woman will tell me not to tell her husband about the abortions she had prior to their relationship because she doesn't want him to know about her sexual history. Through the years, I've heard many women's stories about illegal abortions—some of them painful, and some quite healing. Several women in their sixties, for example, have told me that they were raped by the abortionist before he performed the procedure—"just to relax you," he would tell them. Because they were so scared and so dependent upon his services, they simply went through the humiliation and said nothing about it for decades. Another woman who had gone through an illegal abortion said that she would be forever grateful to the wonderful man who did her procedure. She felt that his gentle touch and medical skill were a godsend to the many unfortunate women such as herself, in a time when choice wasn't available. May we never see that time again.

The physical results of a woman's shame and regret about abortion can live on in her cell tissue for years. Unresolved emotional pain becomes physical and can set the stage for later gynecological problems like fibroids and pelvic pain. Remember, it is the *meaning* surrounding an event or procedure that gives it its charge and potential to harm or heal—not necessarily the procedure itself. Despite the safety of abortion, I believe that repeated abortions weaken the *hara* or body energy center of the female.

The most difficult abortions I ever did were in those women who had already had one or two children and had homes and resources, but who found themselves pregnant at inconvenient times. I told one of these women, whose husband didn't want the pregnancy, that she might well find herself grieving after this abortion, since she herself clearly wanted the child and was having the procedure mainly to keep peace with her husband. She assured me that she had made a firm decision—that she was finished with car seats for infants and diapers and that she wanted to get on with her life. So I went ahead. Exactly one week later, this woman was back in the office crying, "Why didn't you tell me how bad I'd feel? Why didn't you talk me out of this procedure?" She decided that she wanted to get pregnant again as soon as possible, to "relieve her sense of loss."

Time and time again, women have abortions that they don't want because the men they are with insist upon it. Under these circumstances abortion is a self-betrayal, even a kind of self-rape. It can poison the relationship unless the issues are dealt with openly and honestly.

A patient of mine in her fifties developed continual spotting and an abnormal condition in the uterus called cystic and adenomatous hyperplasia of the endometrium, accompanied by pelvic pain (see Chapter 5). This problem, she feels, was triggered by watching her daughter give birth to a girl. This birth experience caused her to feel a great deal of anger at her husband and a sense of deep sorrow—emotions that she couldn't understand intellectually. Later, after letting herself sit with these feelings, she realized that she still had unfinished business about an abortion she'd had years before that she hadn't wanted. Her husband hadn't been supportive of the pregnancy, so she had gone ahead with the abortion. She is now in the process of doing some belated healing.

In the mid-1980s, I stopped doing abortions. I was tired of mucking around in women's ambivalence about their fertility, and I was tired of performing repeated abortions on women who came back every year for the procedure. I needed a break from this arena for a while and preferred to work on other aspects of the problem—like helping women understand their sexuality and their need for self-respect and self-esteem, regardless of whether they had a male relationship.

At this time, many women are simply neither ready nor able to assume dominion over their own fertility and sexuality. We are still evolving on this point. Abortion as a means of contraception will be necessary in this country for a long while to come, and I will support its availability. Still, I look forward to the day when abortion is rare, when women and men in cooperation will conceive carefully, thoughtfully, and purposefully, and every child will be wanted and cared for.

Healing Past Abortion: Thoughts to Consider
- Were you well supported, counseled, and well informed?
- Did you take time off from your daily routine for a day or two?

- Did you grieve at all? Did you feel the need to?
- Did you feel guilty about it? If so, do you still feel that way?
- Did your early religious upbringing reinforce the idea that having an abortion and choosing your own life were wrong?
- Can you forgive yourself now for what you didn't know then?
- Were you able to share the experience with your family or a trusted friend? Did they support you?
- If you had it to do over again, would you?
- Can you reframe the abortion in your mind as an act of courage—an act of reclaiming your power?
- For some women, the choice of an abortion is a celebration on behalf of self. If that is the case for you, congratulations. If not, what did you learn?

Another View of Abortion

I first heard about communication with the unborn from Dr. Gladys McGarey, in her book *Born to Live.* Dr. McGarey writes of her experiences delivering babies both at home and in the hospital for years. Her deeply spiritual approach to medicine and women's health care has been a great comfort and guide to me over the years, particularly as it relates to the abortion issue. She tells the following story: "I can see that abortion is frequently reasonable, understandable, and the 'right' thing to do. The new light dawned with a story one of my patients told me some time ago. This mother had a four-year-old daughter, named Dorothy, whom she would take out to lunch occasionally. They were talking about this and that, and the child would shift from one subject to another, when Dorothy suddenly said, 'The last time I was a little girl, I had a different mommy!' Then she started talking in a different language which her mother tried to record.

"The magic moment seemed over, but then Dorothy continued, 'But that wasn't the last time. Last time when I was four inches long and in your tummy, Daddy wasn't ready to marry you yet, so I went away. But then, I came back.' Then, the mother reported, the child went back to chatting about four-year-old matters.

"The mother was silent. No one but her husband, the doctor, and she had known this, but she had become pregnant about two years before she and her husband were ready to get married. She decided to have an abortion. She was ready to have the child, but her husband-to-be was not.

"When the two of them did get married and were ready to have their first child, the same entity made its appearance. And the little child was saying, in effect, 'I don't hold any resentments towards you for having the abortion. I understood. I knew why it was done, and that's okay. So here I am again. It was an experience. I learned from it and you learned from it, so now, let's get on with the business of life.' "[5]

My own sister, the mother of three strong-willed and active sons, became pregnant inadvertently when she ovulated during her menstrual cycle—a rare event. She knew that the pregnancy was not right for her—in fact, she felt that it was actively *wrong* on all levels. So she began to work on communicating with the unborn baby, asking its soul to leave. She continued this inner work daily for two weeks. Still she remained pregnant. Finally, she called an abortion clinic to make an appointment, a step she had never dreamed that she would make. No sooner had she hung up the phone than the bleeding started. She miscarried later that day.

Stories such as this one shed a whole new light on abortion. Caroline Myss is very clear that the energy of spirits remains behind after abortion and needs to be fully released. Many ancient traditional cultures acknowledge this as well. (See the story of a patient who went to a Native American shaman for healing around three past abortions that were still emotionally unresolved, in Chapter 6.)

In 1985, while I was attending an international meeting of the Pre- and Perinatal Psychology Association, I participated in a healing abortion ritual performed by Janine Parvati Baker, author of *Conscious Conception*. Baker had learned the ritual from a Native American medicine woman. All the women at the meeting who had had abortions and those who had been deeply affected by them sat in an inner circle. Included in this group were a man whose mother had unsuccessfully tried to abort him, and a man whose wife had aborted a child that he had wanted. In an outer circle surrounding this one sat all of us who had ever seen or done an abortion. We were considered the "eyes" that had witnessed abortion. The outermost circle also included people whose friends and loved ones had had abortions. They were the "ears" that had witnessed abortion.

Throughout an entire afternoon and into the evening, both men and women spoke of—and let go of—years of previously unvoiced personal pain surrounding abortion. Baker, representing a conduit between the worlds, helped release the energy of the aborted spirits. For many, it was a step toward healing.

Each woman's situation is unique regarding whether to have or keep a pregnancy, and no one but that individual woman can or should decide. Whatever her choice is, however, there will be consequences. What is important is that each woman be clear that she has a choice.

Conscious Conception and Contraception

If women expect to improve our personal and professional status in the world, we have no choice but to assume responsibility for our creations and to reclaim our power. This is especially true when it comes to having babies. Women have now reached a time in our planetary history when we must learn to procreate from our conscious choice, not just to fill up an empty space inside ourselves or to try to keep a man. These latter reasons for getting pregnant are remnants of an unconscious tribal programming that no longer serves us. Janine Parvati Baker describes herself as both prochoice *and* prolife: When she was seventeen, she made a decision that she was ready to become sexually active. She also vowed that she would never make love with a man whose child she wouldn't willingly bear, should she become pregnant inadvertently. She says that it took her three years to find such a man. Now *that* is an example of taking responsibility for what we create. Baker's story, like the stories of birthing women in Chapter 12, are beacons for how women might be if they loved and appreciated their bodies and their creative capacities.

To my patients who are contemplating pregnancy, I suggest that they spend some time meditating and praying together with their partner for guidance around the prospect of having a child. Traditional Tibetan women have always spent time in prayer and meditation before conceiving. You can do this even if you're considering donor insemination! The important point is to see your body as a channel for a new spirit and to surrender yourself to the experience—to be open to all that it has to teach you.

I prescribe all the currently available methods of birth control—pills, IUDs, diaphragms, and the rest—and I have worked with women who have done very well with each of these methods. (See Table 6.) Unfortunately, many health care practitioners do not present birth control methods objectively. When I was in medical school and residency, there was a tendency to push oral contraceptives as the optimal method of birth control and to "downplay" the reliability of the diaphragm and condoms. Given our cultural approach to control of the female body, this is not surprising. The "pill" is easy to prescribe, easy to take, very reliable, and very convenient. We can use it to manipulate our menstrual cycles, avoiding periods altogether or on weekends. In short, it fits our cultural ideal. The pill is the most studied medication in history.

Most other birth control methods require more education about the body and more active participation than the pill. They are not geared to the average busy doctor's schedule. Many physicians feel that women will not use barrier methods of contraception such as the diaphragm, condoms, vaginal sponges, and contraceptive foam, because they have seen too many "failures." This is true of some women but not all women. The data show that in the women who are "ideal users"—who use the method correctly every time—barrier methods and even "fertility awareness" (natural family planning) can be 95 to 98 percent effective.[6]

It is important to distinguish between the failure of a birth control method itself and the failure of a woman to use it properly. Many women are socialized to be available for sexual intercourse without involving their partners in contraceptive responsibility. Many women are involved with men who will not cooperate with contraception and feel that it is the woman's job. Obviously, it is best for such women to use contraceptive methods that require no planning, preparation, or male cooperation. Such methods include birth control pills, the IUD, Norplant, DepoProvera, and tubal ligation. Methods that require conscious partner participation, such as condoms and diaphragms, simply are not appropriate for these women.

In order to choose the right birth control method for you, you need to decide *honestly* where you are in your own life—and how much responsibility you are willing to assume over your fertility.

Some women don't even want to think about getting to know their times of ovulation and checking their cervical mucus, let alone inserting a diaphragm before each intercourse. That's fine—they often do well on the pill or other "automatic" method. Other women prefer barrier methods, such as diaphragms, and I encourage these methods too—but only in those women who are committed to using them consciously. I've worked repeatedly with women who've had three or four abortions from failure to use "natural" contraceptives; the pill would have been a better choice for these women, given their sexual behavior. But they refuse to put anything "unnatural" in their bodies. I counsel that there is nothing *natural* about abortion, when a woman fails to use her "natural" method of birth control conscientiously. These women, though conscious about food and the environment, often suffer from the mind/body split we've all inherited—that it is part of being a desirable woman to be available sexually, without asking our partners to share in the responsibility.

Intrauterine Device

The intrauterine device (IUD) is a good choice for some women, though it may carry an increased risk of pelvic infection. The data on this are not yet clear. I've worked with women who've done beautifully with the IUD for up to twenty years. IUDs are associated with an increased risk of tubal pregnancy. They work best for women who've had a child. They are also associated with increased cramping and bleeding in some women.

When I was a medical student, I noticed that women with IUDs seemed to get more infections. The manufacturers of these devices and many doctors denied the problem for a while. At that time, Dalkon shields were being touted as *the* contraceptive of choice for young women who'd had no children. The results were devastating for the many women who tried the product and became victims of its side effects.

Oral Contraceptives

Oral contraceptives may contribute to suboptimal nutrition in some women. The pill has been associated with lowered serum B vitamin levels and other metabolic changes.[7] Women who are on the

TABLE 6
COMPARING CONTRACEPTIVE METHODS

Method	Effectiveness*	Requirements	Advantages	Disadvantages
Fertility awareness	98.5%	Conscious understanding of fertility cycle	Maintains natural hormonal/ fertility cycle	Continual conscious commitment
Diaphragm, with contraceptive cream or gel	98%	Fitting by health professional Faithful use at each intercourse	May protect against pelvic infection and abnormal Pap smears Maintains natural hormonal/ fertility cycle	Unacceptable to some people May cause genital irritation
Condom	98%	Conscientious use for maximal effectiveness Faithful use at each intercourse	Protects against STDs Requires male partner to be cooperative	Unacceptable to some people
Birth control pill	almost 100%	Taking a daily pill	Decreases risk of ovarian and uterine cancer Requires no planning	Blocks natural hormonal/ fertility cycle May increase risk of cervical dysplasia May increase risk of breast cancer
IUD (Progestasert, Copper T)	96–98%	Insertion by health professional Annual replacement	Requires no planning	May increase risk of pelvic infection following insertion or in women exposed to STDs
Spermicidal foam	97%	Conscientious use for maximal effectiveness	Provides partial protection against STDs	Unacceptable to some people May cause genital irritation

Method	Effectiveness*	Requirements	Advantages	Disadvantages
Cervical cap	87%	Conscientious use for maximal effectiveness	Requires no planning	Current caps come in only three sizes—therefore accurate fit is not always assured
Contraceptive sponge	83–95%	Conscientious use at each intercourse	Can remain in place for up to three days Requires no planning	Comes in one size only—may be less effective following childbirth
Withdrawal	77–84%	Conscientious use at each intercourse	Requires no planning	May decrease sexual pleasure
Injectable progestin (DepoProvera)	Almost 100%	Monthly shot	Requires no planning	Spotting and headaches
Progestin implants (Norplant)	Almost 100%	Insertion by health professional	Requires no planning	Spotting and headaches
Vasectomy	Almost 100%	No planning	Requires no planning	Irreversible
Tubal ligation	Almost 100%	No planning	Requires no planning	Irreversible

* Assumes ideal user who uses the method properly every time.

pill should take a good multivitamin containing B complex. The majority of women who have serious health problems with the pill are smokers. Smokers should not use the pill after the age of thirty-five. Oral contraceptives are now being used for women right up until menopause, at which time these same women start on estrogen replacement therapy. Such women are on chemical birth control or hormone replacement for most of their adult lives. I'm not completely persuaded that the benefits override the potential health risks, but many women are persuaded—and it is sometimes *right* for them and where they are in their lives. When a woman uses hormones in this way, however, she misses out on the messages she'd normally get from her uterus and ovaries (as discussed in Chapters 6 and 7).

Progestin-Based Contraceptives

I have had less experience with Norplant and DepoProvera, both progestin-based contraceptives. They are relatively new. Norplant is inserted into the arm under local anesthesia. DepoProvera is given as a monthly shot. Headache and spotting are the most common problems associated with them. They are highly effective, however, and are "automatic" compared with other methods.

Fertility Awareness

Over the years I've worked with many women who've managed their fertility very nicely with various types of "fertility awareness." But I, like most OB/GYNs and most women, never realized until fairly recently, how accurate and well-studied the area of natural family planning really is.[8] When most people think of natural family planning, they immediately equate it with the "rhythm" method. Fertility awareness is much more accurate than the "rhythm" method, which is considered outdated.[9] Dr. Joseph Stanford, a family physician and expert in natural family planning, defines fertility awareness or fertility appreciation as "the use of physiologic signs and symptoms of the menstrual cycle to define the fertile and infertile phases of the menstrual cycle. This information can be used for natural family planning or the diagnosis and treatment of infertility." Fertility awareness involves learning how to determine your time of ovulation. This can be done in a number of different ways: cervical mucus checks, observation of vaginal discharge of cervical mucus,[10] or measurement of basal body temperature (BBT). Observation of cervical mucus, combined with BBTs and other symptoms that occur around ovulation, is called the "symptothermal method" of natural family planning. Commercially available ovulation indicators that test urine pre- and postovulation are also available in most pharmacies. Studies have shown that symptoms sometimes associated with ovulation in some women such as breast tenderness, *Mittelschmerz* (mid-cycle pain associated with ovulation), and change in position of cervix are not always accurate indicators of ovulation.

In a comparative study of fifteen different methodologies, including variations of the most common methods used to determine ovulation, it was found that the observation of vaginal discharge alone, known as the Ovulation Method, was the most precise and practical way to determine time of fertility.[11] The addition of basal body temperature graphs did not improve accuracy over the mucus discharge alone.

The advantage of becoming familiar with your fertility cycles simply through the changes in vaginal discharge over the month is that you will be able to tell beforehand when you are becoming fertile. Lovemaking without intercourse is then possible as an alternative at ovulation time—so is using a barrier method at that time. Highly motivated couples work this out together. Dr. Stanford, who has both personal and professional experience with this method told me that "fertility is not a disease, even though it is often treated like one. It is a part of who we are. When a couple uses this method, they often develop a deep respect for each other, for their fertility, and for their sexuality. This enhances all aspects of the relationship. It is a spiritual thing." Though I did not know about the accuracy of the Ovulation Method at the time I conceived my children, I did use basal body temperature recordings to help time the conception of my children. I found it very empowering.

For birth control, I also used a diaphragm or condom combined with knowing my infertile times until I had a tubal ligation. (I have a very regular cycle, which made it easy to figure out my fertile and infertile times.) My husband and I shared the pleasure and responsibility of dealing consciously with our fertility. I would never have taken the pill—it simply didn't feel right to me to mess around with my hormones to that extent. And I wouldn't have used an IUD—I didn't want a foreign body sitting in my uterus. (I don't make the same distinction when it comes to contact lenses, however.) Nevertheless, the pill and the IUD are exactly right for some women.

Fertility awareness techniques (with or without barrier contraceptives during ovulation) can be highly effective birth control techniques. The Creighton Model Ovulation Method has been studied the most rigorously. Three major studies show method effectiveness rates to avoid pregnancy of 99.1 to 99.9 percent, while actual user rates ranged from 94.8 to 97.3 percent. The differences in these figures were attributable to teaching- and using-related errors.[12]

Knowing when you ovulate can enhance chances of conception considerably. It is generally accepted that the probability of conceiving in one cycle for couples with normal fertility is in the range of 22 to 30 percent. But with fertility-focused intercourse, the chances can increase considerably. In one study of couples using fertility-focused intercourse, 71.4 percent of the clients who had a previous pregnancy achieved pregnancy in the first cycle. With those clients who had never had a pregnancy, the rate was 80.9 percent. By the fourth cycle, 100 percent of those who had never been pregnant had conceived.[13]

In couples who are having difficulty conceiving, using the Ovulation Method charting alone without any other testing can considerably enhance the chances of conception. Dr. Stanford notes that "of couples referred to the NFP center at Omaha for inability to achieve pregnancy (for an average of 3 years), 20 to 40 percent have achieved pregnancy within six months of use of the Ovulation Method, before any further medical evaluation and treatment is undertaken."[14] The Ovulation Method also works well for those who have irregular periods, are breast-feeding, or are perimenopausal.

If you plan to use fertility awareness for contraception, work with a teacher who is highly experienced in assisting couples with optimal use. I do not have much personal experience with teaching this method to my patients. Dr. Stanford, who deals with this fertility awareness extensively, always refers his patients to a thoroughly trained natural family planning counselor, because, though the method is simple, it requires support and education, especially in the beginning. He stresses that to use the Ovulation Method effectively, adequate personalized instruction by qualified teachers is essential for the successful use of NFP in general and the Ovulation Method in particular. It is not learned well from a book. The quality of a woman's (or couple's) experience with this method often depends upon the quality of instruction given and follow-up care received. (See page 683 for Natural Family Planning Resources.)

Couples who use fertility awareness effectively throughout their reproductive lives experience no side effects and often find an increased intimacy in their relationships, which includes a shared responsibility for their combined fertility. Though we tend to associate interest in natural family planning with certain religions, many women are drawn to this method because it is, inherently, a holistic approach to fertility. In a random telephone survey of 1,267 women in Germany, for instance, 47 percent of the respondents were interested or very interested in learning about NFP, and 20 percent indicated a high probability of future use of NFP. Religious factors were notably absent as a motivating force.[15] I suspect that if this method was more widely known and supported by healthcare professionals, it would be more widely used. Whether or not you use fertility awareness for contraceptive or conception purposes, it is empowering to know your fertility cycle. Here's a brief overview of the most common methods used.

DETERMINING THE FERTILE PHASE. The egg lives anywhere from six to twenty-four hours after ovulation. Sperm viability depends on the presence of fertile mucus. Sperm can live for up to five days in fertile mucus. Without fertile mucus, they die in a few hours. Therefore, there is about a seven-day time period during every cycle when pregnancy could theoretically occur.

MUCUS CHECKS (THE OVULATION METHOD). Studies have shown that almost all women can easily learn to check for the presence or absence of fertile E-type (estrogen-stimulated) mucus by the routine observation of vaginal discharge at the vulva.[16] As menstruation stops, cervical mucus is at a minimum. You feel dry. There is no mucus in the vaginal opening and no discharge on your underwear. This lack of mucus is associated with being "infertile." These "dry" days are usually safe for unprotected intercourse. The cervix begins secreting E-type mucus about six days prior to ovulation, so, using this method, you will know when ovulation is apt to occur before it happens. When you see mucus on your underwear or can wipe it off with toilet paper, you know your fertile time is beginning. E-type mucus, when looked at under the microscope, contains channels that help the sperm swim up through the cervix. Fertile mucus is similar in feel and quality to uncooked egg white. Some women may even notice that it wets their underwear. You are fertile from the time when fertile mucus first appears until the fourth day after your peak mucus discharge. The last day of any mucus that is clear, stretchy (greater than or equal to one inch of stretch between thumb and index finger), or lubricative is called the "peak" day of mucus discharge. This "peak" mucus day is highly correlated with ovulation, which occurs plus or minus two days from this "peak" day over 95 percent of the time.[17]

G-type mucus (progesterone-stimulated) appears immediately after ovulation. This type of mucus lacks elasticity. It also has an opaque and adhesive quality. G-type mucus, when looked at under the microscope, lacks the channels that facilitate the swimming of sperm. This type of mucus actually blocks the passage of sperm. Following ovulatory mucus discharge, cervical mucus may cease (you become dry) or becomes thicker and more dense (G-type mucus). Either way, the change is distinct and noticeable. Your period will start about twelve to fifteen days after the peak ovulatory cervical flow.[18]

KEEP A RECORD OF YOUR BASAL BODY TEMPERATURES FOR THREE MONTHS TO SEE IF YOU ARE OVULATING. Though learning how to assess your cervical mucus is more accurate, taking your basal body temperature and recording it for a few cycles is an interesting way to learn about your body and its internal rhythms. It may also enhance your ability to correlate your cervical mucus changes with ovulation.

The temperature rise that occurs with ovulation is due to the effect of progesterone. If you become pregnant during the period you have been taking your basal body temperature, you will notice that it stays up and doesn't drop down again. This temperature elevation on BBT is a very early sign of pregnancy. (When women are pregnant, they have a great deal of progesterone in their systems and their temperature is higher than in the non-pregnant state. Pregnancy was the only time I could comfortably swim in the ocean in Maine.)

Take your basal body temperature first thing each morning starting on the first day of your menstrual period. (This is considered day one of your cycle.) Do this for three cycles, and chart each cycle separately. You can then use your temperature graph to record cervical mucus changes. (See Figure 10.) Ovulation is accompanied by a rise in basal body temperature of about 0.6 to 0.8 degrees. Ovulation occurs somewhere between the time when the temperature begins to rise and the highest point that it reaches. Ovulation occurs plus or minus two days after peak mucus flow. The fertile time generally ends the fourth day after the mucus peak or at the end of the third day in a row of elevated temperature. (See Figure 10.)

If your cycles are quite regular you can get a general idea of the length of your fertile and infertile times by charting the following: Record cycle length for at least six months to determine the earliest possible day that your ovulation could occur. The follicular phase of the cycle (from day one of your period until ovulation) is variable in length. The luteal phase (the time from ovulation to onset of your period) is generally fixed at fourteen days. To determine the earliest day of the cycle when you could ovulate, subtract fourteen from your shortest cycle length. Therefore, if your cycle ranges in length from twenty-six to thirty-one days, the earliest you could ovulate is day twelve (26−14=12). Depending upon your cervical mucus, you could probably have intercourse until day eight or nine of your cycle and avoid pregnancy. (In doing these calculations, you can easily see why charting mucus flow is generally more accurate than this "calendar" method.)

FIGURE 10: FERTILITY AWARENESS:
OVULATION AND BASAL BODY TEMPERATURE CHART

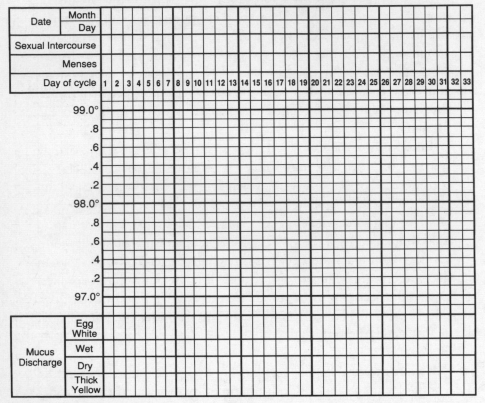

The consistency of your cervix also changes over the monthly cycle. During ovulation, it is much softer and the opening becomes wider than at other times of the month. Some women notice that the position also changes. You can easily feel your cervix by squatting and inserting your index or middle finger into your vagina. You can also do this in the bathtub.

In summary, there is no right or wrong way to work with your fertility. Each of us, however, must look at how deeply programmed we have been to believe that we can't trust our bodies without external hormonal manipulation. When you understand this, you can make a conscious choice. Some of my patients who are in loving relationships with supportive men do not use any contraceptive

FERTILITY AWARENESS:
OVULATION AND BASAL BODY TEMPERATURE CHART

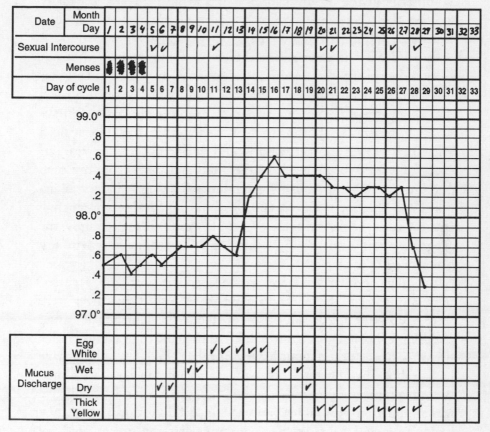

method at all. They simply enjoy sex when they want to, knowing that if they conceive, it will be fine.

Tubal Ligation

Tubal ligation is the most common form of permanent contraception in the United States. Many women are ambivalent about it, however, even when they know intellectually they don't want more children. Most of us value the *ability* to conceive, even if we choose not to use that ability. Permanent contraception closes a door that usually cannot be reopened. For centuries, women were valued solely for of their ability to bear children, and bearing children has been the one socially acceptable outlet for women's creative power. Voluntarily giving up this capacity stirs primitive fears. Yet many women find that being free of the fear of pregnancy is health-enhancing and rejuvenates their sexuality.

Tubal ligation is an excellent choice for some women—but not all! I chose this procedure after waiting until my younger daughter was four. Somehow, though there is no logic to it, this made me feel that she was "safe" and "permanent." At about the age of thirty-seven, my path was split in front of me in terms of childbearing. I knew that having another child would mean another five years of energy diverted to the needs of the child and away from my own pursuits. I still went "mushy" sometimes looking at babies in air-ports, and I harbored a secret fantasy of having "the ideal pregnancy and the ideal labor," in which I would rest and really enjoy the pregnancy *and* the new baby—things I had not done fully with my other two children.

But I had seen far too many women become pregnant "acciden-tally" in their late thirties and early forties, just as their lives were settling down after a decade or so devoted to the demands of raising children. I was at a point in which I had to make a conscious choice one way or the other about having another child. I wouldn't have had an abortion if I became pregnant at this point in my life. (If I had become pregnant during my training years, however, I would have had an abortion without hesitation.) Still, I didn't want a pregnancy just to happen. I wanted to be a conscious decision-maker, not have my life decided by "fate."

My husband assured me that he didn't *need* a son to feel com-plete. Right after I pushed out our second daughter, he had said to me, "You never have to do that again for me." Like many women, I would gladly have had a third child if my husband had wanted to try for a boy. I was and am very pleased to have two daughters. I know I would love them just as much if they were boys, but I don't feel incomplete without sons. But neither my husband nor I really wanted more. We made our decision together, though the final choice was mine. Making the decision to have a tubal ligation was not difficult. I knew that I personally didn't want to bear any more children—so I felt that I should have the procedure, even though vasectomy is technically easier to perform. In the event that I acquired another sexual partner one day through a change of circumstances, I wanted to be sure I would not get pregnant. Besides, I had performed many tubal ligations and felt comfortable with the procedure. (Other couples feel much more comfortable with vasectomy. Studies have shown that it is safer and cheaper than tubal ligation.)

A tubal ligation changes the blood supply to the ovaries somewhat. There may even be a slight risk of an earlier menopause following tubal ligation if the blood supply to the ovary becomes severely compromised, but this is rare. Some women develop "post–tubal ligation syndrome," an ill-defined problem characterized by increased cramping, irregular periods, and heavier bleeding. (Many studies do not show this effect, so its existence is controversial.) I had read the medical literature and knew that the risk of an earlier menopause was very small; from my clinical experience I had concluded that it was mostly a problem for women who had been on the pill prior to their tubal surgery and hadn't experienced natural periods for years. Indeed, they may have developed bleeding problems anyway when they went off the pill, not necessarily *because* of the tubal ligation. A recent study suggests that tubal ligation may even be somewhat protective against ovarian cancer.[19]

I checked with a few medical intuitives to see if they felt that the energy pattern around the pelvic organs could be permanently damaged by a tubal ligation (or a vasectomy). Though some ancient Taoist traditions feel that it interferes with the energy flow of the body, my consultants said that the life-energy around the body simply reroutes itself—that there is no permanent damage to the body after a so-called sterilization procedure. Caroline Myss says that the only problem with a tubal ligation or vasectomy is when the person is ambivalent about it and really doesn't want it done. As with abortion, it's not the procedure itself that can potentially cause problems—it's the *meaning* of it.

I was very clear that the potential problems associated with tubal ligation were *nothing* compared with the disruption that an unplanned pregnancy would cause in my life. So I made an informed choice. Then I called my sister.

Moving into Greater Creativity

My sister Penny had a miscarriage a year before I decided to have a tubal ligation. (We're eleven months apart in age—the doctor asked my mother if she had poked holes in her diaphragm.) After her miscarriage, I said to her, "Why don't you have a tubal ligation and be done with the worry?" She said, "I'll do it when you do." So when I finally decided to do it, I called her up and asked her if she wanted to join me for the event and schedule them at the same time. She said she did. I made arrangements for both of us to have our procedures done in the office under local anesthesia via a technique known as a minilaparotomy (small operation). After I made the appointments, I hung up and experienced about thirty seconds of sorrow about what I had just done. I vowed that if this feeling of loss continued, I'd cancel the procedure. But the feeling passed very quickly.

We decided to make this a meaningful event for both of us. Penny has no daughters; I have no sons. Each of us had to make peace with that. We named our operations and the ceremony we had before-hand "Moving into Greater Creativity" because we saw our lives after childbearing as rich with potential to develop ourselves further. I've always hated the word *sterile* because of its negative connotations—"barren" women are sterile; a bare, cold room is sterile; hospitals are sterile. I didn't consider myself sterile before the tubal ligation, and I certainly didn't see how having my fallopian tubes cauterized would change how I felt about myself. I had simply chosen to be proactive about avoiding future pregnancy.

Our operations were scheduled at nine and nine-thirty on a Friday morning in May. Springtime—a perfect time to celebrate newfound fertility and also, according to Caroline Myss, a good time to have surgery. The energies associated with spring bode well for healing and new growth. The night before, Penny and I participated in a beautiful ceremony—one prepared for us by Judith Burwell, a friend who guides people via ritual through significant life changes. Another friend had made us two exquisite spring flower wreaths to wear on our heads during the ceremony. I felt like a bridesmaid—virginal in the true sense of the word, a woman complete unto herself.

Each of us spoke in turn about how she felt taking this step—and about how, when we make a conscious choice, there's always griev-ing for the choice not taken. Yet we must fearlessly go forth and consciously work with our circumstances to the best of our ability, working to manifest our dreams. In the ritual Penny and I made space to grieve aloud our unborn children—me for my unborn sons, and Penny for her unborn daughters—knowing full well that our Mother Earth doesn't really require more people right now, that that part of Earth's history—the order to go forth and multiply—is over. "For now," I said, "may we go forth and multiply many spiritual children and give birth to ourselves."

The next morning we arrived at the doctor's office, three miles from my house. We had brought a special music tape with us to listen to during our surgery, which was to be performed under local anesthesia with a very light intravenous sedative. My sister went first. I held her hand and checked to see that her tubes were cau-terized in just the right way—not so much that the blood supply would be compromised.

Penny walked into the recovery area, and then it was my turn. It was all quite painless. The doctor at one point said, "Do you want to see your tubes? They are very long and perfect." I said, "No, I'd just as soon have a mind/body split right now." I didn't like the idea of actually burning nice healthy fallopian tubes, something that so many women would love to have. But I had made my choice. If I had changed my mind even *during* the procedure, though, I would have told the doctor to stop.

Afterward, my husband drove us home and fed us lunch and dinner while we rested on the couch, kept ice packs on our lower abdomens, and watched all the episodes of *Anne of Green Gables* on videotape. We developed shoulder pain, which often results when the abdominal cavity is opened and excess gas from room air or carbon dioxide gets trapped under the diaphragm and then is "referred" to the shoulder because the nerves that supply the dia-phragm are connected to the nerves that innervate the shoulder. This gas gets reabsorbed after a day or two, and the pain goes away. The intensity of our shoulder pain was unexpected, but we were very happy with our choice.

The following morning we gathered spring flowers from the yard and floated them in the bathtub while we sat on the side, soaked our feet, and talked about our parents, our childhoods, and how happy we were to be celebrating this momentous event together. Then, while listening to the singing of Susan Osborne, we gave each other a foot massage. Then we rested some more.

Later that afternoon, we drove into Portland to a special store called the Plains Indian Gallery. I bought a piece of art called *Tree Momma*, a magical figure of a woman made out of a weathered wooden branch, fur, and some clay. Penny bought a painting that had deep meaning for her, of two Sioux warriors riding away from a burial platform. These purchases were personal symbols of our conscious choice to shape our destiny by clarity and intent—not chance!

Neither my sister nor I have had any regrets. One chapter of our lives is closed, but we each have opened an entirely new one.

The Trauma of Infertility

Almost all women assume that they will be able to have children someday, even if they're not sure they want to; the potential to have them is important even to women who never intend to use that potential. The ability to conceive and bear children is an almost instinctive birthright of every woman. So when a woman finds that she is unable to have a child, she's often thrown into great despair and feels a sense of injustice: "Why me?" Seeing teenage mothers having no problems getting pregnant becomes almost impossible to bear, unless the woman can find some meaning in the experience and come to terms with it.

One in every six to ten couples has a problem with infertility. Conventional medical wisdom is that about 40 percent of these problems are related to a male factor and 60 percent to a female factor. Statistics show that sperm counts have been gradually falling over the past century. Humans cannot pollute and overcrowd this planet without consequences to our bodies, and infertility is one of them. Conditions on the Earth may not favor fertility the way they used to. It's as though the "collective species brain" were generating a great deal of energy toward making many women and men infertile, due to the stresses of today's families, social environments, and the planet itself. Too many stressful childhoods remain unhealed;

too many children grow up too fast. We're not allowing nature's rhythms to click into gear naturally. The preliminary data on reproductive problems associated with toxic chemicals and with electromagnetic field disturbances around the Earth support the idea that fertility is down.[20]

About 20 percent of infertility has unknown causes—in other words, medical testing cannot explain why a couple is infertile. But the most common factors I see as affecting female infertility are the following:

- Irregular ovulation
- Endometriosis
- A history of pelvic infection from an IUD or other source, causing scarring of the fallopian tubes
- Stress
- Immune system problems—some women make antibodies against the sperm of some men and not others. Likewise, they can make antibodies against the fertilized egg and sperm that is created with some partners but not with others.[21]

A certain percentage of women who've been told that they are infertile for a "medical" reason get pregnant even without treatment. Infertility is never a completely straightforward affair. Many physical, emotional, and psychological factors are involved in conception, so many that it is ridiculous to try to reduce fertility to a matter of injecting the right hormone at the right time. An infertility specialist I met recently said, "I do all the latest high-tech surgery and hormone treatment to try to make someone pregnant. When it is all said and done, I still don't know who will get pregnant and who won't and why. After all my years of training, this area is still a big mystery that I can't control."

The conventional "management" of infertility focuses on the body as a hormonal machine and in large part ignores emotional, psychological, and even nutritional factors that have physical and hormonal manifestations. In fact, most of the studies that link mind and body in infertility were done more than thirty years ago. As our society became more technologically focused, the study of the mind/body connection in infertility, which holds the potential to do so much good for women, has been virtually abandoned, in favor of extremely expensive and invasive technology, the results of which are often disappointing. About $1 billion are spent annually on overcoming infertility.[22]

Psychological Factors

On a personal level, many women do not get pregnant because in their heart they really do not want to—they are afraid of the demands a child will make on them. Caroline Myss explains that women have only so much second chakra energy. If a woman is using her ambition for career success and is already very busy in this area, she may simply not have enough energy circuits available in her body to conceive a child unless she cuts back on her other commitments. Many infertile women are working sixty to eighty hours per week, and are exhausted; then they pursue having a child as though they were writing a Ph.D. dissertation. Conceiving a child is a receptive act, not a marathon event that can be programmed into your DayTimer. Several studies have indicated that excessive focus on the goal of having a child may result in premature maturation of the eggs in the ovary and subsequent release of eggs that are not ready for fertilization![23]

One fascinating study of women undergoing donor insemination noted that after the first several attempts to produce pregnancy, the women, who were previously ovulatory, actually stopped ovulating. The authors concluded that artificial insemination—and any other mechanized, unnatural technique for "forcing" pregnancy—is on some level a traumatizing procedure that leads to the inhibition of the very process it is trying to accomplish. It cannot substitute for the intimacy and the high emotional gratification that occur naturally when two people come together to create new life.[24] Interestingly, orgasm has been found to enhance a woman's chances of conception. Involuntary vaginal and uterine movements that promote conception accompany orgasm. Failure to achieve orgasm may lead to circulatory changes in the blood flow to the pelvis, which can affect fertility.[25] High-tech conception techniques, by their very design, completely ignore this aspect of fertility.

Whenever a woman feels conflicted over birthing, children, or the restrictions that children may impose once they arrive, infertility may result. Several studies have shown an association between infertility and ambivalence toward pregnancy and children.[26] Infertility may result from a woman being treated like a dependent child within her marriage. Interestingly, in several studies the infertile women had resented the onset of their menstrual periods and desired to remain childlike. They often had juvenile faces and bodies, they were parentally overprotected and grasped for sympathy and affection, and they felt inferior about being female.[27]

The relationships between husbands and wives who are infertile have also been studied. Many of the women in these studies had an actual aversion to intercourse; they had low levels of orgasm when they did have intercourse, and they felt a marked sexual disharmony in their partnership. When these women found more suitable partners, however, they became fertile.[28] I have seen this phenomenon repeatedly in my practice. Psychological testing done on 117 husbands of infertile couples indicated that the men had a pronounced lack of self-confidence, were introverted, and had decreased social assertiveness.[29]

Niravi Payne, a therapist in New York City who specializes in infertility, has worked with hundreds of infertile women who unsuccessfully tried to achieve pregnancy through medical intervention.[30] She has found that many of these women have the psychological characteristics already mentioned and have unconsciously absorbed beliefs about pregnancy, sexuality, and having children that are actually blocking their fertility. For example, some women are actually very unhappy with their current partner but are afraid to say so because they feel they have no alternative but to stay with him. Other women were told by their mothers that having babies could ruin their lives. Many of our mothers had no choice but to stay home and raise children, even when they had lots of talent and ambition in other areas. Their daughters often picked up on this and now blame themselves for their mothers' frustrations. They don't want to risk passing this pain on to the next generation. In those women who are willing to come to terms with unconscious beliefs such as these, Payne reports a subsequent pregnancy rate significantly higher than expected.

Artificial and Natural Light

Living in artificial light without going outside into the natural sunlight regularly can have adverse consequences on fertility, because light itself is a nutrient. Far too many people are not only stressed at work, they don't get outside much. When I was trying to conceive my first child, my basal body temperature rose very slowly at ovulation. As I've already mentioned, ovulation causes a rise in basal body temperature of about 0.8 degrees. The ovary produces progesterone at ovulation, which in turn produces this rise in body temperature. I decided to walk outside in the sunlight without glasses or contact lenses for twenty minutes each day. Natural light has to hit the retina in the eye directly. We shouldn't look at the sun directly, but we must be out in the daytime. Within one menstrual cycle, my basal body temperature rose very sharply at ovulation—a big improvement in the pattern. I got pregnant within two cycles of doing this, having tried for five months before. Though this isn't scientific proof of anything, it is an example of a simple change that had immediate measurable effects. The scientific literature on light and human biocycles is extensive.[31]

Nutritional Factors

Nutrients affect every hormonal interaction in the body, and adequate levels of them are clearly important in human reproduction. The standard American high-fat, high-processed-food diet is a setup for suboptimal nutrition at the time of conception. Studies have shown that taking vitamin C (500 mg. every twelve hours in one study) and zinc supplements has helped infertile couples.[32] Other studies have shown a beneficial effect of folate and B_{12} supplementation.[33]

If a woman has been on the pill, especially if she is coming off it to conceive, I recommend that she take a good multivitamin if she isn't already. Given the standard diet today and the stress levels of modern life, a good case could be made for putting all women on a multivitamin and multimineral around the time of conception.

Eating disorders have also been associated with infertility. In one study, the investigators determined that 16.7 percent of their infertile subjects had eating disorders ranging from bulimia to anorexia. They recommended that a nutritional and eating disorder history be taken in infertility patients, particularly those with menstrual abnormalities.³⁴ (See Chapter 17 for more on nutrition.)

Tubal Problems

In order to become pregnant, the fallopian tubes have to be able to pick up an egg and assist its passage to the waiting uterus. This process is dynamic and can be affected by myriad factors. Tubal problems, says Caroline Myss, are centered around a woman's "inner child," while the tubes themselves are representative of unhealed childhood energy. "Blocking the flow of eggs because your own inner being is not 'old' enough or 'mature' or 'healed' enough to feel fertile," she remarks, "can be an energetic pattern behind tubal problems. A part of the woman may remain in prepuberty due to incompletion in her own unconscious mind regarding her readiness to produce life, if, on some level, she's not out of the egg herself."

Women's Stories

GRACE: CHILDHOOD FEARS. Grace was a successful businesswoman from the Midwest at the time when she first came to see me about her infertility. Married for three years, she had been unable to conceive. Like many of my patients, she preferred to avoid extensive and invasive testing to investigate her problem unless it was absolutely necessary. Her reason for this was that she didn't want anyone "mucking around in there."

Grace ovulated regularly, had a normal pelvic exam, and regular pain-free periods. She had no history of infection, IUD use, or prior pelvic surgery. In short, nothing about her history would lead me to think that there was anything wrong with her reproductive system. Her husband's sperm count was normal.

Over the course of her care, she got in touch with a memory from when she was four years old. At that age, she recalled, she had become so ill that she passed out with a high fever and ultimately had to be taken to the hospital. Though she'd felt sick for several days, she had not said anything to her parents until she was quite ill and had developed urinary retention. In the hospital she had to be held down by several nurses and orderlies while they inserted a urinary catheter into her bladder. Her mother felt that this represented very unseemly behavior on her daughter's part.

After Grace's recovery, her mother took her by the hand and made her apologize for being a "bad girl" to each of the nurses and orderlies who had taken care of her. She remembers acutely how ashamed she had felt. She had always felt that she had had a happy childhood, though she admitted that she couldn't remember much about it. But her hospital experience and her mother's abusive behavior had left a very deep wound. I suspect that her childhood was not nearly as happy as she remembers it.

After Grace told me about that childhood hospitalization, her reluctance to undergo invasive testing became understandable. As of this writing, she is working with a therapist and has decided to put her fertility workup on hold so that she can transform her old fears. She recently told me, "I realize I'm not ready to have a child now. I have too much work to do on myself. I don't want to pass my own unfinished business on to a child."

MARGARET: THE OVARIAN WINDOW. Margaret was twenty-seven when she first came to see me. She was not married at the time, but she told me that she wanted children someday and had always dreamed of becoming a mother. From the time she started her menstrual periods, Margaret had had very bad cramps and excessive bleeding, often resulting in missing days of school. At the age of eighteen she decided that she could no longer live with the problem and went to see her mother's gynecologist. He suggested surgery immediately and admitted her to the hospital. He performed major pelvic surgery, removing an ovarian cyst, and he told her she had endometriosis.

Postoperatively in the hospital Margaret developed what is called a paralytic ileus—her bowels wouldn't move. She was given a 1,000 cc. soapsuds enema daily, which she said hurt so much she wanted to die. She also developed a fever that wouldn't go away. She had her mother bring in aspirin to bring her fever down so that she could go home. (She was a nursing student at the time and knew that this would work.) She said that the hospital treatment was so abusive, she wanted to get out of there at any cost. During this time, her parents were going through a divorce—and although they visited her at the hospital, they used her room as a place to fight. Her post-op recovery was far from ideal.

After her surgery, Margaret's cramps lessened a bit, but they were still present for most of her menstrual cycle. This went on for several years and she simply put up with it. At about the age of twenty she had decided to become sexually active and went to a gynecologist for a diaphragm fitting. He told her, "Your pelvis is destroyed. You are definitely sterile. You'll never have kids." She told me that she took in this message "at a cellular level" and that she didn't see another gynecologist for a long time after that. When she finally did see another doctor, he said to her, "Have your children now, or you may never have any." Since she was just finishing nursing school, was not in a relationship, and was in the process of moving, conceiving a child was not high on her priority list at that time.

Around the age of twenty-five Margaret moved to Maine. At a routine gyn exam she was told by a midwife that she had a huge endometrioma (an ovarian cyst filled with old blood from endometriosis). For a second opinion, she saw a gynecologist who was very reassuring and told her her pelvis was normal, which was very comforting to her. But she had by this time gotten a lot of mixed messages. Was she okay or not?

At this time she was a visiting nurse, teaching pregnant teenagers parenting skills and working with many people who had been reported to the Department of Human Services for child abuse. She told me that during this time in her life she simply ignored the issue of possible infertility. It would have been too hard to face, given the suffering she saw every day.

Margaret first saw me when she was twenty-seven years old. We went over her notes from her prior surgery. The ovarian cyst that had been removed was probably a functional cyst from ovulation. Very little, if any, endometriosis had been seen. (If she had had that surgery today, it could have been carried out via laparoscopy, without a big incision. The scarring that she had as a result of that surgery would most likely not have happened.)

Because she was still having pelvic pain, I suggested a vegetarian diet with no dairy food. Within one cycle her pain stopped, and it has not returned. She got married several years later and tried to conceive. After a year or so of unsuccessful efforts, she went to a specialist in Boston, who did a laparoscopy. He told her, "I did the best I could, but I don't think there's much hope. You have too many adhesions in there." Adhesions are fibrous bands that form from inflammation and can block mobility of the organs. (Do you remember using mucilage glue in school? If you put some of this glue on your fingers and then try to pull the fingers apart, little stringy threads of glue form between your fingers. These are what adhesions look like. Some are firm, and some are quite flexible.) Margaret eventually had a second laparoscopy from an infertility specialist to whom I referred her, to see if there had been any improvement in her pelvis. (It is not uncommon for a woman with infertility to have a number of laparoscopies.) We scheduled this surgery at a time when I could be present so that I could support her psychologically and see her pelvis as well. She had *no* endometriosis. Instead, her fallopian tubes were encased in scar tissue, most likely from the prior surgery. But around one ovary and tube was a clear window that was free from adhesions. Under the right circumstances, she had a chance of getting pregnant.

In the recovery room, this fertility specialist told Margaret, "It looks like a bomb went off in there." (Doctors' words are powerful at any time. In the recovery room, when someone is coming out of anesthesia, they are doubly powerful. I was not happy about that comment to her.)

I told Margaret about the adhesion-free window. Later that night, she dreamt that a wise old man came to her and said, "There's a window there. I can see it. It's a window of opportunity. It's all you need to become pregnant." After this dream, she stayed home and cried for three days. Then she went into high gear and called every fertility clinic in the United States, as well as many adoption agencies. She organized and collated a resource book for herself.

About six months later, she decided to do in vitro fertilization (IVF), and she and her husband went to a place in New York. "It was awful," she told me. "I was on Pergonal and Clomid [drugs that make the ovaries produce many eggs]. The scene in the waiting room at the IVF place was crazy. There were fifteen women, all talking about where they were in their cycles and how much money they'd spent already. One woman was on a protocol that cost $30,000 per cycle. She had just remortgaged her house. The other women were talking about what they still had to sell, so that they'd have the money to keep trying. It seemed as though their whole lives were focused on this one issue."

Margaret had been in recovery for a long time for bulimia and compulsive overeating. "There's no question but that infertility treatment becomes an addiction," she says. "You don't know when or how to stop. And you keep hoping that maybe, just maybe, the next drug or surgery will help."

Margaret and her husband had agreed to give the IVF one try. Her husband was, by now, fairly tired of the whole infertility scene, she noted, having to perform "on command."

"I used to get so mad at him," Margaret told me. "Sometimes when I was ovulating, he'd be uninterested in making love. I'd wonder why he couldn't be like all the other men—able to produce an ejaculation at the sight of a *Playboy* pinup. He just didn't like making love on demand. When I asked him what the bathrooms were like at the infertility clinics, he told me about all the pornography at the hospitals and clinics in which he'd given sperm samples by this time."

When Margaret told me this part of the story, I realized once again that with all our high-tech infertility technology, we still need the human mind to produce an ejaculation. Margaret's husband's mind was primed with pornographic images at the time of ejaculation, and Margaret admitted that she played right into this. She wanted a child, and he was her sperm donor. But the energetic quality and even the physiological properties of seminal fluid ejaculated during intercourse with a person a man loves, I am convinced, is entirely different in quality from what he produces via masturbation in a hospital bathroom while reading pornography. How much nicer it would be if ejaculations collected for potential egg fertilization were accompanied by a feeling of deep love in the moment, both for the woman and for potential offspring.

Margaret said that the physician who performed her egg retrieval was "so nasty." She and her husband had been told that there was a 5 percent chance that her eggs wouldn't fertilize. They never expected that they'd have that problem, but nine eggs were collected and none of them fertilized. The technicians said that there might be "antisperm antibodies." So she and her husband went to Boston to have special cultures done to check for this. About this time, she remembers feeling punished. She said, "I felt like kicking and crying. I was mad at God. I kept remembering those teenagers who were pregnant. I was pissed." No antisperm antibodies were found.

During the whole time, Margaret remembers, no one ever talked to her about how she was feeling. From my perspective as a physician, she always appeared to be jovial, in control, and upbeat. But she told me later, "Being in control was my way of avoiding my feelings. I wished so much that someone would sit me down and try to piece the whole puzzle together for me."

Still, Margaret had that "window" around her ovary. She heard of another surgeon in Boston to whom she wanted to talk, and I referred her to him. She found him very respectful and helpful. He performed a meticulous laparascopy, during which he cleared up many of her adhesions. "There was something very special about this surgery," she told me. "This surgeon was a true healer. He was positive. After this surgery, I knew I had done everything that I could possibly do. Now, I was almost ready to turn the whole issue over to my higher power."

By this time, Margaret and her husband had completed their adoption home studies, and in the spring they were told that a baby was available through an agency in Mexico. They adopted a baby boy and have since adopted two more children.

Margaret turned forty this year. Her husband stays home with their three adopted children, all under age three. Though she doesn't want any more children, Margaret once told me, "I miss not being pregnant. I grieve the fact that I may never experience pregnancy and that I may never breast-feed. My cousin was recently pregnant. Seeing her, I longed to have that kind of belly. I keep saying to myself, 'What do I need to learn from this?' I still don't know. When I hear about other people getting pregnant, I still feel bad. Sex is tainted for me, in a way. I still can't separate it from the goal of getting pregnant. My husband and I are in a support group with other parents who've adopted children. People think that now that we've adopted, I'll get pregnant. But statistics show that this isn't any more likely following adoption, though it happens.

"I keep thinking, though I know that it isn't helpful, that if I had done my interpersonal work, I'd be pregnant, and that there must be something I still have to learn from this. I keep thinking that if I could just figure it out, I'd get pregnant. It's as if getting pregnant would be *proof* that I was doing everything right!"

Last year, Margaret went to New York and worked with Niravi Payne. Through insightful work on her family history, she discovered that her mother had unconsciously never wanted children, though she had always said she did. Margaret had picked up on her mother's conflict *in utero* and internalized it. She discovered that her maternal grandmother also had not wanted children. Margaret was now going to break the chain of pain passed down to her. As a result of uncovering and naming the family conflicts about childbearing that she had internalized, she was able to release the whole issue of "longing for pregnancy." She feels free for the first time in years.

I've learned a great deal from Margaret. She told me that none of the books on infertility talk about how abusive the infertility rat race is to one's self-esteem and self-worth. Many infertile couples stay on the infertility quest for *years.* Though our current technology is very costly and complex, the "take-home" baby rate is still surprisingly low. A recent article in *The New York Times Magazine* quoted Alan DeCherny, chief of the department of obstetrics and gynecology at Tufts and a reproductive specialist: "I wish the odds were higher. People think my job must be such a happy one—what could be better than helping an infertile couple have a baby? But the reality is, I'm plagued by my failures. Too many couples fail."[35] The IVF register for the United States records a success rate of only 17 percent per transfer cycle (embryos transferred to the female body)—in couples who are considered "good" candidates. "Success" doesn't guarantee a baby—it only means the ability to produce high-quality eggs, sperm, and embryos.[36] Even with these factors in place, a baby is not guaranteed.

As long as technology keeps holding out yet another chance, infertile couples can't and don't fully grieve their loss and get on with their lives. They're caught in an emotional holding pattern— hostages to their hope. After a time, it is important for their health to move on.

Pregnancy Loss

Miscarriage and Incompetent Cervix

Approximately one in six pregnancies ends in miscarriage. I tell patients that miscarriage is usually God's way of getting rid of conceptions that will not result in healthy babies. Women who miscarry still must grieve the potential child, though, even if they believe the pregnancy wasn't "meant to be." In some cases, they go through as much grief as women who deliver stillborn babies.

After a woman has a miscarriage, her chances of having another one are not increased, but many women nonetheless lose trust in their bodies after a miscarriage. Grieving and learning to trust again are major issues for women following miscarriage. Another major issue is guilt: Many women have the mistaken impression that something they did must have caused the miscarriage. I tell my patients that healthy babies don't just miscarry. (Women who smoke, unfortunately, *do* have two times the normal rate of miscarriage. And it appears from studies on the "products of conception" that these are miscarriages of otherwise normal fetuses.) A recent study by Dr. Claire Infante-Rivard of McGill University in Montreal found that drinking an amount of caffeine that is more than three cups of coffee a day during pregnancy nearly tripled the rate of miscarriage.[37] Though previous studies have not shown this effect as clearly, women would be wise to decrease or eliminate caffeine consumption before conception and during pregnancy. If you've had a miscarriage, don't spend a lot of time trying to figure out *why.* Just stay with what you're feeling, and give yourself time to mourn your loss.

Several studies have indicated that in women who have repeated (three or more) miscarriages, there may be an interplay between emotions and the hormonal systems involved in pregnancy. Dr. Robert J. Weil, a researcher on the emotional aspects of infertility, and C. Tupper write, "The pregnant woman functions as a communications system. The fetus is a source of continuous messages to which the mother responds with subtle psychobiological adjustments. Her personality, influenced by her ever-changing life situation, can either (1) act upon the fetus to maintain its constant growth and development or (2) create physiological changes that can result in abortion."[38] The ways in which a woman's body modulates her feelings about her pregnancy are diverse, but all are mediated by the immune and endocrine systems. Thus, studies have shown that there are endocrinological imbalances resulting from emotional stress in women who habitually miscarry (known as "habitual aborters" in medical circles) and in those who have what is known as an "incompetent cervix," a cervix that dilates too quickly so that the uterus cannot hold on to a baby. Women who habitually miscarry or who have an incompetent cervix sometimes also have difficulty accepting motherhood and their feminine role. Femininity, to these women, means being self-sacrificing, passive, and suffering and having to serve and cater to their husbands (yet control them). They became pregnant "because their husbands want a child so badly." They also feel that "having a child is a woman's main accomplishment and that not being able to have children means being inadequate as women."[39] They frequently choose dependent, nonverbal husbands and have restricted social outlets and low adaptability. Due to their aloofness, they are often unable to take part in life around them. The control group of nonmiscarrying women in these studies had much healthier images of what it meant to be a woman.[40] Another study found that "habitual aborters" basically receive their pleasure in life through fulfilling the expectations of others. They react compliantly to the demands of others, even as tension and hostility build in their bodies. Feeling guilty about directly expressing their anger at other people's demands, their frustration builds until their body responds with a physical illness. Miscarrying the child (the "psychosomatic" or "autoimmune" illness in this case) relieves the tension that has built up in their bodies. Interestingly, when many of these same women later underwent psychotherapy and learned how to deal directly with their anger rather than storing it in their bodies, their success rate for subsequent pregnancy was 80 percent, while it was only 6 percent for those who do not go through therapy.[41]

In one study of women with incompetent cervix who underwent surgical procedure to sew the cervix shut, 89 percent of the patients went on to have postpartum psychosis, compared with only 11 percent of the control group. It is standard procedure to place a purse-string suture in the cervix in those pregnant women who are presumed to have a cervix that can't hold a pregnancy. This procedure is done early in pregnancy. The author of this study concluded that "these women were forced into motherhood." Women who habitually lose pregnancies may have severe emotional conflicts about motherhood. When their emotional issues aren't dealt with, they are exacerbated postpartum via emotional breakdown. Though this is a fascinating study, my experience suggests that the psychosis figure is very high.

A group of pregnant women, mostly in the northeastern United States, were given the hormone diethylstilbestrol (DES) during the 1950s and 1960s. This synthetic estrogen was thought to prevent miscarriage and was widely used by some physicians in women who had spotting during early pregnancy. It was later discovered that this hormone was associated with abnormalities in some female and male offspring who were exposed to it in the early weeks of gestation. The daughters of women who took DES, known as DES daughters, often developed structural cervical abnormalities associated with repeated miscarriage and prematurity. (Some DES sons have mild genital abnormalities, but in general they have not been as severe as those in DES daughters.) Some DES daughters even developed a very rare vaginal cancer, with several deaths resulting. This syndrome was first discovered in the 1970s, when I was doing my residency training. I have followed a number of these women closely since then. Most DES daughters are now in their late thirties and forties. Many have been able to have children, but some have not. This drug and its consequences are a tragic example of a hormonal treatment that turned into a nightmare for both mother and offspring.

Stillbirth

While I was in my residency, a lovely young Catholic woman gave birth to two perfect identical-twin girls. Unfortunately, these twins had gotten their cords wrapped around each other and died just before labor started (a very unusual event). As I was helping the attending physician deliver these two babies, I asked the mother if she'd like to see them and hold them. I had intended to wrap them in baby blankets and spend some time with her after the delivery, sitting with her while she held her babies. But her doctor scolded me, and he said to her, "Regina, it's better if you don't look. We'll just give you something to sleep so you can just get on with your life and get this behind you. It will bother you if you see them." An obedient woman, she complied. As a physician in training, I knew that it wasn't a good idea for me to argue with her doctor.

I knew instinctively that this doctor was wrong and that this mother needed to interact with what she had created, lest she go on to dream for years of babies with no faces. Her babies were in fact beautiful. She needed to see their little hands, their perfect bodies, and their angelic faces—and to know that her body had created them. It is *so* much easier to deal with what *is* than with our fantasies about what is.

Most women need to interact with their "creations"—their stillborn babies. Otherwise, unfinished emotional business may result. When a couple has a deformed baby or a stillborn, they need to look at and touch this being, take pictures, name the child, and perhaps have a ceremony of some kind that acknowledges that this child existed. Many hospitals now provide cameras, so that couples can take pictures of babies who are sick or who have died—so that parents have something tangible to hold on to.

When Dr. Elisabeth Kübler-Ross's work on grief and dying became better known with the publication of her classic work *On Death and Dying* (Macmillan, 1969), hospitals started to realize that avoiding and denying death didn't help the patients' healing process. Far too many women who have lost babies never grieved properly—in fact, they were often told "You have other children at home" or "You can have more" or "You must be strong." Grief was considered self-indulgent.

But that which isn't fully grieved cannot be released. (This is also a problem with infertility.) Healing from the pain of pregnancy loss is a process. It requires time. It requires that a woman give herself the time and space necessary to grieve and heal.

One of my patients, after a long bout with endometriosis, surgery, and infertility, healed herself through a process of writing down her feelings and drawing pictures to illustrate them with her left (nondominant) hand. Drawing with the nondominant hand activates the brain's right hemisphere and facilitates getting in touch with imagery and emotions that are important to integrate consciously in the healing process. Memories from childhood often surface as well, because writing and drawing with a hand we don't usually use puts us instantly in a "childlike" state.[42] My patient's process led to a book that documents and honors her healing process.[43]

As a result of her infertility, however, she and her husband became estranged for a while. She wrote, "Over time, a great abyss and a mountain developed between me and my husband and a gigantic unscalable mountain rose between us. I didn't know how to get over, under, or around these obstacles. I had tried everything that I knew how to do. I had gone to couples counseling and to individual counseling as well. I raged. I was loving. I was rejecting. I isolated myself and went on my own way.

"I created a healing ritual for myself. I made a 'child' from pine branches, spruce, pine cones, and berries. All the beauty of the woods went into constructing that child. She had flowers in her pine needle hair. She was angry for not being born. I gave her my name.

"I sat her [the stick child] next to a tree by the pond. She withered and died. I saw her sometimes when I walked by the lake. Now there is nothing left but her stick-bones.

"She didn't 'live' very long but there was energy and beauty in the brief moments of her life. Her coming and going helped me to face the hurt and sadness I felt because I couldn't have another child.

"I read books looking for role models of women who had to deal with infertility. I didn't find many role models, but in Queen Guinevere I finally found some comfort. She couldn't give King Arthur a child and she suffered greatly. I felt less alone and less ugly when I read that tale. I discovered that not all princesses who get married have children and live happily ever after. There was at least one other woman like me."

Eventually, through her writing and drawing process she began to heal. (See Figure 11.) "I have stopped blaming and rejecting my body," she wrote. "I am learning to love my ovaries, fallopian tubes, and uterus. I drew some pictures honoring my reproductive organs. I noticed that at first they were totally separate from my body. In some drawings, they were yearning for a connection. Then I drew them reaching out to me—seeking connection.

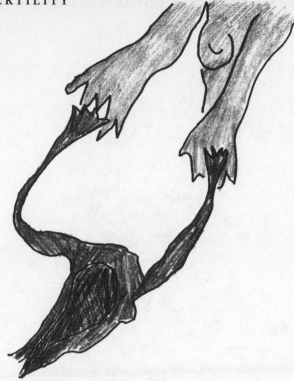

FIGURE 11: SEEKING PARTNERSHIP

"Through this drawing process I began to feel a softening and a tingling in my reproductive organs. Life was returning to my uterus, ovaries and fallopian tubes. They had been feeling dead and hurt for far too long. I named them Queen, Princess, Crowned Jewel, Heart, Warmth, and Love.

"Finally, through seeing how I had separated my uterus, fallopian tubes, and ovary from my body in my drawings, I was able to create a positive and loving image of myself and return my reproductive organs to their proper place, where I look at them with gratitude for giving me a son [from a previous marriage] and making me a woman." (See Figure 12.)

Adoption

Through the years I've worked both with women who have given up babies for adoption and with women who have adopted babies. In the past, adoption agencies operated under the illusions of

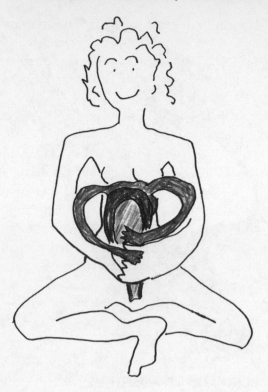

FIGURE 12

secrecy and denial. Now, through the efforts of birth mothers and adopted children alike, natural parents and their adopted-out babies are finding each other, sometimes with joyous results but sometimes also with great disappointment. Both giving up a baby for adoption and adopting one have consequences. Giving up or taking in a child is always emotionally stressful for all parties. Adoption is an area in which society is learning that secrets don't work. They especially don't work with matters of lineage. Blood lines are very powerful— they hold ancient memories. The birth mother and the mother who adopts-in both need to know this. All my patients who have adopted children into their homes have put together as much information as they can about the child's birth circumstances, to share it with the child when the time comes. Most children want to know their heritage. Birth mothers, too, almost always want to know where their children are and if they are all right—even when they know that they themselves are not capable of raising them adequately. In matters of adoption, the only thing that works is honesty.

Currently, a large number of American couples have adopted foreign infants. I can't think of a better way to promote global awareness and intercultural understanding. A patient who adopted two Chinese children told me the following story, which she calls "Listening with the Heart."

In November 1981 Susan and her husband Bob went to Taiwan with the intention of adopting a child. One month later, they returned as a family of four with Anio-Nicholas, almost six, and Shao-Ma Annie, almost four. "Christmas of 1981 was a wonderful celebration of the birth of our new family," says Susan. The following Thanksgiving Susan invited her extended family of origin to share the holiday with her "new" family. Near the end of that day of celebration, Annie, sitting on the stairs, asked accusingly, "*Why* did you come to get us in that taxicab in Taiwan, anyway?" Susan wondered what had prompted that question. Then it dawned on her that for the first time since the adoption, she was sitting in a roomful of people whom she dearly loved, to whom she had been paying a great deal of attention—the kind of attention that up until then Annie had seen her give only to Bob, to Nicholas, and to herself.

Focusing on her daughter's question, Susan told her the truth: that she had had a very happy life, full of friends and family, work and play, but that she had still felt filled with a love that wasn't used up. And so she and her husband had gone looking for someone to love and had found her and her brother. Annie paused, tipped her head pensively to one side, then went off to brush her teeth. Susan joined her for their nightly ritual together. As Annie squirted toothpaste onto both their toothbrushes, she said defiantly, "I want to go back to Taiwan to see my *Chinese* mother"—even though she had been told that there was no record of her mother and that it wasn't known who had brought her to the home. Susan realized that her daughter's desire to go back to Taiwan at that moment was symbolic and important. So Susan asked her, "Would you like me to go with you, or would you like to go by yourself?" Annie answered "By my*self*." Susan was struck by a sense of loss, emptiness, and despair. She later told me, "Welling up in me was the question, 'But what about *me*?' *I* love you and have loved you with all my heart! Isn't that good enough? What about *me*?"

Then she looked at her daughter and knew that her longing for her Chinese mother was simply a natural part of her birth history and who she was. "Annie was, in her love for a woman whom neither of us would probably ever meet, sharing with me her deepest self. I could join her now, at the core of her being, in her love, or I could bar myself from it. And so finally, I, the verbalizer, just listened—actively, achingly—with my heart."

Several Christmases later, Susan and Bob were walking together, with Annie swinging between them, holding their hands. She swung high, and as Bob's and Susan's eyes met over her head, she called out to the sky: "Hello, Chinese Mother! How are you? I am happy and I hope you are too! I love you! Good-bye!"

I once participated in a wonderful adoption ceremony with a couple, long infertile, who had successfully found a child with the help, intent, and prayers of their extended family and community. They brought the baby to a large gathering shortly after the adoption to share their joy with us. I would recommend a similar ceremony to all who are adopting a child. It is a touching and conscious way to bring a child into her or his new community.

In ceremonial fashion, the woman leading the event had the adoptive parents hold up the baby and carry it around to the members of our community to be welcomed. At the same time, she asked those people who had been adopted to please stand in the center of the circle during this ceremony. As we each welcomed the baby, she addressed the people who had themselves been adopted. "As we welcome this new baby and celebrate his birth and his new parents, may this day symbolize for you that you are deeply wanted, that you were always deeply wanted. And from now on, no matter what has happened to you in the past, may you know how meaningful your birth was and, seeing how deeply wanted and blessed this child is, claim the same thing for yourself." This ceremony was a great healing on many levels for many people and was full of wonder and hope.

Fertility as Metaphor

We must deal with the economic and social problems that are the root causes of high fertility rates: widespread poverty and the oppression of women. . . . When women everywhere have control over their own reproductive choices, fertility rates drop.
—The Union of Concerned Scientists

Motherhood is not simply the organic process of giving birth . . . it is understanding the needs of the world.
—Alexis DeVeaux, mother and sponsor of MADRE, a Latin American relief organization

The population of the Earth is growing way beyond our means to support it. We humans have been very clever, producing more and more food from less and less land. The Union of Concerned Scientists writes, "Our species simply cannot survive today's recklessly accelerating population growth, the irresponsible squandering of the Earth's resources, and the continuing destruction of our environment. . . . Every day, there are a quarter of a million more of us than there were the day before. Every week, we must find ways to feed another city the size of Philadelphia. Every month, we must wrest from the Earth additional resources to keep alive another New Jersey. And every year, we are adding another whole Mexico to the burden of this small planet."[44]

The time of endless productivity without replenishing is coming to an end. We as women *must* use our inherent creativity—our womb power—to regenerate our planet as well as to produce the next generation. We can no longer have baby after baby with no thought for the consequences. Many of us already can no longer bear to use disposable diapers because of what we know they're doing to our planet's landfills—but we must also look at the fact that the average child in the United States uses fifty times the resources of a child born in the Third World. Few issues are as controversial as population growth, and I don't intend to go into that controversy here.

In the United States as well as elsewhere, women who have no means of child support bear child after child. All of us in the health care field have personally heard women discuss having another child to get more welfare money. These are the mothers who are most at risk for developing problems in labor, having growth-retarded, premature babies. But these women's problems are *symptoms* of the imbalance in our culture—they are *not* the problem. The underlying problem is society's treatment of women and the cycles of poverty, victimization, and abuse in which these young women stay locked.

Sixty percent of teenage mothers are victims of sexual abuse. Almost instinctively, they mate with men who then abandon them. That is all they know—a premature commitment that keeps them trapped. The only role they perceive as open to them is that of baby carrier. They don't know that they have choices. When they think they can do little else, they have babies. The cycle continues.

But what if we started now to teach our young women that they have inherent worth—and that though they may choose to have a baby, there are many other opportunities open to them as well? What if they knew that their menstrual cycles are part of their sacred connection with the earth and the moon—and that their sexuality needn't necessarily be shared with a man? That they could have it all to themselves if they chose? What if they didn't measure their worth by whose baby they had or whom they were sleeping with? What if they knew that their wombs, whether or not they had children, are their body center for creativity—and that the womb has its own meaning and value, separate from being a potential carrier for children?

We need to expand the meaning of *fertility* and *birth*. We must begin to see female birth power for what it is—the basis of all of creation. When enough women sense this creative female power inherent within each of us—not dependent upon what we produce or don't produce with our bodies, not dependent on who we let into our bodies—the world will change. When women tap into this power, the children, the ideas, and the new world to which we give birth will be supportive of all beings, including ourselves.

Whether we ever choose pregnancy, every one of us has encoded in our cells the knowledge of what it is to conceive, gestate, and give birth to something that grows out of our own substance. You don't have to have a baby to learn how to labor. Labor, whether physical or metaphorical, teaches us not to fight the process of birthing, no matter what we're birthing, even when it hurts and we want to quit.

On some level we all have miscarriages, abortions, dysfunctional labors, and stillbirths, as well as beautifully formed creations. Unfortunately, we've been taught in patriarchy that creations that are not "perfect" are not "worthy." What patriarchy has seen too often as failure is actually part of the whole from which we can learn. We don't need to go through these processes physically to understand them and heal from them—they're inherent processes of nature.

Each woman must find her own truth about how to use her fertility or to heal this area of her life. I do not pretend that I know what is best for another woman—only she can figure that out. What I do hope is that this section has stimulated you to look more deeply into your body's creation experiences and helped you toward understanding and healing.

TWELVE

Pregnancy and Birthing

> For all eternity, God lies on a birthing bed, giving birth. The essence of God is Birthing.
>
> —Meister Eckhart

P regnancy has great consequences for both mother and child. Having a baby is rarely a rational or logical decision and cannot be made with the intellect alone, but it can still be made consciously and with the heart. My wish for all women is that we gain the courage to choose conception consciously and wisely.

When I recall the reasons that I had children, I see how emotional and instinctual, unconscious and "tribal," my decision was. The biological pull is still strong. I and many other women have longed to have another baby even knowing that another child would tax our emotional and physical resources in an unhealthy way. Some women simply love being pregnant. Others adore little babies and want one around all the time. Some women are even addicted to having babies and giving birth—in part because it's the only thing that is totally "theirs" in their family structures. I've worked with many women who have become obsessed with having another child in their late thirties or early forties, partly so that they could put off deciding what to do with their lives for another five years.

Pregnancy can be used as a way to fill a void in a woman's life that another human being can never fill. We must know ourselves intimately before we can ever be intimate with another human being.

When a baby is brought into being to fill the unmet needs of an adult, the child will carry an unfair and often harmful burden of a parent's impossible expectations.

Pregnancy is a miraculous process and should be a time when a woman makes every effort to tune in to her body and baby with the support of her surroundings. For centuries, midwives helped mothers through the pregnancy and birthing processes, standing by them with medical and emotional aid. The very word *obstetrics* is derived from the Latin word *stare*, which means "to stand by." A woman's body knows how to give birth instinctively and will respond in settings in which she is encouraged to move in the ways that feel right and to make the sounds that she needs to make. Modern obstetrics, however, has changed from a natural, patient "standing by" and allowing the woman's body to respond naturally into a domineering and often invasive practice. Women's cultural conditioning causes us to turn ourselves over to pregnancy experts so that most of us have lost touch with our innate birthing knowledge and power, as have most of these experts, who rely on tests and machines to tell them how to help. I had the vaguest sense of this during my training, when I wondered why our cesarean section rate was so high. But only in the last few years—despite delivering babies for almost a decade and having two of my own—have I come to appreciate that most women's experience of pregnancy, labor, and delivery is nowhere near as empowering as it could be.

Our Cultural Inheritance: Pregnancy

Pregnancy as Illness

During my mother's era, pregnant women were not expected to go outside their homes much or to travel. Maternity clothes, which included that anathema, a maternity girdle, were ugly and did not enhance women's body image. Many women lost their jobs if they became pregnant. And for women who didn't lose their jobs, there was no formal pregnancy leave, even as late as the early 1980s. As the first physician in my former practice to have a pregnancy leave, I experienced some resentment from a few of my colleagues, who felt that pregnancy should not be treated the same as a broken leg because it was, after all, a *chosen disability* over which I had some control. We've certainly come a long way since then, but pretending that a pregnant woman is just like everyone else and has no special needs is short-sighted and puts her and her baby's health at risk. Our culture can't seem to find a happy medium.

Pregnancy, whether or not the pregnancy is desired, is a special time that requires a woman to make some arrangements for increased rest and care. Otherwise, she may experience increased fatigue, premature labor, and toxemia.[1] Studies have shown that women who aren't supported or are highly stressed in their pregnancies have a higher incidence of adverse outcomes.

In my view, however, the biggest factor in poor pregnancy outcome (miscarriage, prematurity, toxemia, and so forth) is when the pregnancy is unwanted or not planned. Current data suggest that at least 50 percent of pregnancies fall into this category.[2] At least 50 percent of pregnancies are not planned. It's much more difficult to ascertain which ones are unwanted because many women adjust well to unplanned pregnancies and end up desiring them. Maternal ambivalence about pregnancy is a set up for complications unless a woman can resolve her feelings during the pregnancy. (See Chapter 11.) A woman who feels (usually unconsciously) that she must end her pregnancy as soon as possible to get on with her life, get it over with, or to "get her body back," may go into premature labor or develop another condition that ends her pregnancy sooner. Numerous studies have documented the profound effects of psychological variables on birth outcome, in other words the correlation between poor maternal emotional and physical investment in pregnancy and prematurity.[3] Animal studies have indicated that the death of a baby *in utero* may be related to marked maternal anxiety. In pregnant monkeys, guinea pigs, and rabbits subjected to emotional stress, the uterine and placental blood flow was constricted from adrenaline released in response to the stress. As a result, the fetuses did not receive enough oxygen, and many died of asphyxia. Marked maternal anxiety and stress also cause uterine blood vessels to constrict via hormonal and neurotransmitter release into the circulation. This reduces oxygen to the baby and may well be related to pregnancy complications, such as placental abruption, placenta previa (a condition in which the placenta covers the cervical opening, which can lead to bleeding and/or prematurity), prolapsed umbilical cord, cord around the neck, and breech presentation.[4]

While mothers automatically communicate stresses they feel through their bodies to their unborn babies, they can also learn to communicate healthful emotions to their babies. After all, the baby is a part of a pregnant woman's own body. Getting in touch with her inner guidance system can help her learn how to keep her baby safe and even interrupt premature labor and halt the progression of toxemia. Of course, women who develop premature labor and toxemia also have to be willing to stop work, rest more, and change any harmful patterns of behavior and thought. Toxemia is a syndrome in which a pregnant woman develops swelling, high blood pressure, and protein in the urine. No one knows exactly what causes it, although there are many theories. Women with kidney disease and high blood pressure are more susceptible than others. Toxemia is a leading cause of prematurity and pregnancy disability. If untreated, it can lead to seizures—the condition is then called eclampsia.

Studies of pregnant women with toxemia have shown that they feel less attractive, less loved, and more helpless than do normal pregnant women. They are excessively sensitive to the opinions of others, and they orient themselves to what others expect of them. For these women, pregnancy provides an additional crisis that adds stress to their already overstressed lives. Although they view pregnancy as a crisis, they are ill-equipped to deal with their emotions about it. They are unable to cope with others' perceived expectations, taking to heart minor criticisms and injustices done to them. However, they do not show externally that any of this bothers them. Instead, their body reflects this stress as an increase in blood pressure. They frequently have conflicts with their employer, and their blood pressure often rises when they try to negotiate their maternity leaves. They often try to get everything settled before the delivery. Compared with women without toxemia, these women's emotions manifest physically through the autonomic (subconscious) nervous system: They frequently blush in the face and neck, talk rapidly, and have rising blood pressure, dizziness, and heart palpitations.[5] One study showed that women with a triad of excessive weight gain, premature rupture of membranes (one of the leading causes of premature birth[6]), and toxemia have high anxiety, social seclusion, and hypochondria compared with controls. If a woman understands what it's like to have a baby in the intensive care nursery, she can begin the process of seeing her own body as the best intensive care space possible for the baby, not to mention the cheapest.

The Collective Emergency Mindset

Pregnancy is a time when common sense all too often flies out the window, chased out by a culture that is out of balance. Nowhere is a woman's connection or loss of connection to her inner guidance more evident than during pregnancy. Suddenly, her body is no longer her own. Her entire extended family feels that it is pregnant, and all of them give her advice about what to eat, what to wear, and what to do. I was amazed by how total strangers would approach me when I was pregnant, pat my belly, and offer suggestions. Friends seem to think it their duty to tell pregnant women the worst stories they can think of about cesarean sections, labor pain, and poor outcomes. (This is another example of internalized patriarchy—glorifying pain and destruction over the life-enhancing qualities potentially available through pregnancy and birth.) I felt blessed to be an obstetrician because I was spared hearing all these horror stories. (Perhaps people figured that I had been "socialized" by having already learned these horrible stories.) War stories about the rigors of birth are often passed down from generation to generation. Mothers not uncommonly tell their daughters that "now you'll see how I suffered with you."

At some very deep level, we are all awed by pregnant women and their power. But instead of emphasizing a woman's power, in classic patriarchal reversal our culture attends to the fear that that power brings up. Pregnant women are emotionally more porous and more in touch with their intuition than usual, and they are therefore more vulnerable. They pick up on all the collective societal fear of them.

Media images of pregnant women suddenly falling to the ground during pregnancy and shrieking things like, "Oh, John, the baby!" reinforce in our psyches that pregnancy is a time of great danger and unpredictability. They falsely remind us that pregnancy, like our female body, is a disaster waiting to happen. In every hospital I've ever worked, pregnant women are rushed to the labor and delivery floor as quickly as possible, even if they've come into the emergency room for some other problem. In Boston, the ER crew once sent up a woman in mid-pregnancy who had a broken leg!

This emergency mindset is especially damaging to women who are having babies in their thirties or forties. Most, if not all, pregnant women over the age of thirty are taught by our culture that they are much more at risk for complications than if they were in their twenties. This perception of increased risk is simply not necessarily true and depends on the individual woman's health. I remember the first pregnant woman I ever met who was over thirty. It was in the prenatal clinic at the Mary Hitchcock Hospital during my second year of medical school and I thought that she was very unusual and very brave to be having her first baby at age thirty-two. I remember thinking that she was old for attempting this, although I myself was twenty-three at the time and pregnancy and having children were very far from my personal plans. Looking back, I realize that this woman was at the very beginning of a trend that began in the 1970s and has continued into the 1990s—delaying childbearing until later.

I've always resented the term "elderly primigravida," a term that doctors use for women who are having their first baby after the age of thirty-five, or even after age thirty, depending on the doctor. Whether or not a woman is more at risk in her thirties must be completely individualized. I'd much rather take care of a forty year old in excellent health who had planned her pregnancy than a twenty-five year old who smokes two packs per day and quaffs a gallon of diet Coke daily. Too often the medical profession "hexes" women who become pregnant in their thirties and forties by lumping them into statistically high-risk categories that are not necessarily applicable. Older women who are pregnant, as well as infertility patients who become pregnant, have a much higher risk of a C-section. But in some places, a woman older than forty will be told that she is very apt to have a cesarean because hers is a "premium pregnancy" (as opposed to a pregnancy in the mother's twenties, whose success doesn't "matter" as much because "you can always have another—you have time"!). Premium pregnancy means that because the mother is presumed to be or is more anxious (or is *made* to be anxious by her culture and her doctor!), we should treat her differently. This is a reflection of the health care team's own unfinished emotional work.

In fact, age is not an absolute measure of the intensity or duration of labor. Chronological age (age in years) and biological age (age of one's tissues) aren't necessarily related. My closest friend had her first baby at forty-one. The first stage of her labor lasted only three hours—very short, by any standard. And if her hips hadn't been so narrow, she'd have delivered in a total of four hours. Older women in my practice often have similarly successful pregnancies and births.

One of the nicest things about women having their first babies in their late thirties and early forties is that by then, these women have often established themselves in the outside world of work and career. When they do have babies, they take the time to enjoy them. They already know what it's like "out there." They realize the limitations of the corporate world and are willing to put aside its "benefits" to reassess their lives through the lens of parenting. Many have had time to get in touch with their bodies over the years and are more comfortable with themselves than they were in their twenties. In my mind, these women are actually low risk.

The Transforming Power of Pregnancy

Women should savor and celebrate pregnancy, the gestating of the next generation, as the miracle that it is—a crucial time in their child's development. This doesn't mean that we should think of pregnancy as an illness or as a time for us to be treated with kid gloves. Still, it is a period when we need quiet reflective time to tune in to the baby and to rest. The hormone progesterone, released naturally during pregnancy, has calming and soothing effects. (It also relaxes and slows the bowel, which can lead to constipation in some women.) The body is doing a lot of inner work growing a baby. The tenor of the pregnancy itself contributes to the strength of a child's constitution throughout the rest of his or her life. I'm amazed that this culture has been so unable to appreciate the fact that forty weeks of gestation is a *very short* amount of time in a woman's life, relatively speaking. Yet it is a time that is crucial for the health of the next generation.

Because our culture values women more highly during their childbearing years, and because women tend to take better care of themselves during pregnancy than at any other time, pregnancy is a fantastic opportunity for women to learn more about themselves and their own power. Since the baby is part of their own bodies, positive inner communication between the two translates into a deeper trust of themselves that continues even after birth.

Quality care and education during pregnancy would prevent an untold number of costly problems later, including many cases of prematurity, growth retardation, mental retardation, physical disabilities, and learning disabilities—all of which make the process of parenting much more difficult. The care of pregnant women, who are very powerful and very vulnerable at the same time, should be the highest priority in this country.

An Obstetrician Gets Pregnant

When I became pregnant with my first child, I had recently completed my four-year residency training and had by then worked with hundreds of pregnant women, providing them with prenatal care, labor support, and assistance with delivery of their babies. I had been a proponent of natural, drug-free childbirth throughout my residency, and I was very optimistic about my own. After all, the vast majority of pregnancies end with a normal baby—I had seen the truth of this firsthand.

My attitude toward the pregnancy was one of watching an experiment with my uterus. Wasn't this interesting—to see the changes my body was going through! I realize now that I didn't allow myself what I then considered the *luxury* of excitement and anticipation, though mine was very much a planned and wanted pregnancy.

I had learned very well how to separate my mind from my body, so I decided that I didn't want to "bond" much with my baby until after the pregnancy was well along and I knew that the baby was normal—something I would be assured of only *after* he or she was born. Notice the paradox in my thinking here. I felt strongly that everything would be normal, yet I didn't want to make much of an investment "just in case." I had watched some women furnish entire nurseries as early as their third month of pregnancy, when the risk of miscarriage is still one in six. I didn't want to go through that kind of grief and thought that their emotional investment was premature. Years later, I learned that babies know what's going on *in utero* and can hear, feel, and experience emotions long before they're born. When their mothers are detached and not invested emotionally, babies sense this.

Back then I didn't realize for myself, though I taught it to my patients, that a woman's process of bonding with her baby starts when her pregnancy test is positive. At this point, women usually start fantasizing about the baby, thinking about names, and looking at baby clothes and other items. I had never been very interested in babies and could not understand the behavior of women at baby showers—events that I could barely stand. Oohing and ahhing over baby clothes had never appealed to me.

When the nurses asked me, toward the end of the pregnancy, if I had the baby's room ready, I said, "No, I don't even have a T-shirt." I had no baby stuff at all, not even a diaper. My husband was completing a fellowship in orthopedics and was, as usual, busier than I was. He certainly wasn't up for baby shopping. Although I was clear that I didn't want a baby shower, luckily some nurse friends ignored my adamancy. Though I was mortified at the time, I was grateful later. I didn't have a clue as to how to go about buying baby things.

Rather than read parenting guides, I trusted my ability to mother without question. Sentimentality about babies was not, in my opinion, a prerequisite for good mothering. My own mother had been a "lioness" type, with excellent instincts most of the time. She didn't give in much to "experts"—a trait for which I'll always be grateful.

As my baby grew, I watched my body change with interest. I learned a great deal about morning sickness, pain under the rib cage, constipation, excess gas, and heartburn. I'd heard women complain about these things for years, and now I could see why. Although my husband thought my changing body was beautiful, I wasn't convinced. I was concerned about gaining too much weight. How was I supposed to *enjoy* a disappearing waist, puffy cheeks, and increased fat on my hips in a culture that worships quasi-anorexia!

I now regret that I have no pictures of myself while I was pregnant. I was amazed at my patients in the early 1980s who showed me entire photo albums of themselves during pregnancy and delivery—they were proud and unashamed of their bodies. At the time, these women seemed like specimens from a different planet—didn't they "get it" that the culture (and I) didn't think they looked all that great?

During my second pregnancy, I lost my waist almost as soon as I conceived and looked pregnant almost immediately, a common event. This time, I was busier than I had been with the first, but I remember taking more time to talk to the baby (except that I thought she was a boy and called her William for nine months—she was much more active than my first, so I made a sexist assumption). Toward the end of this pregnancy, I had difficulty walking because of separation of my pubic bone, which happens so that the baby can fit through the pelvis, but by and large, it was a completely normal pregnancy. Though my belly got a lot bigger, I gained the same amount of weight—twenty-five pounds—in both pregnancies.

I recently met a sophisticated professional woman in her late thirties who was in the middle of her first pregnancy. She had finally conceded that she needed to purchase some "ugly clothes" because it had become too hard to "hide" her pregnancy and she had to modify her polished executive look of slim skirts and high heels. Her attitude that pregnancy is something to be endured, ignored, or tolerated is all too common—and I was guilty of it myself to a degree. The less pregnant you look, the better everyone tells you you're doing—"Oh, you're so little, you look great—I can hardly tell!" A prenatal vitamin advertisement in one of the medical journals from the mid-1980s shows a very thin, tall woman who doesn't look at all pregnant, running around taking pictures, working out at the gym, and staying late at the office. The caption reads, "Pregnant, but she won't slow down." The ad reminds me of my own attitude during my pregnancies, when I ran up the hospital stairs to do C-sections or surgery. I didn't want the pregnancies to interfere with my life in any way. Unfortunately, studies have shown that "not slowing down" is sometimes associated with increased health risks. A pilot study of stress and pregnancy in pregnant physicians and nurses showed that certain hormones (urinary catecholamines) produced by the adrenals and other tissue under physical or mental stress increased by 58 percent during work periods, compared with nonwork periods. The pregnant physicians' catecholamine levels were also increased by 64 percent over those of working nonphysicians' control groups of similar gestational age.[7]

When I was pregnant with my second child and had to get up at night to go deliver babies, I was so tired that I occasionally walked into walls while I was getting dressed. (My first child, once born, didn't sleep through the night until she was five, so I was up at night for years, whether I was on call or not!) But no one suggested that I slow down. Besides, I was *still* trying to prove myself a worthy professional—especially now that I'd had children!

> Woman literally illustrates the on-going life pattern of how energy becomes matter through pregnancy, labor, and delivery.
> —Caroline Myss

Our Cultural Inheritance: Labor and Delivery

I worked with pregnant women for six years or so and saw that labor and delivery very often go well. Yet we as a society continue to treat the normal process of birth with hysteria. The high anxiety about pregnancy and birth in this country is partially the result of our collective unresolved birth trauma—nearly every one of us has unfinished business about her or his own birth that we keep projecting onto pregnant women. Most baby boomers, after all, were born drugged and were then whisked away from their mothers to the glaring lights and sterility of the hospital nursery.

In the previous generations of each family there were most likely dozens of women who died in childbirth. The cemeteries of New England, for example, are strewn with the headstones of women who died young, surrounded by the graves of their dead children. Fears of death augment the hysteria we bring to childbirth as another aspect of our collective unconscious.

Ironically, most of these deaths and traumas resulted from poor nutrition, overwork, and lack of maternal support, *not* necessarily from lack of sophisticated medical intervention.[8] Data show that women who are unsupported in labor are at greater risk for prolonged labor and poor outcome. Several excellent studies have shown that the presence of a supportive woman called a *doula* who "mothers the mother" during her labor decreased the average length of labor from admission to delivery from 19.3 hours to 8.8 hours! The presence of a doula also resulted in the mother being more awake after delivery so that she was more likely to stroke her baby, smile, and talk to her or him.[9]

In so-called "primitive" societies, babies are often spaced two to four years apart through such practices as prolonged breast-feeding. In these societies, provisions are made to support a pregnant woman and her labor. The birth is celebrated as a community event. Though I don't mean to imply that childbirth is always a completely risk-free, glorious process, even in those societies in which women have been well-nourished and well-supported, we could learn a lot from the collective women's wisdom of native, nature-centered peoples and combining it with our current medical technology.

Women Labor As They Live

Having participated in hundreds of cesarean section deliveries and other forms of medicalized birth over the years, I've learned that our current dilemmas over birthing start *long before* a woman ends up in Labor and Delivery. It starts years before she even gets pregnant! Each of us carries the seeds within ourselves, and we must look at the ways in which we daily participate in less-than-optimal treatment.

A woman's attitudes about pregnancy arrive with her in Labor and Delivery. One professional woman I know wanted to labor without feeling a thing. She said, "Knock me out—I'm not an Indian." This is the statement of a woman who doesn't understand the power of labor and delivery. It implies that only "primitives" go through labor and that sophisticated intellectuals get babies via technology, keeping their hands clean, their brows uncreased, and their makeup intact.

Studies have shown that women with prolonged labor have certain personality characteristics. They have inner conflicts about reproduction and motherhood and are unable at the time of the labor to communicate and admit their anxiety. These psychological factors may result in inefficient uterine action and subsequent prolonged labor.[10]

Too many women approach labor with the wish, stated or unstated, "Take care of this inconvenience, please. I don't want to feel a thing—just hand me the baby when it's over!" Though what women need most in labor is encouragement and loving support for their abilities to birth normally, too often they don't get this because doctors and nurses hold the same attitudes about labor as they do about a crisis or inconvenience—cure it as soon as possible.

I've learned that a woman's entire life leads up to what will happen in labor. Her deepest fears can play out during labor, not necessarily consciously. Women who have experienced incest or other abuse are prime candidates for dysfunctional labors and subsequent cesarean sections. Many of these women have learned at a deep level how to be victims. This plays out in childbirth—a time when, instead of being a victim of their bodies, they need to be at one with the process. One of my patients realized that she had gotten stuck in labor because at some unconscious level she was afraid of giving birth to her father's child. Another sexual abuse victim came to realize that she had learned the victim role so well that she could not *push* her baby out. Like most people living out of a feeling of powerlessness, she simply turned the experience over to the hospital and the staff. On some level she expected them to birth the baby for her. I've worked with countless women who have learned this attitude.

Other survivors of abuse, however, use control as a survival mechanism. During pregnancy these women often come into a doctor's office with a long list of demands: No IVs, no monitor, no medical students, a limit to exams, and no enemas (despite the fact that we haven't done shaving or enemas for more than a decade). Many obstetricians sense that those women who need to control the birth process the most are often the ones who end up with the most interventions. Any birth attendant will tell you that "the longer the laundry list, the greater the chance of an unplanned intervention, such as a C-section." The reason is that the "laundry list" is often a symptom of the woman's illusion of intellectual control, her at-

tempt to control a situation about which she feels completely ter-
rorized and out of control. By trying to control all the variables
associated with the birthing process, she thinks she can somehow
avoid the terror that she associates with her body, with feeling her
body in general, and with the birth process. The more a woman
operates from intellectual control, the less likely she will be to
surrender to her body's process and the more likely that an intervention will be necessary.

Labor also reveals the bare bones of a woman's relationship with
her husband or other labor support people. Sometimes women
suddenly, when nine centimeters dilated, lash out at their husbands
viciously, simply because they are in transition. I was taught that
this just "happens," but it never made sense to me. I've since learned
that it doesn't just "happen." Any hostility that emerges between
people during labor was already there long before labor began. But
because of the essential primitive nature of the process, all pretense
at socially acceptable politeness gets dropped, and reality shines
through. My father once told me that if I wanted to learn who
someone really was, I should go on a camping trip with them. You
could say the same thing for the labor and delivery process.

Gayle Peterson, in her book *Birthing Normally*, points out that
women labor in the same way they live. Labor is a crisis situation for
most women. They approach it the way they approach any crisis:
Some believe they are powerless, while others try to assume control.
A study of the differences between women who had chosen to
induce labor and those who had chosen to let labor come spontaneously showed that those who chose induction lacked trust in their
own reproductive systems. They were more likely to complain
during their menstrual periods, had more complications in their
obstetrical history, and had more anxiety about going into labor.[11]
Gayle Peterson and Lewis Mehl did a study of pregnant women in
which they were able to predict within 95 percent accuracy which of
them would get into trouble during labor based on the criteria in
Table 7, which is supported by the many studies on individual
complications.[12]

TABLE 7: POTENTIAL RISK FACTORS IN CHILDBIRTH

High-Risk Childbirth	Low-Risk Childbirth
Passivity	Activity
Dependence	Independence
Reliance on others	Self-reliance
Inability to accept support from others	Ability to accept support from others
Rejection of womanhood	Acceptance of womanhood
Repressed sexuality	Healthy sexuality
Self-view as sexual object	Self-view as sexual being
Childlike	Adultlike
Limiting beliefs about birth	Facilitative beliefs about birth
Nonconducive prior acculturation	Conducive prior acculturation
Dishonest, manipulative communication	Clear, honest communication
Spiritual beliefs that interfere with birth	Spiritual beliefs conducive to birth
Self-image of weakness	Self-image of strength
Split of mind and body	Integration of mind and body
Conflictual relationships	Loving relationships
Complete discrepancies in birth plan	Agreement with birth plan
Fear not being worked through	Fear being worked through
Sedentary	Physically active
Frail body appearance	Robust body appearance
Rigid in resisting change and new ideas	Yielding in accommodating to change
Chaotic home	Comfortable home
Does not want child	Wants child
External control of own life	Internal control of own life
Denial of the reality of birth pain	Acceptance of the reality of birth pain

"Rescuing" Women from Labor

Not uncommonly, a woman in labor will demand that her partner do something to rescue her from the "dilemma." How well I remember husbands whose wives sought out their support during their contractions by crying something like, "Jer-ry—*do something!*" These men then yelled at me and said, "How much longer is this going to go on? You'd better take care of this soon, or you're going to hear from me." I've been threatened repeatedly by husbands who wanted me to "fix" their wives' labor as soon as possible—or else!

Unable to control their wives' discomfort, and angry at their own feelings of helplessness in a process about which they can do nothing, these men became abusive to the obstetrician—"End this misery!" Their wives, helpless to continue their usual role as "male emotional shock absorber," watch helplessly or expect their husbands to do their "Mr. Fix-it" role. These women become even further out of touch with themselves. Labor is *not* an ideal time to educate a couple about transformative experiences. However, if a couple can be encouraged between contractions simply to stay with the process, understanding that it is normal and natural and not life-threatening, then sometimes they can be helped to work *with* the contractions and the process of labor, and not against them. My associate, Bethany, reminds the husbands or partners of her patients that they can't have the baby for their wives; nor can they take away the pain. But what they can do is love their partners. This is a very big gift for most women in labor—simply to be loved through the entire process. Women who change their attitude during labor are very often changed forever by the knowledge that they *were* able to go through with it, that they have the inner resources after all. To do this they require constant support. No woman should ever labor without it.

Reversing a lifelong pattern of coping behavior during labor, however, is not always possible. When I was still delivering babies, I found that no amount of cajoling, education, or pleading on my part could reverse many women's inherited belief that they *cannot* give birth normally, that they must have drugs and anesthesia to do it. Five thousand years of programming can't be overturned in a decade.

The medical system participates fully in treating childbirth as an emergency needing a cure. Because of its addictive, patriarchal nature, the medical system becomes the symbolic "husband" for all the women crying, "Jer-ry, *do something!*" And believe me, doctors are trained in many ways to "do something." Each of our doings has a price. Some studies show, for instance, that epidural anesthesia increases the rate of cesarean section. This anesthetic relaxes the pelvic floor muscles, causing the baby to engage with the head in what's called the occiput posterior position—facing up. It's much harder to push a baby out when he or she is in this position; it also slows down the process and may add to the baby's distress. Pain medications cross the placenta and may affect the baby. Forceps, episiotomies, vacuum extractors, pitocin augmentation of labor, and

unnecessary cesarean sections are other interventions that are not
without risk.

When I was delivering babies, I believed that a woman has the
power within to birth normally and that drugs and anesthetics have
potential side effects. I was frustrated by women who had no
intention of delivering normally and I tried to change them. But this
was *my* problem, not necessarily theirs. They wanted all the technology that the hospital could offer. I now realize that it was not my
job to change them or anyone. Each woman must look inside and
see where she is—and be as honest with herself as possible. My job
is to present alternatives in every situation and let each woman
choose. I must also be clear about my own beliefs and agenda.

Birth Technologies

During the great blizzard of 1978 in Boston, when all the roads
were closed and driving was impossible, I skied to a nearby hospital
that did not do obstetrics, to deliver a few babies in the emergency
room. Laboring women during that storm were being brought into
the nearest hospitals by the National Guard. The emergency room
(ER) staff, used to dealing with everything from gunshot wounds to
heart attacks, were nearly undone by these births. ERs by their very
natures are set up to *do something fast.* Births, by their very nature,
require *just the opposite.* They require the qualities of a midwife—
standing by expectantly, supportively, lovingly, while *doing* very
little in the conventional sense. In most cases, it is the laboring
woman herself who delivers the baby, *not* the doctor or staff, who
merely catch it.

Hospitals, however, are set up to accommodate and medicate the
deepest fears of laboring women. Hospital procedures usually do
not address and work through these very real fears, but instead,
medicalize childbirths. They are designed to "save us" from the
discomfort and inconvenience of childbirth, a view of childbirth to
which society collectively contributes. Hospital birth practices flow
seamlessly out of our adoration for technology and our fear of the
process of birth. Doctors have been very willing to use technology
to "improve" outcome in obstetrics because our culture believes in
technology's superiority to the body's natural wisdom. We trust

technology more than a woman's experience of herself and more than the documented benefits of loving human support in labor.

Unfortunately, the beliefs that support hospital procedures are often so pervasive that even those women who enter the hospital wanting natural childbirth often end up with some kind of intervention. This is because a woman in labor is highly vulnerable. If she is not supported in her labor process by people who truly trust labor and see it as normal, she can be talked into almost anything.

Cesarean Sections and Fetal Monitors

There is no more striking example of the overuse of technology in childbirth than the high cesarean section rates at many U.S. hospitals, as a result of the medicalization of childbirth, fueled by fear of lawsuits if a baby is not perfect. The cesarean section rates, however, vary widely depending on the doctor and on the hospital. The average in most teaching hospitals is 25 percent, but in some cities, a white woman with insurance has a 50 percent chance of having a cesarean![13]

During my residency training, when fetal monitoring hit the scene and the cesarean section rate began to soar, I remember thinking, "How can it be that 25 percent of women aren't able to go through a normal physiological event without the aid of anesthesia and major surgery? How could the human race have possibly survived if this many women really need major surgery to give birth? What is going wrong here?"

I was taught that I must treat everyone as though she were going to have a potential complication, as if a normal labor could turn into a crisis at a moment's notice. Whenever a woman arrived in labor, we immediately put in an intravenous line, drew blood, ruptured her membranes—broke the amniotic sac ("bag of waters") surrounding the baby—screwed a fetal scalp electrode into the baby's head, and threaded a catheter into her uterus to measure intrauterine pressure on the fetal monitor. Then, she and her family, the doctors, and the nurses all fixed their gazes on the monitor and pretty much relied on *it* to tell us what to do next. The woman was asked to labor in the position that gave the best monitor tracing—not the one that felt best to her. I recall trying to get these monitoring devices even into women whose babies were about to be delivered when they came through the door. If I didn't have a monitor strip for documentation and there was a bad outcome, I knew that I would be in trouble with my attending physician. Later, studies would show that fetal monitoring did not actually improve perinatal outcome when compared with a nurse listening to the heart rate periodically.[14] What it did do was increase cesarean section rates—a great example of technology "catching on" before all the data were in. (Monitoring has its place—I'm not against it. It simply is *not* a substitute for caring, human interaction, though it is often used as one.)

During my second year of residency, I went to a meeting of the International Childbirth Education Association (ICEA) and learned that membranes don't normally rupture until a woman starts to push, and that babies in whom the membranes have been artificially ruptured have evidence of more stress in utero—the acidity (pH) of their scalp blood samples is lower. I also learned at this meeting that the amniotic fluid is the best "packing material" available. It cushions the baby's body during contractions. Why were we so eager to mess with nature's protection? So that we could put in our technological monitors!

Is it any wonder that when you hook a vulnerable laboring woman up to three or four different tubes and wires, and then rupture her membranes, she, and subsequently her baby, might get a little scared—resulting in some fetal distress? Looking back, I realize that *many* cases of fetal distress could potentially have been reversed by soothing the mother and asking her to focus inside on how her baby is—and send it messages of reassurance. Biofeedback has documented the profound effect of thoughts on body systems such as blood pressure, pulse, and skin resistance. The baby is *part* of a woman's body. She can tune in to it.

Many obstetricians feel inherently that vaginal delivery is just plain dangerous, leading to increased fetal trauma. I've been in discussions with male and female colleagues who believe on some very deep, probably unexamined level that abdominal delivery is the superior mode of arrival.

Approximately 50 to 85 percent of women who've had a cesarean delivery can go on and deliver subsequent babies normally. Though obstetricians used to be taught the dictum, "Once a cesarean, always a cesarean," this is no longer the case. The scientific literature documenting the safety of subsequent vaginal deliveries was available by the late 1970s. We routinely offered vaginal birth after cesarean section (VBAC) as an option during my training. Yet this option is *still* not offered to all women who are candidates for it. And for those women who are candidates, it is often not an option they choose, probably because they are scared. A recent article in one of the OB/GYN magazines was entitled, "When the Patient Demands a C-section." Dr. Bruce Flamm, interviewed for this article, was right on target when he said, "When someone is scared, it is not an indication for surgery. It is an indication for education."[15] Clearly the practice of medicine is a two-way street. One of my colleagues, Dr. Bethany Hays, commented on reading the Flamm article, "This is great. We create the fear of vaginal birth, and then we blame it on the patient!"

C-section rates vary tremendously among individual doctors. Some of my colleagues have personal C-section rates of only 6 percent. These are the same doctors who are highly supportive of midwifery.

Episiotomy

Another procedure that usually isn't necessary is episiotomy. It is estimated that 61.9 percent of all women who delivered vaginally in the United States in 1987 underwent episiotomy, the surgical cutting of the tissue between the vagina and rectum.[16] Nationally, 80 percent of first-time mothers delivering vaginally in the United States undergo this procedure.[17] In many hospitals virtually 100 percent of women undergo this surgical intervention.

Unfortunately, women who undergo episiotomy are fifty times *more* likely to suffer from severe lacerations than those who don't have it.[18] The reason for this is that episiotomy cuts frequently extend farther into the vaginal tissues during the delivery. This surgical cut of the perineum can result in excessive blood loss, painful scarring, and unnecessary postpartum pain.[19] The woman's discomfort may affect her bonding with and nursing of the infant. No long-term benefits have been shown for women who have had episiotomies, although I was repeatedly taught that episiotomy was absolutely necessary to prevent a later prolapse of the uterus and/or excessive laxity of the vagina.

Studies have shown that whether a woman giving birth has an episiotomy is most dependent upon whether she is attended by a doctor or by a midwife. Midwives are taught how to do normal, noninterventional deliveries. Doctors naturally *do* more—that's what they've been trained to do. Letting a woman push her baby out slowly, gently, and without interference is a rare experience in some hospitals.

There are no data to support the need for routine episiotomy, yet it continues to be taught routinely in OB/GYN residency training. (So much for the "science" of medicine.) Episiotomy is, in fact, a telling example of how in clinical practice a belief—"women's bodies can't give birth without intervention"—can actually win out over scientific evidence, which in this case supports *not* doing an episiotomy.

Anesthesia

Modern anesthesia is a godsend in many instances, but in labor it is used far too often. This culture believes that if a little is good, more must be better. So there are now obstetrical services in which almost every pregnant woman, long before she goes into labor, is sold on the virtues of epidurals—"the Cadillac" of obstetrical anesthesia. The seed is often planted during hospital-sponsored childbirth classes: "You don't need to feel a thing." Anesthesia is offered as a panacea to many women. I've heard many women say, "I want that epidural catheter put in during my last two weeks of pregnancy!" But the risks include arrest of the first and second stages of labor, fever, increased forceps use, pelvic floor damage, and fetal distress, with subsequent increase in cesarean section rates.[20]

Supine Position

Women who deliver in a physiologically normal position, such as standing or squatting, are much less apt to have perineal tears and are more apt to have normal, nonsurgical second stages of labor. In fact, lying supine while pushing out the baby is a position that is actually unfavorable for birth because this position favors excessive pressure of the delivering baby into the posterior vagina, and it *decreases* the diameter of the pelvic outlet—a setup for vaginal tears. (Ever try to move your bowels while lying flat on your back?) This position, known as the lithotomy position, was apparently popularized by Louis XIV in France, who was a voyeur and wanted to watch the births of women in his court without their knowledge of his presence. In the lithotomy position, with her skirts hiked up, the laboring woman couldn't see who was watching. This position caught on because it was associated with the upper classes and therefore was imitated.

Probably another reason it caught on was the popularization of obstetrical forceps. Forceps were originally developed in 1560 by Peter Chamberlain, a male midwife who came from a family of male midwives. These tools remained a Chamberlain "family secret" until they were released to the general public in 1728.[21] Training in the use of this instrument was given only to men (usually physicians and surgeons), and they were originally used when all else failed and the woman had been trying to push the baby out for hours. The lithotomy position was the one in which the exhausted woman could rest while forceps were applied. It also allowed the obstetrician maximal control over the process of forcep delivery.

During the second stage of labor, women who squat instead of lie supine increase the size of the vaginal outlet naturally, because this position distributes pressure equally throughout the entire vaginal circumference and helps bring the baby's head down. In the squatting position the anterior/posterior diameter of the bony pelvis (front to back) is increased by a half-centimeter or more.[22] The squatting position also keeps the pregnant uterus *off* the major pelvic blood vessels leading to the heart. The blood supply from the mother to the baby is therefore improved, resulting in increased safety for both. (I've seen countless babies go into fetal distress in the delivery room simply because of the mother's position flat on her back.) Women who are encouraged to touch their perineum and the baby's head get connected up very quickly with their birthing babies and deliver much easier.

Sterilization

The mother's vulvar area is often sprayed with betadine antiseptic prior to birth to "dilute" any possible germs. When I was in medical school, I got the impression that the most important thing that had to happen before delivery was to place the sterile drapes on the woman's legs and abdomen. There was a very precise way this had to be done. (These special water-resistant delivery drapes are the same type used in surgery. Does this fact tell you anything?) When the draping is finished, the perineum and vagina are the only parts showing. (In the 1970s they were arranged so that the mother couldn't see what was going on. Later she could watch in a mirror—yippee!)

The operating site (where the incision would normally be made) is a mother's vagina and perineum. Before the drapes were applied, these areas were scrubbed, then sprayed with the betadine antiseptic. The birthing mother's body, once draped, was viewed as a sterile surgical field. Though many hospitals relaxed the draping procedures in the 1980s, drapes are being used much more now to protect the hospital staff from the possibility of AIDS from the patient's bodily fluids.

When birth technology is truly needed, however, it is life-saving and miraculous. When a physician is in the operating room transfusing a woman whose placenta simply won't separate from the uterus and who is losing blood quickly, she knows that one hundred years ago, her patient would have died. Usually, however, more "high-touch" and less "high-tech" would do the job.

My Personal Story

As a mother and a women's doctor, I have experienced childbirth from both sides of the bed. Every mother has moments that she cherishes from the birth experience and insights and feelings she'd like to share with other women. I'd like to tell you my story and also some remarkable stories of other women.

The due date for my first child was December 7, 1980. I continued my work supervising the residency clinic at a Boston hospital, and I flew or drove to Maine every other week to keep my practice going there. I had watched far too many pregnant women stop work early and then mope around the house eating, waiting for the baby to come, sometimes begging their obstetrician to induce labor. I didn't want to fall into that category. I had also seen dozens of women go overdue. I certainly wasn't going to get excited about labor—at least, not until my due date.

On Thanksgiving we went to dinner at a friend's house. Later that evening, back home in bed, I started to experience very mild, but regular contractions that didn't hurt. Like the good controlled doctor that I was, I went into the bathroom and decided to examine my cervix to see if I was dilating. When I did this, my water broke. I thought, "Damn, now I know this really *is* it."[23] Shortly thereafter, without the natural "padding" that the amniotic fluid provides, my contractions began coming every two minutes and were much more uncomfortable than initially.

I called my mother, who was planning to help me after the birth, and said, "I'm not going to like this." She said that she understood (after six children, she knew) but that it wouldn't last forever. In the 1940s, Mom had always had to labor alone, strapped down in bed with no pain relief or personal support. For each delivery, she had been knocked unconscious by drugs and was handed the baby later by the obstetrician, as though it were a gift from him, and not the fruit of her own labor. Thousands of women like her were never given a choice and didn't even know there were other ways to deliver.

The pain of labor was far greater than I thought it would be. (It's always worse after the membranes are ruptured, a point that doesn't seem to stop some obstetricians from doing it prematurely even when there's no need to.) I had seen hundreds of women in labor after five years of OB training. I had always focused on the women who didn't appear to have any discomfort, and I was so sure I would be one of them. But here I was—stuck. I felt as though I were in a box, and there was no way out except through. My intellect could not get me out of this—and I was determined to go through the process naturally. I already trusted the natural world more than the artificial man-made one. What I didn't appreciate then was the depth of my own programming into and cooperation with that same man-made world.

We called my obstetrician, a sensitive man with whom I had worked in the hospital for several years. He suggested that my husband and I go into the hospital. The only problem was that all I wanted to do was stay on the floor on my hands and knees. Moving *anywhere* seemed to me the most unnatural thing I could think of. It went against every instinct in my body.

I didn't have a bag packed for the hospital, so my husband ran around and put some underwear, a nightgown, and a toothbrush in a bag. Then he tried to get me dressed, out the door, and into the car. He nearly had to carry me. Left to my own instincts, I would never have left my position on my hands and knees on the floor.

When we got to the hospital, a place where I had worked for half a decade, I had to go through the admitting office as a patient. Admissions had lost the correct papers and would not let me go upstairs to Labor and Delivery, where my nurse friends and my doctor were waiting. This was my introduction to the bureaucracy of hospitals, something I'd been shielded from for years. (Laboring in a hospital hallway alone is inhumane; but for thousands of women, it is their experience.) I simply walked out of that room, went to the back hall elevator, got in, and went up to Labor and Delivery by myself.

When my doctor examined me, I was four centimeters dilated. (You have to get to ten to be ready to push.) For the next three hours my contractions came frequently. But I failed to dilate beyond six centimeters, where I remained "stuck" for those three hours. The contraction pattern on the monitor was "dysfunctional." Though the contractions hurt a lot, and I never got much of a break between them, they simply were not getting the job done. I had what is known as hypertonic uterine inertia, which means that the contractions, though present, are not efficient—they are erratic, originating all over the uterus at the same time, like the heart when it goes into atrial fibrillation. (The high heart—in the chest—does the same sort of thing as the low heart—the uterus in the pelvis—sometimes.) Instead of beginning at the top and moving in a wave to the bottom of the uterus, the contractions originated in many places at the same time. Labor didn't progress well. It was like trying to get toothpaste out of a tube by squeezing it in fifteen places at the same time with a little bit of pressure, instead of squeezing firmly only at the back end of the tube so that the paste comes out uniformly.

When my doctor told me that I had made no progress in three hours, I knew what was next. (Remember, my intellect thought it was in control of my labor.) "Okay," I said, "start the IV, plug in the fetal electrode, and hang the pit." Pitocin is a drug that artificially contracts the uterus. After the pitocin was started, the contractions became almost unbearable, going to full intensity almost as soon as they started.

No amount of Lamaze breathing distracted[24] me from the intensity of the feeling that the lower part of my body was in the grip of a vise. At one point, I looked at the clock and saw that it was 11:15 A.M. What I recall thinking was, "If this goes on for another fifteen minutes, I'm going to need an epidural anesthetic." I didn't know that I was in transition—the part of labor that is most intense, just before the cervix becomes fully dilated. Within the next twelve minutes I suddenly felt the urge to push. It was the most powerful bodily sensation I've ever felt, and I was powerless to resist it. The thought flashed through my mind, "If I ever tell another woman not to push when every fiber in her body tells her to push, may God strike me with lightning!"

In two pushes, Ann almost flew out of my body. My obstetrician quite literally "caught her." Though I was laboring in the "birthing room," I wasn't laboring in the "correct" delivery bed, and I barely made it to the delivery bed in time. (Birthing rooms now are equipped with beds that adjust for delivery of the baby, so that moving from one bed to another isn't necessary.)

Ann cried and cried, and though I put her to my breast almost immediately, it still took quite a while to calm her down. I believe this was because the pitocin made for a far too rapid second stage of labor. It was too intense both for Ann and for me. Neither she nor I had much chance to recover between contractions.

A primiparous patient—one having her first baby—usually takes an hour or more to push the baby out. From the time the cervix is fully dilated to delivery—the second stage of labor—I went from six centimeters to delivery in less than one hour; my uterus was being pushed by a powerful drug, a very intense and distinctly unnatural experience.

To this day, my daughter is not particularly "at home" in her body and is afraid to take physical risks, for instance in skiing or hiking. Though there are various reasons for this, I know deep within me that being propelled into the world with so little time to accommodate herself to the process of labor was a terrifying experience for her. She had difficulty nursing, and she was never a good sleeper. Part of the reason is that she was small (five pounds, eight ounces) and early (38.5 weeks), and part is her personality—but another part is how she was born. I've discussed all this with her. I didn't know then what I know now, and I don't for one minute blame myself about how she was born. I do, however, allow myself to feel sadness about the experience, which would be considered a completely normal labor and delivery by most everyone.

After Ann's birth, the cord got pulled off the placenta, so that my placenta had to be manually removed by my doctor. The explosive uncontrolled delivery had left me in tears, so that though removing the placenta was somewhat uncomfortable, nothing could equal the discomfort of those pitocin-induced contractions. I was euphoric to have the whole thing over with. I had had a "normal vaginal delivery" and felt lucky to have avoided a cesarean. Most women obstetricians are automatically treated like candidates for "high-risk" pregnancies and deliveries, because women doctors (and other women who have been highly trained out of their instinctual feminine knowing) often split their intellects from their bodies, mistrust their bodies, and unconsciously set themselves up for the possibility of labor problems. We as a group are also at risk for working too many hours during pregnancy to "prove" that we can "handle it" and compete with the men.

When I look back now, I realize that my being "stuck" at six centimeters was a perfect metaphor for my ambivalence about having a baby and for how I felt during my labor. I had felt "stuck" and trapped by the pain—something my intellect had not prepared me for. My intellect, you recall, thought I was doing an experiment with my uterus. I wasn't very invested in actually having a *baby*. I had made no room in my life for a baby. I had spent the previous decade proving to myself and to the world that I was as good as any man— and men don't do babies.

Another factor in creating my dysfunctional labor was the process of moving off my hands and knees in my house, getting to the hospital, going through admitting, and then answering insurance and medical questions for forms that I had already filled out several times. All those things are interruptions of the inner focus required for normal labor. I didn't really know that at the time, though I'd seen countless women come to the hospital in active labor, only to have the process become slowed down or dysfunctional when they were "processed by the system."

Now it was me having a baby—something that I was determined would not change my life. Too late, I realized that what I needed when I got stuck was a midwife or a doctor with good midwifery skills, preferably some wise woman (or wise man—male midwives and male obstetricians with the souls of midwives do exist) who had been a parent and who trusted the process of labor and the messages my body was sending. I needed someone who would have said to me, "Go inside and talk to your baby. Let the baby know that it's okay to come out, that she will be fine." Then the midwife would have taken me for a walk in the hall—a very effective way of getting contractions back on track. She might even have helped me work through my ambivalence about having a baby.

With my second labor, I did go to a midwife. I began labor at home and spent some time in the bathtub. (Studies done in Sweden have shown that women who labor in warm water dilate much faster.) I didn't want to go to the hospital until I had to. My husband was asleep, and I didn't wake him until I knew that the labor was moving right along, several hours later. When he examined me, I was already seven centimeters dilated. We went to the hospital and my colleague, Dr. Mary Ellen Fenn, met me at the front door and parked my car, a gesture of support that I will always treasure.

When I arrived in the birthing room, I was nine centimeters dilated. I spent the rest of the labor rocking from one foot to the other while standing up. This second baby was a lot bigger than the first—eight pounds, seven ounces. Her head was what is called posterior (she was face-up in my body). I never felt the urge to push, but I pushed her out anyway with a great deal of effort. Even after I was fully dilated, the contractions felt the same as they had at nine centimeters. I didn't have an episiotomy (the surgical cut made in the vagina just before birth allegedly to increase the size of the vaginal opening and avoid tears)—and I didn't tear. My baby, Kate, and I left the hospital an hour after she was born. Kate was calm and collected, and she has been that way ever since. Her personality and body type are entirely different from her sister's.

Having my midwife in the room with me was heaven. I felt so supported. I had much more trust in myself this time—and I had all the baby things ready. I remember thinking during this second labor that every woman deserved this same amount of support. *Every* woman should be able to labor in whatever position her body wants to take. She should be surrounded by beloved friends of her choice (not spectators but supporters—there's a big difference!). Every woman should be massaged and cared for and cherished during her labor.

In this labor I had pain, to be sure, but I went deep down inside myself with it. In my first labor, I had fought the pain and reached out to my husband in desperation—I wouldn't even let him go to the bathroom. But this second labor felt as though it was between me and my baby. I had plenty of time to rest between contractions and to chat with my caregivers. They gave me backrubs that felt fantastic. No drugs interfered with the labor. I learned to trust my body in a letting-go process that feels like a kind of surrendering to a process that *is* you but that is also *greater* than you. I didn't learn any of this stuff in my residency training—I didn't even learn it from watching women in labor, though I believe that it can be learned that way and that I eventually would have. What you have to do is trust nature, expect the best, and get your intellect's death grips off your flesh.

Labor feels very instinctive and primitive, but because our culture teaches us not to trust our instincts, we usually associate the word *primitive* with *ignorant*. The Random House dictionary defines *primitive* as "unaffected or little-affected by civilizing influences." Believe me, that's exactly how labor feels. We cannot labor with our intellect. We women need to reclaim this animal part of us and embrace ancient and necessary wisdom. Although Lamaze seemed a step in the right direction to me at one point because it attempts to help us listen to our bodies, I've started to rethink the prepared-childbirth-class approach. Lamaze breathing, for instance, now seems to me simply another attempt to control our bodies and keep us out of touch. Instead of doing a six-pant blow during my second birth, I now wish I had groaned loudly and let my groans help me expel the baby. But I was far too "professional" (read: out of touch) to do that. I am deeply saddened by all the unnecessarily medicalized births that occur because women in labor don't trust themselves and aren't surrounded by those who could assist them in this process.

Turning Labor into Personal Power

Trusting the birth process and knowing how to tune in to the baby are abilities that enhance labor and make it an experience that offers us the opportunity to empower ourselves. Instead of running from these lessons, we as women could learn a great deal if we were willing to embrace them.

Dr. Bethany Hays, one of my colleagues, is the mother of three sons. She wrote me the following reflections on the pain of labor and how we can best work *with* it:

"I used to think that labor was just a matter of dealing with pain and the fear of pain. I knew that with labor the pain was qualitatively different from any other pain experienced in our bodies. I never subscribed to the punishment theory of labor pain. I was looking for a natural and reasonable explanation. I did not believe labor pain was a whim of Mother Nature any more than it was a punishment from God.

"With all other forms of pain, the pain is there to tell us that something is wrong. 'Stop walking on your foot, there's a piece of glass in it.' 'Don't eat any more chili, it's giving you heartburn.' With labor, I knew that the reason for the pain, at least in most cases, is not related to anything being wrong. The physical process of birth is completely normal and exquisitely planned by nature to ensure the safe delivery of an infant with minimal trauma to the mother. Pain was a part of that plan, and I had but to view it in that context to understand its purpose.

"As I observed women through their pregnancies, I began to understand that nature would have to have a signal to get women to stop what they were doing, to find a safe place to give birth, and to gather people around them to help. For some, nothing short of a sledgehammer would do. It needed to be a signal that no one could ignore but that left the mother able to participate in the birth if there were circumstances requiring her to do so."

Certainly, the pain of labor is a strong signal that says, "Stop what you're doing and pay attention." Instead of the "no pain, no gain" cultural mentality that often leads to self-abuse, gaining from the pain of labor is an entirely different way of being with pain. Once a woman has stopped, gathered support people around her, and gotten herself to a safe place to birth, she has reached the point when she must use the pain for something else. Dr. Hays suggests that at this point the pain is something to allow, and she points out that one of the meanings of *to suffer* is "to allow," as when Christ said, "Suffer the little children to come unto me."

Once settled in, women in labor, then, must *allow* the pain. Thrashing about doesn't help. Going deep within yourself does. Dr. Hays and I were talking recently about the pain of labor and how to help women work with it, and we exchanged a few stories about women who appeared to "go to another place" when they were in labor.

She told me about the wife of a medical student she once worked with who sat quietly in bed with the lights dimmed during her labor and was so focused that her mother and husband figured that she probably wasn't in labor. Not only was she in labor, however, when she finally opened her eyes and spoke, she said, "I think it's time to push."

"After the birth," Dr. Hays told me, "my curiosity prompted me to ask her where she had gone when I instructed her to go 'somewhere else.' [Early in labor, she had seemed to be very disconnected from her body, and Dr. Hays had told her to get comfortable, relax, and just "go somewhere else."] Her answer was totally unexpected. She said, 'Oh, I was concentrating on the pain.' Her answer intrigued me. Could a woman really deal with the pain of labor not, as I had been taught, by distracting herself and concentrating on something else—her 'breathing' or her 'focal point' or her fantasy trip to the Caribbean? Could she, rather, focus on her body—on the work it was doing, on the *pain itself*?"

So Dr. Hays began questioning those women who labored without noise or a lot of activity each time she worked with one. One said, "Well, I was just concentrating on my cervix. You know, letting it open up for my baby's head." The common thread running through all these labors was that the women were *with* the pain.

They were going down inside themselves to the place where the pain was and allowing it.

One of Dr. Hays's patients gave her the following beautiful piece of birth imagery in answer to the question "Where do you go during your contractions?" She said, "Well, you know when you are in the ocean, in a heavy surf, if you stay on the surface you will get thrown about against the reefs and the rocks, and you get a lot of water in your nose and mouth and feel like you're drowning. But if you dive down and hold on to something and let the wave pass over you, you can come up in between and feel just fine. Well, that's what I did during labor. When the contractions came, I dived down and let them pass over me." Water imagery is very common when women describe normal birth.

During my own second labor, I realized that I had *allowed* the process quite differently than I had with my first. Labor is a true *process*—with its own rhythm and timing—and it is a process that is bigger than we are. For that reason, learning to go with it, to let it sweep us along—is something that we never forget. And it is great training for the give-and-take of parenting.

Birth and Female Sexuality

Upon leaving the hospital after Ann's birth (I left about six hours after she was born), it was wonderful to get into bed beside my husband, with our new little daughter sleeping in a cradle right beside my head. She was a gift that the two of us had created together. I felt like making love with my husband in that moment, which we did (avoiding actual intercourse, however).

Many women describe birth in natural settings as erotic. Ina Mae Gaskin, in her classic, *Spiritual Midwifery*, writes that women need to be loved in labor, to be treated like Goddesses. Another provocative piece of writing I once read said that the birth of a baby is the completion of the act of intercourse, conception, gestation, and now delivery. With the birth of a baby, the circle is complete. This book suggested the birth take place between the mother and her mate, with her presenting this baby back to him.

Hospital surroundings, in which complete strangers wander in and out, are not very conducive to a woman being in touch with her deepest self. Nor do they support spontaneous acts of affection between the woman and her mate. Such acts make the staff very uncomfortable because they then become potential voyeurs. A husband holding his wife from behind with his hands under her breasts while she is squatting is a problem for some. Also, many hospital staff and patients are taught to be very concerned about keeping a woman's body covered at all times—despite the fact that in the middle of pushing out a baby, most women could not care less!

Bethany Hays writes, "As I began to reexplore my own births, I realized that I too had made an attempt to go inside to deal with the pain. My own births, however, were filled with great violence. I recently found the five-day diary I had written after the birth of my first child, a birth I have always spoken of with great pride in my accomplishment, the delivery of a nine-pound, six-ounce baby using Lamaze.

"The language I used in those days immediately after the birth, however, was that of physical abuse. 'Just get mad and push that baby out.' I remembered thinking that the birth was a mixture of loss and accomplishment, of joy and trauma. I remember my mourning over the loss of my normal vagina and perineum after a fourth-degree episiotomy [an episiotomy that goes right into the rectal lining]. I remember being surprised at how little actual physical pain that had caused. I remember that every inch of my body felt like it had been attacked 'by a tire tool.'

"I remember wanting to be alone to find some way to reconcile these powerful, joyful, and at the same time threatening feelings. I remember knowing innately that this was related to my sexuality, to my erotic core. But it was many years before I realized that I had rejected my greatest innate ability to deal with the pain of my births: that very well of elemental energy that kept calling me."

Bethany Hays experienced labor as being split into two people: one who wanted to do Lamaze breathing and carry on a rational conversation with her birth attendants, and another who was drawing her into a "pit down inside" that terrified her. I, too, recall feeling split in two with my first birth. Part of me was fighting the pain, and part was reading the fetal monitor with the practiced eye of a physician who knows that despite wide variable decelerations (dips in the heart rate) on the monitor strip, the "beat-to-beat variability" (another measure of heart rate) was excellent. (Now I know that that monitor strip indicated that my baby was scared.)

Bethany told me that she realized that the Lamaze method of breathing had worked for her only up to a point. When the cervix was nearly dilated and it was time for the baby to traverse the pelvis, she was suddenly no longer able to do the ordered breathing patterns that, she thought then, had gotten her that far. When it was time to push, she recalls being in a place she could only identify as "somewhere I could not stay." At this point she said she wanted to get rid of the baby at all costs. (Women sometimes yell at this point "Get it out of there!") For Bethany this included, during her first birth, demanding that forceps be used to accomplish the delivery. (But in her defense, she realized that being strapped to the delivery table flat on her back to deliver a nine-and-a-half-pound baby after one and a half hours of pushing was not ideal.)

In subsequent births she again found herself in that "terrible, unacceptable place" in which she used all her rational powers to "bypass that terrible transit through the pelvis." "Just get tough." "Get mad and get him out!" "Ignore the pain, just push through it." This resulted, she notes, in "considerable pain and trauma to myself." Both of us remember telling similar things to our patients repeatedly: "Just push through the pain—get him out. Get mad!" Labor and delivery staff are trained to do this, too.

Later in her career, Bethany met a woman who taught her—and me—the secret of the second stage of labor, which now seems obvious: Women don't want to push because we feel disconnected from that part of our bodies, and because giving birth is a sexual experience, almost taboo with so many people looking on. Instead of pushing through the second stage of labor as though it were an athletic event, women would do well to let their uterus do the work, while allowing their vaginas to relax into the process.

During my residency training, I was accused of being Dr. Pain by the nurses because I didn't insist on a spinal anesthetic for every delivery. Even then, I knew that pushing the baby out took a relatively small amount of time, and I believed that it was far better for a woman to be alert for her new baby than to have the lower half of her body paralyzed from a spinal so that forceps had to be used to pull the baby out. I witnessed many women who had spinal anesthesia for routine deliveries fall asleep on the delivery table. These women were much less "present" to greet their babies than those who had birthed normally.

Back then, I didn't appreciate the fact that birth is part of the continuum of female sexuality and that by numbing the lower half of the body to feeling anything painful, we were also numbing the possibility for feeling anything ecstatic or sexual.

Women's Stories

REBECCA'S STORY: RECLAIMING BIRTH POWER. The following story is related in the words of Bethany Hays, Rebecca's obstetrician.

"Rebecca was a second-time mother whose first labor had been long, but she did well with the help of her labor support person and a gentle loving husband. Rebecca arrived at the hospital for her second birth already seven centimeters dilated and feeling great. She walked and talked with her team of supportive people, and she sipped fluids. She tolerated our medical intrusions into her birth with monitor, blood pressure cuff, and thermometer.

"After several hours, Rebecca was still only seven to eight centimeters dilated. She was puzzled and frustrated, wanting to 'get on with it.' We discussed her options, including rupture of the membranes, which might bring the baby's head down against the cervix. The cervix felt ready and soft enough to allow the passage of the head, waiting for some unknown work yet to be done.

"After considering the possible negative effects of it, she chose to rupture the membranes. This was done. Now the contractions got harder, but after some time the exam showed that she was not quite fully dilated. The head was still high up in the pelvis. She showed some urge to push when squatting, but she was not pushing effectively. Her monitrice [professional labor support person] reminded me that during the first labor, she had also had difficulty pushing—requiring three hours in the second stage and pressure applied to the posterior vaginal wall to encourage her to push.

"Maybe that would help again, someone suggested. So as Rebecca squatted, I knelt on the floor, placed two fingers in her vagina, and pushed firmly on the posterior wall. Her response was an immediate and reflexive withdrawal. I realized that not only was I causing her pain, but I was triggering some much more serious emotional response. My own reaction was equally strong. 'No,' I thought, 'I will not participate in this abuse. This is sexual abuse of another woman's body, and I will not do it.'

" 'Rebecca,' I said, 'let's try something else.' Now, I have always been touched at the faith (often undeserved) that patients place in me, and I knew that she trusted me. Whatever the new plan was, she would try it. The joke was that I had no plan. I was flying totally by the seat of my pants. I asked her to get comfortable, and she arranged herself semireclining on the bed, with her husband behind her and wrapped around her. 'Now,' I said, 'I just want you to relax and listen to my voice. First, go down inside yourself and find your baby where he is in your body. When you are with him, tell him he is okay, in case he is scared.'

"As we waited, a slow smile came over her face, and I knew that she was with her baby. The fetal monitor no longer disturbed her. It now showed sudden resolution of the small to moderate variable decelerations she'd been having with contractions. [Variable decelerations are heart rate patterns associated with compression of the umbilical cord, which can sometimes produce stress in the baby.]

" 'Now,' I said, 'I want you just to listen. Many of us women have not owned all the parts of our bodies. We have not allowed ourselves to feel our vaginas and our perineums. They have seemed separate and are not within our control. They have negative connotations: pornographic or dirty. In many ways these parts of our bodies are problematic for us. But the truth is that they are ours. They belong to us like our hands and our lips and our minds. This part of your body is yours, and you can reclaim it. Right now. Take it back as the sensual, enjoyable part of you that it really is. Since it is yours, you are totally in control. You can allow your baby to move through this part of you as fast or as slowly as you like. It does not have to hurt you, but you will feel very strong signals from this part of your body that you are not used to feeling. Allow those feelings and celebrate them as the return of a long lost friend.'

"Now we were all watching. Rebecca was totally relaxed, lying in her husband's arms. The room was quiet except for the fetal monitor, which was quietly attesting to the continued well-being of the baby. I was wondering if I was deluding myself—pretty sure that everyone in the room must think I was nuts.

"Suddenly I realized that with each contraction, Rebecca's perineum was bulging—the head was coming down. It was working. Occasionally, Rebecca lost contact with her body, became frightened, and clutched her husband. Immediately when this happened, the baby's heart rate pattern showed prolonged variable decelerations with slow recovery. At these points, I would say again, 'Talk to your baby again, Rebecca. He's scared. Remember, don't go any faster than you want to. This is your body. All of it belongs to you.'

"Once again, Rebecca was quiet, and we saw the baby's head begin to crown [to appear, just before delivery]. Soon, with little or no pushing effort, the baby was born into his mother's loving arms."

After hearing this story, I realized that the second stage of my own second labor might have been different if I'd had a doctor like Bethany Hays. I also realized that I have been involved in the unwitting physical abuse of many laboring women by pushing down on their vaginas to try to help them push, and by encouraging them, like a football coach, to "push him out." I wouldn't have done that if I had known what I now know.

AMANDA'S STORY: A HOME BIRTH. Bethany also attended a birth in which one of her patients went further into herself than either of us had known it was possible to go. Amanda's first baby had been delivered by Bethany by cesarean section. "I thought we had done everything right," Bethany says. "She had been healthy, confident, and wanted a normal birth, including labor without anesthesia. She had labor support, family, and friends. Though it seemed perfect, the baby simply wouldn't come. We did everything I knew to do, which at that time was not a lot. I finally did a cesarean."

With her second pregnancy Amanda returned to Bethany's care and said, "I want to have a normal birth this time." Bethany agreed and told her that she thought that was entirely possible. The women who are most motivated to give birth normally are those who did not succeed in doing so with their first child but hadn't lost the desire to try. Amanda also did not want to have her second baby in the hospital, because she felt that the hospital environment had been part of the problem the first time. Instead, she would have it at home.

For years I've always had a special place in my heart for those women who choose home birth. The reason for this is that these women trust themselves more than doctors and hospitals. Though they sometimes make mistakes, they have something to teach us. My sister had a home birth, and I wish I had had at least one child at home. Though I left the hospital right after both my children were born and neither one of them went to the nursery, I would still have liked the experience of waking up in labor and not having to get into the car and go someplace. Both times it felt like a very unnatural interruption of my process.

Though she wanted Bethany there, Bethany does not do home births. Finally they reached a compromise. Bethany would be there only as a labor support person, and Amanda herself would hire the best midwife she could find. For an OB/GYN to do a home birth is politically very unsafe. Many hospitals will not allow physicians who do home births to have hospital privileges, and most malpractice insurance companies won't insure such physicians. (Many physicians even consider home birth to be "child abuse" because of the potential risks associated with childbirth.) But Amanda was determined to have Bethany present, and Bethany was interested in supporting her, as long as she wasn't responsible for being the caregiver.

Long discussions intervened, regarding risks, uterine rupture, fetal compromise, their likelihood, and what Bethany could and could not do if these problems happened at home. Ultimately, Amanda convinced Bethany that she herself was in charge of the safety of her baby and the integrity of her uterus, and that if she felt she could not do this job, she would let Bethany know and they would all go to the hospital.

The day of Amanda's delivery came. Her early labor was long and painful, but she didn't call anyone. When she finally invited her caregivers to join her, they found Amanda in the rocker. "I feel so great," she said in one breath. And with the next she said, "The pain was so bad this afternoon, I thought I would die." Bethany later told me, "I didn't know how to put those two statements together." As the birth neared, Amanda lay in her king-size bed on her side. "As we tried to keep up with her," Bethany told me, "she circled the bed. Her head remained in the center, and her feet made a full circuit around the bed twice, a maneuver that I had not seen before in the hospital. It was very primitive. Though it was not clear to me what it represented, I trusted her need to move in this way as part of her unique birth process.

"There was little talk. Amanda said nothing and made little noise. She pushed her baby out on hands and knees and then kneeled over her. She was somewhere else. We were all commenting on the baby, but she was not looking at her infant. Her body was in a pose of ecstasy. When spoken to, she did not respond. For a moment I was frightened that she might not come back from wherever she was. Then she looked down at her infant and slowly came back into her body—or was it back out of her body?"

Bethany took a picture of Amanda in that ecstatic state, and she showed it at a recent medical meeting in which we both lectured on women's health. From this and from reading Vicki Noble's *Shakti Woman*[25] I learned that Amanda's experience of ecstasy is potentially available to all women at birth. Since then, I have talked at length with some of my patients who have had home births. One recently told me that during her home birth she "left her body" and became an eagle flying high overhead. She experienced no pain. She had never told anyone about this. From that moment on, however, she trusted her body completely.

Women have learned collectively, though not necessarily consciously, to fear the birth experience, and every obstacle has been put in our collective paths to keep us from experiencing this power. But as Bethany says, "This kind of birth is possible in many environments. It requires a mother who trusts her body and is connected to all of its parts. She must love and want her baby. She must understand that birth is a sexual event and be comfortable with her sexuality. She must feel safe. She needs to know that the people around her accept her body and the sexual nature of what she is doing and are not embarrassed by it and will not interfere with the process. She needs to know that she can go down inside and come back safely. If she has never been there before, she needs the grounding love of family and friends who will, if needed, call her back."

Those women who have already had babies in standard ways should understand that they are not responsible for what they didn't know at the time. I was born drugged, as were all my brothers and sisters. Though we were breast-fed, we were still left in the hospital's nursery for hours while my mother woke up. This isn't the way she had wanted it, but she didn't know she had a choice.

Remember that *being responsible* simply means "being able to respond." No one is guaranteed a perfect birth. In fact, the concept of "a perfect birth" is part of the perfectionism of the addictive system. Sometimes a baby needs to be observed in the nursery right after birth. Sometimes an emergency cesarean is necessary. When this happens, it is not a failure on the woman's part. She is only one part of a complex and mysterious process. The baby herself (or himself) is also an active participant in the labor process. Each baby makes a unique contribution to her mother's pregnancy, labor, and delivery. We can always learn something from it and use the experience for personal growth. But whatever happens, parents should be involved as much as possible, at all stages of pregnancy, labor, and delivery. They need to understand that their input is very important to their baby's health.

Reclaiming Birth Power Collectively

Imagine what might happen if the majority of women emerged from their labor beds with a renewed sense of the strength and power of their bodies, and of their capacity for ecstasy through giving birth. When enough women realize that birth is a time of great opportunity to get in touch with their true power, and when they are willing to assume responsibility for this, we will reclaim the power of birth and help move technology where it belongs—in the service of birthing women, not as their master.

For many women, having a baby is their first experience of being connected with other women and with their vast creativity. It has the potential to transform the ways in which we think about ourselves. As one patient said to me, "I felt at one with every woman who ever gave birth. I felt powerful and in touch with something within me that I never knew was there. I took my place among the lineage of women as mothers."

THIRTEEN

Motherhood: Bonding with Your Baby

Early Touching

*T*he process of becoming attached to a new baby begins long before the actual birth. However, the events associated with birth can have a very powerful effect on a mother's feelings about her new baby. When I was a medical student, a newborn baby was quickly wrapped in a sterile drape, shown to the mother only briefly, as though the baby's life depended on being somewhere else, and then whisked off to a "warmer" in the nursery, while the mother looked on with pleading eyes, aching to hold her creation. Early bonding studies reported that new mothers greeted their babies first by touching them gingerly with their fingertips, then finally holding them skin-to-skin, yet this response was nothing more than a cultural artifact, the *result* of immediate separation. During my residency, we began to place babies on their mothers' abdomens instead of putting them immediately into the warmer. If a mother holds her baby skin-to-skin with a blanket over both, the baby doesn't need a warmer, the mother *is* the warmer—which is as it should be. At a normal birth, the mother swoops her baby into her arms and holds her full frontal against her skin as soon as the child is born. She knows this baby is hers and needs to be welcomed and comforted immediately.

The birth of a baby also has great significance for the baby's father. The more he is included, the better. Margaret Mead once said that the reason so many cultures banned fathers from births was that if they participated, they would be so "hooked" by the experience and the new baby that they would never be able to go out, steel themselves, and "do their thing" in quite the same way. I believe that the increased participation of men in childbirth—not as bosses or saviors, but as witnesses to the awe of the moment—holds great potential for balancing our world.

I never wanted my own babies to go to the hospital nursery, because I was aware of how different the atmosphere in the nursery was from what I wanted for them. They had just spent forty weeks listening to my heartbeat, bathed in warm fluid in a darkened space. In the hospital nursery, they would be isolated in small bassinets, alone, under fluorescent lights that were on twenty-four hours per day, cared for by a stranger. I knew that my entire physiology was set up by nature so that my baby and I could become "attached." The breast colostrum (first milk) contains antibodies optimally suited to protect the baby from germs, and the suckling of the child produces hormones that help the uterus contract. Babies are innately most interested in eye contact at a distance of about twelve inches, the distance between a mother's eyes and those of her nursing infant. Looking into my baby's eyes, having her look back at me, having her sleep close to me skin-to-skin—all of these events have been set up by nature as the "glue" that continues the mother-infant bond that begins in utero. I knew that these experiences were important for both of us.

Too many babies are taken to the nursery to "get cleaned up" after birth (to get rid of all that filthy vagina stuff!). The process of bathing can lower a baby's body temperature to the point that the nursery nurses won't let the baby out of the nursery again to be with the mothers until the temperature is back up! I figured, why bathe the baby and make her cold? Why not just nurse her, keep her near me, and hang out together?

When I had my first baby, I went to the postpartum floor, but I kept Ann with me. When I got up to go to the bathroom, I took her with me. A nurse came in and yelled through the door, "Where is the baby?" I replied, "In here with me." She said, "You're going to have to learn to leave her sometime." I replied, "Not on the first day of her life!"

I was afraid of my vulnerability postpartum. Too many mothers are undermined by the nursing staff, and I didn't want to risk arguing with the nurses or their rules about when I could and couldn't hold my baby. I wanted my own mother to be able to hold her first female grandchild. In those days, the hospital rule was that only the immediate family could hold the baby, as though the hospital "owned" the child. (Though hospital rules have now changed, I had to fight with the nurses back then to let a baby's grandparents, even those who had driven for hours to see their new grandchild, actually hold her. Sometimes, depending on the nurse involved, I didn't get very far.)

Expecting a hospital stay to be restful was the stuff of mythology, I knew. My home was where I wanted to be, so I left the hospital on the day of delivery both times. The first few weeks of life are a crucial time of adjustment for both the baby and the parents. I wish now that I had spent even more time with my newborns. Studies have repeatedly shown that these first weeks of life are crucial to health.

Dr. John Kennell is a pioneer in the field of neonatal (newborn) care.[1] High-risk refers to any baby who requires intensive surveillance at birth and in the first few days, weeks, or months of life. The majority of high-risk babies are born premature. Many premature babies' bodily systems aren't fully developed at birth and this causes them to have an increased risk of lung problems, developmental and feeding problems, and infection. He and another colleague, Dr. Marshall Klaus, later turned their attention to preventing the conditions that lead to babies entering the high-risk nursery in the first place. They found that there is an unusually high percentage of battering among babies who were born prematurely or who were otherwise sick and whose care was taken over by the nursery staff.

Their research, first on mother-infant bonding and then on parent-infant bonding (adding the father), showed that mothers whose babies stay with them from birth onward bond better and are more attentive to their babies' needs than are those whose babies are whisked away to the nursery to be cared for by "experts."[2] These babies are also healthier and more intelligent overall, months and even years later. (Note: The human psyche and soul are very resilient. Separation doesn't necessarily cause irreversible damage.)

Klaus and Kennell's research has shown what should be common sense to everyone—that human touch and concern have a measurable impact on a baby's health. One study on infant touching—known as "tactile stimulation"—indicated that a group of premature infants who were stroked regularly gained weight much faster than those who weren't touched—even when both groups are fed the same diet! And in the study at the University of Miami the touched babies were discharged from the hospital earlier—a cost savings of $3000 per baby![3]

Touching is so simple, so instinctive. Pregnant mothers automatically stroke their bellies, sending love and energy to the unborn and practicing for when the baby is born. How could we ever have devised a system in which babies were separated from their parents' love and touching in the first minutes of life and sent alone to nurseries run by strangers?[4] No mammal leaves its children unattended and unsuckled the way humans do. A mother bear is at her most dangerous when she's protecting her cubs. She won't let anyone or anything come near them. Many women could use a little more bear energy.

Culturally, we've all participated in subtle and not-so-subtle abuse of our vulnerable newborns in the name of science, partly out of fear and doubting of our own natural instincts. Putting burning silver nitrate or erythromycin ointment into infants' eyes to prevent gonococcal infection is one example. Why do this to all babies, even those whose mothers don't have gonorrhea or chlamydia? I signed a waiver to forgo putting anything in my baby's eyes. I knew I didn't have gonorrhea or chlamydia, and I couldn't see why my baby should have to undergo treatment for something I didn't have. The waiver absolved the hospital from all responsibility for my choice, which is as it should be.

Clamping the cord immediately after birth is another example of an overly stressful act against our newborns. When a baby is born, his heart and lungs must go through profound changes relatively quickly. The child goes from a water environment in which he is nourished via his mother's bloodstream to an air environment in which his lungs must expand and begin the process of respiration.

While this changeover is taking place, the umbilical cord still pulsates, even after birth, so that the baby still has his old oxygenation system in place as the new one is getting ready. Clamping the cord immediately after the baby's birth forces the baby to make the switch over to air more quickly than is necessary. Many mothers and doctors feel that this gives the baby a feeling of panic—that there is not enough air. This practice is like shouting a command, "Okay, breathe now—or else!"

After most normal births, the baby can be placed on the mother's abdomen and the cord can be allowed to gradually stop pulsating on its own. Babies often rest very peacefully while this is going on. They breathe gently and don't cry. In fact, mothers and fathers sometimes worry that something is wrong when their babies are calm at birth. They've learned from the culture that a screaming, terrified newborn is *normal*. (Remember, that which is normal in this culture is not always that which is healthy.) A generation ago, a limp, unresponsive baby was considered "normal." A nurse friend of Dr. Bethany Hays recalled that at the first Lamaze birth she ever saw, she thought there was something wrong because the baby didn't cry immediately!

Circumcision

Circumcision of baby boys is another example of a painful procedure that is unnecessary. I've done hundreds of circumcisions—I am incapable of doing one ever again. Though I often used a local anesthetic, even inserting the needle for this caused the baby unnecessary pain and didn't always work very well. In the past, I would ask mothers to come into the nursery to comfort their babies while they were being circumcised, but they wouldn't do it. They couldn't stand the idea. I always made sure I personally took the newly circumcised baby to his mother as soon as I was finished—so that she could comfort her child. I didn't want him wounded and then left alone in the nursery. Circumcision is a perfect example of the triumph of emotion and outdated and unproven beliefs over common sense and scientific data that it is unnecessary. Circumcision makes it easier to keep the penis clean during conditions when bathing is not accessible (wartime), and it may decrease the risk of cancer of the penis (which is very rare). But there is very little medical justification for routinely circumcising newborns. Dr. George Dennison sums up the circumcision issue very nicely: "To me the idea of performing 100,000 mutilating procedures on newborns to possibly prevent cancer in one elderly man is absurd."[5]

The discussion of circumcision is a perfect example of the strength and influence of first chakra tribal programming on our thought and emotional responses. This programming is so ingrained that many people cannot even discuss the subject of circumcisions without guilt, denial, or other strong emotions. I know that even addressing the subject of the baby boy's bodily integrity, choices, and pain if the procedure is done can cause a "kill the messenger" reaction. But first chakra programming can be successfully questioned and worked through, if desired. Many Jewish couples have rethought the entire circumcision issue and have decided not to have it done to their sons. This will certainly not be everyone's choice.

If I had had a son, I would have draped my own body over his to protect his foreskin if necessary. One of my friends had a son recently and didn't have him circumcised. When asked why not, her answer was simple: "Why would you automatically cut off a piece of the body simply because it is there?" Even Benjamin Spock, the baby expert of all time, said that if he had it to do over again, he'd leave his son's little penis alone.

I've seen circumcisions done in the delivery room. Welcome to the world, baby boy—now to initiate you properly, we're going to cut off one of the most sensitive parts of your body with no anesthesia! Circumcision is known to cause sleep disturbances for at least three days.[6] I believe that it also has profound implications for male sexuality that I can't begin to address adequately in this book. In fact, it's a form of sexual abuse. We certainly feel that way about female clitoridectomy, circumcision, and infibulation, but we justify male infant circumcision by pretending that the babies don't feel it because they're too young and it will have no consequences when they are older. I was taught that babies couldn't feel when they were born and therefore wouldn't feel their circumcision. Why was it, then, that when I strapped their little arms and legs down on the board (called a "circumstraint"), they were often perfectly calm;

then when I started cutting their foreskins, they screamed loudly, with cries that broke my heart? In some hospitals, surgery on infants is still carried out without anesthesia because of this misconception! Women who are going through memories of abuse in childhood know how deeply and painfully early experiences leave their marks in the body.

The foreskin is a highly innervated part of the body. There is no doubt that circumcision "toughens" the delicate skin of the tip of the penis. Men who have been circumcised later in life and who therefore know the difference report a decrease in their sexual sensations. One of my friends who is *not* circumcised says that he wonders if rape is less common in countries in which the men are not circumcised. His experience is that having intercourse with a woman who isn't aroused and well-lubricated is as painful for him as it is for her because of the delicacy of the foreskin!

Formula Versus Breast Milk

Artificial infant feeding is another area that requires rethinking. In the 1940s, infant feeding became very "scientific." Mothers sterilized nipples, bottles, and everything else, and the medical profession as a group systematically undermined breast-feeding as inferior. Hard, unyielding rubber took the place of a warm human nipple. Feedings were timed. Even if a child showed a need for frequent feedings, the mother was warned not to feed her before four hours had passed. This information was based on a very early study of dead babies (who had been sick enough to die!) that found that at one, two, and three hours there was still food in the stomach, but that four hours after death the stomach was empty. Like routine episiotomy, the every-four-hour feeding schedule was accepted into the culture and after a while simply became standard practice. The needs of the individual child were sacrificed on the altar of efficiency and "science"—with all its measuring and weighing. Can you imagine the pain of an infant who cries out to be held or fed, and yet the mother does not do so because the "experts" have told her to ignore all her instincts so she won't "spoil" the baby! (Babies were often weighed before and after a feeding to make sure they "got enough"—a practice that does *not* yield reliable data.)

Even now, women ask their doctors, "How will I know if I have enough milk?" It never occurs to them (or to their doctors, in some cases) that if the baby is growing, happy, and healthy, she is getting enough! Since women's trust in themselves has been systematically undermined in every area of their lives for centuries, how could we be expected to trust our bodies' ability to feed our babies? (Thank goodness that over the years a few did!) I don't for a minute expect that every woman will want to nurse her babies. For some, it's too anxiety-provoking, while for others bottle-feeding is the only way they can get child care from their husband, because he will be able to help with the feeding. We all have to start from where we are, but we should start from knowledge—not ignorance.

Nature set it up so that when a baby is put to breast right after delivery, the suckling action causes the hormones oxytocin and prolactin to be secreted by the mother's pituitary gland. Prolactin induces mothering behavior as well as milk production. These hormones set the stage for adequate milk supply. Mothers who nurse right after delivery also have fewer problems. These hormones help contract the mother's uterus, for example, which helps the placenta separate naturally and thus decreases blood loss. In addition, breast milk is different from cow's milk or formula, and it is unique in that its composition changes over time *depending on the needs of the baby.*

Children who have been breast-fed have one-third fewer hospitalizations than those who are bottle-fed, and they have many fewer allergies. Cow's milk is highly allergenic and can cause bedwetting, asthma, eczema, recurrent infections, runny nose, abdominal pain, depression, and other symptoms in allergic children.[7] Frank Oski, chief of pediatrics at Johns Hopkins Medical School, reports that one-third of iron deficiency in a pediatric practice is caused by gastrointestinal bleeding related to drinking cow's milk.[8] Cow's milk can set the stage for later reactions to pollens, dust, and other substances. (My husband, who was bottle-fed and had asthma as a child, is allergic to cats as an adult *only* when he's been eating dairy food. This is true for many people.) Babies who are breast-fed have a more normal dental arch and palate than those who are bottle-fed. One meticulous study even showed that premature babies fed breast milk had higher intelligence quotas, suggesting that breast milk has some beneficial components for neurodevelopment.[9] This study was unusual in that the babies were fed either formula or breast milk by tube, in order to control for the known beneficial effects associated with actually holding a baby close to the mother's body during breast-feeding.

Most women have to go back to work when their baby is six weeks old, making it much more difficult to nurse in an unrestricted way. By *unrestricted*, I mean breast-feeding in which the mother doesn't "time" her feedings but simply responds to the child's needs instinctively. Women who nurse instinctively usually are unable to remember "when they last fed the baby." Mothers have often told me that they did not intend to nurse precisely because they had to go back to work in six weeks. But so what? is my reply. They could nurse for just that first six weeks—or even for the first few days so that the baby could get the colostrum, to give the baby's health a head start that no artificial formula could provide. We only kid ourselves when we think that baby formula can do as good a job as nature. No amount of scientific experimentation can come up with food that is more specifically made for a baby than the mother's milk.

I expressed my breast milk into bottles and froze it so that if I was going to be away, someone else could feed my children with my milk in a bottle. Both children took both the breast and the bottle, so I had a win-win situation. Breast-feeding is also much more convenient than carrying around a bunch of bottles, particularly while traveling. I nursed discreetly in restaurants, medical meetings, movies, and theaters. Usually, no one noticed. Some, like Dr. Bernie Siegel, congratulated me and thought it was wonderful. (Some babies are really loud nursers and sound like little piglets, however, so you have to adapt to their behavior and be considerate.)

Ashley Montagu has said, "We learn to be human at our mother's breast." Breast-feeding is one of the most natural, nurturing things that a woman can do for herself and her baby. Yet we live in a culture in which it's perfectly acceptable to walk down the beach in a string bikini but it is not acceptable to breast-feed an infant in a public place. That is seen as "obscene." Mothers who nurse toddlers are judged as being somehow "unnatural," fostering unnecessary dependence of the child, though it's been shown that people who feel the most secure in later life are those who had a very healthy physical and emotional bond with their mother in childhood. Children who feel most secure in their childhoods often are willing to take the most risks later in life. Only in a patriarchy would we get the idea that it "spoils" children to pick them up when they cry and to comfort them when they need it. (An aside: Why should adults get to sleep with someone, while children have to sleep alone?)

Our culture's priorities are completely reversed from what they should be, especially at a time when it has become so hard for mothers to nurture their children adequately and still make a living. I changed my priorities after my own personal wounding with the breast abscess. On the third day after Kate's birth, I noticed that my milk didn't seem to be coming out of my right nipple. Then the full impact of the damage I had done to myself two years earlier hit me fully. I wanted to sob. I remember sitting on my bed, looking down at my beautiful new baby girl, and thinking, "Here you are, and I can't even feed you properly because I screwed up my body two years ago trying to prove I was a man." I *was* able to nurse but had to supplement whenever I was away from home long enough to miss a feeding. I couldn't maintain an adequate milk supply most of the time and had to supplement with formula.

I came face-to-face with the fact that I had done irrevocable damage to myself. I'd been taught it was "normal" to feel the "baby blues" on about the third day after a baby was born, but my own depression was exacerbated by the knowledge that I wouldn't be able to nurse Kate completely normally. In fact, on her second day of life I had to supplement her diet with formula. I knew that her stools would immediately start to smell bad. Breast-fed stools smell like buttermilk because of the bacterial balance. Changing a diaper is a completely different experience with a breast-fed baby. But once you add other food sources, the bacteria change and the smell becomes putrid!

Even though the medical community has again begun to endorse breast-feeding, the culture often keeps women from breast-feeding with the declaration that nursing will "ruin" their breasts. Some women who've nursed a couple of children do notice that their breasts don't look the same. For a while, they can be quite flaccid and can take several years after pregnancy and nursing to regain their shape. This does usually reverse over time, but that flat appearance, even when it is only temporary, is not what our culture deems attractive. This was illustrated to me once when a friend who had nursed several children told me the following story. She was undressing one night when her four-year-old son walked in. He looked at her chest, then looked up at her and said, "Mom, what happened to your breasts? They died!" Rapid weight loss caused by inadequate food intake while nursing or prolonged nursing without adequate food intake can deplete the fat stores in the breasts and exacerbate this effect. Rapid weight loss also decreases milk supply.

The experience of producing milk, nursing a baby, and feeling the milk "let down" in response to the baby's cries, or even in response to their own thoughts about the baby, is an experience that connects women everywhere. Even years later, I can still feel that tingling sensation in my breasts occasionally. The midwife who delivered Kate used to tell me that she felt her own "let-down" reflex many times when she heard a baby cry or was aware of a child in need— even after her kids were in college. I like this body memory, knowing that even though I'll never nurse a child again, my body still knows what it is to be connected in that way.

When we trust the makers of baby formula more than we do our own ability to nourish our babies, we lose a chance to claim an aspect of our power as women. Thinking that baby formula is as good as breast milk is believing that thirty years of technology is superior to 3 million years of nature's evolution. Countless women have regained trust in their bodies through nursing their children, even if they weren't sure at first that they could do it. It is an act of female power.

Newborns who are treated gently are very beautiful. I've seen in their eyes very wise old souls in tiny bodies fresh from God. I heard the following true story at my office. After one couple had their second son, their four-year-old kept wanting time alone with the baby. They were a bit reluctant, feeling that sibling rivalry might be a factor. But the four-year-old kept insisting. Finally, they let him have some time alone with the baby. Listening quietly at the door, they heard him ask the baby the following, "Please tell me what God is like. I'm starting to forget."

Mothering in the Addictive System:
The Hardest Job in the World

The only thing that seems eternal and natural in motherhood is
ambivalence.

—Jane Lazare

Some women say that the most fulfilling time of their mothering
was when their babies were small. Others find it exhausting. For me,
having young children was—bar none—the most taxing part of my
life, a time that I wouldn't care to repeat again unless I had two
beloved nannies, sisters, or friends living with me full-time to help
with child care. (I might feel differently about this, had my circumstances been different.)

The author Lynn Andrews once wrote that there are two kinds of
mothers: Earth Mothers and Creative Rainbow Mothers. Earth
Mothers nurture their children and feed them—and they thrive on
this. Our society rewards this kind of woman as the "good mother."

Creative Rainbow Mothers, on the other hand, inspire their
children without necessarily having meals on the table on time. I
know that beyond a doubt, I'm a Creative Rainbow Mother. I once
read the cookbook *Laurel's Kitchen* and fantasized about how wonderful it would be to bake bread daily and relish being what Laurel
calls "The Keeper of the Keys"—and to create that ever-important
nurturing home space. But this is not who I am—and to try to be
something I'm not would ultimately do my children and me a great
disservice. I love to be alone. I love to read. I love quiet and music
and writing. My soul is fed by long hours of unbroken creative time.
Young children require a much different type of energy—a type of
energy I don't have in abundance.

When my children were little, I became aware of how difficult it
is for women to do *anything* for themselves with little children
around. Children get and keep our attention through any means
possible. They are phenomenal little energy suckers. (I don't blame
them for this—it's normal. They're developing healthy egos when
they are young. Our culture, however, expects *mothers* alone to
meet all their children's attention needs.)

Roughly one-third of all children in this country—19 million—

live apart from their fathers. "Among the children of divorce," writes Ellen Goodman, "half have never visited their father's home. In a typical year, 40% of them don't see their father. One out of five haven't seen their father in five years.... It is no wonder that the search for a man missing in the action of parenthood is such a recurrent theme in our culture and conversation these days."[10]

Sometimes, a woman with young children needs free time, space, and sleep. But for many, there's no one to take over the burden of raising a child. I once said to Anne Wilson Schaef that I thought the optimal adult-child ratio was three adults to one child. "I think your workaholism is showing," she replied. Then she went on to tell me about an aboriginal culture of Australia where she had recently visited with the tribal elders. In aboriginal societies, all of the mother's sisters—the child's aunts—are considered the child's mothers. All the father's brothers—the uncles—are considered the fathers. If you ask an aboriginal child who her mother is, she will point to not only her biological mother but to all her aunts as well. Same with the father. If her biological mother feels the need to go "walkabout"—a spiritual initiation—she knows that the child always has a place in the tribe and is not dependent solely on her, as she so often is in our patriarchal tribe.

Can you even begin to imagine what life would be like for women if they didn't have the crushing responsibility to provide most of their children's emotional and physical nurturing? What would it be like if we *knew* that our society would care for our child if we had to work late at the office one night? What if our "family" life were not separate from our "work" life? What would it be like if a woman could still pursue art, music, computers, or whatever she wished, even if she had just had a baby? What if we lived in a society in which a woman didn't have to choose *between* her needs, those of her job, and those of her family? Dream on that for a while.

No one, male or female, should have to be a prisoner in their own home caring for young children for hours each day without meeting their own adult needs for rest, conversation, time alone, and creative pursuits. I remember that the best time I ever had with my children when they were little (three months and two years) was when I went to visit my mother while my sister and her children were visiting. My sister was also nursing a baby at the time, so when I wanted to go out for a while, she simply nursed Kate for me as women have been doing for centuries. (Kate looked up at her, wide-eyed, the first time, as if to say, "Who is this?" Then she settled right down to her meal.) Our children played together happily, and I was able to enjoy the company of adults *at the same time* that I was enjoying my children. This was my only experience of what a loving tribe must have felt like.

One widely held misperception about raising children has always upset me. That is the myth that prepubescent and pubescent boys are *inherently* easier to raise than girls, and even many feminists subscribe to this belief. I'm told by many people, "You just wait—you'll see how difficult girls are when they get to be eleven or so." Well, I've had an eleven-year-old girl by now. (She's now thirteen.) I supported her in every way that I could to be strong, even opinion-ated if necessary, and to be powerful. I didn't want her to "dumbify" herself when she became a teenager. She was *not* difficult, and she is not difficult now. (In fact, my thirteen-year-old nephew was much moodier on a regular basis.) That boys are easier to raise than girls might well be the experience of many. But this difference is cultural, a consequence of the differences between the way boys and girls are treated and reared. In her latest book, *Fire with Fire* (Random House, 1993), Naomi Wolf makes a strong case for the fact that all girls are born with a strong will to power that gets turned inward by what she calls "the dragons of niceness." This innate desire to excel and win, when thwarted, gets turned against a young girl.

It makes sense to me that girls would get moody around the age of twelve or so. They can see what's coming. If girls are socialized to be passive and self-sacrificing, their powerful spirits don't like it! (If someone was actively trying to do that to me, I'd be *very* tough to live with.) Instead of attributing this moodiness to the inherent hormonal inferiority of the female, we should be encouraging girls to speak their minds, not to turn their gifts and talents inward. If a teenage girl is taken seriously and encouraged to follow her dreams, she will be no harder to raise than a boy. Young women need to be cherished, honored, encouraged, and praised for their gifts. Other-wise, the world won't benefit from these gifts, and the cycle of oppression will continue.

Each of us mothers must also learn to mother ourselves, or else we can't possibly be good mothers to our children. Self-sacrifice is not a healthy path to motherhood, even though we've been taught to do this for years and have often witnessed the martyrdom of our own mothers. Mothering ourselves takes a great deal of courage, and I encourage you to try it for your health's sake.

The following meditation on mothering well was sent to me by Nancy McBrine Sheehan.[11]

Mothering Myself
In a society preoccupied with how best to raise a child
I'm finding a need to mesh what's best for my children with what's
*   necessary for a well balanced mother.*
I'm recognizing that ceaseless giving translates into giving yourself
*   away.*
And, when you give yourself away, you're not a healthy mother and
*   you're not a healthy self.*

So, now I'm learning to be a woman first and a mother second.
I'm learning to just experience my own emotions
Without robbing my children of their individual dignity by feeling
*   their emotions too.*
I'm learning that a healthy child will have his own set of emotions
*   and characteristics that are his alone.*
And, very different from mine.
I'm learning the importance of honest exchanges of feelings because
*   pretenses don't fool children,*
They know their mother better than she knows herself.

I'm learning that no one overcomes her past unless she confronts it.
Otherwise, her children will absorb exactly what she's attempting to
*   overcome.*
I'm learning that words of wisdom fall on deaf ears if my actions
*   contradict my deeds.*
Children tend to be better impersonators than listeners.
I'm learning that life is meant to be filled with as much sadness and
*   pain as happiness and pleasure.*
And allowing ourselves to feel everything life has to offer is an
*   indicator of fulfillment.*
I'm learning that fulfillment can't be attained through giving myself
*   away*
But, through giving to myself and sharing with others,

I'm learning that the best way to teach my children to live a fulfilling
  life is not by sacrificing my life.
It's through living a fulfilling life myself.
I'm trying to teach my children that I have a lot to learn
Because I'm learning that letting go of them
Is the best way of holding on.

FOURTEEN

Menopause

Like an electrical charge, menstruation and the ebb and flow of
energy is an "alternating current." During menopause, the flow of
energy becomes intensified and steady, like a "direct current." We
are charged with energy to the degree we have opened ourselves to
the wisdom of the Crone.[1]

—Farida Shaw

*M*enopause refers to the cessation of menses. The years surrounding menopause constitute an entire stage of a woman's
life known as the *climacteric*. Many women know the menopause
by the name "change of life." Whatever we call it, no other stage of a
woman's life has as much potential for understanding and tapping
into woman's power as this one—if, that is, a woman is able to
negotiate her way through the general cultural negativity surrounding menopause.

The negativity associated with menopause is currently being
changed as the women of my generation, the baby boomers, are
now entering menopause. Since we baby boomers are approximately five times more numerous than preceding generations, the
climacteric experience will never be the same when we are finished
with it. More books on this subject are now being written by
leading feminists such as Germaine Greer and by doctors and researchers than on any other in the women's health field. Though the
advice about menopause ranges from exalting hormone replace-

ment as a panacea to promoting natural menopause, the important point is that the silence surrounding this process is now being broken by many different voices. The medical profession stands poised to help women through this life stage, and there are even Menopausal Medical Centers springing up all over the United States! Every woman, though barraged with conflicting advice, must listen carefully to her individual inner guidance to hear her personal truth.

Menopause marks the beginning of the second half of life. A woman is apt to live thirty-five or more years following her menopause. The reproductive years, those years when our society thinks women count, only last about thirty years, maximum. Though men may go through a midlife change, with physical and even hormonal consequences, they maintain their reproductive ability until death. We women have to learn entirely new ways of thinking about who we are when childbearing is no longer part of our body's potential.

In her book *Reclaiming the Menstrual Matrix*, Tamara Slayton writes, "The natural expression of personal power and wisdom available to women during [menopause] is thwarted and frustrated in our culture. This surge of energy is subsequently turned inward on oneself and can result in many unpleasant symptoms such as hot flashes, depression, mood swings, and a general feeling of being lost and unable to find a new and vital identity. Lack of support during this time and a tendency toward nutritional depletion in the American diet generates a negative and self-destructive experience of menopause. When women confront the culture's misinformation and address the nutritional needs, unique to females, they have, during menopause, an opportunity to discover a deeper and freer experience of self."[2]

The wisdom years, the years after menopause, when all of a woman's life experience comes together, can be used for a purpose that suits her and at the same time serves others. In Celtic cultures, the young maiden was seen as the flower; the mother, the fruit; the elder woman, the seed. The seed is the part that contains the knowledge and potential of all the other parts within it. The role of the postmenopausal woman is to go forth and reseed the community with her concentrated kernel of truth and wisdom. In some native cultures, menopausal women were felt to retain their wise blood, rather than shed it cyclically, and were therefore considered more powerful than menstruating women. A woman could not be a shaman until she was past menopause in these cultures. "Menopause," observes Slayton, "when understood and supported, provides the next level of initiation into personal power for women. As part of the menstrual taboo which still lives in our culture, the voice of the menopausal woman is feared and denied. She has been made invisible or encouraged to remain forever young through hormone replacement therapy or other medical intervention. This cultural alienation from a vital rite of passage leaves older women feeling useless, isolated, and impotent."

In native cultures menopausal women "provided a voice of responsibility towards all children, both human and *nonhuman*, to the Earth and to the Laws of Good Relationship," Slayton notes. "These older women contained great power and scrutinized all tribal decisions. They were unafraid to say a strong no to anything that did not serve life. They also initiated and educated the younger women into this knowledge and responsibility."[3]

Once a woman understands that the true meaning of menopause has been, like many of the other processes of a woman's body, reversed and degraded, she will be able to make her way through the rest of her life fortified with purpose and insight.

Our Cultural Inheritance

The conventional medical mindset is that menopause is a deficiency disease, not a natural process. Just as women's bodies have become pathologized and medicalized by the patriarchal, addictive system, so too has every function unique to women, menopause included.

Dr. Jerilynn Prior, an endocrinologist and researcher, writes, "Our culture finds it easy to blame women's reproductive systems for disease. Linking the menopause change in reproductive capability with aging, making menopause a point in time rather than a process, and labeling it an estrogen deficiency disease are all reflections of nonscientific, prejudicial thinking by the medical profession."[4] Women's bodies in menopause are commonly described in terms of "production" or "failed production." Since menopausal women are no longer using their energy in childbearing, their systems are described in terms of functional failure or decline; breasts and genital organs gradually "atrophy," "wither," and become "senile."[5] Menopause, viewed through this lens, is the ultimate in "failed production"—a system that is "shut down."

For years the OB/GYN profession has been steeped in lectures and teaching on "managing the menopause." Now a new topic is appearing—"managing the perimenopause." Perimenopause refers to the years leading up to the last menstrual period. I cringe when I read this—yet another normal life stage that requires management and, its subtext, control. In our culture the only ages when females' endocrine processes escape potential "management" are the years *before* menarche and *after* the age of seventy! (These are the years in which girls and women are even more devalued in our culture; otherwise the culture would have figured out a way to manage them then, too.)

Fear of Aging: Symptom of an Ageist Culture

We live in an ageist culture, in which most people believe that it's natural for aging people to become depressed, fatigued, incontinent, forgetful, and senile. Estrogen companies and gynecologists plant in women seeds of fear that as soon as they go through menopause, their bodies will simply fall apart and waste away unless they are on medication, particularly hormones.

• An ad for Premarin (an estrogen made from pregnant mare's urine, hence the name) shows a lovely young woman wearing an exercise leotard. The caption reads, "Aerobics every week, calcium every day, bone loss every year." The implication of this ad is that without estrogen, this woman's bones will dissolve right out from underneath her, regardless of whether she exercises or eats well, unless she takes Premarin.

• An ad for Estratest, a combination of estrogen and testosterone that increases libido (discussed later in this chapter), shows an attractive middle-aged woman leaning back against an Ivy League–type distinguished gentleman in a sailboat. Both are drinking orange juice (or mimosas). The caption reads, "I feel like a woman again." What was she before?

• A more recent Premarin ad shows an attractive middle-aged

woman with a huge grin on her face while a man kisses her neck. The caption under this one is, "You think it's good medicine. *She* thinks it's wonderful."

• On the cover of a magazine called *Menopause Medicine*, a woman stands by an open window with flimsy curtains blowing at her side; only her back is visible. She is looking out on a landscape covered by dead trees and parched dry earth. The caption underneath this illustration reads, "The Fate of the Untreated Menopause."

It doesn't take a degree in psychology to understand how the hormone companies influence the sensibilities of the average doctor. Nor does it take ten years of feminist activism to see how the hormone companies manipulate the stereotypes associated with aging and the deep cultural fears that we women have about them: Without hormones, the message runs, we'll lose our attractiveness to men, we'll dry up, we'll become brittle, like parched, cracked earth, devoid of moisture and nourishment. The values and beliefs of our culture are that women should retain their "fruitfulness" at all costs, and that becoming seeds of wisdom is somehow less than "feminine."

The experience of aging as we know it is largely determined by beliefs that need updating. Though many people *do* decline with age in this culture, this decline is not a natural consequence of aging—it is a natural consequence of our collective beliefs about aging. My mother, who is sixty-eight and has never been on hormones, recently completed hiking the Appalachian Trail, and she skied around the base of Mount McKinley last year. She told me that as soon as she had turned sixty, her mailbox was suddenly full of ads for hearing aids, diapers for incontinence, and various aids for failing vision, none of which she had any need for. She resents the constant barrage of negative messages about aging. No wonder so many women are willing to pay any price to prevent it. Who would want to get old in a culture that holds these beliefs!

Another reason why so many women are afraid of menopause is because of a misunderstanding of the Crone, or Wise Woman archetype. Caroline Myss points out that in fairy tales, and in our collective unconscious, the Crone is often depicted as an old woman living alone in the woods. She is often associated with witches or eccentric behavior.

Caroline notes that this image of a woman alone in the woods symbolically represents a woman who has freed herself from her original tribal programming. She no longer bases her activities, thoughts, and self-image on the approval of her family. She is free to come and go as she pleases and on her own terms. She need not be alone, but her relationships are more likely to be partnerships and mutually satisfying.

Caroline suggests that we very much need a new updated "Aquarian Crone" archetype at this time.

Dr. Deepak Chopra, an endocrinologist, best-selling author, and internationally recognized authority on how consciousness affects our bodies, has reported on an experiment conducted among the Tara Humara Indians in Mexico, a group known for their running ability. Routinely, certain members of the tribe ran the equivalent of a marathon or more every day, and had regular races between groups. The most intriguing aspect of their culture, however, was that they *believed* that the best runners were those in their sixties. A team of researchers showed that the best lung capacity, cardiovascular fitness, and endurance were *indeed* found in the runners in their sixties! Dr. Chopra points out that for this belief to translate into physical reality, the entire tribe has to believe it.

In our ageist culture, many women, instead of believing in their capacity to remain strong, attractive, and vital throughout their lives, instead come to expect their bodies and minds to deteriorate with age. Thus we as a society collectively create a pattern of thoughts, behaviors, and fears that makes it that much easier to manifest the worst physical reality. We can't reverse our collective cultural negativity about menopause and aging overnight. What we *can* do is consider ourselves pioneers in a new frontier, one in which menopause and aging will be redefined. This is clearly possible. For instance, my mother had a health reading from medical intuitive Caroline Myss last year. Though my mother is sixty-eight years old, her body read "energetically" as though she were in her thirties. The more women like my mother ignore what is supposed to happen when we age, the better the chances are that *all* of us will stay healthy.

Many women here in New England have grandmothers in their eighties and nineties who are strong, healthy, and living independently. These women are the best "proof" possible for trusting the body after menopause.

Kinds of Menopause

It is clear that some women really do suffer during the menopausal years. Part of their suffering is due to chronic depletion of their energy during the perimenopausal years.

During the menopause, the ovaries make fewer hormones, including androgens. Since menopausal women's ovaries produce less androgen, it has been suggested that this is why libido levels may decrease in some (not all) menopausal women (see Figure 13). But androgenic hormones are also made by the adrenal gland, the skin, muscle, brain, pineal gland, hair follicles, and body fat. These hormones are also associated with sexual response and libido as well as a sense of well-being. During menopause, these other organs normally take over for the ovaries. Chronic stress over a long period of time leads to adrenal depletion and is a possible setup for menopausal problems. The stronger a woman's adrenals and the better her general nutrition, the easier the transition into menopause. At the time of menopause there is a twofold *increase* in production of androgenic hormones from other sources. What that means is that even though ovarian production is falling, the other androgen-producing sites in the body are taking over. Since androgens can themselves act as weak estrogens, it is clear that the body of the menopausal woman is equipped to deal with the hormonal changes that the ovary is going through. Many women, however, approach menopause in a state of nutritional and emotional depletion and may therefore require hormonal, nutritional, or other support.

The pituitary gland in the brain makes a hormone called luteinizing hormone (LH), which communicates with the ovaries and tells them to increase androgen production. The amount of androgen produced from the other organs in the body depends upon how many building blocks for these molecules are available in those organs and on the nutritional status of the woman.

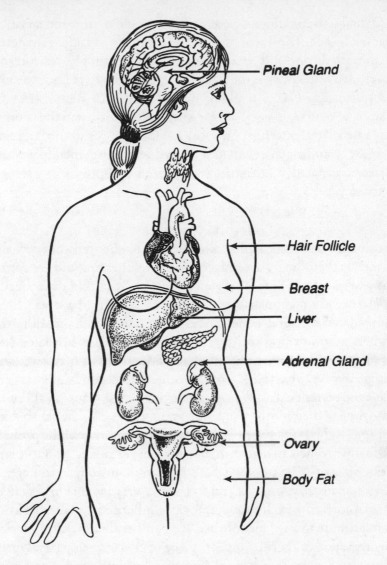

Pineal Gland

Hair Follicle

Breast

Liver

Adrenal Gland

Ovary

Body Fat

FIGURE 13: HORMONE-PRODUCING BODY SITES

Ovarian estrogen and progesterone levels decrease after menopause. Other body sites, however, are capable of making these same hormones, depending upon a woman's lifestyle and diet. The female body, therefore, has the capacity to make healthy adjustments in hormonal balance after menopause.

Overall, the metabolism of androgens does not appear to be affected by age. The liver remains the major site of androgen metabolism both during and after menopause. Interestingly, testosterone secretion by the ovary is the *same* in women who have gone through natural menopause as it is in younger women.[6] Removal of the ovaries, of course, is associated with a dramatic drop in the production rate of testosterone. Surgical menopause results in a greater decrease in androgen production than does natural menopause and is also associated with more pronounced symptoms of estrogen deficiency.[7]

Natural Menopause

Caroline Myss suggests that all of us have inherited the view that women in their forties are finished with childbearing and are getting ready to go into decline. This view inevitably results in the collective experience of menopause at about the age of fifty-two. If we changed our cultural beliefs, Myss maintains, it is possible that women wouldn't stop their periods until their sixties or later.

Currently, the average age of menopause is about fifty-two, with a range of forty-five to fifty-five. Women can go through it as early as age thirty-nine. Most women go through menopause at about the same time as their mothers did, unless they have consciously broken their genetic and unconscious bonds to their mothers. The problem for many women is that their mothers never talked about menopause, so many don't know what their family history in this area is. As with menstruation, many of us have at least two or three generations of foremothers from whom we've inherited a shame-based or silent attitude toward menopause. Remember that the climacteric is a process, not an "event." It takes place over six to ten years. During this process, periods may stop for several months and then return. Periods may get quite heavy or very light. Some women stop their periods for a year, I've seen, only to have them restart a year later and continue every twenty-eight days for a full two years more! Periods tend to change in character during each decade of a woman's life, though this hasn't been well-studied to my knowledge. In my experience as a clinician, women undergo a set of period changes in their twenties, other changes in their thirties, and still another set in their forties. Many women skip a period in their forties or have some other change, such as a different flow. This is *not* menopause—but there is a change in ovulation associated with this change in the menstrual cycle. Many women begin skipping ovulations in their mid to late forties. Many women who come to see me in their late thirties and forties with a skipped period or change in their period are worried that they are starting menopause. Usually, they are at least five years away from the actual last period, but I tell them to think of their forties as a decade of time during which their ovaries are gradually changing from one way of functioning to another.

Menopause is often heralded by the onset of a change in menstrual flow or skipped menstrual periods. Some women simply stop having periods and have no symptoms whatsoever. Others experience hot flashes, vaginal dryness, decreased libido, and "fuzzy thinking." A blood test can be taken to measure the levels of the pituitary gonadotropins' follicle-stimulating hormone (FSH) and luteinizing hormone (LH). These hormones are produced by the pituitary gland to stimulate the ovary to produce eggs. During the years of menstruation, FSH and LH peak at mid-cycle each month at ovulation, which is accompanied by the emotional and physiological changes discussed in Chapter 8. During the climacteric the pituitary gland and the ovaries undergo a gradual change, during which ovulations decrease and the FSH and LH levels gradually increase. This is because when the ovary is no longer producing eggs, the pituitary gland continues to send out LH and FSH because it is not getting the usual hormonal messages from the developing egg to tell it to slow down production. The usual ovarian signal telling the pituitary gland to decrease production of FSH and LH is no longer present. So the pituitary gland *continues* to send high levels of FSH and LH into the bloodstream for reasons that have not been well studied. A blood test can be taken to determine their levels. When these hormones reach a certain level in the blood, they are said to be in the "menopausal" range. In this menopausal range, we assume that the ovary is no longer responding to FSH and LH from the pituitary gland.

I was taught that once a woman's FSH and LH are in the menopausal range, she was indeed menopausal and would stay that way, but I have found that this is not always the case. One forty-year-old

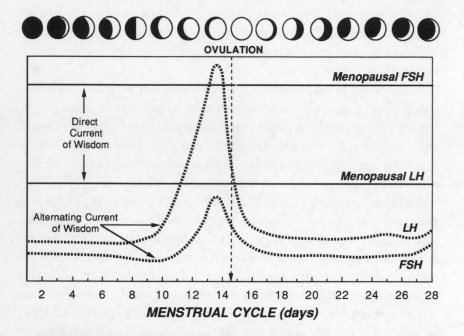

FIGURE 14: CURRENTS OF WISDOM

FSH and LH stimulate ovulation and are released cyclically each month up until the years surrounding menopause. They then undergo a change during which ovulations gradually cease and neurotransmitter levels (FSH and LH) gradually increase. I believe that these high levels have to do with moving from "AC" current to "DC" current. The wisdom that is now available to us most clearly during only certain parts of the menstrual cycle is now potentially available all the time.

woman, for example, who had no periods for six months and had menopausal levels of FSH and LH later went back to having normal periods. A recheck of her hormone levels showed that they went back to premenopausal levels. When I order a test of FSH and LH hormonal levels in a woman who is skipping periods or has stopped her periods for a few months, I tell her that getting menopausal results does not necessarily mean she's completely finished with her periods and is definitively menopausal! A woman can theoretically become pregnant up until one year *after* her last menopausal period. For that reason, I recommend that she continue to use some form of contraception, if applicable, until a year has gone by since the last period.

Premature Menopause

A small percentage of women experience "premature menopause" in their thirties or early forties. If the age of forty is the cutoff, naturally occurring premature menopause occurs in about one woman in a hundred.[8] Premature menopause is, in some cases, an autoimmune disorder.[9] Women who undergo it tend to make antibodies against their ovaries, known as antiovarian antibodies. When the body makes antibodies against itself, you may recall, the immune system may be getting unconscious messages. When a woman's diet has been poor for years or she has been under a great deal of stress, the result may be increases in allergies and systemic yeast problems, which in my practice are sometimes associated with autoimmune disorders. One woman whom I saw with this condition had developed it at the age of thirty-nine after learning that her husband was having an affair.

When a woman loses the ovarian supply of estrogen *too* early in life, nerve cells in a specific memory center in the brain may lose function. There is a body of scientific literature that suggests that women who have a *premature* menopause are more susceptible to developing dementia (a global impairment of cognitive functioning and memory). This is entirely different from the "fuzzy thinking" many women describe during normal menopause. Another woman I know went into early menopause at age forty-three after using the drug Clomid to induce ovulation in an attempt to conceive a child. It is possible that she already had antiovarian antibodies in her bloodstream at the time she started to use Clomid and that the Clomid did not "cause" her premature menopause. It is also possible that she would have gone into menopause at around forty-three in any case.

Artificial Menopause

Hysterectomy with ovarian removal (or bilateral salpingo-oophorectomy, removal of both tubes and ovaries) makes a woman *instantly* menopausal if the surgery is done before her natural menopause. This process is known as surgical menopause and is quite different from the normal climacteric. The symptoms can be severe and debilitating without proper readjustment of hormonal levels.

Menopause may come on more quickly even if a woman has a hysterectomy in which her ovaries haven't been removed.[10] Sometimes, the ovaries will decrease production of hormones for a time following hysterectomy and will later increase production. (Some of my patients have hot flashes after hysterectomy even when they still have their ovaries. These often go away later, presumably after the ovaries have had a chance to recover from the shock of surgery.) There is also some evidence that tubal ligation may bring on menopause or some type of dysfunctional uterine bleeding earlier than normal.

Women who have had chemotherapy are also apt to undergo premature menopause,[11] as are those who have had radiation to the pelvis. It is estimated that 7 to 8 percent of women under the age of forty enter menopause as a result of medical intervention. The women who undergo "natural" premature menopause combined with those who undergo "artificial" menopause adds up to about one woman in twelve facing menopause before the age of forty.[12]

Symptoms of Menopause

Before I get into a discussion of menopausal "symptoms" and their "relief," I want to stress once again that menopause is a normal female process that is not a problem for the majority of women. Unfortunately, the increased media and medical attention to this phase of life, have now led many otherwise normal women to *expect* and *worry about* potential problems. So when a woman asks me, "What can I expect to experience during menopause?" I usually have to spend some time allaying fears that she already has acquired by the time I see her. I can't really say what her individual experience is likely to be except to tell her that it will depend upon her level of health at the time, combined with her unconscious beliefs about menopause.

That is, expectations of problems in menopause *lead* to problems. If a woman watched her mother, or sister, or grandmother, go through hell at this time of her life, chances are that at some deep level, she'll have a belief that menopause is hell! I do not question the fact that many women *do* suffer during the menopausal years, any more than I would question the suffering of women with PMS whom I've treated. But if a woman can change how she thinks about her body and about menopause, and give menopause a new, more positive meaning, her innate healing powers will often be called forth and her symptoms alleviated.

Just as our addictive medical system conducts studies on disease and not on wellness, we have not studied women who sail right through menopause. We don't research those women who *don't* get fractures, depression, or thinned vaginal membranes. We focus on menopause as a problem, and this focus reinforces the problem by creating a self-fulfilling condition for women. Some cultures in which menopause is not considered a problem, however, have been studied. Anthropologist Ann Wright studied menopausal symptoms in traditional and acculturated Navaho women and discovered that traditional Navahos had few symptoms. Wright found that economic ranking and menopausal status were clearly related to women's experience of symptoms. Her study suggested that it is psychological stress rather than physical stress[13] that causes menopausal symptoms. All stress, whether it is physical or psychological in origin, has real biochemical effects on the body.

From an evolutionary viewpoint, prehistoric menopause was most likely an entirely different experience for women from what it is now. For most of human history, women spent more than fifteen years in pregnancy and lactation and just under four years having monthly menstrual cycles. In times past a woman most likely finished nursing her last child and simply did not get another period because the high levels of prolactin and oxytocin associated with nursing shut down ovulations. Thus, moving from nursing to menopause would be a shorter hormonal "leap" than from ovulatory cycles to menopause, and their bodies may not produce hot flashes in response to wide hormonal swings. A study of !Kung women in Africa verifies that this is their most common pattern. In the !Kung culture women's status *increases* after menopause and there is no word for hot flash—even though the vast majority of women in *our* culture get them.[14] Is it possible, then, that the !Kung women don't get them? Or do they experience them but have a different meaning in that culture and therefore experience them entirely differently, as not a problem?

Hot Flashes

Hot flashes, also known as vasomotor flushes, are experienced by 80 to 90 percent of American women during the menopausal years. Hot flashes are characterized by a feeling of heat and sweating, usually involving the head and neck to a great degree. At night, a woman may throw off her blankets, soak the sheets with sweat, then feel cold a few minutes later and need even more blankets. Hot flashes are measurable phenomena. Skin surface temperature increases during a hot flash. Some women experience these for a few months; for some they last a few years; and for a rare group of women, they go on for a decade or more.

Hot flashes are thought to be probably related to norepinephrine metabolism in the brain, related to estrogen deprivation. Norepinephrine is a neurotransmitter, one of those peptides that sends messages from our brains to our organs and immune system, and which the system sends to the brain. Because hot flashes involve the neuroendocrine system, unresolved stress tends to increase them. They can often be treated well with placebos, which underscores the fact that what's in your mind affects them via subtle neurotransmitter changes.

Note that *not* all hot flashes are related to decreases in estrogen. Hyperthyroidism can cause them, as can alcohol intake and out-of-control diabetes. I remember having hot flashes during my pregnancies, and I sometimes have them premenstrually. Many women report similar patterns.

Caroline Myss says that hot flashes are related to blocked kundalini energy and unused sexual juice. They are a classic occurrence for nonorgasmic women for whom sexual pleasure has been limited. The kundalini energy begins to rise naturally around the age of forty, and it "activates" the chakras through which it passes. Any unfinished business residing in the lower chakras will make itself known during the menopausal years.

Some women have hot flashes so continually that they result in sleep deprivation, particularly in interruption of rapid eye movement (REM) sleep, the type of sleep associated with dreaming. This can result in depression.

Caroline Myss explains that depression is a classic first and second chakra energy dysfunction. Since the second chakra is the sexual area, blocked sexual pleasure or unused pleasure can result in hot flashes and depression. One is often linked to the other. Myss says that women who have not fulfilled or expressed their erotic needs on a regular basis are often the ones who have the most difficulty with menopausal symptoms—especially hot flashes. Many women hold the belief that their sexual attractiveness will be gone after menopause and that they will never have a chance for a fulfilling sexual life again. Women who hold this belief often experience menopause as the end or death of the possibility of sexual fulfillment that they may have longed for earlier in their lives.

An alternative way to think of hot flashes is simply as energy that is available to us. One of my patients noted that each time she got a hot flash, it was followed by a flash of insight that helped her in her work. Others have mentioned that they need much less sleep after menopause and are filled with new-found energy. In her book *Shakti Woman*, Vicki Noble notes that high body temperature kills cancer cells and also bacteria, a well-established fact. She feels that hot flashes may be nature's way of killing off latent cancer cells to make women healthier as they move into their wisdom years.[15] When we shut down the hot flash process, we may be interfering with a mechanism developed by the body with our health in mind.

Treatment

ESTROGEN REPLACEMENT. For women who are suffering from a combination of depression, sleep deprivation, and hot flashes, estrogen replacement can be very helpful, and I prescribe it regularly, particularly for women who prefer this type of therapy. At average blood levels of 150 ug/ml of estradiol, a type of estrogen, you get a 100 percent decrease in hot flashes, if they are the result of decreased estrogen levels. It usually takes two to four weeks before estrogen therapy reduces hot flashes, though it may happen as soon as two or three days.

NATURAL PROGESTERONE. Natural progesterone, as a skin cream (absorbed through the skin) or capsule (taken orally and prescribed by a physician), has been used by many women to alleviate menopausal symptoms of hot flashes and headache. Women who are on natural progesterone often find relief from various menopausal symptoms; doses are individualized. Natural progesterone is *not* the same thing as synthetic progestin, though some women have had relief of menopausal symptoms even on synthetic progestins. (See page 124.) Natural progesterone is a precursor molecule that can be converted in the body to androgens, which may be why many women report increased libido when using it.

NUTRITIONAL TREATMENT. Taking Vitamin E in the form of d alpha-tocopherol 400 IU two times per day has helped some women with hot flashes. Eliminating sugar, caffeine, and alcohol is helpful. As always, following a high-complex-carbohydrate, low-fat diet is preferable. Various herbal preparations such as Siberian ginseng, don quoi, fo ti, black cohosh, and wild yam have helped many women with hot flashes and other menopausal symptoms. Vitex Agnus Castii (chaste berry), which is available as a tincture in many health food stores, has helped many of my perimenopausal patients. The complexities of many Chinese herbal remedies for menopausal problems are beyond the scope of this book.

Susun Weed's *Menopausal Years, The Wise Woman's Way*, contains a wealth of information on herbal remedies for relief of menopausal symptoms.[16] Naturopathic physicians well-trained in botanical medicine are another excellent resource.

ENERGY MEDICINE. Since hot flashes are increased by stress, many women have found help through meditation and relaxation, and acupuncture has helped many as well. Homeopathic remedies are also very useful. I am not trained in homeopathy, but often refer my patients to those who are.

Vaginal Dryness, Irritation, and Thinning

Some menopausal women complain of vaginal dryness and thinning, which cause irritation. Vaginal tissue is made of many cell layers. When the vaginal mucosa is well-estrogenized it is called "cornified" epithelium. Cornified refers to cells that are tough and resilient. After menopause, some women literally lose the outer cornified layers of their vaginal tissue. Under the microscope, they have fewer cell layers, which can result in irritation and a dry feeling. These complaints are highly individual and subjective. Two different women's vaginas can look exactly the same to me, and one woman will complain of dryness and irritation and the other won't.

Thinning of the vaginal lining is associated with decreased estrogen levels after menopause. The vaginal mucosa has an outer "cornified" layer of cells, about six layers deep, that is very estrogensensitive, and often becomes thinned when estrogen levels have fallen significantly. In some women, this thinning and irritation is accompanied by an increase in the normally low pH of the vagina. At higher pH levels, bacterial vaginitis sometimes results. Even when vaginal tissues are clearly thinned on physical exam, not all women with thinned tissue will experience symptoms of thinning, which cause dryness, itching, and pain on intercourse. (The patriarchal name for thinning and associated symptoms is atrophic vaginitis.) Diagnosis of this thinning is made by physical exam, but treatment isn't necessary unless a woman is having symptoms.

Vaginal thinning at menopause is *not* inevitable. Many women past menopause—especially those who remain sexually active, with or without a partner—have vaginas that look the same as when they were thirty, even when they are not taking any estrogen! This is especially true in women who are heavier than average because body fat produces the estrogen hormone, estrone.

Urinary Frequency from Urethral Thinning

Urinary frequency is sometimes associated with thinning of the estrogen-sensitive tissue of the vaginal and urethral tissues. The urethra is a tubular structure running from the bladder to the urethral opening just below the clitoris. You can feel it just underneath the vaginal tissue at the top and just inside the vaginal opening. The outer third of the urethra is estrogen-sensitive. Urinary frequency from localized estrogen lack can be very easily alleviated by placing a small amount of estrogen cream directly on the part of the vaginal tissue that covers the outer third of the urethra. The cream is used according to the same regimen as listed below for vaginal symptoms.

Treatment

LUBRICANTS. For some, the use of a lubricant during intercourse is all that is necessary to counteract vaginal thinning. The following lubricants can be used at any time:

- Replens, an over-the-counter preparation that lowers the pH of the vagina and helps provide relief from itching by preventing overgrowth of bacteria
- K-Y or other over-the-counter jelly
- Cold-pressed castor oil
- Vitamin E oil or suppositories
- Sesame or other high-quality oil

These oils can be applied with the fingertips to the external vaginal entrance, where the symptoms of dryness or chafing are apt to be the most severe.

HERBS. Herbs such as dandelion leaf and oat straw have been used successfully to help restore vaginal lubrication. For a full discussion of North American herbs for menopause, I recommend Susun Weed, *Menopausal Years, The Wise Woman's Way*.[17] Many combinations of Chinese herbs can also be used for menopausal symptoms. Because Chinese diagnosis and treatment is completely different from Western symptomatic approaches, I refer women directly to those who are trained in the use of Chinese herbs.

VISUALIZATION. Some of my patients have used the power of their mind *and* their bodymind to reverse vaginal dryness and thinning. One fifty-year-old who had initially seen me for pain with intercourse because of postmenopausal vaginal thinning said recently, "I've finally decided to refuse to see menopause as a time of decay! The truth is, I've never felt better about myself in my life. My youngest child is just finishing high school and I'm finally free. When I finally decided to move forward with joy, my vaginal condition cleared up and I no longer need to take estrogen." She was right. Her entire vagina was completely normal, with no evidence of the inflammation and thinned tissues that I had seen a year before.

Another woman, recently divorced from a husband who had not been sexually available to her for years, was able to reverse her vaginal thinning and dryness by visualizing the area as healthy, pink, moist, and desirable. She was also working on reversing a lot of other problems in her life that had resulted from a sexually barren marriage.

ESTROGEN. Full replacement doses of estrogen (ERT) taken orally usually restore vaginal tissue that has become thinned or dry. ERT will also usually decrease urinary symptoms if these are present. For those women who would like to avoid systemic ERT, a small amount of estrogen cream applied vaginally is all that is needed periodically to keep the area well estrogenized and healthy. Interestingly, even in some women on full estrogen replacement by pill or patch, the vaginal area still becomes dry and sensitive and additional treatment with estrogen vaginal cream is necessary.

I prescribe frequent application of estrogen cream to thicken the vaginal tissue gradually. Once this is accomplished, a small amount applied once per week keeps the tissue in good shape. Systemic absorption at these low levels is negligible after the first three weeks. For the "buildup" phase, breast tenderness, bloating, and other symptoms associated with estrogen may be experienced. These will go away as the doses decrease. In women who have very severe thinning, the use of an estrogen cream may initially be accompanied by a burning sensation. This should go away after a few days. An occasional woman is allergic to the cream base, but this is rare. Vaginal circulation is aided by regular intercourse *or* use of self-love if no partner is desired or available.

Estrogen vaginal cream is available by prescription. Common brands are Estrace, Premarin. The regimen is:

- First week: one-third applicator-full (or smaller amount) two times per day for one week
- Second week: one-third applicator-full once per day for one week
- Third week: one-third applicator-full every other day for one week
- Fourth week: one-third applicator-full every three to seven days thereafter

Most of my patients use the cream only once per week after the initial buildup phase. Some use less than the one-third applicator, with very good results. For those whose only symptom is urinary frequency, a fingertip full of estrogen to the urethra twice a week or so is often all that is necessary for total symptom relief.

Estriol vaginal cream (0.5 mg/gram) can also be used.[18] Usual dosage is one gram (¼ tsp) once daily for one week, then three times weekly thereafter. (See below for further discussion of estriol.)

Osteoporosis

Postmenopausal osteoporosis is the progressive loss of bone mass and bone strength associated with menopause caused by a variety of factors. It is one of the most common and disabling diseases affecting women in North America today. Studies have shown a 2 to 5 percent loss per year in women over a five-year period during the climacteric. After that, the loss levels out on its own. A woman with maximum peak bone mass achieved in young adulthood (peak bone mass means the optimal density of bone that is normally reached by a well-nourished female shortly after puberty) and maintained until menopause is likely to complete this phase of accelerated bone mass with little fracture risk. But if bone mass is low going into menopause or if it becomes low during this time, bone density may have already reached the fracture threshold (which is approximately 30 percent below the average level for a normal twenty-year-old.)[19]

Though most women start to think of bone loss *only* at menopause, it often begins years before. In fact, up to 50 percent of the bone that women lose over their lifespan is lost before menopause even begins. Statistics show that 6 to 18 percent of women between twenty-five and thirty-four years of age have abnormally low bone density.[20] Hip-fracture rates for white women in the United States begin to rise abruptly between the ages of forty and forty-four—much earlier than menopause begins.[21] Since estrogen levels don't fall until *after* menopause, it is obvious that the cause of bone loss is a lot more complex than loss of estrogen only. It is characteristic of our society, however, that it boils this complex problem down to a matter of taking estrogen or not.

Women over seventy-five constitute about 18 percent of the population but represent 58 percent of those who are hospitalized for osteoporotic problems. The lifetime risk of a hip fracture is 15 percent in white women.[22] Osteoporosis is most common in Caucasian women, less common in Asians, and least common in black women. Though some men suffer from the condition, it's much more rare.[23] Statistics show that of all women who fracture a hip from osteoporosis, 50 percent will never walk on their own again and another 25 percent will be dead in one year.[24] The reasons for this are medical complications from hip repair, such as blood clots to the lungs, pneumonia, and overall failure to thrive for reasons that aren't always clear. Many of these women simply stop eating and their will to live declines.

Risk Factors for Osteoporosis

- Lack of exercise or physical inactivity
- High-fat, high-protein diet[25]
- Smoking
- Excess alcohol intake: Alcohol has adverse effects on bone metabolism and it increases the likelihood of falling and subsequent fractures.[26]
- Malabsorption of nutrients as a result of antibiotic use
- Estrogen deficiency
- Progesterone deficiency
- Calcium, magnesium, and other mineral deficiencies from our modern diet of processed foods
- Genetic predisposition
- Nulliparas: Women who've never had a child are also at increased risk. Contrary to popular opinion, having only two or three children does not increase a woman's chances for osteoporosis by depleting her. During pregnancy the body actually increases its ability to absorb minerals from the diet even better than during the prepregnancy state.[27] One study even showed that in some women bone mass increased during pregnancy compared with prepregnancy levels.[28]

Menstrual Disturbance: A Setup for Osteoporosis

Although estrogen deficiency in menopause is an important factor in the development of bone loss and osteoporosis, menstrual cycle irregularities and other hormonal deficiencies are also related to osteoporosis.

Irregular menstrual cycles (ovulatory disturbances) and subsequent progesterone deficiency are very common. Studies have shown that spinal bone loss occurs in women athletes who have irregular menstrual cycles but normal estrogen levels.[29] Finally, stress, nutritional deficiencies, lack of exposure to natural light, as well as other factors in modern life contribute to ovulatory disturbance and bone loss. Clearly modern women are at risk for ovulation disturbance and subsequent risk of osteoporosis.

Although it is frequently overlooked, the role of progesterone in bone metabolism has been well-documented. Estrogen works to prevent bone loss, whereas progesterone stimulates bone formation. Even though scientists have focused mainly on estrogen alone, both hormones are involved in normal bone formation.[30] Moreover, synthetic progestin taken alone, such as Provera, can increase bone density even without estrogen.[31] Osteoporosis has been reversed in patients as much as sixteen years past menopause using natural progesterone (a cream from wild yams) in combination with other dietary factors and exercise. Bone density increased significantly, and the incidence of fracture decreased considerably.[32]

Screening for Bone Density

A quick and easy screening method for osteoporosis is the following. For women over the age of thirty-five, arm span and height should be about equal, give or take an inch or so. Measure your arm span with your arms outstretched, from the tip of one third finger to the tip of the other. Then measure your height. Note: Decreased height doesn't always mean bone loss. Years of being "weighted down" by life's burdens, poor posture, and lack of stretching can decrease height. Some height loss results from shrinking the spaces between vertebral discs, even when bone density is good. My patients who do yoga regularly seem to show the least height loss. I believe that this is because yoga tends to keep the disc spaces between the vertebrae more supple and open.

Another method is dual-energy bone densitometry, a low-dose X-ray technique. This is the best test to determine bone density and monitor it thereafter.[33] I recommend this for those women who need more data before deciding on hormone therapy, who need motivation to change their diets and start exercising, and who have a family history of osteoporosis. It's felt that bone densitometry, though not a perfect test, is as predictive of fracture risk as cholesterol is for determining risk of heart attack. When a woman gets a low reading, I suggest she adopt a regimen such as the one below, or use ERT, depending upon her situation, and then repeat the test in a year.

Although the test itself has limitations, it can be very reassuring for many women. When I send a fifty-five-year-old with a family history of osteoporosis for a bone density test, for example, and the test comes back with a reading that her bones are as dense as those of a healthy twenty-nine-year-old or denser than 99 percent of all women, both of us are pleased and she doesn't worry so much about osteoporosis.

Bone-Health Program[34]

Bone is dynamic living tissue, and therefore osteoporosis—at least in part—can be reversed. For women who are entering or past menopause and don't necessarily want to use estrogen, I suggest that they try a program that includes natural progesterone, dietary changes, and exercise. I consider natural progesterone use for those who are not ovulating regularly long before menopause since they are at a higher risk of having bone loss. There are no side effects of the bone-health program I use. Every woman who chooses to avoid estrogen replacement in my practice understands that estrogen replacement is the only FDA-approved method to decrease osteoporosis risk, despite the efficacy of the other modalities I suggest. Therefore, she is taking responsibility for using an alternative that is less extensively studied.

A HIGH-COMPLEX-CARBOHYDRATE, LOW-FAT DIET, RELATIVELY LOW IN PROTEIN. Limit servings of red meat to lean cuts no more than three times per week. (Red meat is very high in phosphorus, as is soda. High phosphorus intake extracts calcium from bones to keep calcium/phosphorus levels in balance.) Concentrate on eating dark green leafy vegetables such as kale and collards.

PROGESTERONE CREAM. Apply one-third to one-half 2 oz. jar per month. Apply one-quarter to one-half teaspoon to the face, neck, inner arms, abdomen, inner thighs, or soles of feet daily for thirty days, then at least two weeks out of the month thereafter. Alternate sites where the skin is softest. The reason for this is that the progesterone is absorbed into the fat layer underneath the skin. If you use the same site all the time, the fat will become saturated in that area, and you won't get optimal absorption. Note also that if the amount of cream on the skin is absorbed quickly, this empirically suggests that the body may require more. (Progesterone cream comes in several different brands and strengths. Dosage depends upon which product is used.)

STOP SMOKING. Smokers, along with those who take in two or more alcoholic drinks daily, are at highest risk for osteoporosis. Smoking literally poisons the ovaries and decreases production of all the ovarian hormones chronically.

NO COLA OR ROOT BEER DRINKS. These are too high in phosphate, which directly interferes with calcium absorption.

WEIGHT BEARING EXERCISE. Do walking, biking, weight training, NordicTrack—anything that puts weight on the bones, twenty minutes five days per week, or thirty minutes three times per week.

VITAMIN C. Take 2000 mg. per day. Vitamin C is involved in collagen synthesis and repair. The work of Dr. Linus Pauling suggests that vitamin C intake should be relatively higher than we've been taught. An orange provides only 60 mg. per day. Dr. Pauling's evidence is quite convincing that vitamin C is beneficial and has no side effects at levels around two grams per day.

MAGNESIUM. Take 300–800 mg. per day, depending upon the quality of your diet. Magnesium is a constituent of bone and is essential for several biochemical reactions that are essential for bone-building. The standard American diet is low in magnesium. A diet low in magnesium and relatively high in calcium can actually contribute to osteoporosis. Though blood levels of magnesium are often normal, this is misleading. A more accurate test is red blood cell magnesium, which is often low in cases of depression and fatigue. Overconsumption of processed food is usually the culprit in magnesium deficiency. It is found in organically grown vegetables, whole grains, sea vegetables, and meats such as turkey.

CALCIUM. The usual dose recommended is 1000–1500 mg. per day. This advice is based on calcium requirements for those who are on high-protein diets. The World Health Organization recommendation for calcium is only 400 mg. per day for most of the world's population. This is because, when the diet is relatively low in protein, much less calcium is necessary. When the diet is relatively low in protein (about one and one-half ounces per day for a nonpregnant, nonlactating woman), then calcium needs are *easily* met from food alone. A cup of cooked collard greens, for instance, contains about 300–400 mg. of calcium.

BORON. Take 2–12 mg. per day. Boron is a trace element found in fruits, nuts, and vegetables. It has been found to reduce urinary calcium loss and to increase serum levels of 17 estradiol (the most biologically active estrogen),[35] both of which help bone health. The minimum dose of boron needed (2 mg.) per day is easily met with a daily diet rich in fruits, nuts, and vegetables.

VITAMIN D. Take 350 IU per day. Note that a thirty-minute sunbath will provide 300–350 units of vitamin D, but most people don't get outside enough and leave too little skin exposed to the sun when they do. For the average Caucasian living in the United States, exposing the hands, face, and arms for 15 to 20 minutes to midmorning or late-afternoon sun three days a week provides sufficient vitamin D March through October.

BETA CAROTENE. Take 25,000 units per day (15 mg.). Beta carotene is converted into vitamin A in the body. Vitamin A promotes a healthy intestinal epithelium, which is important for optimal absorption of nutrients, and it also promotes strong joints. It is found in abundance in yellow and orange vegetables such as acorn squash and carrots and also in dark green leafy vegetables.

For those women who continue to suffer from vaginal dryness or hot flashes despite this regimen, estrogen can be used in addition. When progesterone levels are adequate, however, a much lower dose of estrogen will give the same beneficial effect.

Sexuality in Menopause

What we believe about sexuality and menopause has a lot to do with our sexual expectations and experience. A very common misconception about menopause is that sexual desire and activity significantly decline during this period, but the gynecological and psychiatric literature fails to support this belief. Because our society views menopause as "failed productivity" and associates reproductive capacity with sexual capacity, many women have "bought" the belief that their sex drive is supposed to go away. But in humans, the capacity for sexual pleasure and the capacity for reproduction are two distinct functions. We can always have one without the other.

Some women truly do notice a decline in libido at menopause. One of them told me that her lack of libido is not a problem for her, personally. But she does worry about her husband getting enough sex. I suspect that this concern is shared by many. I suspect that one of the reasons that libido falls after menopause for some women is that their "life-force" or *chi* is simply exhausted from years of stress and they have nothing left over for sexual desire.

But for other women, the climacteric and postmenopausal period is associated with heightened sexual desire and activity. For many women, it is the first time that they are truly free from the fear of unwanted pregnancy.[36] Many physicians mistakenly believe that as women become older, they refrain from sex. But women who are not sexually active do not lack sexual desire. Studies have shown that the reason they are not sexually active is that they have no partner, or their partner is ill, or they have vaginal thinning leading to pain with intercourse. For some women, the availability of a suitable partner is more important to their sexual interest and desire than any other factor. Of greatest importance to continued sexual desire and interest is marital happiness.[37]

At least 50 percent of menopausal women report *no* decline in sexual interest, and fewer than 20 percent report any significant decline. Masters and Johnson have shown that the sex drive is *not* related to estrogen levels and therefore should not automatically decline with menopause.[38] Androgens are the hormones associated with libido. Many of my menopausal patients who left unsatisfying marriages and remarried more compatible mates have better sex lives than ever. Particularly striking was one very proper seventy-five-year-old woman who always came in dressed formally in blouses with high lace collars. She was having a problem with some vaginal dryness and was worried that she'd have to stop her sexual activity. Newly married, she was regularly having seven orgasms per lovemaking session with her husband, after being anorgasmic for her entire forty years of marriage with her first husband. She told me that she had had no idea how wonderful sexual activity could be. All she needed was a bit of estrogen cream and some reassurance that she was normal.

Another woman, age fifty-five, was at her most sexually fulfilled when she began a relationship with a man fifteen years younger than she. There is some evidence that in prepatriarchal times, the older women initiated the younger men in sexual learning that would be especially pleasing to women. The combination of an older woman and a younger man in this regard makes perfect sense—though it goes against everything that our culture has taught us! (No one blinks an eye when a fifty-five-year-old man marries a twenty-five-year-old woman, however.) Sexual preference may also change at midlife. Several of my patients found themselves sexually attracted to women after menopause, although they had defined themselves as heterosexual beforehand.

A big problem for many heterosexual women is that their male partner's ability to get and maintain an erection may change as he ages. If the male perceives this as impending impotence, he may avoid sexual activity altogether. Many women have told me that they would like to enjoy regular sexual activity, but their husbands won't participate anymore because of their fear of impotence. Because these women are afraid of offending their husband's ego, however, they keep quiet instead of getting help. Usually all the help the men need is a bit of education. Still, antihypertensive and other medications can interfere with erection and even orgasmic capacity in some men. Lifestyle changes such as weight loss, a low-fat diet, and increased physical activity can reverse hypertension in those who are motivated to make them.

Ancient Taoist cultures taught exercises (like "ovarian breathing" exercises in Chapter 7) to the women of royal families, who were reported to have retained their youthful appearance and sexual potency long after menopause as a result. These exercises all involved using the mind to flow life-force energy throughout the body. Especially important to these practices was (and still is) the rerouting of potent "ovarian energy" to other organs of the body. Mantak Chia, a master teacher of these techniques, writes, "With the Ovarian Kung Fu method as it is now taught, a woman can continue sexual activity for as long as she desires because no energy is lost; in fact, energy is gained through the transformation of her sexual energy." He adds that many Taoist women consider the results of these exercises to be the best cosmetic in existence.[39]

Treatment

Treatment for lack of sex drive must be highly individualized. Some women report feeling more like their former selves on ERT. Others note an increase in libido following the use of transdermal progesterone cream. This progesterone-containing cream is absorbed "transdermally" across the skin, the same way as scopolamine patches for motion sickness and nitroglycerin patches for angina. It may work, in part, because natural progesterone is a precursor molecule, and when the body requires it, it can be turned into androgens and even some types of estrogen. Testosterone is the major androgen associated with libido. In those women who don't seem to be able to produce enough of their own androgens, testosterone, in the form of a skin cream, a gel, or a capsule can be given. The usual dose is 10 mg. per day and is available by prescription from many pharmacies. (See Resources for source.) The hormone dihydroepiandosterone (DHEA), which is a precursor of testosterone, can also be given orally.[40] The usual dosage starts at 5 mg. per day. When given with progesterone, it appears to enhance well-being in those women who don't respond to progesterone alone. The side effect of too much testosterone or DHEA is a slight increase in hair growth on arms and legs. Estrogen combined with testosterone can also be taken in a widely available form known as Estratest. Other women have done well with homeopathic remedies. There may be a placebo effect on the libido from "doing something" about it. Remember, sometimes it's not your hormones—it's your *life* that needs "medicine."

Mood Swings and Depression

Research shows that menopause itself does not contribute to poor psychological or physical health. It has found that menopausal women aged forty-five to sixty-four actually have a significantly lower incidence of depression than younger women. Moreover, the major stress in the lives of menopausal women is most often caused by family or by factors *other* than menopause.[41] For example, approximately 25 percent of women in the menopausal years are caring for an elderly relative, according to some studies, which certainly can be stressful.[42] Dr. Sonja McKinlay, an associate professor of community health at Brown University who researched a group of healthy menopausal women who were not seeking medical advice, says, "For the majority of women, menopause is not the major negative event it has been typified as. That is basic mythology." She noted that only 2 to 3 percent of the women in her study expressed any regret at moving out of their reproductive years. One unique feature of this study is that it was done on healthy women who were *not* seeking medical advice. Clearly, many physicians have a negative view of menopause based on their biased population.

Some women, though, find that going through menopause brings up the same stormy emotions that they experienced in adolescence, for menopause is the other end of that process. Some women even feel as though they have a PMS that lasts for months but is never relieved by getting a period. Most of us haven't lost that rebellious eleven- or twelve-year-old who felt she had to make a choice between pleasing herself and appearing selfish—or pleasing others and getting cultural support. Menopause is a time when we are preparing to move into our wisdom years, and we may come up against the "unfinished business" that we have accumulated over the first half of our life. We may find ourselves grieving for losses never fully grieved, longing to get a college degree that we never completed, or longing for another child or a first child. All the unfinished business of women's lives comes up at menopause to be reexamined and completed, as if we have gone down into our basement and found boxes and boxes of stuff to be sorted and weeded out. If a woman is willing to deal with her own unfinished business, she will have fewer menopausal symptoms. She will find that her symptoms are messages from her inner guidance system that parts of her life need attention.

Treatment

When a woman is willing to resolve the unfinished emotional business of her life, no "treatment" of her mood swings is necessary. Dietary improvement and exercise can work wonders. So can the inner work described in Part Three of this book. Other women will need physical support of their endocrine, energy, and emotional systems, through ERT, homeopathy, acupuncture, and other approaches.

Fuzzy Thinking

Many women describe a perimenopausal change in their thought processes: They feel as though they can no longer think straight. Marian Van Eck McCain, in her book *Transformation Through Menopause*, calls this "cottonhead" or feeling unable to use the left brain or intellect for such tasks as balancing the checkbook or getting organized.[43] I have asked many women about this and have found it to be common. Many are very relieved to find that it is normal because they are afraid they are getting Alzheimer's disease. There is no evidence to support the commonly held myth that women as well as men normally lose their memory or get "senile" as they age.[44]

After I read about "cottonhead," I realized that I felt this same way after having my children. I seemed virtually unable to concentrate on linear tasks. My brain felt fuzzy. I wanted to watch movies, be with my baby, and not have to think, at least in the limited way that our culture defines thinking. The way I understand this "cottonhead" state is that it forces us into our right brains and out of our former "logocentric" way of being. We now have a chance to think with our hearts. If we allow it to unfold, if we don't fight it or see it as a dysfunction, it can be an initiation into a whole new way of experiencing the world, a far more intuitive way. For many women the ability to express themselves in art, writing, or sculpting comes from allowing their "cottonheadedness" to center them and help them withdraw from the world ruled by the steely organized intellect.

When Peggy, a fifty-eight-year-old kindergarten teacher, went through menopause, she began to experience an inability to concentrate in her classroom. "After thirty years as a teacher," she said, "I couldn't remember the names of the kids in my classes, and sometimes I couldn't even remember how to spell words." Every fiber of her being told her to take a sabbatical from teaching to give her inner life some attention. Her "thinking" problem became so bad that she eventually started crying in front of her classes. She realized that she needed a change. She left school, traveled to California, and lived in a small cottage near the beach for a year. During that time, she began to knit. She found that the knitting was exactly what her brain needed for meditative activity.

On a hunch, Peggy began to teach senior citizens the knitting techniques she was learning. She mailed a beach chair to me. She had handknit the seat and the back in beautiful and unusual designs. She found that her skills were in great demand. In addition to her knitting, she allowed herself to grieve fully for the end of her marriage ten years before. She forgave herself for the impact that it had had on her son. By the time I saw her a year later, she was a healed woman with a great deal of trust in life. She had accepted the challenge of menopause, moved into her intuitive side, and begun a whole new life. She now spends half the year in California and half the year in Maine. She is back to a small amount of teaching, on her own terms. She no longer forgets names or class plans.

Estrogen Replacement Therapy (ERT)

A Brief History

The history of ERT is another example of the connection between science and culture. During medical school, when I was doing a family practice rotation at a small hospital in Vermont, I found Robert Wilson's book *Feminine Forever* in the medical library and did a report on it. This book, written in the 1950s, endorsed the wonders of estrogen replacement as a youth pill that would rescue women from all the horrors of old age. I was oblivious to cultural influences and knew nothing about menopause, being only in my mid-twenties. I embraced the book and its message with great enthusiasm, as did countless other doctors and patients throughout the United States.

What I and my colleagues didn't know at the time was that estrogen replacement, used in the way it was then used, led to a tenfold increase in cancer of the uterus. When this information became available in the mid to late 1970s, estrogen replacement therapy (ERT) fell rapidly out of favor. Doctors and patients alike were afraid to use it. Then, in the late 1970s, studies began to associate ERT with reduced fractures from osteoporosis, the decline in bone density associated with menopause. Osteoporosis itself was halted by the use of estrogen, and subsequent fracture rates went down as well. When these studies first started appearing, my husband and I did a joint presentation on the subject to the department of obstetrics and gynecology at Tufts. Some of my professors at the time said that they didn't care what the data showed, they were afraid to use ERT because of the link between estrogen and uterine cancer. But over the next decade, the attitude of the medical profession once again began to swing back to a pro-hormone position, spurred on by the research on ERT and pushed by the drug companies.

Estrogen was again prescribed much more commonly, but for those women with intact uteri, synthetic progestins such as Provera were now added to the hormone replacement regimens to reduce the risk of excess stimulation of the uterine lining resulting in endometrial cancer (cancer of the lining of the uterus). Excess stimulation of the uterine lining is a direct result of estrogen replacement.

Some subsequent studies have shown that women who take ERT with a progestin added have a risk of uterine cancer that is *even lower* than in women who take no hormones at all. This is because the progestin uniformly sloughs off the endometrial lining at regular intervals. In women who are not on hormonal regulation, the endometrial lining is subject to fluctuations in estrogen and progesterone levels based on dietary fat levels, stress, and other variables.

In the 1980s and now in the early 1990s, the hormone companies have funded study after study that shows the benefits of ERT, to the point that some gynecologists are now saying that *all* women past menopause *need* this therapy for optimum health. Though ERT has been approved by the FDA *only* for the prevention of osteoporosis, the list of *possible* benefits resulting from use of ERT are the following:

- Decreased risk of fractures from osteoporosis
- Prevention of vaginal thinning and dryness
- Possible prevention of cardiovascular disease, including heart attack
- Improved elasticity of the skin
- Amelioration of hot flashes
- Increased libido
- Decreased depression

Seeing all these "benefits" listed at once, what woman *wouldn't* be interested in ERT, especially if she believes that menopause is a disease and that it is just a matter of time before *her* bones start dissolving and *her* vagina starts thinning? Is it any wonder that ERT is the choice for many women? Approximately 50 percent of my postmenopausal patients are on an ERT regimen. I'm not *against* it in any way, but it needs to be kept in perspective. ERT is *not* the only way to alleviate the problems that *some* (not all) women experience menopausally.

Bias in Hormone Prescribing

All studies on hormones are biased in favor of their use to some degree. In the office setting, whether a woman gets ERT depends very much on how much she and her doctor believe in its benefits. Most physicians tend to give hormones to healthy people and not to women who have already established medical diseases such as heart trouble and migraine headaches or a strong history for stroke.[45] In many medical circles, it is now considered "standard of care" to put *all* women on estrogen replacement at menopause. Doctors routinely warn women about the risks of *not* using it, convincing them that osteoporosis and heart disease are inevitable without it. So great and so pervasive is the magnitude of the pro-ERT rhetoric at this time that I am often powerless to change a woman's mind about it. By combining so-called medical "fact" with fear, an entire new generation of women is being brainwashed that ERT is the gold standard—"Don't leave menopause without it." The current "medicalization" of menopause has been so successful that most women's own menopausal wisdom and trust in their bodies to remain healthy during this natural life-stage is almost nonexistent. Therefore, since I don't believe that menopause is a deficiency disease, a woman's desire to try ERT is the number-one reason I prescribe it.

The rare woman who wants to get through menopause *without* estrogen replacement now has to fear that she may not be making the right choice. She doesn't get the cultural seal of approval that she would get if she were on ERT. Women may feel better on ERT in part because they are doing the culturally approved "right thing." This can be comforting and health-enhancing in and of itself.

Yet it is intuitively obvious that nature would not set up our lives so that the majority of women would deteriorate with disease following menopause. If we lived according to our faith in our inner guidance and our bodily wisdom, menopause would be, for the majority of women, what it was meant to be—a safe transition into our wisdom years. But given the current link between research funding, drug company profits, and the medical profession, we are not likely to get the kind of "proof" we require to assure ourselves that we can remain healthy without hormones. Because most of the scientists now working on menopause see this life stage as a disease, their studies will find disease. Much more research is necessary.

Because we have no large-scale, unbiased medical research studies on healthy women who do not take ERT, I cannot cite research to help women make the choice to avoid or go on ERT. I have only the "anecdotal" experience of caring for the women in my practice who have decided to avoid it with my support. I find myself on the horns of this dilemma every day. Ultimately, after giving a woman the facts as I know them, I refuse to try to *convince* her, if she is drawn to it, that she *shouldn't* take ERT, when all current conventional medical opinion suggests that she would be a fool not to. On the other hand, I fully support those women who want to avoid it. Each woman must tune in to her own inner guidance on this one. Currently, approximately 50 percent of the women in my practice are on some form of ERT and 50 percent are not. I also offer a wide array of alternative hormone combinations such as estriol and natural progesterone that are often better tolerated than conventional ERT regimens.

Breast Cancer

I am very concerned about the risk of breast cancer in ERT. I am especially reluctant to put any woman with a family history of breast cancer on conventional ERT. (Some still want it, even knowing about the risks.) Every published paper on breast cancer shows that estrogen is somehow related to breast cancer. Since breast tissue has estrogen receptors in it and is estrogen sensitive, it makes sense that in a woman potentially at risk for breast cancer, ERT could start a tumor growing that might otherwise have been dormant. The now-famous Bergkvist study in Sweden showed an increase in breast cancer after seven years of estrogen use.[46] Several other studies have linked ERT with increased risk of breast cancer, though not all studies support this link.[47]

Approximately twenty-eight studies have looked at the relationships between estrogen replacement in the form of estradiol or conjugated estrogens (such as Premarin), and, through a statistical test known as metanalysis, they have suggested that estrogen replacement therapy is associated with an increase in the risk of breast cancer ranging from 1 to 30 percent.[48] However, none of these studies showed that the increased risk was statistically significant. I'm still concerned because even a small increase in risk with conventional ERT could result in a very real increase in breast cancer cases. Dr. Alan Gaby, a well-known expert in the field of nutritional medicine, writes, "Given a one in nine (11.1%) chance of developing breast cancer, a 30% increase in risk (the highest number reported in the metanalysis) would increase the overall breast cancer to 14.4%. If this worst-case scenario is accurate then for every 1,000 women receiving ERT, there would be 33 more cases of breast cancer (above and beyond the 111 already expected)."[49]

Yet many medical experts downplay the risks, and some even say that there is probably no medical reason why women who have had breast cancer can't safely go on ERT. The main reason it isn't prescribed in these women is the fear of a lawsuit if the cancer recurs.

Even though many more women die of hip fractures and heart

disease than breast cancer overall, most of my patients are much more frightened of breast cancer than of either osteoporosis or heart disease. Breast cancer kills more women than AIDS and is the leading cause of death in women aged forty-five to fifty-five, but heart disease and osteoporosis are far more common causes of death in women overall than either breast cancer or AIDS. Statistics don't change behavior—emotions do. We stay away from what seems the most fearful to us.

Heart Disease

Heart disease is the number-one killer of postmenopausal women overall. (Breast cancer may be the number-one killer of women aged forty-five to fifty-five, but heart disease is still much more common overall.)

The cause of heart disease in women over fifty-five is commonly thought to be estrogen "deficiency," and estrogen replacement therapy (ERT) is thought to be the answer. Merely linking cardiovascular disease with lowered estrogen levels implies that cardiovascular disease is *caused* by lowered estrogen levels. But this theory has never been substantiated. Based on the more "scientific" lectures that I hear, I often get the feeling doctors see estrogen as a panacea for menopause. As in osteoporosis, physicians have taken a multi-factorial disease like heart disease and decided that for all women there is a single treatment or cure—estrogen replacement. Cardio-vascular disease is epidemic in this culture in part because of lifestyle and diet, not estrogen deficiency. The addictive system is fascinated by the "fix" of a prescription, rather than looking at people's life-style. (I mean this collectively, not necessarily individually.)

Several studies have indicated that women on ERT have a de-creased risk of dying from heart attack. Unfortunately, no one has studied a group of older women who are *not* on ERT and who *do not* have heart disease. I have many of these women in my practice. Estrogens and synthetic progestins (the hormones most often used for ERT in women with an intact uterus) have complicated effects on cholesterol. Numerous studies have shown that hormonal treat-ments, ranging from birth control pills to various kinds of ERT, have an effect on lipids—some positive, some negative.[50] Right now, there are no convincing data showing that menopausal women with the same age and risk factors have more heart attacks because of their menopausal state.[51]

I suggest that all women have a lipid profile, to find out what their risk factors for heart disease are—at least, the ones associated with cholesterol levels. I like to see the total cholesterol below 200, though some studies suggest that women can have a cholesterol above 200 and not be at high risk for heart attack, as we previously thought from studies done on men. Throughout the world heart disease is associated with a refined-food, high-fat diet, smoking, and a sedentary lifestyle. Therefore, there is much that a woman can do besides ERT (or in addition to it, if she prefers) to decrease her risk of heart attack. I've come to believe that the best way to protect the heart is to live with passion and joy, so that the energy of the fourth chakra is available throughout the body.

Other Problems with ERT

Many American women have had too much estrogen and not enough progesterone during their entire reproductive lives. Putting them on conventional ERT regimens with synthetic progestin simply re-creates this imbalance during a time when their own bodies are trying to make an adjustment. Because estrogen stimulates breast, uterine, and ovarian tissue, ERT can cause uterine cramping, heavy menstrual periods, headaches, sore breasts, bloating, and weight gain for some women. In general, the more body fat a woman has, the more circulating estrogen she will have. These women can often reach hormonal balance by taking natural progesterone only or by making simple dietary improvements such as a low-fat, high-fiber diet.

Certain types of ERT also put a burden on the liver because this organ must break down hormones metabolically. This increases a woman's need for the B vitamins and some minerals. Since many menopausal women are already nutritionally compromised, ERT puts an added burden on the system.

I have a real concern that the natural brain changes that are supposed to accompany menopause may well be interrupted by introducing estrogen postmenopausally. Higher estrogen levels during the menstrual cycle are also associated with focusing our attention "outward" rather than "inward." What insights might women be losing when they interrupt the natural hormonal state associated with menopause? If a woman takes ERT, might she be sabotaging a part of her wisdom?

Integrative Treatments for Menopause Problems: Unproved Doesn't Mean Ineffective

There are a number of ways in which menopausal women can accomplish symptom relief, maintain a healthy heart, and keep their bones strong without conventional estrogen replacement if they are motivated to do so. Dietary change, exercise, classical osteopathy, acupuncture, and homeopathic and herbal remedies are some of the ways in which my patients have supported their transition through menopause. Many also add small amounts of hormones such as natural progesterone, androgens, and estrogens as needed. Because I do not have long-term clinical data on the use of any one regimen, my experience is considered "testimonial" or "anecdotal," not "scientific," and is often scorned in medical circles. Nevertheless, it makes perfect sense that healthy, well-nourished women can have a satisfying and enlightening transition through menopause and that each woman's treatment must be individualized.

Phytoestrogens: Natural Hormones in Food

Specific foods contain compounds that have estrogenic activity. Phytoestrogens (plant-derived estrogen) are present in soybean products such as tofu, miso, and the beans themselves. One study of Japanese women suggested that a high intake of these products was the reason why they had so few hot flashes or other menopausal symptoms.[52] Other foods that contain significant amounts of phytoestrogens are cashews, peanuts, oats, corn, wheat, apples, and almonds.[53] Because plant estrogens are weak estrogens only, they appear to block the effects of excess estrogen stimulation of organs such as the breasts and uterus and may well be protective.

Treatment of Surgical Menopause

Currently, one out of every four American women will reach menopause through surgery. In 1975 alone, 725,000 hysterectomies and

471,000 oophorectomies were performed, more than half of both in women under age forty-five.[54] Because surgical menopause is very different from natural menopause, I believe that hormone replacement—at least for several years, depending upon the age of the patient—is very important for these women; otherwise the surgery and hormonal change all at the same time produces a type of endocrine "shock" in the body, which isn't healthy. Because normal menopause happens around age fifty-two, ERT should probably continue at least until then. The ovaries produce androgens to some extent as well as estrogens and progesterones, so some women feel better on an estrogen-androgen preparation such as Estratest, along with natural progesterone.

Estriol: An Estrogen That Deserves Attention

There are three separate types of estrogen: Estrone (E1), estradiol (E2) and estriol (E3). Estradiol is the type of estrogen produced directly from the ovary. Estrone is formed from conversion of estradiol. Estriol is also produced by the ovary but in much smaller amounts than the others. Estriol levels are particularly high during pregnancy when it is produced in large amounts.

The type of estrogens used in conventional ERT are estrone and estradiol. These are also the estrogens that have been implicated in breast cancer. Estriol, on the other hand, a somewhat weaker estrogen, since it must be given in higher doses to achieve the same effect, may well have a protective effect against breast cancer.

Over twenty-five years ago a study showed that estriol inhibited the breast cancer–promoting effect of estradiol in mice.[55] In two studies, one in mice, and one in rats, the animals were treated with chemicals known to induce breast cancer. In the animals that received estriol, breast cancer development was inhibited.[56] Dr. Henry Lemon, impressed by the beneficial effects of estriol in animal studies, investigated the effect of estriol in relationship to human breast cancer. He developed a formula called the "estrogen quotient," which is the ratio of the cancer-inhibiting estrogen (estriol) to the cancer-promoting estrogens (estrone plus estradiol) in an individual woman. His theory was that if the estrogen quotient was high, then a woman's body was producing a large amount of estriol relative to the amount of the other estrogens. In these women, the risk of breast cancer would presumably be reduced. If the estrogen quotient were low, however, then very little estriol would be present compared with the other two estrogens. These women would be expected to have a higher risk of cancer. To test his theory, Dr. Lemon measured the different types of estrogen present in urine samples from both healthy women and women with breast cancer. He found that the average estrogen quotient in healthy women was 1.3 prior to menopause and 1.2 after menopause. Only 21 percent of the healthy women in his study had estrogen quotients that were below normal. But in the twenty-six women with breast cancer who had not received hormonal therapy, the average estrogen quotients were from 0.5 to 0.8. Sixty-two percent of the women with breast cancer had values below normal.[57] Dr. Lemon's results suggest, then, that women with breast cancer do indeed have a low level of estriol relative to the other estrogens. Epidemiologic studies have supported Lemon's findings. Women in countries with a low incidence of breast cancer have high levels of urinary estriol excretion compared to the urinary estriol levels of women in countries with high rates of breast cancer.[58] Dietary factors can also clearly influence estriol levels. A study showed that vitamin E administration was able to reduce the incidence of chemically induced breast cancer in rats[59] while in another study in women with mammary dysplasia (often characterized by sore tender breasts with dense irregularities throughout the breast tissue) vitamin E therapy resulted in an 18 percent increase in their ratios of estriol to estradiol.[60] The protective effect of early first pregnancy on the incidence of breast cancer may also be related to higher estriol levels in women who have had their first child before the age of thirty.[61]

Because of the relative safety of estriol, Dr. Lemon and his colleagues conducted a study in women who already had breast cancer that had spread (metastasized) to other areas of the body. One group was given estriol, and another was not. The estriol dosage range was 2.5 to 15 mg. per day. At the end of the study, 37 percent of those women who received estriol had either a remission or an arrest of their cancer. Given the natural history of metastatic breast cancer, these results were much better than expected.[62] Right now, the drug tamoxifen, which blocks the effects of estrone and estradiol on breast tissue, but which is known to increase the incidence of uterine cancer, is being given to women at high risk for breast cancer in order to try to decrease their risk of getting the disease. Estriol, a natural, safe hormone with almost no side effects, might well accomplish the same thing with fewer side effects.

Estriol also appears to have a much safer effect on the lining of the uterus than do the other estrogens since studies have shown much less endometrial build-up when estriol is used for ERT compared to the other estrogens. In one study of fifty-two women on doses of estriol as high as 8 mg. per day, no cases of breakthrough bleeding or endometrial hyperplasia were found.[63] Estriol also has been shown to have the same beneficial effect on the collagen layer in skin as the other estrogens.[64] Vaginal estriol cream is highly effective in alleviating vaginal and urinary symptoms in postmenopausal women.[65] Rather high doses of estriol (12 mgs./day) appear to be required for the prevention of osteoporosis. Given the multifactorial nature of osteoporosis, however, this may not be the case if a woman is adequately nourished and has enough natural progesterone.

Whether or not estriol has the same potentially protective effects against heart disease as the other estrogens has not been determined. In a study comparing the risks and benefits of several different ERT regimens, estriol did not produce any changes in total serum cholesterol, triglycerides, or HDL cholesterol. In comparison, those women who were treated with estradiol (E2) and a synthetic progestin showed a decrease in both total cholesterol and HDL and an increase in LDL cholesterol. As with the more conventional estrogens, more studies are required before estriol's effect on heart disease can be ascertained.[66]

Estriol, which is derived from plant sources, is considered generic and unpatentable.[67] It has been safely used in Europe for years and is available by prescription in the United States at many pharmacies. (See Resources section.) Dosage of estriol must be individualized.

Deciding on Menopausal "Treatment"

Now, you have read the pros and the cons, as I see them, of various treatment regimens. You've probably already read other things as well. If you still can't decide whether to go on ERT, I suggest you sleep on it. Let the decision come to you in dreams or another form (see Part Three). In general, women who have individuated the most from their original tribes and who trust their bodies are the ones who are most comfortable with going through menopause using less conventionally well-studied methods of menopausal therapies.

A Trial Run

Consider doing a trial run. In women who can't decide and who are having symptoms, I often prescribe such a trial run. I start with the lowest dose of estrogen that works, and I give it daily. I add either a synthetic or a natural progesterone during the first twelve days of the month in every woman who has a uterus so that excess buildup of the uterine lining from the ERT will be avoided. There is no reason why a woman needs a "break" from estrogen (that is, taking estrogen on days one to twenty-five, then off five days). I used to prescribe estrogen in this way and many physicians still do. Because ERT regimens vary widely among doctors, there is no "one right way" to do it.

After three months on any ERT regimen, I ask my patient to come back. We then review how she feels, do an exam, and check her blood pressure. If she's happy with how things are going, we review the ERT situation yearly thereafter—paying attention to her dreams, her feelings about ERT, and other indications or messages from her body wisdom. Unfortunately, many OB/GYN physicians tell women that once they're on ERT, they must stay on it for good. I don't know where this recommendation comes from or what evidence it is based on. I suspect it has to do with that ugly word *compliance* and the fact that a woman must stay on a regimen to receive the purported benefits of that regimen.

But as I've already pointed out, the human bodymind is not static over time. We are an energy system that is constantly changing. What works one year may not work the next. Like everything else, a decision to take hormones can be changed. If you're seriously considering ERT, why not try it for a bit and see what your body thinks? If it doesn't work, you can always stop or try another type.

Estrogen Choices

These are the forms in which estrogen is available.

- Conjugated estrogens (Premarin), taken in a dose of 0.3, 0.625, or 1.25 mg. per day
- Estradiol (Estrace), taken in a dose of 0.5 or 1.0 mg. per day
- Estradiol transdermal patch (Estraderm), taken in a dose of 0.05 mg. to 0.1 mg. every three and a half days

The patch is ideal for some women. I liken it to an ovary that sits on the skin and gives your body estrogen. Estrogen that enters the body through the skin (transdermal estrogen) need not be metabolized by the liver. (For that reason, its critics argue that transdermal estrogen doesn't have the same possibly beneficial effects on cholesterol.)

- Estradiol and estriol are also available as skin creams that can be used with or without added progesterone.

The patch is worn on the lower abdomen, buttocks, or thighs. An occasional patient will change her patch every four or five days, though these lower doses are not felt to be as protective for the heart and bones as "full replacement doses." Using the lowest dose possible is fine with me. Some of my patients are on half the amount of estrogen listed. Each woman's situation *must* be individualized. Fifteen percent of women have itching at the site of the patch and discontinue it for that reason.

- Estriol. The recommendations I've given here are based on my clinical experience to date. There are many other effective regimens in wide use. In fact, a survey of 283 gynecologists in the Los Angeles area found that the doctors used eighty-four different patterns of estrogen replacement. The main patterns were: 1) cyclic estrogen alone, 2) cyclic estrogen plus cyclic progestin, 3) continuous estrogen alone, 4) continuous estrogen plus cyclic progestin, 5) continuous estrogen plus continuous progestin, and 6) progestin alone, either cyclic or continuous.[68] The doctors surveyed were prescribing only the standard, conventional forms of ERT in this study. When one

takes into consideration an integrated approach that includes
options such as DHEA, natural progesterone, and estriol, the
possible combinations are endless.

At this time I have limited clinical experience with prescribing
estriol. I am very impressed with the research data, however, and
plan to prescribe it much more commonly.

One of my colleagues, Dr. Jonathan Wright, a well-known expert
in nutritional medicine, has been using estriol since the early 1980s.
He has found his patients do best with estriol when it's combined
with small amounts of the other estrogens, estrone and estradiol.
The reason for this is that some women require very high doses of
estriol to relieve their symptoms. The side effect of these high doses
is nausea.

Dr. Wright developed a formula that increases the benefits of
estrogen while minimizing the risks. His formula consists of a
combination of 80 percent estriol, 10 percent estrone, and 10 percent
estradiol. This formula is known as triestrogen. Usual starting dose
is 2.5 mg. triestrogen per day. This can be increased to 5 mg. per day
as needed. Triestrogen is given for 25 days each month with natural
progesterone added during the last 12 days of each cycle. (This
could also be added during the first 12 days.) Many other estriol,
progesterone, estradiol, and estrone combinations can be prescribed
either orally or via skin creams.[69]

Natural Progesterone and Synthetic Progestin
in ERT Regimens

All women on estrogen replacement who have a uterus need a
natural progesterone or synthetic progestin to counteract the possible excess buildup of tissue that estrogen may cause in the uterus
(see Chapter 5 for difference between synthetic and natural progesterone). The progesterone or progestin needs to be given for ten
to twelve days each month to adequately counteract the effects of
the estrogen. I usually prescribe it starting on the first day of the
month. Thus, a woman takes her progestin or progesterone on days
one to twelve of each month. Natural progesterone (200-400 mg. per
day taken the first twelve days of the month) is preferable for some
because it is exactly the same as what the body produces, has fewer

side effects such as bloating or depression, and has less adverse effects than progestin on blood lipids. If a woman is on a synthetic progestin or prefers this, I use the lowest dose of synthetic progestin that protects against excess buildup of the endometrium. There are fewer side effects that way. (The dose is usually 2.5 mg. to 5 mg. per day for twelve days.) Some women feel fine on doses as high as 10 mg. per day. Most women will have a light period on this regimen. In most there is no need for 10 mg. doses—the normal dose given in the past. The dose of natural progesterone needed to accomplish the same thing is 100-400 mg./day depending upon dosage of estrogen.

The ERT regimen I have prescribed most frequently in the last few years was developed by Dr. Joel Hargrove at Vanderbilt University, who studied the use of oral natural progesterone (100 mg. daily) combined with estradiol (0.5 mg.) in the same capsule as a daily ERT regimen.[70] This is an ideal regimen for many women, since there are no adverse effects on blood lipids, the estrogen is low dose, and women don't get their periods after the first three months on it. Giving estrogen and progesterone at the same time keeps the lining of the uterus stable. Women also get the beneficial effects of natural progesterone without the side effects of progestin on this regimen.

ERT: Only *You* Can Decide

One of my patients, a longtime feminist writer, experienced a great deal of fatigue and withdrawal from her family during menopause that was alarming to her. She never expected that she would take ERT—she had been politically against it for years. But her symptoms became so severe that I suggested she give it a try. She went on the patch and took natural progesterone by capsule. Her body loved it, and she has felt much much better. She said to me, "Well, my intellect would never have believed this, but my body loves it and said yes." I saw her recently and we both decided to try estriol and natural progesterone as a skin cream. Her heart and bones are in excellent condition. So are her emotions and her spirit.

Other women, after their three-month trial or even before, notice that their bodies say a clear no to ERT through messages of swollen breasts, heart palpitations, and many other symptoms. There is no way to know for sure what your body will or won't do. You must trust your inner guidance here and listen to your body.

When patients ask me if I'm going to take estrogen after menopause, I say, "I don't know yet. I'll have to see how I feel at the
time." So will you.

Coming Off Estrogen: How To Do It

If you've been on ERT for a number of years and have decided to
get off it, you should do this *very slowly* to allow your body time to
readjust. To decrease ERT or to get off it, cut down very gradually
over a six-month period. One month you can drop your Sunday
pill; the next month drop the Monday pill; and continue very slowly
until you are off it. Or, consult with your doctor about establishing
your own regimen. When you do it this way, your body can readjust and hot flashes usually won't come back. Some experts are now
advising women to come off conventional ERT after eight years or
so.[71] *No one* has the final word on this. Those on estriol are probably safer to continue.

Self-Care During Menopause

Ask yourself the following questions and answer them truthfully.
Your answers will provide you with the guidance you need to make
personal choices during menopause.

- Do you believe that your body knows how to be healthy
  during and after menopause?
- Do you feel obligated to take hormones after menopause?
  Why? Why not?
- Who are the role models you have had for menopausal
  women? If necessary, are you willing to change your family
  script about menopause? Does your mother or grandmother
  have osteoporosis? What happened to your mother at menopause? Your grandmother? Your aunts? Do your close family
  members all have heart disease? Is there anyone close to you
  with breast cancer? Why are you afraid you will get it? What
  are your true beliefs about this time of life? Are you willing to
  look at what you are doing that might be contributing to
  continuing your family patterns?

- Would you feel better if you knew what your bone density was right now?
- What is your cholesterol level? Do you know about your own lipid profile and your heart disease risk?
- Are you doing work that you love? Do you routinely block your passion, or do you express yourself joyfully?
- Do you believe that your sexual desirability will decrease after menopause?
- Does a period of celibacy at menopause feel like a good choice for you?
- Do you believe that you will be alone in your old age?
- Do you exercise regularly to keep your bones healthy?
- Do you nutritionally support yourself by eating whole, delicious, fresh foods?
- Are you willing to allow your intuition to speak to you clearly as you become a "seed" for your community?

Many menopausal women have dreams of giving birth. These birth dreams are important—they signify that there is much within us that needs to come forth. In this culture, women who are about to go through menopause or who are already in it need more than ever to reach deep within themselves and give birth to what is waiting there to be expressed. We can no longer afford to let our culture silence the wisdom of the wise woman—the woman who contains her sacred blood.

Susun Weed writes, "The process of menopause—not the last menses, the last drop of blood, but the entire thirteen-year menopausal process—sets the stage for initiatory ritual the world 'round. Just as menstruating women's natural needs/abilities became the basis for all other initiations.

"During the process of menopause each woman finds herself immersed in and creating the three classic stages of initiation: isolation, death, and rebirth. . . . our female bodies insist on completeness, wholeness, truth, change. Much as any woman would like to deny her shadow-self, her body will not let her. Menopause brings the individual woman and thus the entire community face to face with the dark, the unknown."[72]

With or without the help of hormones, every woman will benefit if she enters menopause consciously, ready to gather the gifts available at this stage of life. What we have to lose is not nearly so valuable as what we have to gain, finding our own voices and the courage to speak our own truth. When women do this, they are truly irresistible in their power and beauty.

In the story "The Dancing Grandmas," Clarissa Pinkola Estes tells of four old women refugees who wore black, had red hands and ruddy cheeks, and whose "entire history was in their forearms." At a family wedding, these four danced beautifully and powerfully, "lifting their skirts to display piano ankles wrapped in Ace bandages." As was their tradition, they danced to exhaustion, all the young men, including the groom, as a way to test their stamina. And at the end of the evening "Everyone had been inoculated with the power of age. No one could ever become sick from age, or made ill by the idea that aging was a pathetic time. Everyone knew a good and decent, deep life awaited them in later years."[73] We've been too long without those powerful, honest, wise women of old—too long without images of their beauty, power, and strength. Welcome them back. They are inside each of us—waiting to be born through the initiation of menopause.

PART THREE

Choices for Healing: Creating Your Personal Plan

As long as you think that it's somebody else's problem, you'll never get better.

—Annie Rafter

*T*here is power inherent in committing yourself to the process of creating health in all levels of your life. Once you've made a commitment to heal your life, you will discover that guidance and information from many different sources becomes available to you. Commitment engages your will, the power to hold and direct thought into its desired physical manifestation. Making a commitment to healing involves two steps: The first is admitting that healing is necessary, and the second is opening yourself to the information that you begin to attract following the commitment.

Goethe said it best.

Until one is committed, there is hesitancy, the chance to draw back, always ineffectiveness. Concerning all acts of initiative [and creation], there is one elementary truth the ignorance of which kills countless ideas and splendid plans: the moment one definitely commits oneself, then Providence moves too. All sorts of things occur to help one that would never otherwise have occurred. A whole stream of events issues from the decision, raising in one's favour all manner of unforeseen incidents and meetings and material assistance which no man (or woman) could have dreamed would come his [or her] way. Whatever you can do or dream you can do, begin it. Boldness has genius, power, and magic in it. Begin it now.

Problem-solving, whether through drugs, surgery, or herbs, is entirely different from creating health. Creating health requires making a paradigm shift, or systems shift, to a new way of thinking about and being in relationship with our bodies, our minds, our spirits, and our connection with the universe. Very few people maintain or regain health and wholeness until they make this shift.

Creating health means accepting that there are events in everyone's lives that cannot be explained or changed, and at the same time realizing that each of us has conscious input into our state of health through choosing relationships, thoughts, foods, and activities that support and nourish us fully. The following chapters will provide you with ideas, examples, and healing programs for the body, mind, and spirit. They have assisted many women in their journeys toward health.

FIFTEEN

Steps for Healing

*T*he steps in this chapter have proved helpful to women who want to become more deeply in tune with the inner guidance of their bodies, minds, and spirits. By going through this chapter mindfully you will be practicing preventive medicine at its best, whether or not you are currently being treated for anything.

Step One: Get Your History Straight

You need only claim the events of your life to make yourself yours. When you truly possess all you have been and done, which may take some time, you are fierce with reality.
—Florida Scott-Maxwell

It is helpful for each woman to get her medical, social, and family history straight. At Women to Women, our patients fill out an extensive questionnaire that covers not only their medical history but their family history and a "daily living profile" in which they check off the effects of their living situation, job, relationships, and other factors on their health. (See the Women to Women Intake Form on pages 488–93.) Many of our patients find that taking the time to pull all this information together enables them to see patterns that they had not seen before. One woman pointed out, "Until I filled out this form, I never realized how much alcoholism was in my family. I also didn't see that my fibroid uterus started to grow

485

right after I had that second abortion." Some women realize the significance of virtually every woman in their extended family having had a hysterectomy before the age of fifty—thus creating a self-fulfilling medical family prophecy around the uterus.

Because conditions such as alcoholism and depression are often denied within a family system, the form specifically asks about these things. Through this form, we also pick up on habits and conditions that patients are tempted to downplay. ("I'm not really an alcoholic, I'm just a heavy social drinker.") Also, the emotional impact of a history that includes the premature death of a parent, loss of a beloved pet, or loss of a significant relationship, is frequently denied. This, too, is often revealed in filling out the form.

Lois, a forty-three-year-old woman with a history of early cervical cancer and pelvic endometriosis, said recently, "I was a battered wife five years ago and finally got out of that marriage; then, my daughter was in a car accident and I had to take care of her for months. Then, this summer I was in another accident and sustained a whiplash injury. I seem to want to cry, but I keep pushing it down. It gets harder to do, though. Is this from early menopause?"

Going over Lois's intake form with her, it was easy to see that she had been through a very significant amount of change and loss in the past decade, which she'd tried to deal with by keeping everything in order, going to work daily, and appearing cheerful. She admitted that it seemed to be harder to keep her house in order these days, and that even though there was no current crisis, she still felt inefficient and emotional. In fact, her back pain from the whiplash was gone, her daughter was now in college, and her job was going quite well. What she realized she needed to do was acknowledge the losses she hadn't grieved and give herself the necessary time and space for this.

What Lois was experiencing was what I call Break Down to Breakthrough. She needed to feel what she was feeling. She took a week off from work and family, went to a small country inn, and spent the next week mostly in robe and slippers, reading, crying, drinking tea with the lady who runs the inn, and gradually getting back in touch with parts of herself and feelings that were long denied. When I next saw her, she looked fifteen years younger. "Now I know that those feelings you mentioned don't come up when you want them to," she said. "They come when they come. It took me three or four days of being quiet and by myself before I could really cry. But I also learned that I can get off by myself when I need to in order to do this for myself. My relationship with my husband [she had remarried] and daughter is better than ever. I learned that *When I take care of myself, everything else takes care of itself.*"

Women To Women

Confidential Health Inventory

GENERAL INFORMATION:

Date:_____

Name: _____ Age _____ Birthdate: _____
          LAST   FIRST   MIDDLE

Address: _____
            CITY   STATE   ZIP CODE

Mailing Address (if different from above)_____

Home Phone No.: _____ Work Phone No.: _____ SS# _____

Occupation: _____ Employer: _____ Address: _____

    Employment Status: ❏ Full-Time ❏ Part-Time ❏ School ❏ Retired ❏ Unemployed Other _____

    Living Situation: ❏ Alone ❏ Friend(s) ❏ Partner ❏ Spouse ❏ Parents Number of Children _____

    Names and ages of those living with you: _____

_____

    Pets: _____

Status: ❏ Single   ❏ Married   ❏ Divorced   ❏ Widowed

Name of Partner/Spouse/Parent: _____ Occupation: _____
                      CIRCLE ONE

In Case of Emergency Notify: _____ Phone No.: _____

Religious/Spiritual Preferences: _____

Educational Background: _____

How did you hear about Women To Women: ❏ Phone Book   ❏ Ad _____ Another Patient_____

    Course/Seminar Taught By _____ Physician/Professional _____

    Articles Written By or Referring To _____ Other _____

INSURANCE INFORMATION:

Name of Insurance Co.: _____

Address: _____ Phone: _____

Contract No.: _____ Group No.: _____

    Other Medical Insurance: _____

FINANCIAL AGREEMENT

I claim full financial responsibility for services rendered at Women To Women for _____
                                                           PATIENT

and understand that payment is required in full at the time of service.

_____   _____
   SIGNATURE—PATIENT OR PARENT OF MINOR   RELATIONSHIP TO PATIENT

AUTHORIZATION TO RELEASE INFORMATION AND ASSIGN BENEFITS

I hereby authorize the release of any medical information necessary in the processing of my claim. I also authorize payment directly to Women To Women for the surgical/medical benefits.

Date _____ Signed _____
                                  PATIENT, OR PARENT OF MINOR

INTENTION FOR THIS APPOINTMENT:
_____
_____
_____

ALLERGIES
Drug allergies (penicillin, etc.): _____
_____

Allergies to foods, pollens, etc.: _____
_____
_____

MEDICAL STATUS
General Health: ❒ Excellent ❒ Good ❒ Fair ❒ Poor
Medications (vitamins, prescription or otherwise): _____
_____

Have you ever had your cholesterol level checked? _____ Date(s) _____ Results _____
Have you ever had a mammogram? _____ Date(s) _____ Results _____
Do you do self-breast exams? _____

HOSPITALIZATIONS/OPERATIONS

Dates	Hospital	Diagnosis/Operation	Doctor

PREGNANCIES (including miscarriages and abortions)

Dates	How far along	Sex	Weight	Problems

CURRENT/RECENT HEALTH CARE PROVIDERS

Name	Dates	Care Provided

Do any health care providers request follow-up on your visit here? _____ If yes, name: _____
address: _____

OTHER PAST MEDICAL CONDITIONS

Childhood diseases: ❑ German measles ❑ Chicken Pox Other _____
❑ Heart trouble: _____ ❑ High blood pressure ❑ Stroke ❑ Varicose Veins ❑ Phlebitis
❑ Clotting defects   ❑ Bleeding tendencies   ❑ Blood transfusion   ❑ Diabetes   ❑ Kidney trouble
❑ Rheumatic fever   ❑ Jaundice/hepatitis   ❑ Epilepsy   ❑ Fractures _____ ❑ Cancer _____
❑ Arthritis ❑ Colitis ❑ Asthma ❑ Chronic Fatigue/Epstein Barr ❑ Eating Disorder Other _____

HABITS

Dietary preferences/restrictions: _____
Sample of day's menu:
    Breakfast: _____
    Lunch: _____
    Dinner: _____
Routine physical exercise: Type of exercise: _____
For how many minutes? _____ How often? _____
Tobacco use (how much): _____ Previously? _____ How much? _____ How long?_____
Alcohol use (how much): _____ How often? _____
Caffeine use (how much): _____ Mood altering substance use (i.e. marijuana, cocaine—past and present):

STRESSES

Stresses (family, work, self, etc.): _____
_____
_____
_____

FAMILY HISTORY

MEMBER	LIVING?	AGE?	IMPORTANT DISEASES Alcoholism, High Blood Pressure, Cancer, Diabetes, Heart Disease, Osteoporosis, other addiction, other illness	CAUSE OF DEATH & AGE
Mother				
Father				
Sister(s)				
Brother(s)				
Maternal Grandmother				
Paternal Grandmother				
Maternal Grandfather				
Paternal Grandfather				
Paternal Aunt(s)				
Maternal Aunt(s)				
Maternal Uncle(s)				
Paternal Uncle(s)				

GYNECOLOGICAL HISTORY

Date last period began: _____   Date of last pelvic exam: _____

Date prior period began: _____   Date of last Pap smear: _____

Age at first period: _____   Were the above normal? _____

Have you ever had an abnormal Pap? _____ When: _____ Results: _____

Treatment: _____

Are you sexually active? _____ Do you have intercourse? _____ Do you practice safe sex? _____

Are you trying to get pregnant? _____ How long? _____

Current birth control method: _____ How long? _____

   Problems with it: _____

Past birth control methods: _____

Normally (not on pills), the number of days from the start of one period to the start of the next: _____

Number of days of flow: _____

   Amount of bleeding: _____ Amount of cramps: _____

   Premenstrual symptoms: _____

   Starting when? _____

Any current changes in your normal pattern? _____

Any bleeding between periods? _____ When? _____

Any unusual pelvic pain, pressure, or fullness? _____ When? Describe: _____

Any unusual vaginal discharge or itching? _____ Describe: _____

How long? _____ Past treatment: _____

Any sexual concerns to discuss? _____

Any past history of tubal infection? _____

Any past history of sexually transmitted disease? _____

Any history of DES exposure? (DES was a drug taken by mothers during pregnancy to prevent miscarriage.) _____

Other: _____

REVIEW OF SYSTEMS

Check any symptoms of **present** significance. (If any past problems, please note under Past Medical Problems on Page Three.)

GENERAL PHYSICAL

❒ Fever or chills ❒ Hot flashes ❒ Unusual hair growth ❒ Skin eruptions ❒ Weight change

ABDOMEN

❒ Bloating ❒ Heartburn, indigestion ❒ Cramps or pain ❒ Nausea or vomiting ❒ Change in bowel habits ❒ Bloody or tarry stools ❒ Diarrhea ❒ Constipation ❒ Hemorrhoids ❒ Flatulence

HEAD

❒ Headaches ❒ Dizziness ❒ Visual defects ❒ Hearing defects ❒ Sinus trouble ❒ Fainting spells

BLADDER

❒ Frequent urination ❒ Painful urination ❒ Blood in urine ❒ Inability to hold urine ❒ Inability to empty bladder ❒ Need to get up at night to urinate

CHEST

❒ Chest pain ❒ Shortness of breath ❒ Heart murmur ❒ Mitral valve prolapse ❒ Palpitations ❒ Chronic cough ❒ Coughing up blood ❒ Wheezing

BREASTS

❒ Lumps ❒ Bleeding ❒ Discharge ❒ Tenderness

COMMENTS OR OTHER CONCERNS: _____

DAILY LIVING PROFILE

Please read the following statements which relate to your current life at home and work, and indicate whether each statement does or does not describe part of your current life by placing an "X" in the "yes" or "no" box at the right of the statement. This questionnaire is designed to increase your awareness of the effects of your life-style and stresses on your physical well-being.

NEIGHBORHOOD STRESSES
1. My neighborhood is too noisy .... ❐ Yes ❐ No
2. My neighborhood is too crowded .... ❐ Yes ❐ No
3. My neighborhood is too quiet .... ❐ Yes ❐ No
4. I do not have enough friends/neighbors .... ❐ Yes ❐ No
5. It is a dangerous neighborhood in which to live .... ❐ Yes ❐ No
6. Having so many household tasks irritates me .... ❐ Yes ❐ No
7. The weather here bothers me .... ❐ Yes ❐ No
8. I'm new to this area .... ❐ Yes ❐ No
9. Other neighborhood problems .... ❐ Yes ❐ No

    (if yes, describe): _____

_____

FAMILY STRESSES
10. I am recently married .... ❐ Yes ❐ No
11. I am recently divorced or separated .... ❐ Yes ❐ No
12. I am recently moved or am planning to move .... ❐ Yes ❐ No
13. I am alone too much at home .... ❐ Yes ❐ No
14. I am concerned about my relationship with my partner .... ❐ Yes ❐ No
15. I am concerned about my relationship with another family member
    (parent, child, brother, sister) .... ❐ Yes ❐ No
16. I feel I was raised in a dysfunctional environment .... ❐ Yes ❐ No
17. There is a new baby in our family .... ❐ Yes ❐ No
18. I or one of my family members is having legal problems .... ❐ Yes ❐ No
19. There was a recent death of a family member or close friend .... ❐ Yes ❐ No
20. There is a serious illness in my family .... ❐ Yes ❐ No
21. I am worried about one of my family members .... ❐ Yes ❐ No
22. Someone close to me drinks too much .... ❐ Yes ❐ No
23. One of my children has moved away from home recently .... ❐ Yes ❐ No
24. My partner has recently retired .... ❐ Yes ❐ No
25. Other concerns about home _____

_____

WORK STRESSES
26. I am bored with the work I do .... ❐ Yes ❐ No
27. Other people make too many demands on me .... ❐ Yes ❐ No
28. I have too little control over my own work .... ❐ Yes ❐ No
29. I am not satisfied with the work I do .... ❐ Yes ❐ No
30. Often I feel overwhelmed by my responsibilities .... ❐ Yes ❐ No
31. There is not enough time to finish my work .... ❐ Yes ❐ No
32. I just began a new job .... ❐ Yes ❐ No
33. I just lost my job .... ❐ Yes ❐ No

34. I don't get along with my boss/employees .... ❏ Yes   ❏ No
35. I am having problems with people I work with .... ❏ Yes   ❏ No
36. Other work-related concerns (describe) _____

_____

PERSONAL STRESSES

37. I worry about money a great deal .... ❏ Yes   ❏ No
38. I feel lonely .... ❏ Yes   ❏ No
39. I am bored with my life .... ❏ Yes   ❏ No
40. I am generally concerned about my health .... ❏ Yes   ❏ No
41. I think a lot about dying .... ❏ Yes   ❏ No
42. I have particular concerns relating to my religion .... ❏ Yes   ❏ No
43. Other personal concerns (describe) _____

_____

STRESS EFFECTS

44. I have difficulty falling asleep .... ❏ Yes   ❏ No
45. I have difficulty staying asleep .... ❏ Yes   ❏ No
46. I have difficulty staying awake .... ❏ Yes   ❏ No
47. I feel tired when I wake up in the morning .... ❏ Yes   ❏ No
48. I feel nervous most of the time .... ❏ Yes   ❏ No
49. I often feel depressed .... ❏ Yes   ❏ No
50. I worry a lot .... ❏ Yes   ❏ No
51. I am ill frequently .... ❏ Yes   ❏ No
52. I have considered committing suicide .... ❏ Yes   ❏ No
53. I have some sexual problems .... ❏ Yes   ❏ No
54. I sometimes feel weak or light-headed .... ❏ Yes   ❏ No
55. I often have pains in my shoulders, neck, or back .... ❏ Yes   ❏ No
56. I often feel like crying .... ❏ Yes   ❏ No
57. I drink too much coffee .... ❏ Yes   ❏ No
58. I smoke too much .... ❏ Yes   ❏ No
59. I often drink too much alcohol .... ❏ Yes   ❏ No
60. I eat more than I used to .... ❏ Yes   ❏ No
61. I eat much less than I used to .... ❏ Yes   ❏ No
62. I am concerned about my weight .... ❏ Yes   ❏ No
63. I lose my temper more than I used to .... ❏ Yes   ❏ No
64. I think I might be helped by counseling .... ❏ Yes   ❏ No
65. Other concerns (describe) _____

_____

66. Do you have any personal matter you wish to discuss only with your
    practitioner? .... ❏ Yes   ❏ No

Please use this space to add any other information about yourself that you think will be of help to us.

_____

Last, please circle the answers to any statements or concerns that bother you a great deal.

THANK YOU.

© 1991

Step Two: Sort Through Your Beliefs

Commit yourself to setting aside some time to answer the following series of questions. You might want to do this with a friend or in a group. Your answers would make an excellent starting place for a personal journal that you can update regularly as new insights come to you. Writing your answers down is, in itself, a significant commitment of your time and energy toward creating health. You will learn a great deal about yourself and your relationship with your body. *Note: This is health care that won't cost you a penny.*

Do you understand how inherited cultural attitudes toward our female physiological processes such as menstruation and menopause have contributed to the illnesses suffered by our female bodies? What are the attitudes that you are conscious of?
If you've grown up believing that your menstrual period is "the curse," for example, it's quite likely that your attitude toward your female physiology is less than optimal.

To what extent have you internalized these values?
One of my patients became menopausal following chemotherapy for Hodgkin's disease at the age of twenty-seven. Though she had gone on estrogen replacement therapy for a few years, she eventually stopped it because "the thought of getting my periods back was chilling and repugnant to me," she said. I found her statement of disgust and its implications about her attitude toward her body equally chilling, but such attitudes are all too common.

Do you believe you can be healthy?
Women who have grown up in a household where the norm is to go to the doctor for sleeping pills, anxiety, headaches, and the common cold often internalize the belief that the human body is meant to suffer from all manner of ills and that there's a pill for every ill. Enjoying ill health is the norm for some people. The possibility of a sound body that isn't susceptible to every germ in the environment is inconceivable to them.

What were your childhood/family woundings?

Have you looked at these problems and tried to understand how they have consciously and unconsciously affected your life? These wounds would include history of incest, chronic illness in a parent, unresolved losses such as a divorce in the family, or having a parent abandon the family. Many women's fathers left them when they were children and never returned. Other women have never talked openly about a parent's death. Though the impact of these events is as variable as our fingerprints, there *is* always an impact. How we deal with the emotions surrounding such losses can be a factor in our physical health. Recall that this information is directly related to the health of our first three chakra areas.

One of my patients, for example, developed panic attacks and severe PMS around her fortieth birthday, several months after her father was diagnosed with bowel cancer. Her mother had died suddenly from a reaction to penicillin when my patient was four years old. She was sent to live with an aunt with no explanation, and she was never given permission to speak about it or grieve her loss. She related that she was never really told what had happened to her mother, that no one had cried, and that she got the idea that she was never supposed to mention it. Now with the possible loss of her father, all those long-buried emotions are working their way to the surface—hopefully this time to be expressed in a healthy manner and released.

What purpose does your illness serve? What does it mean to you?

A forty-two-year-old woman, recovering from a car accident, told me that there was no question that before the accident, the pace of her life was moving way too fast. To pay attention to her needs, she literally had to be forced to lie and stare up at the ceiling for several months, as she was now. She regards this accident as a very positive turning point in her life. Leslie Kussman, a film-maker[1] who has multiple sclerosis, said that during one of her morning meditations it occurred to her that perhaps we need to rephrase the question from "What purpose does your illness serve?" to "What is the illness that will serve your purpose?"

Illness is often the only socially acceptable form of Western meditation. Our society is set up such that taking a nap or meditating in the middle of the day to recharge and renew ourselves is frowned upon as hedonistic or irresponsible, but getting the flu is a socially accepted way to rest.

Without slipping into self-blame, think back on the last time you had to miss work because of illness. Was the illness a satisfying break from your routine? What did you get out of it? What did you learn from it? Do you see any way that you could get the same rest without being sick? A young female doctor developed breast cancer while she was pregnant with her third child. As a result, she changed her diet, her work schedule, and her life. Two years later she told me, "My life has never been better. Every day is a joy. I'm glad I had cancer. It saved my life."

If you only had six months to live, would you stay at your current job? Would you stay with your current partner? Would it take a serious illness for you to begin making beneficial changes now?

Are you willing to be open to any messages that your symptoms or illness may have for you?
Before you begin working with this question, please note that a willingness to be open to the message is entirely different from a need to control and figure out the meaning of an illness exactly, especially while it is happening. The former is associated with healing. The latter is just manipulating yourself and is part of our illusion of control. As they say in twelve-step programs, "Whying is dying." Being open to meaning means that you allow the illness to speak to you, often through the language of emotion, imagery, and pain. Your intellectual understanding of your situation may well come only after an illness is over with.

Back in the 1980s, when our culture was learning about the mind/body connection, people would actually ask questions like, "Why are you needing to create cancer?" as though the intellect could figure that out through cause-and-effect thinking. These addictive questions keep the intellect running in circles and can lead to "thought" addiction. Being open to meaning is an attitude, a process. As Anne Wilson Schaef says, "It's 'waiting with,' not 'waiting for.'"

When faced with an illness, what is your usual reaction?

Learning the meaning behind the illness is a process that doesn't lend itself to questions like "Why me, why now?" Evy McDonald writes, "Don't get caught in the tangling web of why. The search for the explanation and meaning of your illness can lead to frustration and desperation and can paralyze your ability to make decisions and take action."

In the days of the ancient Greeks, a messenger would be sent to the leader with news of the current battle. If the news was bad, the messenger would be killed. Your task is not to kill the messenger of illness by ignoring it, complaining about it, or simply suppressing the symptoms. Your task is to examine your life carefully, observing and searching for those discordant areas where harmony, fulfillment, and love are lacking.

What is preventing you from healing yourself?

"Waiting with" this question is a good meditation. Don't expect an answer to spring forth immediately, though it sometimes does. Back in the 1980s, I repeatedly asked myself what changes I needed in my life and what I needed to do next. The answer that kept coming was simple: *Rest. You're burned out.* Taking *action* on that insight took over a year. It was, and always is, a process.

Some people never heal because they believe that if they were healed, they would be alone and abandoned. Being sick in this culture can be a very powerful way to get our needs met legitimately. Saying to someone, "Please hold me—I feel ill" is quite different from saying, "Please hold me—I want to be held because it feels good and I like it." The first sentence uses illness to justify the universal human need for closeness. The second sentence simply states the need clearly. Many of us don't know what intimacy would be without using our wounds to get it, are brought up to be ashamed of our needs, and learn very early to bond with each other via our wounds.

During my residency training, I was very proud of the way I had handled a certain woman's care, and I decided to tell one of my nurse colleagues who also knew this patient well and who could celebrate with me. When I told her, she said, "Don't break your arm patting yourself on the back." I was stunned. I had simply been expressing a natural human need to share my success with a colleague who would understand its implications. When I was growing up, my parents had always believed that each of us children needed his or her "place in the sun." We were routinely recognized for our gifts and achievements, and we felt good about ourselves and each other when these were shared. But my nurse colleague had obviously learned that it was "not okay to blow your own horn." Often, the only time good things are said about the life of another person is at their funeral. This is tragic. Each of us needs to accept that no matter how strong, independent, and healthy we become, we will always need others for companionship, celebration, and joyful living.

Do you still take on everyone else's problems and put yourself last? This is the classic dilemma for women. Feeling the need to be the healer and peacemaker for our entire family or place of work is a pattern that many of us learn in childhood. To create health, a woman must face this tendency squarely and commit to changing it.

Here's an example: Last year, my children (ages ten and twelve at the time) were complaining repeatedly about one of my colleagues who is a good friend of mine. This woman has helped with the research for this book and has been a very entertaining companion for me during the process. My children perceived that my friend was taking up too much of my time and that I was not as available to them as they would like me to be. I noticed, however, that when Ann and Kate were playing with their friends, reading, or living their own lives fully, they ignored me for hours, even days on end. And during the many days and hours when my friend wasn't around, my children came and went as they pleased focusing on their own needs. They were not necessarily interested in my companionship if they had other things going on. They became extremely interested in me, however, the moment my entertaining friend walked in the door.

To deal with this situation, I initially spent hours listening to Ann and Kate's complaints and trying to negotiate only *their* needs. Then I realized that, on an unconscious level, they didn't expect *me* to have any needs for friendship, laughs, and companionship *separate* from them. When I realized this, I let them know very clearly that I also had needs—individual needs that were as important (not *more* important—*as* important) as theirs. I came to see that I had to take a stand for my own needs as well as the needs of my children. Together, we began working on becoming conscious of the ways in which they, unconsciously, didn't expect me to have a life separate from them, and the ways in which I have been socialized to sacrifice my life for their needs.

When I became clear about this situation and what needed to happen, I had a dream about being given a red 1950s-style gas pump that pumped milk. The name painted on the pump was "The Mother." I had to keep the pump refrigerated so that the milk wouldn't spoil. I kept trying to think of who I was going to give the milk to. My family didn't need it—we don't drink milk. When I woke up, I realized that the pump represented me and that it was now time to let go of an obsolete kind of mothering (a 1950s gas pump that could service only one car—perform only one role—at a time).

Do you fully understand the workings of your female body and how intimately your thoughts and feelings are connected to your physical health?

Your body experiences every thought and sensation as a "physiological reality." By thinking of the taste and smell of chocolate, you trigger many of the same physical reactions as when you actually eat a piece. Our bodies are not static structures. The amount of sunlight shining on us in a day affects our physiology. The quality of the sounds we hear affects our physiology. The quality of the relationships we have with others affects our physiology.

Many women don't understand not only how intimately our bodies are affected by our environments but the basic anatomy of our bodies. Many women who have had surgery don't know exactly what was taken out and what was left in. Yet knowing precisely where the organs in our bodies are is very reassuring. During my residency I once did an emergency appendectomy on a woman. She also required removal of her uterus and ovaries because of a life-threatening infection. Several days later, I learned that she thought her appendix was as big as a large melon and that now her entire lower abdomen was completely empty because we had removed it. I explained to her that her large and small intestine completely filled her lower abdomen despite the loss of her pelvic organs, which was very helpful information for her in her recovery because it helped her feel that the loss was less overwhelming. Showing her drawings of her anatomy was also helpful—she learned that her appendix was smaller than her little finger.

One woman said to me, "Oh, my pelvis is being taken care of by the Lahey Clinic!" Instead of believing that the Lahey Clinic is responsible for her pelvis, she would be much better served by assuming responsibility for her pelvis herself.

Many women feel much more confident about their bodies when they have all their records in hand, having read and understood them. At Women to Women any patient who wants copies of her records, including pelvic exam results, Pap smear and mammogram reports, and reports of any surgeries is welcome to have them. We decode medical language for them as necessary so that they know exactly what is going on. We encourage women to get personal copies of all their records from other health facilities, particularly reports of any surgeries they have had, so that they know exactly what is going on inside their bodies, how things look, and what is left. Keeping copies of her own records can also expedite a woman's health care if she is traveling or has to make an emergency room visit. On the other hand, some women won't feel compelled to do this if they are comfortable with the care they are receiving and have no trouble yielding to the care of others.

Like many health care providers, Women to Women keeps mirrors in all exam rooms so that women can see their cervixes and watch their Pap smears being taken if they wish to. Not everyone wants to do this, but we offer the choice. Many physicians will also provide patients with videotapes of their surgeries.

Do you know where your organs are? If not, consider looking through an encyclopedia or standard anatomy guide. Get to know your body in health, not just in sickness!

Are you following your life's purpose?

Our bodies are designed to function best when we're involved in activities and work that feel exactly right to us. Our health is enhanced when we engage in deeply creative work that is satisfying to *us*—not just because it pleases our boss, husband, or mother. This work can range from gardening, to computer programming, to welding.

Unfortunately, our culture doesn't believe that creativity is valuable for its own sake. To be considered worthwhile, an activity must be associated with tangible rewards or productivity. We consider the worth of an activity to be how much money is associated with it. For many people, going to work is more like "making a dying" than "making a living." People often put up with very unsatisfactory work environments because of the "benefits." I call this "dying for our benefits." Financial and gynecological health are intimately connected. The second chakra area of the body (uterus, tubes, ovaries, lower back) is affected by financial stresses. Health in this area is created when we tap into our ability to be creative and prosperous at the same time.

Becoming both creative and prosperous often involves as a first step a change in our attitude toward money and work. To do this, we need to understand the dynamics of work and money— areas long dominated by men. We must be very clear on our culture's belief in the zero-sum model and how this affects us. For instance, many people believe, "If I am doing well, someone else has to suffer. There is only so much to go around." Or vice versa, "If someone else is doing well, then there is no chance for me to do well also. There is no way to get ahead." Each of us must see how deeply these beliefs are embedded within us and how completely they will control our financial realities until we decide to change them.

The headlines daily tell us how many people are out of work and how bad the economy is. This affects us all, and it's clear that we're in the middle of a major economic shift. At the same time, I see women daily who have had their most profitable year ever, using their gifts and talents. When we allow the media to discourage us from dipping into the creative well inside us to come up with ideas that can support us, we give our power away—and become part of the problem.

The work of Joe Dominguez, a former Wall Street analyst and co-author with Vicki Robin of *Your Money or Your Life*, is a good place to start examining these destructive beliefs and turning them around.[2] From Joe and Vicki, I learned that money is the substance for which we exchange our life-energy. The first thing you must do to heal your relationship with money is to figure out how many hours you have left in your life—your total life-energy. Then you calculate how much your work actually costs you in terms of your life-energy. If you work so many hours that you require expensive vacations and frequent illnesses to balance the energy drain of work, you may well find that your work is worth much less per hour than you are actually being paid, once you factor in the "hidden" costs of vacation and illness. The program then helps you balance your relationship with money by determining how much fulfillment you get out of every purchase, compared with how much it has cost you in terms of your life-energy.

Your next step is to consciously make a decision to spend more money on the things or activities that bring you the most fulfillment and less money on the stuff that ultimately has no meaning. What happens is that eventually your expenditures decrease and the fulfillment that you derive from them increases. When you begin to look at money in this way, your entire relationship with it changes. You begin to see that it is not necessary to put off doing what you've always wanted to do until "later." Some of my greatest pleasures, such as walking on the beach, reading, and going to movies, cost almost nothing. It need not cost you much money to begin living your life in a more fulfilling manner. By going through the Dominguez-Robin program, I realized that my free time was priceless to me and that I would never again be able to work in any job, regardless of high pay and good benefits, if the job didn't also fulfill my soul and give me ample time to create my life on my own terms.

Currently, the work of nurturing (not figured into the gross national product) is not acknowledged, rewarded, or shared equally between the sexes. A friend of mine has started to rectify this situation on a personal level by drawing a "salary" from her husband for her daily work as a homemaker, mother, and social secretary. For my part, I'm starting to teach my daughters the importance of financial independence from men. Every woman needs to consider how she can contribute to changing this cultural mindset.

Have you designed your life in a way that fulfills both your innermost needs and your desire to be of service to others?
It is entirely possible to develop yourself fully, meet your innermost emotional needs, and at the same time work with others for the common good. Our culture has taught women just the opposite: that they must sacrifice themselves and their needs for the good of others. But you cannot quench the thirst of others when your own cup is always empty. Many studies have shown, for example, that women who are at risk for breast cancer sacrifice work they love and optimal self-development in order to nurture others. It is not the sacrifice alone that creates the health problem—it is the unexpressed resentment that results from it. When a woman doesn't believe that she has a right to self-development, she won't even allow herself to acknowledge her resentment. Her body wisdom must then bring it to her attention so that she can make a balance.

Do you regularly acknowledge your strengths, gifts, talents, and accomplishments?
A large part of creating health—or anything else—is giving ourselves credit for where we are now. Learning how to take in praise—to let ourselves really *feel* success and completion physically—is a skill that can be learned. Annie Gill O'Toole, a business consultant who has worked with us at Women to Women, and helped us create new forms and structures that serve our goals, points out that a big reason why people get stuck and can't create better lives is that they don't give themselves credit for what they *have* created. If you chronically skip this step of acknowledging your creations and continue to focus only on what you have yet to accomplish, then your subconscious hears only "You are not enough. You haven't done enough. There is so

much more to do. You will never be enough"—instead of "Good job. You've come a long way."

Many women live with the belief that there is too much work to do, that they will never be finished, and that therefore they can never rest and appreciate themselves. This belief comes directly out of our cultural obsession with productivity and the belief that our worth depends upon what we can produce for others, whether this be children or goods and services. Operating under this belief system, we create more and more work that doesn't feel complete or fulfilling. But optimal ovarian health, for example, requires that we acknowledge our creativity as an outward manifestation of our deepest inner need for self-expression. This creativity need not be measured in dollars or productivity to be a valuable contribution to our health and that of others. When we allow others to exploit, judge, and control our innate gifts and talents, we put our health at risk.

One of my medical colleagues learned this lesson well when she developed an ovarian cyst while working on the faculty of a major medical center. Florence had originally gone to work in this center because she didn't believe that she had the skills necessary to start her own practice on her own terms using her creativity to the fullest. Following her ovarian removal, however, Florence knew intuitively that she needed to leave her workplace, that it was somehow dangerous for her to stay. In this work environment, others did not value her innate feminine creativity and as a result she didn't value it herself when she was there. Florence knew that she was not yet strong enough to hold her own feminine viewpoint without at least some support from others, but the ovarian "sacrifice" really got her attention and mobilized her to make a change. She left the medical center and started her own highly successful practice. Only years later, after learning about ovarian wisdom, was she able to appreciate how profoundly her creativity had been at risk in her original work setting.

Women's skills and voices need to be heard throughout all areas of endeavor: in industry, education, medicine, and other professions. Women must start by listening to themselves and hearing their own voices. Our self-development is a planetary priority. We have much to contribute but too often we are unsure of ourselves.

Think of one thing that you're proud of that you've accomplished today, this week, or this year. Feel your accomplishment(s) fully. Take it in, until it's more than just intellectual knowledge. Take yourself right into your heart. If we can't feel good about our skills and accomplishments, no one else can, either.

If you were in optimal health, what would your life look like?
(Answer this one in the form of an exercise.) Sit facing a friend who fully supports you. Have this person ask you the following: If anything at all were possible, quickly, easily, and now, what would your life look like? Who would be in it? What would you be doing? Where would you be living?

Begin answering your partner out loud. Give yourself two or three minutes to do this. Don't think about it. Pretend you're a child, creating your life exactly as you want it, as if anything at all were possible, easily, quickly, and *now*—no holds barred. How would your life be? Your inner guidance knows exactly what your heart's desire is. When you open your mouth and remove the brakes—and get the judge out of your head for a minute— your inner guidance will come up with the right answers.

After you have completed the first part of this exercise, imagine that it is one year from today. You have been able to create everything that you wanted, plus more. Everything that you dreamed could come true is now true. You are celebrating and looking back over this phenomenal year. You've created all of it almost magically, through the power of connecting with your inner guidance and wisdom. Tell your partner in detail about everything that you've created, share how excited you are, and invite her or him to celebrate with you. After you feel this scene fully, begin talking and keep talking for two to three minutes without censoring yourself. Just let it flow—like a child playing make-believe.[3]

You could also write this exercise, but many people associate writing with school and formal education and "getting it right." If this is the case for you, writing your answers may stifle your inner guidance.

Imagine back to when you were eleven. What did you love to do? Who were you? Who did you think you would be? Imagine yourself now, telling the world who you are—and who you are going to become, no holds barred. Speak it into a tape—tell it to a friend or to the wind. Call that eleven-year-old back, now. She's got something to tell you.

Step Three: Respect and Release Your Emotions

The investigation of suffering is the path to joy.
                                                    —Stephen Levine

Emotions are a vital part of our inner guidance. Like our illnesses, our dreams, and our lives—our emotions are ours, and we must own them and pay attention to them. We must learn to feel our emotions, release our judgments about them, and be grateful for their guidance. They let us know how we are directing our life-energy. Chronic anger or sadness, by the law of attraction, tends to attract situations to us that are filled with anger or sadness. Daily doses of joy and appreciation of ourselves and others tend to attract joy and appreciation into our lives.

Children automatically know how to feel their emotions and then let go. When they're hurt, they stop and cry. After just a short time, they're back out playing again. Elisabeth Kübler-Ross points out that a child's natural anger and emotional outburst around it lasts about fifteen seconds. Shaming or blaming the child for that anger, however, often blocks its natural release. The child's natural emotion may get stuck and become a form of self-pity that remains with the person for years! Kübler-Ross points out that people who weren't allowed a natural expression of anger are often "marinated in self-pity" as adults and are difficult to be around. This self-pity is the same thing as self-centeredness. It takes a great deal of energy to hold in our natural emotions. In fact, it's exhausting. If we haven't felt our feelings regularly during a period of personal crisis or change, we often have a backlog of sealed-off emotion stored up in our bodies.

Emotional suppression is a pattern that gets passed down from generation to generation. Many women have natural rage that's been held in check for decades. They hold in oceans of tears that are yet to be shed. One very overweight woman in my practice told me that her mother and grandmother had taught her how to gorge on chocolate whenever their husbands were out of town and they were feeling lonely. The fat on her hips, she told me, represented three generations of stagnated emotional energy held down with chocolate.

Emotional release, or what I've already called emotional incision and drainage, is an organic healing process that is completely natural and safe.[4] When I first went to an intensive workshop and sat with people who were doing deep process work, I felt as if I were in Labor and Delivery—standing by, allowing people to give birth to themselves. All of us have this ability within us. Dorothy's ruby slippers could get her home to Kansas all by herself—she just didn't know it. She thought she needed the wizard.

Making sounds is an important part of emotional release. Myron McClellan, a musician specializing in the healing power of sound, says that "singing is part of the emotional body's digestive system." Singing is one form of healing sound. Wailing or deep sobbing is another. Anne Wilson Schaef teaches that these sounds are like grappling hooks that go through the body, cleaning out toxins and old debris.[5] A woman recently wrote me, "I have taken several months of training in the martial arts simply to help release some of the tensions and muscular inabilities that I have felt in my body. An interesting by-product is that I have found my voice. In the process of learning tae kwon do, I had to be able to give a huge yell with the punches and the kicks that are part of the practice. I had never before in my life been able to make a noise with that much authority. As a child, I learned that if one didn't make noise, then one could possibly avoid aggravating or irritating one's abusers and, possibly, avoid abuse. I have carried that legacy with me for many years, even silencing my grief when my husband was killed. In other cultures women are traditionally taught to keen loudly to express grief, sorrow, and rage at death. I had never made that kind of sound, though I certainly have wanted and needed to do so. Not until now, six years after my husband's death, have I been able to make those sounds. They came, not only because of the karate yell, but as a result of the deep healings to my respiratory tract that I have been able to accomplish through macrobiotics and oriental medicine."

In many ways, the year or two *after* a traumatic experience are more difficult than the experience itself—possibly because we have support for crises in this culture but are then expected, both from within ourselves and from outside, to get on with it when it's over. But this can only happen once we've allowed ourselves the space and time to work through our emotions.

A young woman who had recovered from Hodgkin's disease with the help of a bone marrow transplant a year before came to see me recently. The chemotherapy had caused an early menopause, and we were working with estrogen replacement therapy to help her hot flashes. She was having problems with fatigue and weakness, but there was no sign that the cancer had returned. In going back over her history, she burst into tears in my office and told me that she'd never cried once during the year in which her diagnosis was made or during her entire chemotherapy experience. She had not allowed herself to experience her fear. She had simply gone through it as best she could.

A year later, there was no crisis in this woman's life. Her body was well, but she still didn't feel better. She didn't have the energy to exercise, and she didn't want to cook nourishing meals for herself. After sitting with this for a while, she realized that she needed time to process her recent experience emotionally.

When I first visited an acupuncturist, she told me that in Chinese medicine, emotions such as anger are viewed simply as *energy*. Many women have a problem with the direct expression of their anger and use it to manipulate others instead. But anger can be a powerful ally. When we feel angry, the anger is always related to something we need to acknowledge for ourselves. It is not necessarily about the situation or person that evoked it. It is always a sign that we have allowed ourselves to be violated in some way. That's one of the reasons why anger is so often part of PMS.

All women must learn that no one can *make* us angry. Our anger is ours, and it is telling us something we need to know. Eleanor Roosevelt once said, "No one can make you feel inferior [or angry, or sad] without your permission." Anger is energy—our personal jet fuel. It is telling us that something needs adjustment in our lives.

It is telling us that there is something we want that we don't know we want. Next time you get angry, say to yourself, "Ah! My inner guidance is working. What is it I want here? What do I want to have happen here?" Anger is often an expression of the energy required to make that adjustment. This emotion is only dangerous if we deny it and stuff it in our bodies. Anger and all other "negative" emotions can serve us well when we don't turn them in on ourselves as depression or lash out with them against others.

Step Four: Learn to Listen to Your Body

Learning to listen to and respect your body is a process that requires patience and compassion. You can begin this process by paying attention to your body as you read through the following list. Go slowly and come back to it as needed.

• Make note of those things in your life that are difficult, painful, joyful, and the like. As these things come up, notice your breathing, your heart rate, and your bodily sensations. What are they? Where are they?

• Pay attention to what your body feels like. Do certain parts of you feel numb? tired? Do you feel like crying? Do parts of you feel like crying? These feelings are your body's wisdom. They are part of your inner guidance system.

• What is your image of yourself? How do you think you look to the world? To yourself? Do these images match? Many women, through years of chronic dissatisfaction with their bodies and chronic dieting, develop an unrealistic image of themselves. Some feel much heavier than they actually are. But women who are in touch with their inner guidance will often appear taller and more imposing physically than their actual body size indicates.

• Notice how you routinely talk to your body. What happens when you look in the mirror each morning? Do you criticize your face, your legs, your hair? Do you routinely apologize to others for how you look? Or do you give your body positive messages, such as "Thank you very much for digesting last night's dinner without any conscious input from me"? Cultivate the link between your mouth and your ear—and the rest of you—so that you get used to hearing yourself. Barbara Levine, in her book *Your Body Believes Every Word,* told of a friend who always developed rectal pain during her period. Levine asked her if she thought of her period as a "pain in the ass." The woman gasped and admitted that that was exactly how she felt about it.

• Pay attention to your thoughts and observe how they affect your body.

• Notice what your body needs on a daily basis. Are you hungry? Do you have to go to the bathroom? Are you tired? Do you routinely ignore your body?

• Understand that your health is at risk if you are constantly undermining certain parts or functions of your body. If someone at work has a cold, you automatically undermine your body's ability to stay healthy by obsessing about how many germs you've been exposed to. Instead, say to your body, "Don't worry—I know that you have the ability to stay healthy when I nourish and rest you optimally."

• Notice what fears you hold about your body. Do you avoid touching your breasts because you are afraid of finding lumps? Instead, learn about breast anatomy and learn to touch your own with respect and love. You can transform and heal your entire relationship with them.

• Notice whether there are parts of your body that you have disowned. What are they? Do you consider parts of yourself "unacceptable"? A patient of mine had frequent abdominal pain until she was thirty-five. In her family, she learned that it was completely unacceptable for a woman to pass gas, even though it was okay for her father and her brothers. Thus, instead of allowing routine intestinal gas to leave her body as necessary, she literally held on to it with resulting abdominal pain. Once she realized that she had disowned an entire natural body function, she learned how to allow this function and became free of abdominal pain.

• When you experience a bodily sensation such as back pain, "a gut reaction," a headache, or abdominal pain, pay attention to it. Are emotions such as anger or fear connected with certain parts of your body? When a sensation arises in your body, stop what you are doing, lie down, breathe, and *wait with* your symptom, emotion, or feeling. You may be surprised at what other feelings or insights come up.

• Stand in front of a mirror regularly, and thank your body for all it has done for you. Notice what comes up when you do this. Write the following sentence down on a piece of paper and tape it to the mirror: *"I accept myself unconditionally right now."* I often write it on a prescription blank and hand it to my patient with the following instructions: "Say this sentence out loud to yourself in the mirror while gazing into your eyes. Do this twice per day for thirty days." You can *learn* to accept your body unconditionally *right now,* regardless of where you are starting. When you do this exercise, you will learn a great deal about the "inner critics" that live within you. Give them a name, such as "Esmeralda" or "George," so that you won't take them so personally next time they put you or your body down. When you don't take their criticisms personally, you can tell them to be quiet. Or you can even choose to laugh at them.

• Remember always that 90 percent of your bodily functions take place without your conscious input. Who keeps your heart beating? Who metabolizes your food? Who tells you when you need to replenish your fluid intake by drinking water? Who heals your skin when you cut yourself? Who tells your ears to listen to beautiful music? Who tells your eyes to see beautiful sunsets? Acknowledge that your body is a miracle.

Step Five: Learn to Respect Your Body

Almost all women in the United States have a body image distortion because of the millions of images of "perfect" airbrushed women that the media flash at us continually. We begin comparing ourselves with these icons of perfection even before puberty. Thus, we often relate to our bodies via negative comparisons: "My hips are too fat, my breasts are too small, my knees are ugly, my hair is too thin."

Our cultural obsession with thinness really "clicked in" for me when I was visiting a friend at her beach house. Many of her other friends were there as well, most of them involved with the fashion or entertainment industry and thin, tan, and very fashionably attired. When we went swimming, I was amazed to find myself feeling fat, dumpy, and short (compared to all of them). I thought that I had successfully dealt with all of these issues long before. I simply allowed myself to feel these feelings of inferiority for a while, without trying to change anything.

I gave up weighing myself several years ago, and I regard myself as strong and capable. Though my body is *not* the type that one would see modeling clothes in magazines, every year I'm more and more at peace with that, though I know that I'm not immune to the adverse impact of the media on the body image of average women.

When I arrived home from that visit, I realized a few things:

- Even after years of awareness that a "perfect," thin, model's body is often destructive to women (and men) on many levels, the desire to have this body is deeply embedded in our minds.

- The desire for what society believes is the "perfect body" is completely understandable. I could even respect myself fully for my humanness in having this desire. I am powerless over it. (By this, I mean that the desire rises up unbidden. I have no control over it.) I *do* have control and power over what I choose to do with a thought or desire, however. This is why it is so important to begin to hear ourselves and our thoughts.

- The culturally induced desire for a "perfect" body doesn't have to ruin my respect, caring, or love for the body I have. And if I don't respect, care, and love the body I have, no one will or even *can*. I vow to treat myself and my body with kindness in the future, especially when "putdowns" and comparisons come up from deep inside.

Articles in *TV Guide* and *People* magazine have documented that most media personalities have had or will have plastic surgery at some point in their careers. The models of perfection who beam into our global living rooms every day set up a standard that is impossible for most to aspire to without resorting to measures such as surgery.[6] In a way this is comforting. They are human, after all, just as we all are—subject to the same wrinkles and sags as the rest of us. But their industry standards demand a certain image, and so they meet it through surgery and constant exercise and diet. On the

TV or movie set, someone follows them around the studio all day with a blow dryer, people a friend of mine refers to as "the beauty police." On some level, almost all women would look their very best (or at least their culturally determined best) if they devoted the same amount of time, energy, and money to their appearance as our cultural media icons do.

Michael Marron's *Makeover Magic* shows before-and-after pictures of famous women such as Shirley Jones and Phyllis Diller.[7] In the "before" photos, the women are entirely devoid of makeup. They look like ordinary women—in most cases, one wouldn't even recognize them on the street. The "after" pictures, taken after their makeup has been applied and their hair restyled, are entirely different. These are the stars we recognize. A woman looks strikingly different after her face has been "made up" by an artist. This book is very healing because it shows that the standard held up for us women is impossible to meet not only for us, but for the famous women themselves.

Yet the ancient arts of adornment can be part of caring for ourselves. Wearing makeup and nail polish are healthy choices for many women, not a sellout at all. They're not choices everyone is comfortable with, but all nonharmful modes of self-expression should be honored.

Our approach to dressing, makeup, hair, and personal care can be well served by the wisdom of Dolly Parton, who said, "Find out who you are, then do it on purpose." If we can find out who we are on the inside, we can then express it on the outside. As Coco Chanel once said, "Adornment is never anything except a reflection of the heart." I've decided that I like to wear skirts that are long and warm, and I don't care what the season's lengths are. I've developed a personal style in clothing that suits me and that is not subject to the whims of fashion designers. I've healed my relationship with fashion, clothing, and style by first becoming comfortable with who I am. I call this "fashion from the inside out."

If we believe that in order to look good, we must be uncomfortable, we are in danger of losing touch with real life. I won't wear clip-on earrings or high heels for this reason. If we're dissatisfied with ourselves when we're not wearing makeup or dressed in the latest fashion, we're not creating health or balance in our lives.

We're in danger of what Anne Schaef calls "romance addiction"—always requiring our bodies, our homes, and our lives to look "just right" like a movie set. Some women's husbands have never seen them without makeup. Some still dress behind closed doors so that their partners won't see their bodies in broad daylight, when the imperfections catch the sunlight.

The next time a friend comes to the door unexpectedly, *don't* apologize for the way you or your house or apartment looks. Chances are theirs looks the same way. Just invite them in, and ignore the toilet paper or whatever else is sitting in the middle of the dining room table. They came to visit *you*, not your spotless kitchen or your perfect image. Notice what you learn from not apologizing.

Step Six: Acknowledge a Higher Power or Inner Wisdom

> There is an unseen force, a spiritual dimension, guiding our lives like a loving parent guiding its child.
>
> —Pythia Peay[8]

Our bodies are permeated and nourished by spiritual energy and guidance. Having faith and trust in this reality is an important part of creating health. When a woman has faith in something greater than her intellect or her present circumstances, she is in touch with her inner source of power. Each of us has within us a divine spark. We are inherently a part of God/Goddess/Source. Jesus said that the kingdom of heaven is within, and we can make this spiritual connection through our inner guidance. We need go no further than ourselves to find it.

Learning to connect with our inner wisdom, our spirituality, is not difficult, but neither our intellect nor our ego can control either the connection or the results. The first step is to hold the intent to connect with divine guidance. The second step is to release our expectations of what will happen as a result. The third step is to wait for a response by being open to noticing the patterns of our lives that relate to the original intent.

Each of us has a guardian angel available for guidance. But we have to ask for it. Guidance is always available, but we have to be open to receiving it. Seeing the patterns that connect is a way of looking at life. This is the paradigm shift I mentioned before. Understanding the big picture doesn't mean getting stuck in the particular moment. Gaining access to spiritual guidance means looking at the pattern of our lives over time. As David Spangler said, "Dreams, events, a book, the words of a friend: all of this might be *one word* from an angelic being."

About two years ago, I was standing by my bed on a sunny Friday morning, getting ready for the day. I read through my favorite meditations that I've written down in a small book made of hand-crafted paper. I decided to say aloud a statement taken from Frances Scovell Shinn's book, *The Game of Life and How to Play It*.[9] I spoke it out loud clearly with sincere intent: "Infinite spirit, give me a definite lead, reveal to me my perfect self-expression. Show me which talent I am to make use of now." That very afternoon I received a call from an acquaintance who is a literary agent. "I think it is time you wrote a book," he said. It wasn't until much later that day that I put those two events together. Sometimes the guidance comes easily and quickly. When it does, though, you sometimes have to go through the part of your intellect that tells you you're making it up and are crazy for believing this stuff.

Though each of us is part of a greater whole, we are also individuals. The unique part of this whole that we each embody must be expressed fully in order to create health, happiness, and spiritual growth for ourselves and others. The way to best express this divine part of ourselves is by becoming all of who we are. Our bodies direct us toward full personal expression by letting us know what feels good and "right" and what doesn't. Illness is often a sign that we are somehow off track from our life's purpose. That is why Dr. Bernie Siegel says, "Illness is God's reset button."

Many doctors are open to this realm of mystery, too, but they don't dare to say anything. A highly skilled intuitive here in southern Maine once said to me, "Someday I'm going to have a cocktail party at my house and invite all the doctors in this area who've come to have readings. You will all stand around and be amazed at how many of you there are—and also at who is here."

When we invite the sacred into our lives by sincerely asking our inner wisdom, or higher power, or God for guidance in our lives, we're invoking great power. This can't be taken lightly. The reason people are cynical about this and make fun of it is that they are afraid. When you sincerely invite in the sacred (your inner guidance or spirit) to assist you with your life, you are granting permission for your life to change. Those areas of your life that no longer serve your highest purpose may start to disintegrate—and this can be frightening. Caroline Myss says, "Wiping out a marriage or a job is a day at the beach for an angel."

Believing in angels, having your astrological chart done, or getting an intuitive reading doesn't excuse anyone from the work of healing and becoming whole. Remember that anything can be used addictively—even so-called spiritual pursuits. Too many people use their "spiritual practices" to avoid addressing the difficult areas of their lives. Using crystals, New Age music, and astrology, while drinking four ounces of alcohol every night, will not help you heal. Doing meditation faithfully twice a day and being beaten up by your husband every night will not keep you healthy. All the "spirituality" in the world won't do your human homework for you. Only you can take the action necessary to compose your life. As one of my twelve-step friends told me, "God moves mountains— bring a shovel."

To reconnect with their innate spirituality, many women have to get past years of religious abuse, particularly if they've been victimized by organized cults or patriarchal religions. It's no wonder that being angry with God and struggling with the concept of a "higher power" or "inner wisdom" is a reality for so many, when God has been portrayed as a vengeful, righteous being outside of human ability to understand or know. Some women are stuck at a very childlike stage in which they feel, "If there was a God, *he* would never have let this happen to me." One of my colleagues says, "If I make God something separate from me and outside of myself, then I get to accuse God of punishing me whenever my life doesn't go well."

We are all spiritual beings. Connection with spirit is inherently part of being human. For centuries our culture has tried to control our inherent spirituality via religion. Though some women may gain access to their spirituality through organized religions, too many religions rely on static dogma and rules that serve to split us from our daily spirituality. Spirituality is free-flowing and ever-changing. Though it is clear that most religions were originally based on the immediate and profound spiritual insights of their founders, most organized religions today lack the flexibility and ongoing evolution necessary to truly be spiritually connected.

Partly in response to so many years of male-based religions, many women today are drawn to different aspects of "the Great Goddess." As women we need "a sexually affirming image of power and beauty as a focus for prayer and meditation," says Patricia Reis.[10] Having internalized God as male, the Goddess images that are now rising represent much-needed balance.

I have personally found the Motherpeace Tarot cards to be an extremely helpful intermediary step for getting in touch with my inner guidance. The Motherpeace deck is a set of seventy-eight original images, created by Vicki Noble and Karen Vogel, that incorporate visual images drawn from myth, art, and theology.[11] The Motherpeace images are based on women's culture throughout history. Because the images are archetypal and have universal symbolism, they reflect our unconscious patterns back to our conscious minds. The accompanying reference book and guide to the meaning of the images, *Motherpeace: A Way to the Goddess Through Myth, Art, and Tarot*,[12] includes a great deal of scholarly research that supports women's wisdom. When I am struggling with making a decision or faced with a dilemma that has no easy answers, I will often spread out my Motherpeace deck in front of me. After quieting myself, I ask the question: "What is the highest teaching available to me through this situation?" Then, I draw a card. Recently I was trying to decide whether to do a video project on women's health with a producer in California whose work I admired and who wanted to create something with me. A very small part of me was hesitant to go ahead, and I drew a card for guidance around this issue. The card I drew, "the Hierophant," shows two young girls kneeling before a male priestlike figure clothed in some of the garb associated with the Goddess. It is symbolic of the way in which women's power has been usurped through the ages by the male priesthood. To me, the card meant either that I was putting the producer on a pedestal, or that producing the video might put me on a pedestal as an authority for other women. Since the essence of my teaching is that each of us must become her own authority, drawing the Hierophant served as a caution sign from my inner guidance. It confirmed the subtle hesitation I had already felt about moving forward with the project. Some aspect of either me or this project had to change before I could go ahead with it.

Regardless of what you believe about spirituality, it is important to bring a sense of the sacred into your everyday life. Spirituality pervades all that I do. My spirituality is not set aside for special days such as Christmas, in special buildings called churches, synagogues, or temples. My spirituality is every part of me. On some level I feel part of God/Goddess/All That Is—not separate from it. When I'm filling out insurance forms, I'm in touch with my spirituality (sometimes). When I'm in the operating room, I'm very much in touch with my spirituality. I'm especially in touch with my spirituality when I'm assisting women in opening to their inner guidance system. This is because reaching out to another to help her heal and connect with her spirituality also helps me heal and connect with mine.

Like many women, I feel a deep spiritual connection with nature. Many people find peace and comfort in a special place, a place that they may have gone to as children to feel held close by the nurturing qualities of nature. Women often tell me about special trees, rocks, hills, or other places that connect them very strongly with their own spirituality. Time spent alone in a natural setting is often a catalyst for connection with your spirituality.

A powerful way to tune in to the natural world is to notice what phase the moon is in and see if this natural waxing and waning has any effect on your body, emotions, or perceptions.[13] Notice what effect the seasons have on you. Does the coming of autumn wake up your senses and find you braced for new beginnings—or does this happen for you in the spring? Find out when the equinoxes and solstices are. For centuries, people felt that more spiritual power was available to them at these times. All major religious holidays are held around these times. You don't have to study anything—just be aware of the moon and the rhythms of nature. I live on a tidal river and enjoy the changing water levels outside my window, knowing that, like my body, they're connected with the phases of the moon.

When I was growing up, my father used to go to church on

Sundays because he liked the church and his family had always gone there. My mother, on the other hand, often went for a walk in the woods. "He has his church, I have mine," she said. Each woman must find her own spiritual center and her own inner guidance. And for each woman it will be different.

Regardless of whether we believe in angels, God, Jesus Christ, the human spirit, the Blessed Virgin, the Great Spirit, or the Goddess Gaia, being in tune with our spiritual resources is a vital healing force. Committing ourselves to remember our spiritual selves and receive guidance for our lives is part of creating health.

Step Seven: Reclaim the Fullness of Your Mind

Women need to know that they are capable of intelligent thought, and they need to know it right now.

—Adrienne Rich

The positive thing about writing is that you connect with yourself in the deepest way, and that's heaven. You get a chance to know who you are, to know what you think. You begin to have a relationship with your mind.

—Natalie Goldberg[14]

If we are to reclaim the wisdom of our bodies, we must also reclaim our intellects, our minds, and our ability to think. Once we have experienced how intimately our thoughts and bodily symptoms are related and how intelligent we are, our thinking is less distracted by cultural hypnosis and we trust our inner voice. We question our assumptions more critically, thus freeing ourselves from the mental habits of a lifetime.

Journal writing, writing practice, and meditation are methods that many have used to successfully get in touch with their inner voices and get to know their minds. Proprioceptive writing (PW) taught me to trust my mind and inner wisdom. Originally developed by Dr. Linda Trichter Metcalf, this writing process engages the intellect, the intuition, and the imagination simultaneously and is done to baroque music.[15] (Baroque music has been found to synchronize brain waves at about sixty cycles per second, a frequency associated with increased alpha brain waves and enhanced creativity.)

I learned through my writing that my thoughts have order, direction, and intelligence, and that these are all related to my well-being. More than that, my thoughts are deeply connected with my feeling self. I learned that I use words to express, create, and explore all the relationships and emotions that give my life meaning. When I was in junior high school, I had difficulty writing papers. My teachers told me that I wasn't sticking to the point and that my thoughts were too "scattered." I was taught that in order to succeed, I would need to organize my thoughts in a linear, cause-and-effect way, listing my points in order of importance, first to last. I needed to make only one point with every paragraph and then develop only that point before moving on to the next point. I was taught that ideas should come one at a time and that they should always have some concrete obvious relationship to each other. (That was never obvious to me.) But my mind didn't work in a linear, nonemotional fashion then, and it doesn't work that way now.

When I write or think of a word or concept, my mind immediately goes in several directions at once—all of them rich with emotional content, and all of them related to each other equally, nonhierarchically, and nonlinearly. Thus, my natural thinking process is circular and multimodal, as it is for many women. If I write the word *bra*, for example, my mind goes off in all the following directions almost simultaneously. I think of a woman's relationship with her bra, how she purchased her first bra, what it was like for her, what that means about her relationship with her breasts, whether she's ever used an underwire bra, what her breasts mean in this culture, whether she was breast-fed, and so on.

If I simply wrote down my thoughts as I listened to them, at first they seemed random and without order. But as I continued the process, I saw that my thoughts were weaving a web of interconnected meaning that was going in a certain direction. My job was simply to go along for the ride and record what I heard or felt. I would always come back to my initial point of departure, but with a deeper understanding of my beliefs and wisdom.

Through writing I have come to see that every word that comes into my mind has meaning and that this meaning is connected to my entire being. I've come to appreciate that my ideas, thoughts, and wisdom come from all of me—my brain, my uterus, and my higher power—and that they may originate in any one of the numerous interconnected aspects of me. I have learned to trust my thoughts. Women's (and some men's) ways of knowing are not the logocentric left-brain approaches taught in our schools and universities. It's staggering to realize how many highly intelligent women feel that they are stupid because of this training.

To become free of thoughts and beliefs that don't serve you, you must first be able to *hear* them as they arise. Writing practice is a profound tool for learning how to hear ourselves and to appreciate the multimodal nature of our thoughts. Everyone has this ability, but it is devalued and therefore underdeveloped in our culture. It teaches us that the way in which we talk to ourselves inside is exactly the way we will be perceived by others. We don't speak to others in a way that's any different from the ways in which we speak to ourselves inside our own heads. For years, the word *worthy* came up in my writing because on some deep level I didn't feel worthy. I spent hours asking myself what I meant by this word. Images of school, authorities, tests, and church always arose around this word. Eventually, my meditation on the word *worthy* led me to a break-through understanding of the original sin of being female. How could I have felt worthy, given my cultural programming?

If a word or phrase continually comes into your mind, it is important—it has meaning for you. Explore it. Write about it. Meditate on it. If a thought comes into your mind, learn to accept it without judgment. It will have meaning for you, no matter what it is. It is there for a reason. Linda Metcalf says, "There are no tourists in the mind."

I had always believed that for us to change the conditions of our lives outside, we must make a change inside. Proprioceptive writing is a tool to explore what is inside. After all, if we don't know where we are, how can we ever expect to get anywhere else? What I discovered within me were layers and layers of *shoulds, oughts,* and other impedimenta of my educational and cultural indoctrination. Metcalf describes these as a "mangrove swamp, with all the roots twisted around each other."

Through weeks, months, and years of writing, I gained direct experience of my own indoctrination—and eventually came to hear my true self emerging—my own voice. But I also ran smack up against my guilt. This guilt seemed to be a part of who I was, neatly installed years before. (I also experienced how I had split spirituality from anything political. Now I know that we cannot separate the two.) Guilt is a fantastic tool for keeping women in their place. It is a form of internalized oppression that serves to maintain the status quo. I realized that if I continued to wallow in my own guilt instead of examining its voice within me, I would forever be ineffective at doing the work I am best at—and which I love the most. How could this possibly help me, or anyone else? When I reclaimed my work as political and let go of guilt, I broke free from a set of health-destroying beliefs. Very few in this culture are free from guilt, since it is part of the self-centeredness of the addictive system.

My writing was vital in helping me break free from those parts of my life that no longer served me. However you do it, you too can learn to respect your intellect, your mind, and the fullness of your intelligence.

Dialogues with the Body: Listening to the Mind of the Cells

I often ask patients to carry out a dialogue with their bodily symptoms or with the organ that is giving them problems, through writing, meditation, or drawing. Sitting with your journal open while being receptive to your thoughts, ask your body what it needs or what it is trying to tell you.

One of my patients, who was experiencing heavy menstrual bleeding and a fibroid, asked her pelvis to speak to her. In her journal she wrote, "What is the wisdom you are trying to convey to me through my bleeding and my fibroid?" Over the next several days, she "waited with" this question for about ten minutes per day.

The answer that eventually came was, "Your periods are symbolic of the way you give yourself away too freely. The heavy bleeding represents your own life's blood draining away. You do the same thing in your relationship with your boyfriend. This is related to your relationship with your father."

Another patient told me, "You asked me to have a dialogue with my cervix. [She had had an abnormal Pap smear.] It's all about shame, it's all about deprivation, it's all about not being good enough. I think I need to listen some more."

Many fine publications have been written, and workshops offered on how to do journal work, or other forms of introspective dialogue. I recommend Natalie Goldberg's books on writing practice, *Writing Down the Bones* and *Wild Mind*.[16]

Working with Dreams: A Dream Incubation

> The night dreams speak Wild Woman's language. She is there
> broadcasting. All we have to do is take dictation.
> —Clarissa Pinkola Estes[17]

You can learn to work with your dreams actively and learn to consult them about specific problems in your life. The process of asking for a dream for guidance is known as dream incubation.[18] To do this effectively you must be willing to be 100 percent honest about the circumstances of your life. Here's how to do it.

Choose a night when you have some energy and focus to devote to the process. Spend ten to twenty minutes writing in your journal concerning the particular issue you want to focus on. Address the following questions within yourself, and be open to other input from your inner guidance:

What is the cause of my problem?
What possible solutions come to mind about my problem right
    now?
Why aren't these solutions adequate?
How am I feeling right now as I work on this?
Does it feel safer to live with the problem than to resolve it?
What do I have to lose if I solve the problem now?
What do I have to gain if I solve the problem now?

Write down a one-line sentence or request that deals with the problem as directly and simply as possible, and keep your question gently in mind as you drift off to sleep. Have a paper, pen, and flashlight, or a tape recorder handy at your bedside, and write down any dreams you remember. Sometimes insights will come to you at

3:00 A.M. or anytime you might awaken to go to the bathroom. If you don't write down at least the pertinent details of your dream, you are likely to forget it by morning. This process may take several nights before a clarifying dream arises.

Betty, one of my friends, found herself in a painful social situation in which she felt two of her colleagues were blaming her for the fact that they were being passed over for job promotions. Betty is very bright and creative and is always able to come up with new approaches to her work that are fun, innovative, and productive. Her colleagues through the years have often been jealous of these abilities. Because she loves working with people and has great difficulty with interpersonal conflict, this latest situation was very painful for Betty. She contemplated quitting her job and moving across the country, even though her work was very fulfilling. When she became aware of the hostility of her colleagues in this current situation, the feeling this evoked in her was old and all too familiar. She had been unfairly "blackballed," "picked on," and "scapegoated" similarly by others. It had happened over and over again at other jobs and in several other settings both personal and professional. Completely fed up with being thus victimized by others, she wanted to choose another way to live with her gifts and talents. She decided to do a dream incubation to ask for guidance in changing whatever unconscious patterns kept attracting situations in which she ended up as the victim of other people's inadequacies. After noting all the different situations in which she'd been victimized and allowing herself to feel fully how disgusted she was by the whole thing, she asked for a dream that would help her clarify her situation. She wrote, "Why do I keep re-creating situations in my life in which people pick on me?"

That night she had the following dream: A very good friend was seated to her left. The friend reached over to help a porcupine, and the porcupine shot its quills at her. Betty's friend took the quills and embedded them in Betty's arm—then looked in her face to see what her reaction would be. Betty simply sat there and allowed the quills to be painfully embedded in her arm. So now, the same friend took a handful of needles and pins and began sticking them in Betty's arm. Meanwhile, Betty continued to say nothing—simply sitting there with the pain of this. Finally, Betty decided to do something about her pain. She began taking the needles out herself. When she did this, a great deal of blood started pouring out of all the needle holes in her arm. Overwhelmed with the pain and the extent of the bleeding, Betty then decided to complain to her friend, telling her it was not okay to stick quills and needles in her arm.

Betty then looked to her right side and saw her mother, father, and sister all sitting there. She realized that throughout her childhood, these family members had insulted and physically beaten her. Betty had never complained and had never said anything. Instead, she fixed the pain herself and allowed herself to bleed.

When Betty awakened, she realized that she could no longer allow psychic, emotional, or other barbs to accumulate without saying anything. She knew that she had come to point that she was "bleeding to death" from the accumulation of a lifetime of hurts that she had never acknowledged or complained about. Because of her upbringing, she had been led to believe that if she complained, she simply got beaten more. Now Betty realized that she had to stand up for herself at the first sign of discomfort in her relationships. She saw how deeply the "victim" mentality had been drummed into her in childhood. She had used her considerable gifts and talents to escape her family of origin—only to have the original family pattern recur in all her later relationships. Having become very clear about her part in creating "victim" situations by refusing to defend herself, Betty now speaks up for herself at the first sign of discomfort. She also realizes that if a colleague has problems with her abilities, this is not something that Betty has to fix. The colleague herself must deal with her own inner sense of jealousy and inadequacy to see what it is teaching her. Betty cannot do this for another.

Step Eight: Get Help

> Asking for help doesn't not mean that we are weak or incompetent. It usually indicates an advanced level of honesty and intelligence.
>
> —Anne Wilson Schaef

We do not believe in ourselves until someone reveals that deep inside us something is valuable, worth listening to, worthy of our trust, sacred to our touch. Once we believe in ourselves we can risk curiosity, wonder, spontaneous delight or any experience that reveals the human spirit.

—e. e. cummings

Setting aside the time and money to go and talk with a skilled listener can be invaluable. This person may be a therapist, a minister, or other trustworthy individual. These sessions can be a way to stop, reassess your life, and give yourself a much-needed focus on a regular basis. Many therapists have helped people begin to look at their lives differently and effect change. A good therapist should be like a midwife, standing by while someone gives birth to what's best in themselves. Linda Metcalf, my writing teacher, was everything that a therapist should be. Linda witnessed my growth and prodded me to explore my thoughts further. Our work together was a structure in which I could explore more of myself.

When I was about fourteen and upset about something that I can't even remember now, my father told me how important it was to express what I was feeling and "get it off my chest." (The phrase "get it off your chest" is an accurate anatomic description of dealing with fourth chakra issues such as sadness, which tend to affect the shoulders, breast, and heart.) He told me, "I notice a tendency in you to clam up and not say what's going on. When you do this, you prevent others from helping you." It was good advice. We all can use a reassessment of our lives and a skilled listener on a regular basis. Support of this nature should be built into the culture. Community has been largely lost in the industrial revolution and the ensuing split between work, home, private, and public. In an ideal world it wouldn't be necessary for us to go to individual therapists or to create separate support groups for those with cancer, those suffering from loneliness, or even those who want to create health. Native cultures have lived for centuries without all the therapies that have evolved to fix a society whose basic worldview promotes the myth of the rugged individual who needs no one. No wonder so many people seek support from therapists!

The sexual/power dynamics of the culture potentially impact all of our relationships, including those that are "professional." Thus, many women have also been sexually exploited by therapists. *Sex in the Forbidden Zone* by Dr. Peter Rutter documents therapists, ministers, and other trusted confidants who've been sexually involved with their clients.[19] Rutter also documents the behavior of the women who were involved, many of them survivors of childhood sexual abuse. Currently, 10 percent of psychiatrists admit to having had sex with a patient. Figures on other specialties are harder to come by. A woman who has been an incest survivor will often adopt seductive behavior as a way to win approval from her therapist or minister—a relationship that is valuable to her. If her therapist takes this as an opportunity for a sexual encounter, however, he damages not only her but himself (or herself).

My Women to Women associates and I have worked with a therapist regularly since we began our business to learn how to talk openly and honestly with each other—and to deal with emotions that women aren't supposed to have, like anger. Our therapist has never tried to change or "fix" us. He has simply provided a safe place for us to say what we have needed to say to one another— without our thinking we had to take care of the feelings of the person we were angry with at the same time. In the early years of Women to Women, we honestly didn't know that we were capable of a perfectly functional relationship with each other even when we expressed our anger or disappointment. And we had no skills for breaking through our old habits of "being nice." Having done extensive codependency (relationship addiction) recovery work, we now see that those early therapy sessions were crucial for our ability to be honest with each other. In the past two years we've required many fewer sessions. Our group "therapy" (now called "team building" in the therapy profession) helped us create independence. We have been able to take what we learned and internalize it, and we can now communicate among ourselves without an outside person assisting.

There are many different kinds of therapists. The entire field has been changing in response to evolving knowledge about addiction and recovery. Therapy is not something that should go on for years, in my view. When it does, it can become an addictive process in and of itself—not much different from the alcoholic-enabler duality. All relationships, therapeutic or otherwise, work best when the participants see each other as essentially whole beings with inner resources and strengths, though sometimes in temporary need of assistance. A full discussion of therapy is beyond the scope of this book; I refer you to Anne Wilson Schaef's *Beyond Therapy, Beyond Science*, the most enlightened discussion of this issue I've read.[20]

Though individual therapy is often a first step for many women, group work of some kind, such as a twelve-step group, can be powerful in it helps us see that our problems are shared by so many others. A member of Overeaters Anonymous once told me, "Addiction recovery is God's answer to community." Group work certainly is one answer that is helping millions. The practical wisdom contained in the Twelve Steps of Alcoholics Anonymous are a blueprint for how to live a life based on inner guidance. Many of those in Twelve Step Fellowships simply take out the word "alcohol" or "alcoholic" if it's not applicable and substitute something more relevant. The program and the program's literature is still highly relevant and helpful. Groups help rid us of our "myth of terminal uniqueness," as a therapist friend calls it, while individual therapy for wounds such as incest can isolate a woman further because it "privatizes" what is in fact a cultural and even global problem. Part of the wounding of addiction, incest, or other sexual abuse is its hiddenness. Imagine the relief of participating in a group of women in which all of them are saying, "That happened to you, too? I always thought I was the only one!"

Using the basic twelve-step recovery approach and attitudinal healing, people with chronic or life-threatening illness also come together regularly to share not only their tears, but also their joy and their laughter. This grassroots movement throughout the country has been a source of growth, comfort, and hope to many. I regularly refer people to support groups of all kinds in our community, and participate myself.

For many women, it is important to spend time regularly in women-only settings. When we gather together as women, we each hold a piece of the whole story. Together we heal faster than we would if we remained isolated and separate, and group members hold up a mirror for us so that we can see ourselves more clearly. Anne Schaef puts it this way: "If one person calls you a duck, don't worry about it. If two call you a duck, give it some thought. If three people call you a duck, start looking for tail feathers!"

In the early stages of self-awareness, women often don't tell the whole truth if there's even one man in the room. The same may be true for men. We've been socialized to tailor our conversations to accommodate the other gender. In order to become self-aware, we need environments in which we can truly be ourselves. For many, that means women-only settings for a time.

Annie Rafter, a nurse practitioner and one of the original founders of Women to Women, told the following story: One summer she and a group of women friends crewed together on a sailboat and participated in races. They began to notice that if a man came on their boat, they automatically deferred to him—handing him the tiller or expecting him to chart the right course—before they knew whether he was even a good sailor.

Noticing this behavior in themselves, the women decided that for one season, they needed to sail with no men on the boat so that they could become a cohesive crew. So for that one season, they stuck by their agreement and learned to trust each other. By the next sailing season, it didn't matter who came on the boat—the women crew trusted themselves, each other, and their sailing skills. They no longer automatically deferred to men.

In the early days of Women to Women, we often referred back to Annie Rafter's story about "no men on the boat." Like her crew, we needed to learn to trust each other and to learn how to maintain that trust, no matter who came into the building. I find that working in a women-only environment gives me the time and space to talk out my problems in a way that simply doesn't work with my husband. We women have been taught that our mates should be our best friends and our primary source of emotional support. Occasionally, this works, but not often. When we rely on men to support us emotionally, we often end up disappointed. By the time I get home at the end of the day, I've had my "process" time, and I don't need my husband to be there for me to go over the details of my day and give me advice or support. We meet as peers and share the events of our day in a way that's totally different from the way I would share them with one of my woman friends. By having plenty of women-only time and support, I don't burden my primary male-female relationship with needs that probably weren't meant to be filled in that relationship in the first place.

Meetings and support help people to get out of denial. Twelve-step and other programs have helped millions of people recover inner strength and serenity—this should be the first step in moving on in their lives. In order to heal fully, however, each of us must get to a point in which we're not overly identified with our wounds. This is not easy because "we learn the language of wounds as our first language and we use our wounds to create intimacy," as Caroline Myss says. People don't heal fully and move on with their lives as long as they continue to take what has happened to them too personally and identify themselves solely as victims. When a woman sees herself solely as a victim, she too often *becomes* a perpetrator. She may lash out at anyone who dares to suggest that she has the inner wisdom to change. Eventually, we must take responsibility for our lives and stop laying blame for the conditions of our lives on everything from addictions and incest to the political system. Seeing our dysfunctional patterns, working on them, and letting them go is a process.

Step Nine: Work with Your Body

Rolfing is psychotherapy for the body.

—Paulanne Balch

For some women, talking things out is simply not enough. "I know all of the things that happened to me as a child and with my husband," said one woman, "but talking about it just doesn't change a thing. I seem to be going in circles." When this happens, we often obsess and seem to spin our wheels. It's easy to get locked into "thought addiction"—a kind of gerbil wheel in the brain that keeps us going around in circles.

Much of the information we need to heal is locked in our muscles and other body parts. Getting a good massage will often release old energy blockages and help us cry or get rid of chronic pain from "holding the world on our shoulders." There are many types of bodywork, ranging from polarity therapy to Feldenkrais, that are beneficial. Bodywork can be divided into two different types: physical bodywork (like rolfing, classical osteopathy, and massage), and energetic bodywork (like Reiki, acupuncture, and therapeutic touch). Though I will not be discussing these separately, I want to make this distinction.

Work on and with the body can be an opportunity for understanding and experiencing the unity of our bodymind. These therapies are often deeply relaxing and give our bodies a chance to rest and sleep, a time when much of the body's repair work goes on. Acupuncture works well for all kinds of problems that aren't easily treated through conventional means. I would like to see it and the many other kinds of physical and energetic bodywork used in conventional hospitals.

I refer dozens of patients for bodywork of different kinds and am very gratified with the results. I personally get a full body massage once or twice a month. I regard it as part of my general health maintenance program.

Schedule at least a shoulder or foot massage sometime this month. You can also trade massages with a friend. Eventually, work up to a full massage regularly.

Step Ten: Gather Information

Currently, more books of interest to women are available than at any other time in history. Though we used to maintain a reading list at Women to Women, we found that it was nearly impossible to keep up with all the information being published. So now we simply share with our patients our favorite books on any given subject and they, in turn, let us know what they've been reading. (See Resources section, page 674, for some of these.) Many books and articles are brought to our attention by our patients, a constant exchange of new information and thoughts that is a cherished part of our extended community. Since books of special interest to women abound, I recommend going to your bookstore or library and using your inner guidance to help you make a choice. Acknowledge that you have the wisdom to choose the right book at the right time. Just sit with the books for a while and look over a few titles. See which ones speak to you. Choose the ones that feel right and have appeal. You cannot make a mistake.

It is a powerful experience for women to begin to reclaim our forgotten history by reading about our bodies, menstruation, childbirth, and goddesses, all written from a woman's point of view. One of the greatest gifts of the feminist movement of the 1970s was the deconstructing of the patriarchal mindset, which was seen for centuries as "the truth" or "just the way it is." Ursula LeGuin points out that 50 percent of writers are women, but 90 percent of what we call "literature" is written by men.

Books ranging from *Our Bodies, Ourselves* by the Boston Women's Health Book Collective, a book that heralded a much-needed reevaluation of women's healthcare, to *The Chalice and the Blade* by Riane Eisler have helped a whole generation of women rethink our history and how it has affected our lives.[21] Through the power of the pen, we receive support for our journey together.

The many new volumes on the bodymind connection are also of great help to women in reinforcing their own experience. Books are great companions for many otherwise isolated women who have not yet found each other or come together in communities. Reading and gathering information is a very nonthreatening first step on the healing journey. Many of my patients spent years reading everything they could get their hands on before they felt ready to join a group or seek other support and sisterhood.

Step Eleven: Forgive

> We must let ourselves feel all the painful destruction we want to forgive rather than swallow it in denial. If we do not face it, we cannot choose to forgive it.
> —Kenneth McNoll, *Healing the Family Tree*

Forgiveness frees us. It heals our bodies and our lives. But it is also the most difficult step we must take in our healing process.

It takes a great deal of energy to keep someone out of our hearts. The twelve-step approach teaches that we make amends for ourselves, not necessarily for the other person. But when we make amends to those who have hurt us, both of us are freed. Forgiveness and making amends are completely linked. Holding a grudge and maintaining hatred or resentment hurts *us* at least as much as the other person.

Forgiveness moves our energy to the heart area, the fourth

chakra. When the body's energy moves there, we don't take our wounds so personally—and we can heal. Forgiveness is the initiation of the heart.

When I think back on my breast abscess, I feel great compassion and forgiveness *for myself*. How could I have known what I was doing? I had no role models of women in OB/GYN for balance between work and motherhood. I have forgiven myself, and because of that I have also forgiven my colleagues at the time. I've spent about six years coming to grips with the concept of forgiveness. When I first wrote this chapter, I didn't even think of putting this step in, because the concept of forgiveness is very misunderstood and misused; the misapplication of forgiveness can keep women sick. When we forgive someone because we think it is the right thing to do, we're merely jumping through a socially acceptable hoop that changes nothing. Alice Miller notes that when children are asked to forgive abusive parents without first experiencing their woundings and their personal pain, the forgiveness becomes another weapon of silencing. Leaping to forgive under these circumstances is not really forgiveness—it is just another form of denial. Many women think that forgiving someone who hurt them is the same as saying that what happened to them was okay and that it didn't hurt them. Nothing could be further from the truth. Many women have been brainwashed into submission by the misunderstanding of forgiveness. To get to forgiveness, we first have to work through the painful experiences that require it.

I recently saw a woman with migraine headaches that were becoming increasingly severe. She also had chronic vaginitis, multiple allergies, and a host of other problems too numerous to mention. A perfectionist, she routinely took on too much at her job. When she spoke, she formed her words in a careful and controlled way—and her face twitched in an exaggerated way. On her intake form, she noted that her father, maternal grandfather, paternal grandfather, three brothers, and all her uncles were alcoholic and that her mother had expected her to be an adult almost since birth. "I was never allowed to play. I had to keep the house neat," she wrote. She firmly believed that "none of these alcoholics had any effect on me during the time I was living at home." Her denial was very clearly in place, while her body was screaming to get her attention. Forgiveness of her parents would be ridiculous in her case. It would simply be used to build up another layer of intellectual armor. This woman first has to acknowledge that she was adversely affected by her parents' behavior. Forgiveness is completely premature when a woman doesn't even acknowledge that she *has* an emotional abscess, let alone that it needs to be drained.

True forgiveness, on the other hand, changes us at a core level. It changes our bodies. It is an experience of grace. As I write about this concept, I'm moved to tears by the holiness of what forgiveness really is. I experienced this profoundly a number of years ago when I was reported to the medical board in Maine by a general surgeon. One of this man's patients had come to me for a consultation. Three months before, she had gone to this surgeon because of abdominal pain, weight loss, and narrowing stool caliber. He had attempted a colonoscopy (a test in which a fiber-optic scope is put into the colon to examine the inside and check for conditions such as cancer), but he had been unable to get the instrument all the way up her colon. He told her that she would need to have surgery to remove part of her colon since he was virtually certain she had a cancer that was causing her symptoms.

She had gone home, changed her diet completely to a macrobiotic approach, and over a three-month time period regained the weight she had lost, was free of abdominal pain, and had normal stools once again. All of this had taken place before she saw me. When I first saw her, she was healthy, vital, and committed to avoiding surgery. Since she was so much better, she wanted to know if I thought she still needed the surgery.

I told her that no one could be sure if she did or didn't have cancer without further testing. She had already taken a risk by not having the surgery earlier, but on the other hand, the actions she had taken had certainly reversed all the symptoms for which she had initially sought care. It was possible that she didn't have cancer and that her symptoms had been from diverticulitis (an infection of the colon that can mimic cancer) that was now healed. She decided to continue doing what she was doing with her diet, then have her colonoscopy repeated in a few months. After all, it was her body and she was feeling better than she had in years.

She understood that this decision was in direct conflict with what her surgeon had suggested, but at this point he wasn't aware of her striking improvement. I felt sure that once he saw her, he'd agree to postpone her surgery and repeat her tests. Because I believe that people do best when they are cared for by a medical team that is informed, I sent a copy of our discussion to her surgeon.

As it turned out, he was furious with me for not "forcing" her to have surgery, and so he reported me to our state medical board. I had to submit a report of my end of the story and wait for the board to call me forward for a hearing. They met only every three months, so I had plenty of time to stew about this situation. I felt sure that a doctor-initiated complaint against me would be taken quite seriously, and I was terrified.

This event was the most difficult learning I'd experienced in my career. I had spent my whole life in the pursuit of good grades, respectability, and worthiness. I came from a family tradition of "good doctors." Yet here was the manifestation of my worst fear: The authorities were going to say that I was a "bad" doctor and that I couldn't practice medicine in a way consistent with my own beliefs about healing, and worse, that my patients didn't have that choice with their own bodies, either! I worked with and felt my fear daily for weeks. If I could change how I felt on the inside, I knew, something would change on the outside in the world. This had always been part of my belief system. Now I had to put it to a very practical test.

Part of any healing is "letting go," relinquishing the illusion of control. For me, the letting-go was this conclusion: If I couldn't practice medicine in a way that was consistent with the healing power of the human body and individual free choice, then I would willingly give up my license. I was helped and supported during this process by colleagues and patients who told me that they'd willingly accompany me to my hearing if necessary. Dr. Nancy Coyne told me that if I had to go, she'd make sure that the place was "packed with feminists" in support of me. For that, I will be forever grateful.

One day while doing my writing, I spontaneously began a letter to this surgeon who had reported me: "Dear Dr. M, I know your fears. I know why you are upset. . . ." As I continued, I felt compassion for this man. I knew who he was. I felt him as a frightened man fighting for control—and I forgave him. As I continued writing, I felt the fear in my solar plexus lift for the first time in weeks. It was a physical feeling, not an intellectual exercise. And at the same time, I *knew* that everything would be all right, *regardless of the decision of the board*.

The next day, one of my colleagues who serves on the board saw me in the hospital and told me, "By the way, the board unanimously decided to drop your case. They felt that that surgeon was way out of line!" I never had to go before the board or plead my case in any way. They had upheld my patient's right to informed care, and my right to give it.

My ordeal was over. The most striking thing about this experience was the physical feeling of release in my solar plexus area when my fear finally healed and I felt compassion for my adversary. From this I learned that forgiveness is organic and that it is physical as well as spiritual and emotional. My intent had been to heal my own situation, not necessarily to forgive the surgeon. But I subsequently learned that *the only way to heal the situation* was to withdraw my energy from it and to forgive my accuser. I learned that forgiveness comes unbidden, by itself, when we are committed to healing. To experience forgiveness, however, we must first make a commitment to healing and to making amends, when they are needed.

I never *intended* to feel compassion and forgiveness toward that surgeon. What I *did* want to do was get rid of the knot in my solar plexus. This I did by being willing to stay with the knot, to be in dialogue with it, and to learn from it. I believed at a deep level that I could learn from this experience, and that in fact I *must* learn from it, so that I wouldn't have to repeat it, in another way or another form.

Though I don't recommend being reported to a medical board for personal growth, it was one of the most freeing experiences of my life. I had faced one of my worst fears, stayed with it, and transformed it. The patient's tests were repeated at another hospital two months later. Her colon was perfectly normal, with no sign of a tumor. She had probably never had cancer in the first place, just an inflammation of the colon. She continues to be well. My husband later suggested that I report the surgeon to his board in Massachusetts and ask if it is the standard of care in his state to remove a normal colon. I said, "No. The war needs to stop somewhere. It's stopping with me." I did, however, write Dr. M a note with copies of the patient's normal tests and remarked, "Isn't the healing ability of the human body miraculous?"

Stephen Levine teaches us that the quality of forgiveness is miraculous for bringing balance. Most of us, he reminds us, have been given nothing in our training to work with resentment. Levine has given us the following meditation.[22] Try incorporating this meditation into your life in a daily meditation session. It works—try it yourself. Read it very slowly to yourself, or have a friend read it to you.

> Close your eyes. . . .
> For a moment just reflect on what the word forgiveness might really mean. What is forgiveness?
> And now, very gently—no force—just as an experiment in truth— just for a moment—allow the image of someone for whom you have much resentment—someone for whom you have anger and a sense of distance—let them just gently—gently, come into your mind— As an image, as a feeling.
> Maybe you feel them at the center of your chest as fear, as resistance. However they manifest in your mindbody, just invite them in very gently for this moment—for this experiment.
> And in your heart, silently say to them, "I forgive you."
> "I forgive you for whatever you have done in the past that caused me pain, intentionally or unintentionally. However you have caused me pain, I forgive you."
> Speak gently to them in your heart with your own words—in your own way.
>
> In your heart, say to them, "I forgive you for whatever you may have done in the past, through your words, through your actions, through your thoughts that caused me pain, intentionally or unintentionally, I forgive you. I forgive you."
> Allow. . . . Allow them to be touched . . . just for a moment at least . . . by your forgiveness. Allow forgiveness.
> It is so painful to hold someone out of your heart. How can you hold onto that pain, that resentment even a moment longer?
> Fear, doubt . . . let it go . . . and for this moment, touch them with your forgiveness.

"I forgive you."

Now let them go gently, let them leave quietly. Let them go with your blessing.

Now picture someone who has great resentment for you. Feel them maybe in your chest, seeing them in your mind as an image—a sense of their being. Invite them gently in.

Someone who has resentment, anger—someone who is unforgiving toward you.

Let them into your heart.

And in your heart, say to them "I ask your forgiveness, for whatever I may have done in the past that caused you pain, intentionally or unintentionally—through my words, through my actions, through my thoughts. However I caused you pain, I ask your forgiveness. I ask your forgiveness.

"Through my anger, my fear, my blindness, my laziness. However I caused you pain intentionally or unintentionally—I ask your forgiveness."

Let it be. Allow that forgiveness in. Allow yourself to be touched by their forgiveness. If the mind rises up with thoughts like self-indulgence or doubt, just see how profound our mercilessness is with ourselves and open to the forgiveness.

Allow yourself to be forgiven.

Allow yourself to be forgiven.

However I caused you pain, I ask for your forgiveness. Allow yourself to feel their forgiveness.

Let it be.

Let it be.

And gently . . . gently . . . let them go on their way in forgiveness for you—in blessings for you.

And turn to yourself in your own heart and say, "I forgive you" to you.

Whatever tries to block that—the mercilessness and fear.

Let it go.

Let it be touched by your forgiveness and your mercy.

And gently, in your heart, calling yourself by your own first name, say, "I forgive you" to you.

It is so painful to put yourself out of your heart.

Let yourself in. Allow yourself to be touched by this forgiveness.

Let the healing in.
Say, "I forgive you" to you.

Let that forgiveness be extended to the beings all around you.
May all beings forgive themselves.
May they discover joy.
May all beings be freed of suffering.
May all beings be at peace.
May all beings be healed.
May they be at one with their true nature.
May they be free from suffering.
May they be at peace.
Let that loving kindness, that forgiveness, extend to the whole
planet—to every level of existence, seen and unseen.
May all beings be freed of sufferings.
May they know the power of forgiveness, of freedom, of peace.
May all beings seen and unseen, at every level of existence, may they
know their true being.
May they know their vastness—their infinite peacefulness.
May all beings be free.
May all beings be free.

Step Twelve: Actively Participate in Your Life

By pursuing your allurements, you help bind the universe
together. The unity of the world rests on the pursuit of passion.
                                                    —Brian Swimme

Believe in Yourself. Someone has to make the first move.
    —found on a Salada tea bag during a conference on self-esteem.

When my elder daughter was nine, she reminded me how beautifully we are equipped with the innate capacity to live life fully, appreciating it as we go along. On Easter Sunday, she came bounding downstairs and exclaimed, "Don't you love it when you feel good, and you look good, and your room's clean, too?"

Watch children for a while, and you will begin to see what qualities you need to embody to wake up your soul and your immune system regularly. Most young children know exactly what they want. We are all born with an innate ability to know what we want. We are then socialized to believe that we can't have what we want, and so we gradually dismiss our innermost desires, our life's passion, to avoid disappointment.

David Ehrenfeld wrote in *The Arrogance of Humanism,*

> Our civilization is coming to equate the value of life with the mere avoidance of death. An empty and impossible goal, a fool's quest for nothingness, has been substituted for a delight in living that lies latent in all of us. When death is once again accepted as one of the many important parts of life, then life may recover its old thrill, and the efforts of good physicians will not be wasted.[23]

Get out a piece of paper and write on the top of it, "I intend to receive . . ." Then write in what you want. For example, "I intend to receive a strong, healthy body." Notice that the word *receive* indicates that you don't have to "work" for this. You just have to allow it to come. This is the feminine receptive mode, so often lacking in our culture. Now write down exactly *why* you want what you want, so that you can literally *feel* the excitement generated by your enthusiasm. It is the feeling and the vibration of the feeling that has the power to attract circumstances to you. In one example: "I intend to receive this because I want to feel powerful. I want my body to be an instrument that is highly attuned to my needs. I want a body that is a reflection of the beauty that is inside me. I want a body that is capable of getting me where I want to go. I want a body that has lots of energy and stamina so that I may enjoy my life more fully."

The positive emotional energy generated by this experience literally begins to draw the experience of health to you. Focus on and think often about what you want, and you will be setting up an invisible magnetic field that begins to draw it to you (unless you keep blocking it with other thoughts such as "Well, I want it, but I'll never get it").

Every day, spend just a few minutes focusing on what you *do* want and how it will feel to have it. You will never be able to feel happy or fulfilled in the future unless you can feel how that would feel right now. Your thoughts and your emotions need to line up on this one. If you say you want a healthy body, but deep inside you don't feel that you are worthy of it or that illness is a punishment of some kind, you will be creating a mixed message, and your results won't be nearly as good.

For thirty consecutive nights, just before falling asleep, say to yourself, "I am intending vibrant health." During sleep, the intellect is quieted and your inner guidance takes over. Your intent to attain or maintain health will be programmed into your bodymind as you sleep. Just try this and see what happens.

Intend to receive joy. Intend to receive comfort. Intend to receive support. As you move through your day, use the power of intent to clear a path for yourself.

Notice during each day how often your thoughts about what you want turn to the negative. Gently bring them back. Make it a habit to concentrate on what is working in your life. Cultivate the habit of noticing what is good and appreciating it. A teacher named Abraham says that "Appreciation is the strongest emotion we have for attracting what we want."[24] When you look for people, places, and things to appreciate and learn to appreciate all of the aspects of your life that are working well, you'll attract more of what you like and less of what you don't. Start noticing little things, like how good the bed sheets feel on your toes at night or how good the pillow feels under your head.

I strongly recommend avoiding watching the news on television, hearing it on the radio, or reading about it in the papers for at least thirty days. Wake up to music instead of the news, or to people talking on the radio. When you do this, you will be removing a major impediment to tuning in to your inner guidance—negative information overload. Human beings were never designed to act as receiver sets for the bad news from around the entire planet. For most of us, our own daily lives and those of our families and co-workers offer quite enough opportunities for helping and healing. In this sphere we can make a difference. And if each of us took care of our immediate families, jobs, and communities, the planetary community would take care of itself. We cannot do this adequately if our thoughts are continually overwhelmed with bad news that we can do nothing about. Consciously avoid information overload until you can watch the news without feeling bad, scared, or agitated. Otherwise, you could be putting yourself at risk.

If you wake up to soft music or silence each morning, you will be better able to remember your dreams. Over time, you will notice that you don't miss much by avoiding the news. The culture being what it is, someone will always tell you what is going on "out there." You'll always find out what applies to you and what you need to know. But you'll have the advantage of a much more intimate relationship with yourself than most people have. I have been on a mostly news-free diet for well over a year now. I cannot believe the difference it has made in my thoughts, dreams, and general state of well-being.

Write down your lifetime goals. Over the past ten years, I've written down my goals for the coming year every New Year's Eve. I have written down a five-year plan and a ten-year plan at the same time. My family now does this as an annual family ceremony. When I look back, the amazing thing is that I've accomplished almost every one of my goals—even the ones I later forgot about. The very process of writing them down and thinking about them sets something magical into motion. That magical "something" is the power of intent—the power of our thoughts to create.

Get in the habit of noticing what you want—that is how you find your passion. Maybe you need to wear skirts that swing more, walk in the sun more, dig in the dirt more. Most people find that when they have enough joy, their life is filled with abundance. I guarantee that somewhere inside you, you already know what it is you need and want. If anything at all were possible, how would you live your life?

You are now finished with the smorgasbord of steps for creating health. Some will appeal to you, and others won't. Trust what you're feeling. Give yourself credit for staying with it. Here is a summary of the steps for your convenience:

Steps for Healing
Step One: Get Your History Straight
Step Two: Sort Through Your Beliefs
Step Three: Respect and Release Your Emotions
Step Four: Learn to Listen to Your Body
Step Five: Learn to Respect Your Body

Step Six: Acknowledge a Higher Power or Inner Wisdom
Step Seven: Reclaim the Fullness of Your Mind
Step Eight: Get Help
Step Nine: Work with Your Body
Step Ten: Gather Information
Step Eleven: Forgive
Step Twelve: Actively Participate in Your Life

I hope that going through this section has

- jogged some stuck places in you that needed readjustment
- reassured you that you are right on track
- touched your anger
- brought up tears
- made you laugh
- inspired you

That's what life is—growing, changing, moving, creating—every day.

Maybe you need to sing—maybe you need to run. Don't wait. This life is not an emergency, but it also doesn't offer any guarantees about going on forever. How do you want to feel? Imagine feeling that way often. What action do you need to take right now to live your life more fully? ... Got it?

Now take a step toward it!

Blessed be.

SIXTEEN

Getting the Most Out of
Your Medical Care

Choosing a Health Care Provider

O ne of the most powerful tools for your healing is to develop a working partnership with a health care team in which all members respect the body's ability to heal and maintain health, and are willing to work together to facilitate this process.

Health care providers must be aware of how powerful their words are. The cloak of the shaman rests on their shoulders whether they realize it or not. Their words have the power to heal or to destroy—partly because of the vulnerability associated with illness and with our bodies. Professionals' words must be truthful and at the same time chosen to support healing. As Norman Cousins wrote, "The doctor knows that it is the prescription slip itself, even more than what is written on it, that is often the vital ingredient for enabling a patient to get rid of whatever is ailing him. Drugs are not always necessary. Belief in recovery always is. And so the doctor may prescribe a placebo in cases where reassurance for the patient is far more useful than a famous-name pill three times per day."[1] The placebo effect is *physical*.[2] The effect of working with a healer you trust and believe in is also *physical*, as much a part of your healing as the mode of treatment you actually choose. People have described their doctor's words as burning right into their souls. You must choose a health care provider carefully and deliberately.

I once had a patient with breast cancer who told her doctor,

"Coping with the cancer is no problem, but recovering from my visits with you takes me about two weeks." She was referring to his detached manner and her perception that he didn't care. She didn't expect a miracle, but she longed for some reassurance and an occasional touch. After she conveyed this to him, their relationship improved. This improvement often happens when you give your doctor or other health care provider a chance. When the patient-doctor relationship is supportive and mutually respectful, it is a powerful force, supporting healing.

When the provider is aloof, trying to be objective—giving only facts—only the intellect of the patient gets taken care of, and that is not enough. One of my patients who recently came in for a checkup complained about her doctor in Boston. "She doesn't think she can take care of me without filling the pages with all these little numbers," she said. "I know she's a good technician, but I don't feel heard." Unfortunately, fixing a patient through the manipulation of blood chemistry or the repair of broken bones is the main focus of allopathic health education. It is what medical students get graded on—not how well they communicate with the patient. Though this is changing in medical schools today, most doctors now in practice were taught the skills of curing, not caring.

One of the most common questions I'm asked is, "Is there a doctor like you in New York?" or California, or elsewhere. Many patients value an approach that honors their inner wisdom, acknowledges the message an illness holds, and complements conventional medicine with other modalities. A new "third line" of health care providers is emerging who are open to this approach. My colleagues in the American Holistic Medical Association, M.D.s and D.O.s (doctors of osteopathy), share my approach and my training. Many others, trained in different disciplines, also share this approach.

There are scores of deeply committed, caring physicians practicing in the United States who don't necessarily call themselves holistic. The vast majority of family practice physicians I know are inherently holistically oriented and open to new ideas. This is because family medicine training emphasizes the importance of the family system to health. This orientation quite naturally leads to an openness to explore hidden aspects of illness and the mind/body connection.

The doctor you're working with now may well be open to your ideas about your illness and may be willing to follow along with you. I see many women with large fibroids, for example, who do not want surgery. They need physicians who will examine them every six months or so. For these women, asking for this service is the first step in creating a partnership with their doctor. And they must be willing to take some of the responsibility. By the same token, if a woman with a large fibroid doesn't want surgery, coercing her into it against her will once she's fully informed is not healing practice. Since I believe that the body knows how to heal and because I've seen women heal from many so-called chronic conditions, I'm very willing to work in partnership with them, sharing my expertise along with their faith.

The average OB/GYN in this country has been sued for malpractice at least twice. I am no exception. The emotional toll of this experience is heavy and has served, unfortunately, to put doctors and patients at odds. It makes some physicians less willing to go against standard treatment. One of the ways to get around this is for women to include a signed statement in their medical chart releasing the physician from any potential litigation should they choose alternatives to standard conventional care. Though this is not an ironclad guarantee against a lawsuit, it helps many physicians feel more comfortable with approaches that weren't covered in medical school. If we are to get to a partnership between doctors and patients, we have to start where we are and both sides have to be honest about their needs and fears.

Because of my willingness to avoid surgery, I've had the experience of watching ovarian cysts go away, with such things as emotional and dietary change. I've learned many things about the female body that were not included in my training. My general optimism, coupled with the courage and forthrightness of my patients, have allowed us both to collect a body of clinical information that many gynecologists wouldn't necessarily see. I can only do this, however, with courageous women patients who are truly willing to take responsibility for themselves and their choices.

Changes in the medical system will come about as all of us begin to take responsibility for the part of the problem we're creating. In the meantime, although medical training and the mindset it often engenders can be frustrating, it's good to have a competent doctor on your side when you need her or him.

Patients who want to play an active role in their care are a blessing. When I was president of the American Holistic Medical Association, we came to the conclusion after years of debate that holism is a way of being in the world, whether or not one uses the label. The American Holistic Medical Association is the organization where I've learned most of what I know about alternatives. It is an organization of doctors who, as I see it, represent the "soul" of holistic medicine. Many of my colleagues in southern Maine are holistic in their orientation, but they know very little about alternative treatments. As one family doctor said to a mutual patient who was using castor oil packs, "I don't understand what it is you're doing, but it's working and I support you." This kind of physician is great to work with—open, honest, and nonthreatened by things they weren't taught in medical school. These doctors are true scientists—they're open to new thought.

Women must assume responsibility for their own experience in the health care interaction by being prepared with questions when they visit a new doctor and setting up an interview first, if they have any doubts about their choice. At our center a prospective patient can make an appointment for a fifteen-minute interview, to make sure our practice is a good match for her. This costs much less than a new patient appointment.

Understand that different physicians often have very different training and interests. As a physician who "walks between the worlds," I see the good that's done by a variety of approaches. The patient herself must become her own authority and understand how to get information from various sources. If patients could understand the amount of disagreement among the OB/GYNs in Portland, Maine, about how to treat a certain condition, they would appreciate how vital their own input is in creating an optimal outcome.

Do You Need a Female Doctor?

Though Women to Women is an all-women setting, there are scores of male physicians who are compassionate and highly skilled. Many women physicians and patients will tell you that going to a woman is no guarantee that you'll be treated better than you would be by a man. Sometimes you'll be treated very poorly. The reasons for this are many. To succeed in medical school, women often devalue their own knowing and try to become distant and objective—like some of their male or female role models.

A male physician who is a real healer can do at least as much to help women as a female physician could—sometimes more. If a woman is an incest survivor, for example, and has the mistaken idea that she can't trust men, her entire worldview could be nicely healed by a caring interaction with a male physician who demonstrates to her that not all men are dangerous. One of my patients had been operated on for endometriosis during her teenage years. She was left with a pelvis full of scar tissue and had become infertile. I referred her to an infertility surgeon who is not only highly skilled as a surgeon but is an extraordinarily caring man. My patient told me later that having a man help her heal her pelvis was very precious to her. As she put it, "A man wounded me as a child and set up the conditions that led to my pelvic problems. It is a big healing for me to have a man assist me in healing this part of my body."

Women who think that only women are really healers and that only men can be skilled surgeons miss out on a great deal that could help them. At this time in history, we need some women-only places to heal, but true healing goes way beyond whether we are male or female. Each of us has the capacity to wound each other. We also have the capacity to heal.

Healing the Pelvic Examination

A pelvic examination need not be a painful or dreaded experience if you know what to expect and are prepared to communicate openly with your health care provider. Far too many women have had unfortunate and painful experiences during their pelvic exams and come to expect the pain as an inherent part of the experience. One of my medical student friends told me that she hadn't had a Pap smear for more than ten years because when she had had her first exam during college, it had hurt so much, and the doctor had been so rude, she was too scared to go back. When she finally came to see me for an exam, she was amazed that the exam was not uncomfortable or painful in any way, even though she had been bracing herself for the pain! I have heard this same kind of story repeatedly throughout the years of my practice.

A pain-free pelvic exam includes the following requirements:

• To women who are having their first pelvic exam, the exam should be explained thoroughly beforehand, with visual aids of the body if necessary, so that the patient can see exactly where cells for the Pap smear are coming from, and exactly where her uterus and ovaries are. The patient should be shown all the instruments that will be used including the speculum and brush or swab used to take the Pap smear.

• A compassionate health care provider who appreciates how vulnerable some women feel during their pelvic exams, especially when their feet are up in stirrups.

• During the exam, the health care provider should explain in detail what she is doing to you as she is doing it. You should have the option of viewing the exam with a mirror, if you so desire. For example, the practitioner should tell you when she is going to put in the speculum, where you will feel pressure, what part of you she is checking as she is touching or checking you, when she is taking the smear, when she is going to feel for fibroids, when she will remove the speculum.

• You should know that you can tell the practitioner to stop at any time and that your request will be respected. When I'm examining a patient who is very anxious, I always tell her that she is in the driver's seat and can tell me to stop at any time.

• You should have the option of having a support person of your choice with you during the exam if you wish to hold someone's hand, ask questions for you, or simply to stand by.

• The practitioner should use the smallest speculum that will give an adequate view of the cervix and vagina. (The type of speculum that usually works the best is a medium Pedersen, though some women require a long, narrow Pedersen. The larger Graves speculums are needed only occasionally in a small number of women.) At many of the hospitals where I've worked over the years, the standard speculum that is provided for an exam is far too large for many women, especially those who haven't had children or who do not put anything in their vaginas during sexual activity.

• The speculum should be warm. At Women to Women, we keep the speculums on heating pads in the drawer of the exam table so that they are always at a comfortable temperature. Some practitioners warm them under warm water prior to inserting them.

• I take all Pap smears with a small, soft brush known as a Cytobrush. Most women don't even feel it when I take the specimen. I also tell women what their cervix looks like as I'm doing the exam. One patient told me, "How lovely it is to hear every year that my cervix looks very normal, pink, and healthy!"

• Once the Pap smear is taken, the speculum is removed, and the practitioner examines the uterus and ovaries by inserting one or two fingers in the vagina and pushing up on the uterus behind the cervix while at the same time sweeping the other hand down the lower abdomen beginning at the belly button. In this way, the uterus, ovaries, and the areas surrounding them can be felt between the examiner's two hands. Once again, I always tell the patient what I am feeling as I am doing this. If a woman has a uterus that is easy to feel through the abdominal wall, I will ask her if she wants to feel where her uterus is relative to her pubic bone. Many women who have fibroids are very reassured by realizing that they can often feel the fibroid uterus themselves and can therefore tell whether or not it's growing, staying the same, or shrinking. (Not all fibroids are in locations that a woman can feel through her abdominal wall.)

• After the first two steps of the bimanual exam are done, a third step in the exam is the recto-vaginal exam. During this part of the exam, the examiner's index finger is inserted into the vagina while the middle finger is inserted into the rectum. The entire area behind the uterus can be examined best in this way. I have often felt ovarian cysts, and even rectal abnormalities during this part of the exam that I would have missed without it.

• If I find an abnormality, such as a new fibroid or ovarian cyst, I draw a picture of it for the patient or show her a picture of a finding similar to hers. This information is always helpful because it helps keep the abnormality in perspective. For some women, what they imagine is going on is far worse than the reality. I also generally order a pelvic ultrasound to confirm my findings.

• Some women carry a great deal of chronic tension in their pelvic musculature and must learn how to relax enough to allow a small speculum or examining finger into their vaginas. Otherwise, they themselves create a chronic pain cycle during which their own muscles tighten around even the smallest speculum, causing pain. Many of these women, after getting into recovery from childhood issues, have told me that they literally "leave their bodies" during pelvic exams or other stressful events.

When a woman with this problem learns how to control voluntarily the degree of tension and relaxation in her muscles, she can often allow an instrument or examining finger to enter her body without distress. In severe cases, I refer her to a biofeedback therapist for relaxation training if appropriate. In others, I simply move very slowly through the pelvic exam, point out the PC muscle (see Chapter 8 for how to locate) and suggest that the patient simply lie on the table for a moment or two, breathing regularly. I always check every step of the way to see if she wants to continue with the exam. I also tell her that if she finds she is becoming distressed by the process, she must tell me to stop.

I then have her tighten all her pelvic muscles as tight as she can, then release them fully, visualizing her buttocks sinking into the exam table. Usually, after a few cycles of contraction and relaxation, she will be able to feel the difference enough to allow an exam. If she is too anxious for a complete exam, she always has the option of rescheduling. I always tell my patients that if the idea of having a pelvic exam feels like rape to them, unless they have an urgent gynecologic problem that requires immediate attention, they should wait before having one. Many women practice relaxing their pelvic muscles at home, sometimes by inserting a finger into their vaginas while bathing, or by slowly learning how to insert a tampon.

Choosing a Treatment: From Surgery to Brown Rice

If you are sick, treat the critical symptoms first, by whatever means is the most appropriate for you. Look for insights later. Conventional medicine is unparalleled in its ability to deal with emergencies and severe symptoms. Though I use many alternative treatments in addition to drugs and surgery, conventional medicine is necessary and helpful.

To approach illness without using the diagnostic tools of modern medicine where they are appropriate is as dualistic and harmful to patients as saying to someone with arthritis, "We've completed your tests. You have arthritis. It is a lifelong chronic debilitating disease, and you might as well learn to live with it"—without exploring nutrition, work stress, or lifestyle. Because mystery is a constant part of life, we can never be sure how anything will turn out; we can never be sure that a medical condition is hopeless.

Once a thorough assessment of a patient's situation has been made and she has been informed of the standard recommended treatments for her situation—like hysterectomy for a large fibroid uterus—I then present her with the alternative treatments that I've worked with over the years. The patient herself then decides what "feels" right. For one, the choice will be a hysterectomy. Another with the same problem might be more comfortable with dietary change or castor oil packs. Many women who have had excellent, standard medical care in other settings come to me specifically *for* alternatives to drugs and surgery. Having already had routine testing done and standard recommendations made, they've thought about their options and are very well-informed.

Once a treatment program has been recommended to you, regardless of what it is, let the information "sink in" for a few days or more. See if it feels right in your body. If it doesn't, give it more thought, get another opinion, ask for a dream, or turn it over to your inner guidance. If surgery has been recommended, I'm a very big fan of second and even third opinions. Very few conditions are such an emergency that you have to make a decision on the spot. If you "sit with" a decision for a while, you'll be much more trusting of your instincts if a real emergency does occur.

Which Treatment Is Best?

How a woman chooses to treat a condition will depend on her own needs at the time. I say this while acknowledging the power of the medical-pharmaceutical industry to sway public opinion and the cultural biases which I've already explored. (See Chapter 1.)

People often have prejudgments about treatments. Those who are oriented toward natural therapies sometimes see surgery or the use of drugs as a failure, and the use of vitamins for the same problem as a triumph. To those who are more familiar with conventional drugs and surgery, the very notion that an herb or dietary change could help seems preposterous. I teach women that there are many choices and they need not exclude entire categories that could help them—either conventional or alternative.

Eating brown rice and vegetables is appropriate for some women who want to decrease symptoms related to excess estrogen, for example, while taking a progesterone preparation is the best option for others with the same problem. Sometimes I suggest both. Many women are confused about these points and need to understand that they have options.

A thirty-eight-year-old artist came in for her annual check-up about one year ago. She had been trying to decide whether to go on Prozac, an antidepressant, for her periodic depressions. Philosophically she didn't like the idea, but her condition wasn't getting any better. She had an intuitive reading with a well-respected person in our area who had encouraged her to try the drug. She finally decided that the only way to know whether the drug would help was to give it a trial. She released her judgment and started to take it.

When I saw her three months later, she said that she was feeling wonderful and that the drug seemed to be a "missing link" for her. "I can't believe how my life has changed around," she reported. "Now the universe seems to be providing for me. My artwork is selling well, and I am much more creative. I'm also claiming my own power and energy as my own and am not nearly so worried about what other people think or whether I'm better than or worse than anyone else [as an artist]. I have more energy than I've ever had before." Taking the drug became a turning point for her, but before she could accept it, she had to release her prejudice about it. Though the drug definitely helped, she didn't ignore the issues from her past—

childhood sexual abuse—that were core issues in her depression. She told me, "One of the most helpful things about coming to you was to tell you about my intuitive reading and to tailor my medical care around how I was feeling about that information. That you were willing to listen to all the different parts of my story is precious to me."

Six months later, she stopped taking Prozac because she felt that it was creating "an artificial euphoria" that didn't feel right to her. What had worked well at one point was no longer appropriate. She continues to feel well, powerful, and creative without the drug.

There are many ways to heal. The right way for you is the way that feels best for you at a particular time. We must learn to see ourselves as processes—changing and growing over time. *Eventually, any externally imposed guidelines for how to become well must be consistent with our own inner guidance system. Eventually, we must learn to support ourselves through self-respect—not through restrictive regimens filled with "shoulds" and "oughts" that feel punitive.*

Externally imposed regimens such as dietary improvement are often a first step in healing. These regimens often help women feel good enough to get on with their real work of finding out both about their deepest woundings and about what is most nourishing in life that will help them heal their wounds. These two quests go hand in hand. We can't skip over the parts of our lives that hurt or are disturbing in an attempt to "follow our bliss."

Thought Addiction: A Common Obstacle

We are running around looking for knowledge, but we are drowning in information.

—Karl-Hendrick Robert[3]

Information-gathering is only a first step in creating health. Many people, equating techniques, medicines, and even vitamins with health, stop at this level. I've seen women with a variety of different conditions go to scores of health care practitioners of all types but come no closer to healing than they were before. Often, the more facts they have, the more confused they become. This information dilemma is common and can immobilize us.

Some people can get into thought addiction by looking at a menu and trying to decide what to eat: "Well, I want the chicken, but we're having chicken tomorrow, and besides I'm not sure if it will have too much fat in it, and whether or not I like the sauce. What do you think, Mark? Should I have the chicken?" and so on.

Another example is the following: In people who are trying to heal a condition with diet, there's a time when trying to control the amount and quality of everything they put into their mouths dominates their lives: "How many greens should I have? One cup or a half cup? Should they be cooked? How about my bowel movements—should they sink or float? If they sink, does it mean I should add bran? What about water—two glasses or three? And is it okay to have an orange? How many? One a day or two?" This is an example of taking the dualistic model and transferring it to everything we do.

As Anne Wilson Schaef has pointed out, one of the myths of the addictive system is that it's possible to know and understand everything. This approach becomes very problematic when we are dealing with a living, breathing, ever-changing human body.

Estrogen replacement therapy is a common situation in which women can work themselves into a real frenzy if they rely on intellect alone. No amount of studies on estrogen replacement, calcium intake, or exercise will ever be able to take into account all the variables that affect a woman's life around menopause.

Sometimes we have to take a step back from our intellect and laugh at it, running around in circles, chasing its tail. Writer Natalie Goldberg calls this "monkey mind." Regardless of what the issue is, once you've read all the books and consulted all the experts, only your inner guidance, of which the intellect is only a part, can give you the right answer.

Creating Health Through Surgery

At some point in their lives, many women are faced with the prospect of surgery. I've watched many women put their lives on hold for months or even years while trying to cure "naturally" a condition that is very amenable to conservative, organ-sparing surgery. Surgery to repair the pelvis is totally different from surgery to remove everything in the pelvis. Surgery should always be considered along with other healing modalities. I like to help heal the negativity often associated with surgery by renaming the experience Creating Health Through Surgery. I print that in big letters on the postoperative instructions that I give out after surgery when I'm going over details for home care once a woman leaves the hospital. Surgery can be approached as a healing ceremony. Jeanne Achterberg and Barbara Dossey give full instructions for how to do this in their book, *Rituals of Healing*. Linda Paladin's *Ceremonies for Change* is also full of practical and inspiring advice.

The Second Opinion

Before having any surgery, I advocate getting a second opinion. I see many women for second opinions regarding hysterectomy. The second opinion gives women time to think about their decision, and it exposes them to the vast differences in thinking that exist within the medical profession about treating a particular problem. Some women see as many as five or six different specialists before they decide on a course of action. Ultimately, they have to tune in to their inner guidance to come up with the best answer for them, since no doctor can provide it.

Often when I render a second opinion, I agree with the referring surgeon's rationale for the hysterectomy; heavy, irregular bleeding that has resulted in anemia, for example, is a conventional reason for hysterectomy. If surgery feels like the right solution to the woman, my opinion supports her needs. If, on the other hand, she is open to alternatives such as dietary change, I provide her with this information. She then realizes that the first doctor wasn't wrong but that she has more choices than she had been aware of.

I enjoy working with women who have taken the time to read and gather information. When they finally do embark upon a course of therapy or a surgical procedure, they do so from a place of strength and knowledge, not because some authority figure said they should. No one should ever have elective surgery if they feel they don't have permission to speak up, disagree, or get more information.

Surgery Is Not Failure but a Healing Opportunity

Too often, women think they've failed if they require surgery for their problem. This is another example of the dualistic thinking we've all inherited from the addictive system. One woman with a fourteen-week-size fibroid uterus said to me through tears, "I'm so ashamed. I keep thinking that I should have been able to prevent this or at least to have made it go away by myself." Further questioning revealed that she had the type of family background in which she had repeatedly heard the phrase, "Don't cry, or I'll give you something to cry about." She felt shamed for asking for help and for having needs. She realized that her fibroid was connected to grieving for the childhood she had never had.

Gail, whose ovarian cyst healing was covered in Chapter 7, said, "As a good 'New Age person,' surgery was my last resort. With classic New Age hubris, I felt I should have been able to heal myself, and if I chose surgery, I was a failure. So I tried a gamut of holistic approaches—acupuncture, herbs, castor oil packs, working with a friend who is a channel, and visualization. All of these methods were helpful and were surely healing on certain levels. But I realized that this cyst was too dense, both physically and spiritually, to be melted even by acupuncture needles. It needed to be cut out."

Another patient of mine, June, had a persistent ovarian cyst and very much wanted to avoid surgery. She spent three months doing visualizations, emotional cleansing, and dietary change to heal her cyst. I told June that I felt that surgery was her best option. Her cyst was large—10 cm.—and had failed to go away on its own after three months. Though she wanted to believe that the cyst was gone and that she could avoid surgery, she had had the following dream: "I went to get my car from the repair shop, and it wasn't ready yet. This dream recurred several times. I started to wonder if the cyst was indeed gone. I never had felt that the cyst posed any real danger to me, but even though I felt that I had completed my work"—she had developed a great deal of clarity about what the cyst represented in her life and had experienced a great deal of grieving and sadness about this—"I wondered if maybe the cyst were still there. I rarely admitted that thought to myself at all, choosing instead to think positively that it must be gone because I had completed what I thought was my healing work."

A few weeks before her scheduled surgery, June had dinner with a woman she had just met who was fascinated with myths, dream-work, and art therapy as tools to help people heal themselves.

"When she heard about my car dreams," June later wrote, "she started to push hard. She asked if I knew what was wrong with my car. She said I should have found out what was broken and called in a specialist to tell me how to fix it." This was to be done in dream state. "She was horrified that I was going to let someone take my ovary without trying harder to keep it. The implication was that if I did not try things her way, I wasn't trying hard enough. I answered her questions seriously. The questions felt so heroic,[4] so guilt ridden. I am responsible, and this cyst must be what I want. After I left her place, I felt dirty, sort of emotionally raped. Later I realized that searching endlessly for a nonsurgical cure is addictive, that I could keep the cyst and be addicted to the process, or I could just let it go and be done with it."

An Opportunity to Heal Old Fears

For many women, particularly those who are drawn to natural methods of healing, surgery is terrifying. Sometimes, it brings up childhood memories of hospitals—either of having been hospitalized themselves or having had a loved one hospitalized. I not uncommonly hear women voice abandonment fears based on having been left at the hospital for weeks during the 1940s, 1950s, or 1960s, when parents were told not to visit because it would undermine the child's care. Since most of us baby boomers were children during this era, it is little wonder that fear of the hospital is so prevalent among our generation.

My patient Gail, after her cyst surgery, said, "That cyst helped me uncover several powerful patterns I hadn't been aware of. My terror around my body, disease, doctors, and hospitals was a result of my mother's long mysterious heart disease, which led to her death. Throughout parts of my childhood she was in and out of hospitals, never seeming to get better and the doctors never seeming to know what was wrong with her. What caused even more suffering on my part was the feelings everyone in my family was experiencing around her illness that were never discussed."

Many of my patients have transformed their fears of the hospital and surgery, however, by using such experiences as a "spiritual initiation"—a time to face their fears and walk through them, as well as a chance to reverse old patterns that no longer serve them.

Gail wrote, "As I contemplated my upcoming surgery it was absolutely clear to me that I had a wonderful opportunity to confront my childhood terror of hospitals and all they represented. I could experience that my story was totally different from my mother's story. I learned some wonderful lessons. Reversing my family pattern, I shared my fears and concerns with my husband and dear friends and asked for their support. Their outpouring of love and support was a precious gift that I shall treasure for a long time."

Giving yourself permission to let another individual help you can be a profoundly healing experience. When surgery is the best treatment choice, surrendering to the skills of the anesthesiologist, your surgeon, your nurses, and your inner guidance can be a true growth experience. If you received the message in childhood that your physical and emotional needs for support and comfort don't deserve being met, asking for support during surgery or a hospitalization is an opportunity to reverse this message.

I remind my patients that healing energy is available in hospitals, and that they might consider looking upon the nurses and staff as healing angels. The people who work in hospitals—whether they be nurses, nursing assistants, or orderlies—are often in these settings because they are naturally drawn to healing. When you stop fighting those who are there to help, it's quite a relief.

Many of my patients have a friend or family member come with them for their preoperative visit if I'll be doing the surgery. Their friends then accompany them to the hospital to meet the anesthesiologist and go through the pre-op phase in the hospital setting. After surgery, these friends or others provide support at home through cooking, cleaning, or backrubs. Women must learn how to ask for this support. Getting it is a skill. Sometimes we need help learning this.

June wrote the following about getting support: "On my way home after finding out that I needed surgery, I knew I could not be alone that whole weekend, so I stopped at my friend Carol's house. I think Carol became afraid when she saw how depressed I looked. She delivered a strong lecture about how important I am to my son, and to her, and to many other people. I never had acknowledged my importance to any of those people except my son. She made a very strong case for going forward and letting myself be supported by my friends. She told me that I was to recover at her house so that I wouldn't have to cook or shop, or do any other of those details for myself. She helped me immeasurably."

In preparation for her surgery, June went to see a hypnotist and had three sessions. Her hypnotist produced two tapes for her to use—one to prepare her for a healthy experience and a quick recovery, and a second to help her move on afterward. She used these tapes many times during the next two weeks prior to surgery.[5] She also began work with a physician who understood and taught Chi Kung. (Chi Kung is an ancient Chinese art that teaches us to circulate our life-energy through movement, massage, and the breath.)

Practical Tips for a Healthy Surgery

I encourage patients choosing surgery to do the following:

• Understand that this surgery is a choice. If they want to cancel at the last minute because they've rethought the whole thing or it suddenly feels wrong, they should go ahead and cancel it. There are two times when a woman needs full permission to change her mind: One is at the altar before her wedding, and another is before having elective surgery. (This doesn't apply to life-saving emergencies.)

• For a major surgery (like a hysterectomy or myomectomy), donate two units of your own blood (unless you're too anemic), in case there is any risk of blood loss requiring transfusion.

• Take the following supplements daily one month before your surgery and one month after (dosages are approximate): vitamin C complex, 2000 mg.; zinc picolinate, 100 mg.; magnesium, 800 mg.; and B complex, about 50 mg. of each. These supplements have been shown to promote wound healing.

• Postoperatively, apply vitamin E oil (d alpha tocopherol) onto the incision daily, as soon as the surgical dressing is removed (if your surgeon agrees that there is no contraindication to this). This speeds healing and decreases scarring. Some women prefer aloe vera gel, calendula ointment, or other herbal treatments for this purpose.

• Make arrangements for rest, food, and emotional support for at least four weeks postoperatively, so that you will be free to use the post-op period to listen to your body and its needs more closely than you normally might. You'll be in a very receptive "porous" state, during which you can learn a great deal about yourself.

• Notice and acknowledge whatever feelings arise after surgery. When a part of your body is removed or when the integrity of your body surface is marred through an incision of any kind, you may need to grieve the loss of your former state.[6] None of us like surgical scars on our bodies. It matters little whether you ever did or ever will wear a bikini. We *all* care about how our bodies look, on some level.

• Old memories may surface after surgery that have been stored in the tissue itself. Surgery has the potential to bring cellular memory to conscious awareness. Incest or other abuse memories may arise in the recovery room or in the days or weeks following surgery. These memories won't surface until you're ready to deal with them, so you need not worry about this. The body's wisdom about when to release information is exquisite.

Acknowledging grief and loss is only one part of creating a healthy surgery. Another equally important step is looking forward to a life free from the problem that required surgery. Think of the surgical loss as a cutting away of the old so that there is space for the new to grow.

Allowing yourself to feel emotions connected with surgical removal of tissue is important. Caroline Myss teaches: "When you pull cell tissue out before any of the data has been finalized, the body gets out of synchrony." Many people have most of their energy tied up in the past and very little available in the present for healing. When an organ or cell tissue is removed and the body messages associated with it are not acknowledged or processed, then part of our energy will remain in the past like an unpaid account—a part of our personal unfinished business. So if any emotions or other data surface before or after surgery, feel them fully and let them work their way through your system.

When one of my patients had her fibroids removed, she wanted to be awake during the procedure, so she was given a spinal anesthetic. It turned out that she had severe adenomyosis, a benign condition in which the endometrial glands inside the uterus grow into the uterine wall, causing excessive bleeding. A hysterectomy was the optimal treatment for this. Her doctor gave her the choice of stopping the operation and leaving the uterus in since there was no malignancy (cancer).

She had been chronically anemic from her condition and experienced some pain. She had tried dietary change and acupuncture without much success. As a mother of three relatively young children, her time for taking optimal care of herself was limited and so she wouldn't have time to prepare again for a further surgery. She realized that it was time she "let go" of trying to save her uterus.

Before the uterine removal began, she asked the staff to hold up a mirror for her so that she could see her uterus. She then thanked it for providing her with three healthy children, blessed it and *herself* for trying to preserve it—then said good-bye. Only then did her surgeon begin the hysterectomy. She later told me that the process of letting-go and being able to thank her uterus were a key part of her healing. She ended up feeling empowered by this surgery, not devastated.

June, who had the ovarian cyst, also had a spinal and was awake during her surgery. "The operation took less than an hour," she wrote. "I had a spinal block so that I could be fully aware during the surgery. I had a mirror hooked up so that I could watch. It was fabulous. My body is healthy looking and young for my age [forty-two]. Being able to see the very good condition of my body did me a lot of good. I had lost a lot of confidence in my ability to assess what was going on in my body. [This was because she hadn't realized that her cyst was growing larger. She couldn't feel it.] This showed me what was right about it. My body is in good shape, and the cyst was just not something dangerous that could bring me to the point of surgery. The cyst was almost as large as a softball, but instead of being inside my ovary, it was just on the outside wall. Chris said my ovary looked perfect, and asked me if I wanted to try to save it. She did."

June had prepared a dedication for her left ovary that she could say at the time we removed it. I had a copy in my pocket ready to read in case she was unable to do so. I planned to have one of the operating room staff people read it to her when the time came. She had written the following to make closure around the sacrifice of her ovary:

Thank you, ovary, for helping me become aware of my anger
—my misplaced love
—my disappointment in men.
—and my conflicts
As you leave my body I pass through this stage of holding onto anger,
   disappointment, and conflict.
And I pass into a life of feminine creativity and beauty.

The vacuum that forms in your absence becomes the feminine vessel.
—It fills with healing
—It connects with my Qi [life energy]
—And it provides beauty and creativity for the rest of my life.

As it turned out, we didn't have to remove the ovary. I was able to remove the cyst and then repair the ovary. The scrub nurse handed her the cyst, which she wanted to touch and feel, still warm from her body. She later wrote: "When Chris gave me the cyst to bless, I had a hard time. The dedication that I wrote and had memorized was to my ovary, not my cyst. And I was so ecstatic that she had saved my ovary, I almost didn't care. I recited the relevant parts and left the rest out. I'm not sure it made much sense, but I wasn't performing so it doesn't matter."

Postoperatively, June's friend Carol spent the day and evening with her. June wrote, "She was so supportive and caring. I am so glad she was there. On her way out, she gave me permission to cry. And I did. It was great."

After two and a half weeks of recovery at Carol's house, June's body yielded yet another piece of healing information. She wrote: "Finally I made it home. I still had one more related realization to make and feel. One night I was touching the numbness above the incision, feeling unspeakably sad about the loss of feeling, when I started to cry. Chris had said that if this should happen, to stay with it and explore the feelings. I was crying about the feeling that no man has ever loved me for being the person I really am. Suddenly I realized I was crying about my father. The only two men that have ever loved me for the real me are my cousin and my father. And it was my father who was always there for me. I had never grieved this loss when he died. So I did."

Another patient of mine, a highly intuitive artist, had a hysterectomy for a large fibroid uterus when she was about forty-four. She had visualized the energy in her pelvis and fibroids as very erratic and unhealthy. Postoperatively in the recovery room, she told me that she realized that the static energy in her pelvis was gone. In its place she sensed an even spiral of healthy energy, a vortex in her pelvis. This surgery was a healing for her.

But I Had Surgery Years Ago and Didn't Know About This

If you've had surgery in the past, reading through this chapter may cause you to feel sad for missing the opportunity to be more fully involved in your healing process. (Stay with this feeling—it is not too late.) Many women who have had hysterectomies had few choices available to them for alternative treatments. The choices for treatment that I've mentioned were not nearly so available even a decade ago as they are now. Each year anesthesia becomes safer, and the techniques to preserve pelvic organs have improved—largely through infertility surgery techniques.

It is natural for women who have had unavoidable surgery in the past to feel some loss, especially now that things have changed. I can't prevent you from feeling grief over events that are past and organs that have been removed. I do know, however, that it's never too late to grieve properly and fully over your loss, if this comes up for you. If you are feeling sad now, stop reading, lie down, and see what comes up. Stay with your emotions or whatever you are feeling in your body. This is the way you heal—this is the way you process data in your body and bring all of your cells into the present. Remember, part of what keeps us stuck in our lives is thinking that we should have known years ago what we now know—and beating ourselves up for not knowing it at the time.

Removing an organ doesn't necessarily heal the energy blockage associated with the problem in the first place, though it can be a step in the right direction. Some women, years after surgery, still have energetic attachments to tissue that was removed and have not grieved fully. This attachment can still be read in their energy field. The electromagnetic field of the body contains a pattern of the whole, even after a physical part is gone.

Our healing ability is not limited by time or space. We can heal our past at any time, even fifty years later. Our past waits in our bodies until we're ready. Occasionally a woman will tell me that learning about the female energy system in the body has brought up delayed feelings that she never dealt with at the time of her hysterectomy. Better late than never.

That's the nice thing about understanding energy and medicine. Healing on the energetic level is always a possibility, regardless of what has gone on at the purely physical level and regardless of how long ago it happened. So if you have had or are having surgery, know that this too can be part of creating health. Stay with whatever comes up, and plan to make your surgery a healing opportunity.

Many health care options and choices are available to you. Know that there is no one monolithic "right" way to care for your body. Most important, I hope I have encouraged you to listen to your inner guidance when choosing partners in health care. Albert Schweitzer once said, "It's a trade secret, but I'll tell you anyway. All healing is self-healing."

SEVENTEEN

Nourishing Ourselves with Food

If women are truly to enjoy food, it must become one of life's freely experienced sensuous pleasures. By eating well, women take care of themselves on the most basic level.

Dr. Karen Johnson[1]

*E*ating healthy, high-quality food is one of the easiest and most powerful ways to create health on a daily basis. Since we women do most of the food shopping and preparation in this country, we can have a significant impact on our and our family's health when we improve our diets. Individual food choices also affect the health of our planet overall. Consider that approximately 60 million people could be fed adequately with the grain that would be saved if Americans reduced their meat intake by 10 percent. Our national meat-eating habit also contributes to rainforest destruction in that 55 square feet of rainforest are consumed to produce every quarter pound of hamburger imported to the United States from Brazil. Our bodies evolved over millennia to assimilate foods that are found in the natural world. Therefore, we function at our best when we eat these natural foods much of the time, not imitations. In the process of improving our diets, we all have an opportunity to increase our respect for our own bodies, as well as the body of the planet as a whole, through nourishing ourselves optimally with high-quality food.

Our Cultural Inheritance

Food is an emotional issue particularly for women in our culture; food addiction is rampant. "When I begin to have anxiety," said one woman whose father was an alcoholic, "I go for pastry. As I swallow, I can almost feel my emotions going back down into my gut. Food is my friend. I use it to comfort myself whenever I am lonely." Obviously, placing this woman on a whole-food diet without addressing her other needs would cause her enormous stress. That's one reason why weight-loss diets fail again and again. They simply don't address the reasons people overeat in the first place.

Another part of the problem is that many foods are very high in addictive potential themselves: Sugar, caffeine, and refined foods are common culprits here. I believe that most women in our culture have potential or full-blown eating disorders. Our culture almost demands it. Here's my own definition of the characteristics of an eating disorder:

- Denying yourself food that you really want
- Continuing to eat even after you are full
- Eating even when you are not physically hungry
- Being constantly concerned about your weight
- Using exercise, diets, laxatives, vomiting, or food restriction regularly to control your weight

Our entire culture promotes dietary schizophrenia. Women's magazines tell us how to "Take 10 Pounds Off Fast" in the same issue in which they print "Five Chocolate Recipes Your Family Will Love You For." An insatiable market looks weekly for the next diet, because the real issues underlying why they overeat are never addressed. Happily, prominent women such as Oprah Winfrey and Roseanne Arnold are now telling us the truth about their own dieting failures, which I hope will help other women on the diet merry-go-round.

Food and emotions are very deeply linked in human beings for reasons far older than our current obsession with thinness. For centuries, the human race was able to survive because we ate the things that tribes said were okay to eat. We avoided the poisonous berries and ate what Mother said was safe. Food has always been an essential part of the daily ritual of living, and the foods we were fed in childhood have left a very deep impression on us. At an unconscious and conscious level, they *help us feel* safe and cared for.

How strange it is for our childhood emotional values to have fast-forwarded into twentieth-century adult lives. Women's roles as traditional mothers—providing the "tribal foods"—are out of date. Women need no longer think of themselves as the sole providers of food for their clans, but these roles are still deeply ingrained nonetheless. A number of vegetarian patients of mine have mothers who *still* present roast beef as a special meal when they come home. For these mothers, "the roast" is symbolic of love and caring. The conditioning that says a woman should serve abundant high-fat food to her family to ensure their survival runs very deep. We must become conscious of these patterns now. We now know that our traditional family foods—steak and ice cream—are not healthy. What once ensured our survival is killing us.

Susie Orbach's *Fat Is a Feminist Issue* documents how tied up with food women are because it is our cultural imperative to feed everybody.[2] Though my mother was way ahead of her time in many areas, she was still a product of her culture when it came to food preparation. As soon as the breakfast dishes were cleared, my father would say to her, "What's for lunch?" She used to tell me not to ask my father anything important or controversial until after he had eaten his dinner, which taught me that my job was to feed men, because a hungry man was supposedly unpredictable. At the end of the afternoon, around the time my father came home from work, my mother used to set the table even if she hadn't started dinner, so that my father would *think* that dinner was under way and that she had been busily preparing it for him for hours. A physician friend of mine said that *her* mother used to begin frying onions just before her father arrived home. The house would smell as if dinner were cooking, even though it hadn't been started. Her father would say, "Smells great, honey!" She'd then start the meal, having already produced the illusion that the meal preparation was long under way.

Both my mother and my friend's mother were operating under the 1950s and 1960s imperative that the woman's job was to feed the breadwinner when he came home, regardless of her own needs or her own schedule. This imperative to feed hungry men also operates in the sexual arena, I believe. Women have been brought up to believe that men have "sexual needs" that a woman must fulfill. It's *her* job and *her* duty to satisfy his sexual appetite as well as his nutritional appetite. If she doesn't do it well enough, he's justified in seeking fulfillment for those *male* needs outside the home. Despite the fact that nobody ever died from lack of an orgasm, the cultural mythology of the past several centuries has been that if a man isn't happy in his marriage, it is the woman's fault. My grandfather left my grandmother, I was told, partly because she wasn't "woman enough" for him. (We can only guess what that means.)

Many women have told me how when they were young their dinnertimes were orchestrated around their father's arrival home. If he was late, they waited one or two hours, while the mother tried to keep the food appetizing and calm the hungry children into waiting so that they could all sit down to a "proper" family meal. Mary Catherine Bateson's book *Composing a Life* documents that the presence of a man in a household increases the workload significantly—not because he leaves that many more dirty socks around but because of the *expectations* that he has of those around him and that *those around him have of themselves.* "Women are taught to deny themselves for the sake of the marriage," she writes; "men are taught that the marriage exists to support them."[3] We have the power to change this situation—first by noticing how we ourselves perpetuate it.

Many women have told me how much easier life is when their husbands are gone on a trip and they don't have to arrange their eating, cleaning up, and recreation schedules around his. Having been indoctrinated for a lifetime that their worth is tied up with cooking for men, many women *don't cook for themselves at all* when there's no man to please. Deep inside they've learned that only *he* is worth the effort; not themselves. And they've resented this in silence for years.

Many men's nutritional and emotional needs have been met by women since birth. When they marry, their wives often take over where their mothers left off. When a man cooks or takes care of the children, it's not culturally expected, and so it is almost always regarded as a gift, as something extra that he does for the family.

When a woman tells me that she cooks three separate dinners every night because of all the various preferences in her house, I immediately prescribe for her a book or meeting on codependency. Cooking three separate meals for people who don't appreciate the effort—and who in fact pass negative judgment upon it—is classic relationship addiction. (If, on the other hand, she's well-rewarded for her efforts, loves to cook, and she and her family have all agreed on the arrangement, no problem.)

My mother and thousands of other women employed strategies like cooking onions to give the illusion that dinner was cooking in order to survive—and then they passed these subtle dishonesties down to us. Only in the last five years or so have I become aware of how far I've come in my own deprogramming from these early messages. On a day when I'm home and my husband is not, I'm very aware of my personal programming that the house should be picked up before he arrives home from work and that dinner should be started. I'm aware of it—but I don't necessarily take action on it anymore, unless I want to. I encourage you to review some of the subtle and not-so-subtle ways in which you have been conditioned.

Bringing Our Food Preparation *Shoulds* and *Oughts* to Consciousness

Meal preparation is a minefield for many women. You cannot make a dietary change until you've mapped out your personal minefield (from childhood to the present) and have honestly examined your assumptions that you are the chief cook and bottle-washer or that you cannot take the time to prepare and enjoy good food for yourself. Especially now that the vast majority of women are working full-time outside of the home, our expectations of ourselves about food preparation need considerable updating from our mothers' day.

Ask yourself the following questions:

Do you feel personally responsible for thinking about, shopping for, and preparing the family meals? If the refrigerator is empty when family members are hungry, do you feel guilty? Inadequate? Have you ever discussed this with your spouse? Your children? Your other loved ones?

Before I became aware of my unconscious inner *shoulds* and *oughts* about food preparation, which I brought into my marriage as surely as I brought my hopes and dreams, I sometimes got resentful when my husband would innocently ask me, "What are we doing for dinner?" I used to think that he was *making* me plan the meals, shop for food, and prepare the meals. He didn't understand why I became irritable. For a while, neither did I. Then it became clear to me that I was automatically assuming that feeding him was my responsibility, even though we both worked long hours at the same job! Once I became conscious of my programming, I didn't blame him for *the fact that I felt compelled* to cook and clean against my wishes. At the same time that I was becoming conscious of my *shoulds,* he also began to take a look at his— with some help from me. He came to see that he *expected* me to do the jobs that his mother had always done. Once both of us made conscious our unconscious expectations about food, cooking, and cleaning, our relationship improved in this area. (In most relationships the unspoken *shoulds* and *oughts* for both members need to be articulated—I don't pretend that this is easy.)

Now ask yourself:
Do you enjoy preparing food? Do you prepare delicious meals for yourself even when you're alone? If the answer is no, do you make healthy choices when you eat out or when others prepare food for you?
For me, a vacation is not worth it if I have to cook three meals a day. We once rented a cabin on an island nearby, and it seemed that all I did was cook and clean up. The kids were looking for snacks constantly but weren't old enough to get them for themselves. I was not relaxed at the end of that week—I was angry. Vacation cooking can be fun, however, when the activity is shared with others.
My mother recently said, "It's no wonder retirees like to eat out so often. Many of those women have had to prepare three meals a day for over forty years. No wonder they're sick of it." And although the food on airplanes is not very healthy, I prefer being served by someone else rather than carrying healthy food with me. I believe this stems from being a mother and having to serve

others, while excluding myself, for so long. I enjoy being served and not having to clean up afterward.

Reframing Self-Nourishment

To nourish ourselves optimally, we need to expand our concept of nourishment considerably. Nourishment is not just the food that we put in our mouths. It is also the environment around us, the people we're with, the sunlight and starlight from the skies, and the color of our walls. When we expand the concept of nourishment to all levels and learn how to do it for ourselves, our struggles with physical food decrease considerably. Body weight will take care of itself. It sounds simple, but it is not easy.

Taking nourishment just for ourselves and not to please others is uncommon for women. Women are socialized to interact with others and demonstrate our love for them through shopping for, preparing, serving, and cleaning up food every day. When relationships at home or at work are not completely fulfilling and nourishing, women (and men) try to fill the hole we feel at our center with food—a hole that no amount of food will fill. Because of the massive cultural forces "out there" that keep us stuck in a pattern of eating to fill our inner emptiness, your attempts to improve your diet will be sabotaged until you become aware intellectually and emotionally of why you overeat, or don't eat, or eat only food low in nutrient value. Only we ourselves can take the first step toward breaking free of these influences. When enough women do this, the culture, too, will change.

At the same time that you're exploring your eating behavior, it's important to realize that a meat-based, refined-food diet *itself* is partly responsible for imbalanced eating and overeating. A diet that lacks whole grains, beans, and fresh vegetables almost *guarantees* food cravings. Refined foods encourage binge eating because they are not "whole." The body knows this, and it grazes, seeking the micronutrients, fiber, and vitamins that are missing.

Around 4:00 P.M., the part of our energy system known as the "emotional body" becomes the most active. For this reason, many women overeat starting in the late afternoon through the evening. If I allow myself a rest in the late afternoon, I don't "graze" until dinnertime. For years, especially during my residency training, I ate as a way to nurture myself when what I really needed to do was rest. My experience suggests that many other women do the same.

Dietary improvement and exercise programs are doomed to failure unless they're accompanied by a great deal of self-love, humor, and personal flexibility. Any hint of self-blame when you eat ice cream is a personal setup for failure. One of my patients who was using a macrobiotic diet to heal her fibroids learned that when she said "I love and respect myself," her cravings resolved. The better she felt about herself, the more she felt like eating in a healthy way.

What Should I Weigh?: Rethinking the "Diet" Mentality

Excess weight is dreams in storage. There's a myth that we can store up time. Primitive cultures store up for the winter. We store up time in our hips.

—Paulanne Balch, M.D.

Countless women over the years have asked me, "How much should I weigh?" Though all of us have been weighed and measured since birth and compared with "the cultural ideal," each individual woman must find her own *natural* weight, a weight that may not match the weight tables of any insurance company or doctor's office. The concept of an "ideal" body weight is extremely destructive for many women—and it keeps changing! The average Miss America's weight dropped from 134 pounds in 1954 to 117 pounds in 1980. The ideal fashion model twenty-five years ago weighed 8 percent less than the average American woman at that time, but today, the ideal fashion model weighs 25 percent less than the average American woman.[4] Thus, the current media image of the "ideal" body is unachievable for most women—unless they take laxatives daily, are anorexic, or use exercise addictively as a form of weight control.

Life insurance tables that give an ideal weight range depending on a woman's bone structure and height (always while wearing two-inch heels) can be misleading and are also subject to change. They do not address the biological variability among women and the fact that an individual's body might "know" what is the "correct" weight for her—and might even fluctuate with the seasons and during the month.

Magazines written for teenage girls are full of dieting and weight information and simply serve to "hook" young women into a lifetime obsession with weight and food that keeps their energy and their power tied up until they finally find the courage and the guidance to get off this road to nowhere, freeing up enormous creative energy in the process. The statistics on eating disorders speak for themselves. Currently, 1 percent of the female population has full-blown anorexia nervosa.[5] Bulimia, which consists of binge eating, self-induced vomiting, laxative use, diuretic use, or exercise to try to lose weight, is present in up to 20 percent of college students. It occurs mostly in young women age thirty or younger. Less than 5 percent of cases are in males.[6] Even so, most bulimics don't lose excessive weight but weigh slightly more than they would like to.

The medical profession reinforces these addictive behaviors by serving as "weight police," having women weigh in and admonishing them to lose weight year after year without addressing the complexities of self-nourishment for women. Because most doctors are men, their internal image of the "ideal" female is influenced heavily by the media. The male experience of weight management is often used as a model for women. One of my colleagues was an oarsman in college on the "lightweight" crew. His weight has always been about 160 pounds, and he's six feet tall. When his weight was a bit higher than the limit for crew the week before a race, he simply stopped eating desserts for a few days and ran a little more. Weight management was always easy for him—it wasn't a "moral" issue, at all. His personal weight experience taught him that "all you need to do is cut down on desserts and exercise a bit more." His approach to weight issues is the norm in the medical community: Losing weight, women are told, is simply a matter of self-discipline and willpower. Therefore, if you can't get your body where you want it (or where society thinks it should be) you are weak and have no self-control.

Most women have bodies that are meant to be larger than the cultural ideal. Women's bodies have more fat on them than men's, nature's way of assuring that the nutritional needs of childbearing will be met even during times of famine. Testosterone, the male hormone, contributes to a leaner body for men and a much higher metabolic rate than women have. Men also have proportionately more muscle than women, which leads to a higher metabolic rate. Since cultural expectations of women are that we can never be too thin, and since being thin is associated with self-control, a lifelong struggle with food and body weight is a cultural norm. Our bodies and their weight are the barometers by which society measures how good we are, how attractive we are, how worthy we are.

How much self-control and body-abusing must women go through before it dawns on us that there is something deeply wrong with our entire approach to the "weight problem"? Will-power and self-control are exactly the opposite of what we need. Even women with culturally "perfect" bodies tell me that they're not happy with themselves. Regardless of our body size, self-respect and self-acceptance are the starting points for making peace with our weight. We must know that we have the power to get off the weight treadmill and start enjoying our life, no matter where we are now.

Do You Have a "Diet Mentality"?

- Are you so afraid of gaining weight that you routinely avoid food you really love?
- Do you avoid eating all day so that you can binge at dinner?
- When you're standing before a buffet, do you routinely tell yourself that you can't have what you really want?
- Do you routinely weigh yourself after exercise?
- If you step on the scale and weigh a pound or more than usual, do you routinely beat yourself up for it? Do you let it ruin your day and influence what you eat?
- Do you allow yourself to get so hungry that you gulp whatever is available, rarely even tasting it?
- Do you say, "I'll eat this now, but I'll start on a diet on Monday," or after New Year's?
- Do you routinely drink coffee or caffeinated diet drinks during the day as a substitute for food?
- Do you routinely remove half the bread from a sandwich in order to "reduce" the calories?
- Do you know the calorie count of almost every food?

If you answered yes to any of these questions, you probably have inherited the "diet mentality." Bob Schwartz, author of *Diets Don't Work*, did a study of people who had no problems with their weight or with their food intake to determine whether the "diet mentality" could be created by food restriction.[7] The study subjects were placed on weight-loss diets to lose ten pounds each. In the process of dieting to lose weight, many of these formerly "diet-free" individuals actually developed a "diet mentality." They became obsessed with food, often for the first time ever. After losing the required ten pounds, many gained back not only the weight that they had lost but an additional five pounds besides. This additional five pounds was even harder to lose than the original ten had been. By the very process of food restriction and dieting, these formerly thin people had been transformed into people with a weight problem.

After reading about this study, I finally understood why I had been fighting the same ten pounds since I was thirteen. My very first diet had firmly implanted the "diet mentality"—and my body had rebelled, making each later attempt at restriction that much more difficult.[8] I vowed then and there to stop and I haven't weighed myself, except for an insurance physical, since then. If I were going to trust my body to know what I should weigh, I thought, I had better give it a chance. Because stepping on the scale was too loaded for me, I knew I had better avoid it until I could step on the scale and have it *not* affect me emotionally in any way, good or bad. The scale was not my friend (and still isn't). I had allowed the numbers on a bathroom scale to tell me that I was good or bad and allowed it to determine the entire quality of my day. If I weighed less than 125, it was a good day—if I weighed more than that it was a bad day. Now the scale doesn't come between me and my experience of my body.

All of us have been taught that excess weight is not just unsightly but a health risk. Studies have associated excess fat with high blood pressure, heart disease, and cancer, for example.[9] Obesity is defined as 20 percent over a person's "desirable" body weight. By this definition, 27.1 percent of all women between the ages of twenty and seventy-five are obese.[10]

Some women require big bodies—for reasons that are mysterious to me. In certain large women, their bodies—all of them—are filled with energy and vitality. They like themselves, and this self-love permeates their flesh. I doubt that these women, if they were to be studied separately, would have increased risk for disease. Interestingly, a study done by Dr. Margaret Mackensie, a social anthropologist in Western Samoa, where body fat is *not* considered undesirable in any way, showed that the fat women have no more or different health problems from the rest of the community.[11] Clearly, excess fat is not a health hazard in all women. Dr. Karen Johnson, a psychiatrist specializing in women's issues, writes, "A woman's constant quest to control her desire for food connects with our culture's constant fear of women becoming 'too big.' "[12] When I sense that a woman's energy is *big* and that she seems to require a big body to contain it, I tell her so. Culturally, we often appreciate big men who have some excess fat—why not big women?

There is no doubt that for many overweight women, excess fat represents armoring against pain they've avoided experiencing. The pain of sexual abuse and incest are especially common root causes of overeating. Given the incidence of these endemic crimes, it's no wonder that so many women eat to cover their pain. When fat is used as armor against the world, it is indeed a health risk since it has become symbolic of an unlived life—dreams in storage. Research is beginning to document the link between early abuse and later obesity.[13]

Changing Your Mindset to Create a Healthier Body

Only a small percentage of women achieve permanent weight loss by dieting, despite the multibillion-dollar diet industry. Yo-yo weight loss and regain may in fact have negative health consequences independent of one's actual weight.[14] But no matter what your weight and food history have been, you can maximize your ability to reach and maintain your *natural* weight by changing your relationship with self-nourishment and learning how to rehabilitate your metabolism. Your natural weight is the weight at which your body comfortably stays when you are eating according to your appetite and exercising regularly. As you allow your body to "find" its natural size, I would recommend that you throw your scale away and rely instead on how your clothes fit and how your body feels.

To reach your natural weight, you must also rehabilitate how you have been programmed to think about your size.

Reaching your natural weight and rehabilitating your metabolism happens in your mind and body simultaneously. The steps listed below work best when you intend to use them all. As with other health issues, a woman must change her way of thinking about food while she is changing her behavior around it so that she is truly creating health—not participating in addictive behavior. You can begin at least a part of this program now even if that means only taking a walk once a week, enjoying your breakfast more slowly, or starting a vitamin supplement. Each step you take will make it that much easier to begin the next one.

When women change their body weight slowly over time, they have a much better success rate in maintaining this weight loss because they have had time to integrate their new size into their overall self-concept. People who have been obese their whole lives and then lose weight quickly often continue to have a distorted body image and literally can't see what they really look like even after their size is normal.[15]

STEP ONE: STOP USING FOOD ADDICTIVELY, AND BE COMPLETELY HONEST ABOUT WHAT YOU ARE EATING. Look honestly at how you use food and how much of it you really eat. Include when, why, and how. If you really want to come to terms with your eating, for two weeks or more, write down everything you eat, where you ate it, and how you were feeling at the time. This exercise breaks through denial and will help you come to terms with how well you nourish yourself with food.

If you eat for emotional comfort, you may not want to give that up right now. That's okay. One of my patients who was obese until the age of twenty-one told me that she always knew she would lose weight once she moved away from home and stopped caring for her mentally ill mother and younger siblings. Though her parents took her to doctor after doctor and she was put on a series of diets, she knew that she required food to keep from feeling the pain of her circumstances. Once these changed, she lost weight.

We cannot apply *any* information about improving nutrition

until we've looked squarely at our issues around food and have committed to making peace with them. For that reason, you might address the steps to healing in Chapter 15 before or at the same time as you decide to improve your nutrition.

STEP TWO: EXAMINE YOUR REASONS FOR WANTING TO LOSE (OR GAIN) WEIGHT. The only reason to improve your nutrition or start an exercise program is because you want to nourish your body more fully—for you. Don't do it so that your husband will love you more, or so that your mother will be pleased, or because you have a high school reunion coming up. (It can't hurt, though, to let your family know that you will no longer participate in serving foods that are wrecking their health—because you care too much. Dietary improvement decreases the major health risks for men and children as well—it's very win/win.)

STEP THREE: DON'T RELY TOO MUCH ON THE ADVICE OF OTHERS TO TELL YOU WHAT YOUR BODY NEEDS. As long as my patients put me or anyone else in the "food police" role, they will never be able to tune in to their bodies' unique nutritional needs. They will forever be fighting an authority figure whom they set up as "the answer," because they don't know that "the answer" is inside—not outside.

STEP FOUR: EAT WHAT YOU WANT, WHEN YOU WANT IT. RESPECT THAT SOME OF YOUR FOOD CRAVINGS MIGHT BE PART OF YOUR INNER GUIDANCE SYSTEM. To tune in to your inner guidance about nourishment and weight, you must first begin to uncouple food and weight. In other words, don't automatically censor your food desires because of your preconceived notions of how they will affect your weight. Every time we restrict food we really want, we automatically set up a later binge. In other words, your body will automatically binge in direct proportion to how much and how long you restrict food. This restrict-binge cycle appears to be almost a law of physics.

Eat whatever your body wants, if you're not out of control with food. If you crave an oatmeal raisin cookie, get the best one you can find, then eat it slowly. Usually this will end the craving. If you're going to eat chocolate, don't go for the cheap stuff. Make it an event. Savor it slowly and fully. When you do this, you will decrease your need for that food and probably won't want it again for weeks. The point here is to change your consciousness around food. Eat on purpose, bringing your full self to the table.

Commit to trusting that your body knows what it needs when you give it a chance and start listening to it. Sometimes a two-week "intuition-cleansing" diet of whole foods only will give your body a chance to start responding.

STEP FIVE: RESPECT YOUR BODY REGARDLESS OF ITS SIZE, OR NOT ONLY WHEN IT WEIGHS A CERTAIN AMOUNT. Learn to respect the body you have, one day at a time. A commitment to body-respect is an essential step toward feeling and looking your best. Women who like themselves are irresistible and fun to be around, regardless of their size.

STEP SIX: SHARE YOUR NOURISHMENT DILEMMAS WITH OTHERS WHILE RECEIVING AND GIVING SUPPORT. To keep yourself on track, consider joining a support group that is dealing with food, weight, and emotions, such as Overeaters Anonymous. Read *Why Weight? A Guide to Breaking Free from Compulsive Eating* by Geneen Roth, and go through the exercises that apply to you.[16] Many other excellent books are available to lend support as well. Understand that the vast majority of women have issues around food, for all the reasons I've explored. You are not alone.

STEP SEVEN: EAT WHEN YOU ARE HUNGRY AND STOP WHEN YOU ARE FULL, KNOWING THAT YOU CAN EAT WHENEVER YOU NEED TO. You must become your own mother in the area of food and nourishment. Learn to tune in to your body and feed yourself whenever you are physically hungry. Sometimes I've eaten when I'm not hungry so that I wouldn't be hungry later. This pattern probably comes from a childhood of having to wait for "proper" meal times, regardless of my body's needs. I've noticed that my children sometimes think they're hungry when in fact they are bored. I've asked them to check in with their bodies so that they know the difference. When their hunger is physical, they can eat right then. I don't require them to wait until dinner.

Stop when you are full—but not bursting. You can return to eating anytime you're hungry again, regardless of when it is or who is watching. A good way to do this is to stop when you still want a bit more and commit to waiting fifteen minutes. It usually takes about that long for the brain to register fullness. My sister used to say, "My stomach is full, but my mouth still wants more." That fifteen-minute wait will often link the mouth and the stomach.

STEP EIGHT: EAT MINDFULLY—ENJOYING YOUR FOOD FULLY.
Most diet books tell us to eat only when we are sitting down. Though I personally find this difficult when I'm busy or at work, it is nonetheless an excellent way to become mindful about eating slowly and enjoying my food thoroughly. We are being disrespectful to ourselves and to our deepest needs when we gulp food on the run. When we don't take the time to taste food, savor it, or assimilate it as well as we might in a different atmosphere, we are often tempted to eat more—to fill up the "nourishment void" that results. When eating on the run becomes a habit, it is no wonder that our bodies keep screaming for more—they rarely have the experience of being nourished fully.

We can also nourish ourselves more fully by allowing ourselves to be only with the food when we are eating. Try eating a favorite food without reading or watching TV. Don't talk with food in your mouth. Consider the fact that you can enjoy only the food that is in your mouth this moment. If you are thinking about dessert or your next meal or the show on TV, your body will not be fully engaged in the process of self-nourishment and your food will be metabolized in a different way than if you were fully present with it.

This step may be difficult at first, but it will force you to pay attention to the taste of food and the experience of eating. You will give your body time to *experience* the act of physical nourishment. Cravings will decrease. Women who would like to gain weight often notice that slowing down and fully enjoying their food helps them reach their natural weight as well.

STEP NINE: FORGET ABOUT WEIGHT LOSS AND CHANGE YOUR DIET TO BECOME HEALTHIER. Far too many women associate food with its potential either to put weight on or take weight off. Whether a food is low in calories becomes more important than whether it can create health. When we decide to eat for health and become aware of how food makes us feel, we can often break old destructive dietary patterns for good.

A thirty-nine-year-old artist improved her diet to help heal her chronic vaginitis. She said to me, "I feel lighter when I eat this way—and cleaner. My nose doesn't run all the time. And I've lost eight pounds since I last saw you. I don't feel deprived at all. I know that I can eat whatever I want. You told me to experiment after avoiding all meat and all dairy food for one month. So I went back to eating cheese after about one month, but I found that I didn't like the way it felt in my body. I stopped eating it, and I feel better. *Increasingly, what I want is also what makes me feel best.* This isn't a punishment—it's just a different way of looking at things. It's a complete change of philosophy for me."

This patient underwent a paradigm shift in the way she looked at food. Weight loss was a side effect. She changed her diet to create health—not to lose weight. By changing her diet to create health, she not only lost weight but eventually came to the point where the food she wanted the most was also the food that made her feel the best. She is now in tune with the wisdom of her body, and her former "war" against herself is over.

STEP TEN: SPEND TIME WITH PEOPLE WHO HAVE NO ISSUES WITH FOOD OR WITH THEIR WEIGHT AND THEREFORE EAT NORMALLY. Many of my patients reevaluate friendships that support unhealthy eating. If they always spend time with those who use eating to stuff their emotions or as their only form of entertainment, they quite literally feel and act heavier around these people. You may need to make some new friendships.

STEP ELEVEN: REHABILITATE YOUR METABOLISM AFTER THE YO-YO DIETING CYCLE. Some women find that they can't seem to lose any weight regardless of what they eat but can gain weight on as little as 1,200 calories a day. Such a woman probably has a very slow metabolism resulting from years of dieting and food restriction. When she was in her twenties and thirties, she probably had no problem losing five pounds fast, on whatever diet she chose.

But now, after years of dieting and bingeing, her metabolism may be slowed down permanently unless she makes some adjustments. After each loss/gain cycle, a woman's proportion of body fat increases. Regardless of whether she has been a yo-yo dieter, as a woman ages, her muscle mass is gradually replaced by fat.

All of this can be reversed. To speed up your metabolism, you must decrease the amount of fatty tissue in the body and increase your muscle mass. Muscle has a much higher metabolic rate than fat, and it burns more calories even when we are sleeping. Muscle also weighs more than fat, another reason why body weight has very little to do with health. A woman who has a body fat content of 35 percent may weigh much less than a woman whose fat content is only 20 percent!

• Exercise. As women age, muscle mass is often replaced by fat gain because of lack of exercise. Exercise reverses this fat gain–muscle loss trend no matter what age you start. Women who exercise regularly can look forward on average to twenty more years of productive living than those who don't. To be effective, aerobic-type exercise must last at least 15 to 20 minutes three times per week. (Aerobic exercise means vigorously enough so that your heartbeat increases to your target rate for at least fifteen minutes— see Chapter 18.) The more exercise you do, the faster your metabolism speeds up. Fast walking works very well. (Watch it— exercise taken to extremes can also be a form of addiction.) The increase in metabolic rate with exercise lasts even after the exercise is finished.

• Reduce Dietary Fat Consumption. Fat in the diet becomes body fat faster than any other food. Fat gram counting is a breeze. After about two days, you'll get the hang of it. You'll also find that you can eat more food than you ever imagined if you have a calorie-counting mentality. Buy a fat gram counter at a supermarket or bookstore, and learn the fat content of food. Cut dietary fat to under 40 grams per day.[17] You can increase the fat amount after a 2-

week trial until you find a level that suits you. For some it's as high as 60. For others, as low as 25. Throw away your calorie counter for good. Read labels in the grocery store. Fat grams are listed there for most common foods. More low-fat or no-fat items are available now than ever before. If you splurge on a high-fat dessert once in a while, you can easily make adjustments later.

• Increase Dietary Fiber. A diet based on whole grains (like brown rice, millet, barley, and oats), beans, dark green leafy and other vegetables, and fruits is automatically low in fat and high in nutrients. Learn to use meat as a condiment only. This type of diet has also been shown to decrease cancer risk. When I changed my diet to mostly vegetarian in 1980, I did so because I loved the food.

A lovely side effect was that I no longer lost and gained weight depending upon what I had just had for breakfast or dinner. A grain and vegetable–based diet is so centered in its carbohydrate/protein ratio (about seven to one) that cravings for foods that are unbalanced diminish greatly.

• Use Mineral and Herb Supplements. The mineral chromium has been found to increase the metabolic rate. Chromium is in short supply in nine out of ten American diets[18] and it is absolutely essential for normal insulin function. Ingestion of 200 mcg. of chromium daily has been shown to result in significant fat loss, while muscle tissue has been spared or increased.[19]

At Women to Women we have found that certain herbal preparations combined with chromium also help decrease sugar and fat cravings.[20]

STEP TWELVE: NAMING COMPULSIVE EATING AS A PROBLEM AND TAKING ACTION. If a woman's compulsive overeating is out of control, she may want and need a structured food plan for a while. The plan works as an external control system as she learns what her internal triggers to overeating are. Many women have not yet established the link between their emotional pain and how they are using food to control it. Others may have so much stress in their lives that their immune and metabolic systems are adversely affected. For these women, even small amounts of sugary sweets, yeasty foods, or salty or fatty foods set off binge eating. Most women will fall into one of two broad categories: those who binge on fat-laden sweets such as ice cream and those who binge on salty, fat-laden foods such as potato chips. For these women, sugary or salty, fat-laden food is like alcohol to an alcoholic. Sugar-addicted women have told me that they become light-headed, feel drunk and disoriented, and develop an insatiable desire to eat more and more sugary foods, once they start. (The same thing can apply to fatty and salty binge food.) When women avoid these "trigger foods," their eating returns to normal.

I have noticed that women who come from alcoholic families or who are or have been alcoholics themselves are often very prone to food addictions: You probably know already if you have this problem. You will not be able to stop eating after two spoonfuls of ice cream or chocolate chip cookies or after two potato chips or corn chips. Until you regain some sobriety around these foods, which may take months or years, you will have to eliminate them from your diet completely, so that they will not serve as "triggers" to binge eating. Continuing to eat such trigger foods will keep you out of touch with your inner guidance and with your emotions, such as anger.

Women who binge are often deficient in the B vitamins and magnesium[21] as well as chromium. A dietary supplement of 200 mg. of chromium daily can provide nutrient support for optimal blood sugar metabolism.[22] For this reason I often recommend a good multivitamin-mineral supplement for all women who have a history of binge eating, bulimia, yo-yo weight loss and gain, or anorexia.

Opinions on the effectiveness of food restriction vary. Some women feel the need to be on a food plan for years. Some Overeaters Anonymous (OA) meetings use food plans that restrict all refined flour and sugar products, as well as nuts and salty foods such as potato chips. Others don't. Some women, once they deal with the emotional issues that lead to bingeing, have no need for the food plan as an "external authority." If refined foods send you off the deep end, it is prudent to avoid them and see how being free from these substances affects you.

You will know what plan is right for you by checking in with your inner guidance. See which plan feels right emotionally. Don't go with the one you *think* you *should* be on. Go with what feels generous and kind to your body. Marcelle Pick and Susan Doughty, two of my associates at Women to Women who are registered nurses, have prepared sample food plans, guidelines, and suggestions for making friends with food that we use at our office and in our classes. (See the Appendix.)

Food and Energy

A highly refined, sugary, fatty diet promotes food addiction. On the other hand, it is very difficult to binge on whole food. Have you ever been able to eat eight apples when you've been upset? Three pieces of cheesecake, in contrast, go down quite well. A number of studies have documented the link between food, behavior, and mood. Religious orders, particularly in Asia, have noted that a vegetarian diet promotes inward spiritual attunement, while eating red meat produces more aggressive tendencies. Many of my patients feel calmer when eating a diet based on grains, beans, and vegetables, but are very apt to have violent dreams and anxious feelings after eating red meat. My husband has noticed this, too, and avoids red meat because of it. Experiment with this yourself to see how the energy of food affects you. A number of scientific studies have documented the link between violence, high dietary cholesterol, and triglycerides. The most common source of these high levels is dietary fat from meat consumption. A recent study in *Lancet,* for instance, indicated that high serum triglyceride levels in men were associated with aggression, hostile acts, and a domineering attitude independent of cigarette smoking and alcohol consumption. In women, high serum cholesterol levels were associated with denigratory behavior toward others.[23]

Studies on schoolchildren and the observations of many parents have supported the fact that foods that are low in nutrients and high in sugar, caffeine, and food additives sometimes produce erratic behavior. Alexander Schauss has documented the link between diet, crime, and delinquency, showing the connection between diets high in sugar and preservatives and subsequent erratic behavior.[24]

Years of clinical practice have convinced me that the energy of food has emotional and psychological consequences. Foods aren't broken down completely into anonymous fats, carbohydrates, and proteins when they're digested—they retain some of their original energy. Like humans, food is more than the sum of its parts. It is affected by the way it is raised, processed, handled, and cooked. In short, food has its own unique energy field—*prana* or *chi*. In ancient monasteries, only the most enlightened monks were allowed to cook and handle the food because it was felt that their energy field affected the food. Food has effects other than simply those related to its digestive end products of fat, carbohydrates, and proteins.[25]

Vegetables, whole cereal grains, and beans are centering foods, while meat and refined sugar are on the opposite ends of the scale. In a macrobiotic sense the "balance" for meat and cheese is sugar. Meat is regarded as very contracted and dense or yang, whole sugar and desserts are very expansive or yin.[26] Using this view, the Standard American Diet is balanced but not centering. Eating meat leads to a craving for sweets, and vice versa. A primarily grain, bean, and vegetable-based diet is more centered and leads to fewer cravings. (See Figure 15.)

Grains, Beans, and Health: Macrobiotics

Scientific studies show that a mostly vegetarian, low-fat, whole-food diet is preventive medicine at its finest, whereas the high-fat, high-protein Standard American Diet is dangerous to health.[27] A body of evidence suggests that our current epidemic of heart disease began in the last seventy years, when hydrogenated fats, the food containing them, and refined food devoid of antioxidant vitamins were introduced. Despite our cultural beliefs, a mostly vegetarian, grain-based diet is completely adequate to meet nutritional needs. When I began to learn about macrobiotics, I had just completed eight years of training in a worldview that sees disease as the enemy—to be cut out, suppressed, or eliminated. I then learned about a system that sees disease as the result of imbalance. This system addresses the imbalance, not just the symptoms that result from it.

Michio Kushi, using Oriental diagnosis theory, showed me the energy meridians of the human body and how an imbalance in one system causes imbalances in another. Macrobiotics teaches that we

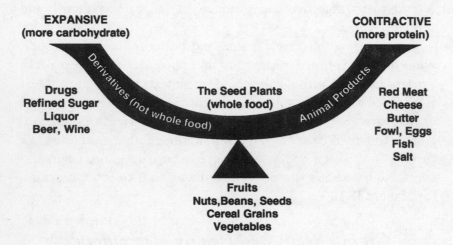

FIGURE 15: THE ENERGETICS OF FOOD

cannot give a drug or suppress symptoms in one area without consequences somewhere else. Inherent in this approach is respect for the body's natural healing ability, once it is given the necessary conditions. A key prescription for health in this system is a grain-based diet supplemented with locally grown produce and other traditional foods, such as miso soup. Yoga, shiatsu massage, time spent outside daily, and a reverent approach to life are also advocated. The common nutritional causes of women's health problems are said to be excess consumption of dairy food, sugar, and meat.

Individuals who follow the macrobiotic diet and lifestyle changes carefully over the course of two to three months and who seem committed to this new way of life experience changes in physical appearance that are astounding. They often look ten or twenty years younger in a very short period of time. Bridget was thirty-five when she was diagnosed with thyroid cancer. As part of her healing, she came to the Kushi Institute for dietary advice. She followed the prescribed strict macrobiotic healing diet precisely for three months. When she returned, her skin was glowing and she had lost twenty pounds effortlessly. Most striking, however, was a complete change in the energy coming from her. She seemed not only younger but wiser—as though she were illuminated from within.

In others, a macrobiotic diet has cured chronic diseases such as scleroderma, Crohn's disease, and even some cancers. The people cured said they had never felt better in their lives. One thirty-two-year-old nurse named Cindy had sought dietary consultation following her diagnosis of Crohn's disease. Standard medical treatment for this inflammatory bowel condition is steroid medication. Cindy knew well the side effects of this drug and therefore she sought alternatives. Within one month of changing her diet, all her bowel symptoms cleared. She also looked vibrant and healthy—healthier, in fact, than she had looked for a decade. All of her colleagues wanted to know what she was doing. As long as she avoids refined foods and dairy products and stays on a mostly grain and vegetable diet, she is asymptomatic. Her follow-up biopsies have been negative, showing no evidence of Crohn's disease. I had not seen this kind of physical transformation very often after conventional medical treatments for the same types of illnesses.

Based on this experience, in my own practice I began prescribing simple dietary changes for those who were open to this approach, often with good results. I noticed that stopping caffeine, dairy food, and refined sugar products often cured headaches, vaginal infections, and PMS.

Most important, I found that the macrobiotic dishes to which I was introduced said yes to my body. The food was nourishing, delicious, and calming. I changed my own diet slowly and took a series of cooking classes at the Kushi Institute. Whole grains, beans, and vegetables have been our family's staple foods ever since. Macrobiotic cuisine, well prepared by someone who knows the foods, is as delicious and gourmet-tasting as anything else and is my favorite way to eat. I'm *not* referring to a macrobiotic healing diet, which is very strict and should be tried only under the care of someone who is skilled in this approach. My family and I didn't begin this way of eating because we were sick, however. Our diet is about 80 to 90 percent whole foods. The rest consists of the highest-quality vegetarian or fish dishes we can find in restaurants, at the hospital, and while traveling. We've been known to stop at McDonald's in a pinch (though not for hamburgers), and I continue to wish it were easier to eat healthfully while traveling. We often go out to dinner on weekends and enjoy living in the world. Too often I've seen dietary rigidity come between people. There's nothing worse than someone who is overly righteous about food choices. (Self-righteousness is probably more harmful to health than all the hamburgers in the world.) Once at a macrobiotic summer camp, I was eating a fresh peach. A young man came up to me and said, "That's poison." From his point of view, the peach was too yin (expansive) and didn't meet his criteria for a "centered" food. His viewpoint will make sense to those who are following a strict healing diet, but for most it is simply too judgmental.

Macrobiotics in the broadest sense is a holistic philosophy and way of life, not just a diet. *Macrobiotic* means "big life"—a way of life that is intended to keep us in balance with our environment by balancing the energies known as *yin* and *yang*. The purist macrobiotic diet is one in which we eat what is locally grown whenever possible. The theory is that to be present in the here and now, we should eat what is available in the here and now. Thus, for an Inuit, a macrobiotic diet would include seal meat and whale blubber. For a Native American from the Northeast, it would include deer and corn.

Macrobiotic cuisine also changes with the seasons. This makes a great deal of intuitive sense: Cool salads (yin) are served most often in the summer when the weather is hot (yang), while hot stews (yang) feel better in the winter when the weather is cold (yin).[28] Meals are arranged according to the four seasons, so that we can easily get a grasp of how to vary our cooking to be in tune with the changes in the seasons. This approach acknowledges and strengthens our link to the earth and to its natural rhythms. To enjoy optimal health, we quite naturally want to eat differently in the summer (salads and cooler foods) than in the winter (stews and heartier fare). To be present in the here and now, it's helpful to eat what grows around us locally, according to the season.

Back in the 1960s, when many young people first turned to more vegetarian diets, doctors warned that they might not get enough protein, calcium, or vitamin B_{12}. Because most Americans have no tradition based on vegetarian eating, this concern had some justification. Vegetarian eating for some consists of french fries, salad, cola, and a half-pound of cheese per day. When I order a vegetarian meal in some establishments, I get a large platter of overcooked vegetables. No grain or bean dish is even considered. No wonder vegetarian diets have been so misunderstood. Our culture has forgotten that the staple food of almost every civilization has been grains and vegetables—not meat.

As I began to apply what I was learning about nutrition in my practice, I saw that nutritional improvement and regular exercise are powerful ways to create health. (See Table 8.) Most women are amazed by how much better they feel when they eliminate most refined foods, meat, dairy products, and caffeine from their diets. The link between diet, fat, and female organs, as we saw in Part Two, is impressive. Our fat-rich, fiber-poor diet is part of the reason that breast cancer, endometriosis, and uterine fibroids are on the increase, affecting millions of women. Sixty percent of all cancers in females (breast, ovary, and uterus) are related to the level of consumption of dietary fat.[29] Both benign and malignant conditions of the ovary, breast, and uterus are related to estrogen levels that are too high.[30] A diet high in a variety of vegetable fibers may lower a woman's estrogen levels, therefore decreasing her risk of breast cancer. Vegetable fibers change the metabolism of estrogen in the bowel. Less is available for absorption into the bloodstream from the bowel and more estrogen is excreted.

Women who start their menstrual cycles (undergo menarche) earlier and their menopause later are at greater risk for breast cancer. American women's menarche is characteristically early (at age twelve or thirteen) and their menopause late.[31] But women who follow low-fat vegetarian diets, such as the Chinese and the !Kung, typically start their menstrual periods at age sixteen or seventeen. They also begin menopause earlier. Their breast cancer rates are very low.[32]

TABLE 8: BENEFITS AND RISKS OF DIETARY CHOICES

Low-Fat, Mostly Vegetarian Low- or No-Dairy, High-Fiber Diet	High-Fat, High-Protein Standard American Diet
reduces risk of bowel cancer	increases risk of bowel cancer
reduces risk of breast, ovarian, uterine cancer	increases risk of breast, ovarian, uterine cancer
reduces risk of cardiovascular disease	increases risk of cardiovascular disease
reduces risk of varicose veins	increases risk of varicose veins
reduces risk of gallstones	increases risk of gallstones
reduces constipation	increases constipation
reduces risk of osteoporosis	increases risk of osteoporosis
relieves heavy menstrual bleeding	exacerbates heavy menstrual bleeding
relieves endometriosis symptoms	may exacerbate endometriosis symptoms
reduces fibroid symptoms	increases fibroid symptoms
reduces breast tenderness	increases breast tenderness
reduces breast cysts	increases breast cysts
relieves polycystic ovary syndrome	exacerbates polycystic ovary syndrome
promotes natural body weight	promotes excess body fat
promotes emotional well-being	may exacerbate mood swings and depression
relieves PMS	exacerbates PMS

Note: Benefits can be significantly decreased when alcohol, refined sugar, caffeine, or tobacco are used addictively.

Breast tissue is exquisitely sensitive to high-fat diets and raised estrogen levels, as we saw in Chapter 10. High-fat diets stimulate breast tissue through excessive estrogen production, resulting in breast pain and cyst formation in many women.[33] Many breast cancer tumors are stimulated by hormones such as estrogen. Tamoxifen, a drug used to treat breast cancer, works by lowering estrogen's effect on breast tissue. The higher the body fat and dietary fat, the higher the estrogen levels and the greater the risk for breast and other gynecological cancer.[34] Body fat itself manufactures estrone, a type of estrogen, through the conversion of cholestrol to androsterone.

As you can see, the diet-fat-female link is impressive. Dr. Dean Ornish has impeccably documented reversal of coronary artery disease in the "high heart" through diet, exercise, and emotional support.[35] And as you will recall, what is good for the "high heart" is good for the "low heart"—the uterus and ovary area. The same diet that reverses or prevents heart disease also works well for common gynecological problems that are *related to* excessive estrogen stimulation: ovarian cysts, breast tenderness, benign breast lumps, heavy menstrual cycles, fibroid tumors, and endometriosis.[36]

Clearly, the primary motivation to change your diet may be to relieve health problems. Simply decreasing the fat in your diet to 20 to 40 grams per day, without necessarily stopping meat or dairy food, may help reduce breast tenderness or uterine problems such as heavy menstrual bleeding or pressure from fibroids. Studies show that people who reduce their intake of animal protein and fat in general are healthier than those who don't, even when fat levels are not lowered. In general, the more we restrict fats, refined foods, dairy food, and meat, the faster and more dramatic the results. (Caution: It is possible to do anything addictively. Don't go overboard, and don't do this without sound nutritional planning.) Here's an example of one woman's healing evolution through dietary change.

When Melanie, a physical therapist, first came to see me in the mid-1980s, she was anemic and had had several D&Cs (dilation and curettage of the uterus) for heavy bleeding. The results of these were benign (no cancer). Her well-meaning doctor at the time had told her she must eat lots of good red meat, which she did almost daily. But her uncontrollable bleeding became worse and finally a hysterectomy was recommended. She came to me for a second opinion.

When I examined her, her uterus was enlarged to the size of a fourteen-week pregnancy from fibroid tumors. The spongy consistency of the uterus also suggested adenomyosis, a condition in which the glands inside the lining of the uterus grow into the muscle wall of the organ. This creates "lakes" of blood inside the uterine muscle wall and can lead to very heavy menstrual periods. Based on her history and physical exam, I told Melanie that hysterectomy was certainly a reasonable option for her. But if she were interested in alternatives and would like to save her uterus, I'd suggest a low-fat diet as a trial. I stressed that she could always have the uterus removed if the diet didn't work or if she hated doing it. I explained to her that excess fat and cholesterol (her cholesterol was elevated to 298) produce excess estrogen, which can produce abnormal fibroid-type tissue. (See Figure 7, page 169.) Hysterectomy might well be necessary, I said, unless she were willing to completely change her diet to one based on low fat and nondairy foods.

Melanie was more than willing to try this and wondered why she had never been given information on the link between diet and fibroids before. She sought a consultation with a macrobiotic dietary counselor, which led to a change in her diet and in her whole family's way of life. Along with a strict healing macrobiotic diet, her counselor recommended hot-tub soaks (known as hip baths, with water just covering the hips) five times a week, with sea salt and seaweed water added to the tub water. (Seaweed is soaked in boiling water, and then this water is strained into the tub water. Seaweed water combined with sea salt creates a very mineral-rich solution for the body to soak in.) Following this, Melanie was told to lie down for twenty minutes. She found herself looking forward to these baths and rest periods. Before, she would not have afforded herself the luxury of time devoted only to herself. This time devoted to relaxation and meditation resulted in a whole new way of being for her. She became more peaceful, centered, and aware.

The macrobiotic diet was not a complete revolution for Melanie or her family. They had never used sugary foods and had always gardened and eaten fresh vegetables. But like most Americans, they had eaten a great deal of cheese and red meat. Melanie's husband joined her in cooking classes and helped her prepare meals. She had also been interested in natural and spiritual healing for years and did yoga occasionally. But now these activities became part of her daily life. She and her husband grew closer. His workaholic nature calmed, and he became less stressed. Her daughter, seeing the changes in Melanie, joined her parents for a few cooking classes. She soon adopted the diet herself to improve her own health.

Within eight months Melanie's uterus decreased from fourteen weeks' size to eight weeks' size, and the bleeding and anemia resolved completely. After two years, her uterus returned to essentially normal size. Admittedly, all this took tremendous focus and discipline, but she told me that the feeling of well-being, vibrant health, and energy that resulted helped keep her on track.

About five years after Melanie healed her bleeding fibroid problem, her mother died—her coronary arteries were completely clogged with cholesterol. Melanie realized that had she opted for the original solution of hysterectomy, she would probably be well on her way to a similar fate. "Treating one small aspect of my body with wisdom," she says, "brought healing and understanding that went beyond myself to my family to my relationships with my patients as a physical therapist, and immeasurably to every aspect of my life. Each part of us is, after all, a piece of the whole, ultimately extending to the total of all life."

If you, like Melanie, are drawn to macrobiotics, I'd recommend working with a cook or counselor who has had training in the philosophy and application of macrobiotic principles. Though it is relatively easy to change your diet by following recipes in a book, it is much more satisfying to have help putting the whole thing together. A dietitian can help you put together a low-fat plan, if that is the change you feel most comfortable with right now.[37]

It is completely possible to be healthy on any number of dietary approaches and individual variations abound. I have had the most experience with a macrobiotic approach, and also find it the most delicious and versatile of the mostly vegetarian options. (See Table 9.)

Common Concerns

AM I GETTING ENOUGH PROTEIN? When we changed to a mostly vegetarian diet, my husband worried that our children would not be getting enough protein. I hear this question repeatedly, though information to the contrary has been available for years. Nutritionists originally thought the nine amino acids that

TABLE 9:
NUTRITIONAL APPROACHES FOR WOMEN

Health-Creating

Disease-Promoting

Standard Macrobiotic Diet

50% whole cereal grains, 10-20% beans, 20-30% locally grown organic vegetables and fruits, sea vegetables, nuts, seeds. Includes traditional foods such as tempeh, tofu, miso. Occasional fish, meat, and eggs, depending upon level of activity and personal constitution. Diet is inherently low-fat, high-fiber, low-protein. Foods and cooking methods vary with seasons. Minimal caffeine, alcohol, refined sugar, refined flour.

Vegan Diet
Grains, beans, vegetables, fruits, nuts, seeds. No animal food of any kind (no eggs, milk). Inherently low-fat, low-protein, high-fiber. May require B_{12} supplementation.

Low-Fat, Low-Protein Diet
May include either vegetarian or animal foods. Dietary fat 40 grams or less/day. Dietary protein no more than 50 grams/day. Generally high in fiber.

Vegetarian Diet
Grains, beans, vegetables, fruits, nuts, seeds, dairy products, eggs. Excludes meat, poultry, and fish. Usually high-fiber.

High-Fat, High-Protein Standard American Diet
Meat, poultry, eggs, high-fat cheese and dairy food, processed meats, high-fat meats, minimal vegetables, and fruit. Generally high in refined sugar and refined flour products. Usually low-fiber, high-fat.

are the building blocks for protein had to be present *in the same meal eaten at the same time* for all of the protein in vegetarian food to be utilized by the body. We now know that this is not true. "You might once have learned that 'complete proteins,' with sufficient amounts of all amino acids, are not found in vegetable foods, or that you have to make careful combinations of foods such as beans and rice in order to make the protein complete. Fortunately, scientific

596

studies have plainly debunked this complicated nonsense," writes John McDougall.[38] The protein from the oatmeal that you ate in the morning will be able to combine with the protein from your lentil soup at lunch to give you your essential amino acids. In other words, most vegetarian diets contain adequate amounts of protein.

Traditional ethnic food automatically contains complementary amino acids, such as beans and corn, rice and soybeans, lentils and couscous. *For most of the world's population meat is a condiment only—not the main course.* Women may start decreasing meat in their diets by thinking of it as a condiment. A grain or other vegetarian dish should be the main course. Though many women know this intellectually, they don't practice it when it comes to meal preparation—old tapes take over, and they feel required to make "nice meaty sandwiches."

Most Americans eat more protein than they require anyway. (See Table 10.) A comprehensive study by T. Colin Campbell, a nutritional biochemist at Cornell University, compared American with Chinese diets. It found that protein consumption, especially from animal sources, is linked to chronic disease. Campbell found that only 7 to 10 percent of the protein eaten by the Chinese comes from animals, compared with 70 percent for Americans. The highest rates of heart disease, cancer, and diabetes—the Western diseases of affluence—are found in areas of China where people eat the most protein.[39]

TABLE 10:
AMERICAN WOMEN'S NEED FOR, AND CONSUMPTION OF, PROTEIN

Age	RDA (grams)	Average Consumption (grams)
11–14	46	66
15–18	44	63
19–24	46	65
25–49	50	55
70+	50	49

Source: HHS, *Nutrition Monitoring in the U.S.* (1989) and *Nutrition Action Newsletter*, June 1993.

Commercially produced chicken has as much hormonal and pesticide residues as does beef, pork, lamb, and veal (red meat). On the other hand, the effects of low-fat beef on blood cholesterol and other lipids are no different from those of fish and chicken.[40] The problem is that most commercially produced beef is heavily marbled with fat.

For most women, becoming overnight vegetarians is asking too much. So a bit of chicken and fish is fine, as are lean cuts of red meat. Ann-Louise Gittleman points out that some women need a bit of red meat now and again for optimal functioning.[41] Game such as venison, buffalo, elk, and moose is generally very low fat and in some locations is becoming more commercially available.

AM I GETTING ENOUGH VITAMIN B_{12}? The vitamin B complex is important for immunity and may help prevent cancer.[42] This nutrient group also helps estrogen metabolism[43] and bowel function.[44] The B complex occurs naturally in many foods in their natural state. The milling of grains into refined flour results in the loss of much of the B vitamins. Vitamin B_{12} is found to some extent in tempeh, sea vegetables, and animal food, but the highest sources are red meat, fish, eggs, and dairy products. Yet most cases of vitamin B_{12} deficiency are in meat-eating people, not vegetarians. Some scientists believe that subtle B_{12} shortages can cause psychiatric symptoms, including mood disorder, psychosis, violent behavior, and dementia.[45]

The amount of B_{12} one has in her body has little to do with whether she is a vegetarian or not. It has more to do with her overall intake of this nutrient, combined with her ability to absorb and metabolize it. The issue of vitamin B_{12} speaks to the enormous biochemical individuality among people. Some people's bodies can make this vitamin sufficiently that they don't need to get it from dietary sources, whereas others can't seem to absorb enough from their diets.[46] For most vegetarians, adding small amounts of animal food in the form of some fish, lean red meat, or an egg occasionally takes care of the requirement for vitamin B_{12}. Others prefer a supplement.

BUT PEOPLE *NEED* MILK, DON'T THEY? Like most Americans, I was taught to consume excessive dairy food, even though three-quarters of the world's population manages to maintain health without drinking milk after infancy.[47] Stopping dairy food often improves menstrual cramps, endometriosis pain, allergies, sinusitis, and even recurrent vaginitis. Because an entire generation of baby boomers has been raised on cow's milk instead of human milk, the cow at some deep level is now associated with "mother" and "nourishment." The very notion of eliminating dairy products causes heart palpitations in some of my patients. They cannot conceive of it—"But don't I *need* milk?"

As a gynecologist, I also see many problems associated with dairy food: benign breast conditions, chronic vaginal discharge, acne, menstrual cramps, fibroids, chronic intestinal upset, and increased pain from endometriosis. I can't help but think that there might be some correlation between overstimulation of the cow's mammary glands and subsequent overstimulation of our own, resulting in benign breast conditions. Nursing babies as well as their mothers are affected by what the mothers eat. They sometimes develop symptoms of cow's milk allergy when their mothers are consuming a lot of cow's milk.

High-fat dairy food consumption has been implicated in both breast and ovarian cancers.[48] With the excessive number of women currently getting breast cancer, women should question continuing a high-fat, high-protein diet.

BUT WHERE WILL I GET MY CALCIUM? Women can get their calcium from the same place that cattle get it: from grains and dark green leafy vegetables such as kale, collard greens, and broccoli. Most of the world's population, including China, which has almost no breast cancer and no osteoporosis in rural areas, gets its calcium from greens. T. Colin Campbell's studies also show that while the Chinese consume only half the calcium of Americans, osteoporosis is uncommon in China despite an average life expectancy of seventy years—only five years less than ours.[49]

African Bantu women eat no dairy foods, but they consume 150 to 400 mg. of calcium daily through the food they do eat. This is half the amount of calcium consumed by the average American woman. Yet osteoporosis is essentially unknown among the 10 percent of the female Bantus who reach more than sixty years of age. Genetic protection was considered the reason but has been ruled out. When relatives of these same Bantu people migrate to more affluent societies and adopt rich diets, osteoporosis and diseases of the teeth become more common.[50]

The calcium supplement and dairy industries have been so effective at offering us an osteoporosis "fix" that we think we can reduce the complexity of bone physiology to a formula as simple as taking calcium pills. But bone is affected by a whole host of factors (see Chapter 14), and bone health is profoundly affected by our daily food and exercise choices.

The current recommended daily allowance (RDA) for calcium *in the United States* is 800 mg. a day for women aged twenty-five and older. Fully 50 percent of American women do not consume this RDA and are thus felt to be at increased risk for osteoporosis.

The current World Health Organization recommendation for calcium intake is 400 mg. per day—half the amount recommended in the United States. For most of the world this is adequate. The average Chinese, who has a very low risk of osteoporosis, consumes 544 mg. of calcium each day, versus 1,143 per day for the average Westerner.[51] If our diets were mostly whole grains, greens, beans, and vegetables, our bones would be more apt to stay healthy on relatively less calcium, as long as we also exercised and got out in the sun for Vitamin D. (See Figures 16 and 17.)

IF I TAKE MORE CALCIUM, WILL IT PREVENT OSTEOPOROSIS?
Women today are commonly advised to drink even more milk and/or consume all manner of calcium supplements or antacids such as Tums to prevent osteoporosis. But osteoporosis is a multifactorial problem in which calcium intake plays a relatively small part. Therefore, the osteoporosis discussion should not be limited to calcium alone. Osteoporosis prevention is *much more complex* than a simple matter of increased calcium intake.

Bones are made of much more than calcium.[52] Magnesium is in much shorter supply than calcium in our diets because of poor dietary choices (refined grains and too few dark green leafy vegetables), soil depletion from erosion, and overuse of chemical fertilizers instead of organic farming methods. We should be supplementing our diets with magnesium, too, not just calcium,

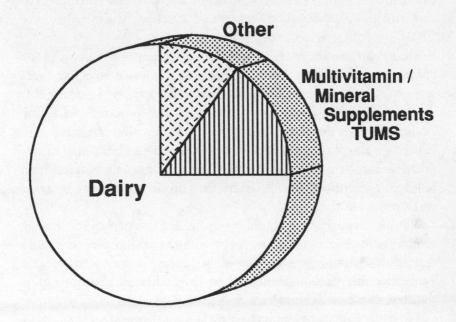

FIGURE 16: CONVENTIONAL AMERICAN APPROACH TO
CALCIUM INTAKE

because the balance between calcium and magnesium is very important.[53]

When our diet is too high in protein, the process of protein
metabolism creates a slightly acidic condition in the blood. To
balance this, the body breaks down bone and uses the calcium to
buffer the blood. Since the average American diet is too high in
protein, all of us, not just menopausal women, are in danger of
developing osteoporosis.[54] A diet high in fat also sets the stage for
osteoporosis by contributing to *decreased absorption of calcium*
from the diet. (Americans still eat far too much fat. In the Chinese
diet about 15 percent of the calories come from fat, compared with
almost 40 percent in the United States.) Other American staple

substances such as caffeine, alcohol, and cigarettes also contribute greatly to osteoporosis. Antacids like Tums decrease the acidity of the stomach, which actually contributes to *decreased* absorption of calcium. One lecturer at our center calls calcium "the laetrile of the 1980s."

Colas and root beer also contribute to osteoporosis because the coloring agent and the phosphorous used in these drinks interferes with calcium metabolism.[55] In our addictive society, a leading soft drink manufacturer soothes our fears of this practice by adding calcium to their diet drink. Many women maintain their weight by drinking a six-pack or more of diet cola per day and skipping meals. Chronic stress is also a contributor to osteoporosis because high levels of epinephrine, produced by the adrenal glands, can increase calcium loss in the urine.[56]

The best approach to building bone health is a holistic one in which we look at all the dietary, environmental, and genetic factors related to osteoporosis development. Eating a balanced, mostly vegetarian diet rich in greens such as kale, collards, and broccoli is the first step (see Table 11).

Note the following points about calcium sources:

- Nutritional content of food is dependent upon where the food was grown, when it was harvested, the quality of the soil, and so on.
- There can be wide variation in mineral content of foods, depending upon soil mineralization.
- Organically grown vegetables have higher nutritional content.
- The figures presented in the table represent average amounts of calcium found in the foods that were analyzed at the time of data collection.
- Calcium is only one of the minerals needed for optimal nutrition.
- Nondairy sources of calcium are particularly rich in the *other* minerals needed for health. Some argue that plant oxalates found in spinach and some other greens interfere with calcium absorption. The same argument has been used for phytates in grain. Newer data suggest that this absorption issue has been highly overemphasized and is not very significant.[57]

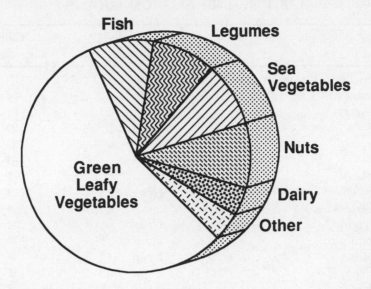

FIGURE 17: BALANCED APPROACH TO CALCIUM INTAKE

GREEN LEAFY
VEGETABLES
collard greens; wild
greens (lambs
quarters, wild onions);
spinach; turnip greens;
broccoli; kale; beet
greens; bok choy;
mustard greens;
watercress; rhubarb
stems; parsley;
dandelion greens

NUTS
almonds;
sunflower;
brazil nuts;
hazelnuts;
sesame seeds

FISH
sardines;
salmon;
oysters

SEA
VEGETABLES
hijiki; wakame;
kombu (kelp);
agar-agar
(Kanten flakes);
dulse

LEGUMES
tofu-firm; tempeh;
garbanzo
(chickpeas); black
beans; pinto beans;
tortillas; corn

DAIRY
milk (skim, whole);
cheese; ice milk;
nonfat yogurt;
cottage cheese

OTHER
mineral waters (Perrier,
Mendocino, San Pellegrino,
Apollinaris, Contexeville);
molasses; orange juice
(calcium fortified); calcium-
rich herb infusions

TABLE 11: HIGH CALCIUM FOODS[58]

Food	Amount	Calcium (mgs.)
Green Leafy Vegetables (cooked, unless specified)		
collard greens	1 cup	300
wild greens		
(lambs quarters, wild onions)	1 cup	350
broccoli	1 cup	150
kale	1 cup	179
spinach	1 cup	278
turnip greens	1 cup	229
beet greens	1 cup	165
bok choy	1 cup	200
mustard greens	1 cup	150
rhubarb	1 cup	348
watercress (raw)	1 cup	53
parsley (raw)	1 cup	122
dandelion greens	1 cup	147
Sea Vegetables (cooked, unless specified)		
hijiki	1 cup	610
wakame	1 cup	520
kombu (kelp)	1 cup	305
agar-agar	1 cup (dry flakes)	400
(Kanten flakes)	(16 tablespoons)	
used as a thickener for sauces,		
etc.		
dulse	1 cup (dry)	567
Fish (bones: the major source		
of calcium in fish)		
sardines	3½ oz. can	300
(with bones)	(drained)	
salmon (canned)	1 cup	431
oysters, raw	1 cup	226
Beans and Legumes		
tofu-firm	4 oz.	80–150
tempeh	4 oz.	172
garbanzo beans	1 cup (cooked)	150
(chickpeas)		
black beans	1 cup (cooked)	135
pinto beans	1 cup (cooked)	128

Food	Amount	Calcium (mgs.)
tortillas, corn	2	120
Nuts and Seeds		
sesame seeds	3 tablespoons	300
(must be ground for absorption)		
almonds	1 cup	300
sunflower seeds	1 cup (hulled)	174
brazil nuts	1 cup	260
hazelnuts	1 cup	282
Other Sources		
blackstrap molasses	1 tbspn.	137
orange juice	1 cup	210
calcium fortified (Minute Maid)		
Mineral Waters		
Perrier	1 liter	140
Mendocino	1 liter	380
San Pellegrino	1 liter	200
Apollinaris	1 liter	91
Contexeville	1 liter	451
Dairy		
milk		
skim	1 cup	300
whole	1 cup	288
cheese (American, Swiss, cheddar)	1½ oz.	300
ice milk	1 cup	204
nonfat yogurt	1 cup	294
cottage cheese (low fat)	1 cup	150

Calcium Rich Herb Infusions
   Old "Sour Puss" Mineral Mix à la Susun Weed[59]
   1 tablespoon supplies 150–200 mg calcium
Choose one or more of the following herbs (these grow all over the United States and are very easy to identify):

   Yellow Dock (*Rumex*) leaves/roots;
   Dandelion (*Taraxacum*) leaves/roots;

Plantain (*Plantago*) leaves;
Nettle (*Urtica*) leaves;
Raspberry (*Rubus*) leaves/canes/berries;
Mugwort (*Artemisia vulgaris*) leaves;
Comfrey (*Symphytum*) leaves/flower stalks
Red Clover (*Trifolium pratense*) blossoms
clean eggshells/bones

Fill a quart/liter jar with fresh herbs. Pour apple cider vinegar over herbs until jar is full. (Vinegar dissolves calcium and other minerals and holds them in solution.) Cover with a plastic lid and let sit for 6 weeks. To use: Pour on your salad, put on your beans, add to soup, or dilute 1 tablespoon in 1 cup of water and add 1 tablespoon of blackstrap molasses, which adds 137 mg. of calcium.

Bonny Bony Brew
(1 cup contributes 300 mg calcium)
Nettle (*Urtica dioica*): 1 oz/30 g dry
Horsetail (*Equisetum arvense*): 1 tablespoon dry/2 grams
Sage (*Salvia officinalis*): 1 tablespoon/2 grams dry

Crush sage between palms and drop into quart/liter container with other two herbs. Fill with boiling water, cap tightly, and let brew for 4 hours. Strain. *Red clover, oatstraw,* or *raspberry* may be substituted for the nettles.

Note: Think of herbs as mineral-rich dark green leafy vegetables. These recipes are very easy ways to add minerals and other nutrients to your diet.

SHOULD I USE BUTTER OR MARGARINE? Essential fatty acids, the building blocks of fat, are necessary for health, but they are often lacking in our diets. One of the reasons for this is the introduction of hydrogenated fat. The damage that fat does to arteries is caused largely by unstable molecules known as *free radicals.* A diet high in hydrogenated fat and low in antioxidant vitamins increases the production of free radicals, which are implicated in cellular damage leading not only to atherosclerosis but to cancer. Partially hydrogenated fats, in fact, are associated with higher cancer rates than are saturated fats.[60]

Partially hydrogenated fat (a trans fatty acid) is an artificial product produced by a chemical process in which hydrogen is added to naturally occurring polyunsaturated fat at extremely high temperatures. The resulting fat has an extremely long shelf life but is not found anywhere in nature. Our bodies haven't evolved to deal with it, yet it is now added to just about everything you can think of and forms the basis for margarine. Start reading labels. You'll see that partially hydrogenated fat is added to almost all prepared cookies, crackers, and baked goods. It's even added to baby formula!

Hydrogenated fats often replace foods in which naturally occurring essential fatty acids are found. These artificial fats also inhibit normal fatty acid metabolism in our bodies and have therefore contributed to widespread deficiency in the essential fatty acids that are necessary for health. Essential fatty acids occur naturally in unprocessed seeds, nuts, and their oils.

Essential fatty acids are especially important for their role in the synthesis of the hormones known as the prostaglandins. Excess dietary protein, saturated fat, stress, alcohol, and inadequate levels of magnesium, zinc, vitamin B_3, vitamin B_6, and vitamin C are all factors that inhibit the conversion of fatty acids to essential prostaglandin hormones that the female body requires for optimal health. This can result in water gain (edema), increased blood clot formation, and increased uterine cramps.[61] Lack of essential fatty acids has also been implicated in breast pain, menstrual cramps, and a host of other problems.[62]

By adding essential fatty acids to our diets, we can protect ourselves somewhat against the deleterious effects of hydrogenated fats. Naturally occurring fat, especially the unsaturated type, is healthier than margarine—a hydrogenated unnatural product of the chemical industry. Borage oil, oil of evening primrose, flaxseed oil, black currant seed oil, and cold water fish (cod, mackerel, sardines, salmon), or ground-up flax seeds (one tablespoon per day) are good sources of the essential fatty acids. In fact, the essential fatty acids found in evening primrose oil, flaxseed oil, black currant seed oil, and borage oil have been shown to reverse the cancer-causing effects of radiation and carcinogens.[63] These specific dietary oils may also inhibit the development of breast and other forms of cancer by regulating immune system function in the body.[64] In one study, patients with multiple sclerosis who remained on a diet high in naturally occurring polyunsaturated fats and low in saturated fats had only minimal disability for as long as thirty years. In contrast, in those patients who discontinued this therapeutic diet, their disease was reactivated and their symptoms increased dramatically.[65]

Essential fatty acids also decrease hardening of the arteries by reducing the "stickiness" of blood cells to artery walls.[66]

A full discussion of the complicated and fascinating subject of dietary fats and their effects is way beyond the scope of this chapter.[67] For practical purposes, one should use only those oils that *require* refrigeration. Avoid baked goods made with hydrogenated oils whose shelf life is longer than your current life expectancy. Because this isn't always possible, I often prescribe a supplement of essential fatty acids. For cooking, I recommend corn, sesame, or safflower oil. In general, use oil only sparingly.

SHOULD I TAKE NUTRITIONAL SUPPLEMENTS? I often recommend nutritional supplements and micronutrients to women who travel frequently, rarely cook, eat out a great deal, or for whatever reason cannot meet their optimal nutritional needs from food alone. Food, however, is still the best source of nutrients for the body. It is the source your body was designed to handle, and it is cheaper than high-quality supplements.

Women who eat mostly organically grown produce, have a diet rich in organically grown grains and beans, and supplement their diets with nutrient-dense foods such as sea vegetables and collard greens usually do not need additional supplements. These women are rare.

The RDAs for vitamins were developed to keep large populations from getting gross deficiency diseases. RDAs were developed only after large-scale refining of flour became the norm, and deficiency diseases began to affect whole populations who no longer ate whole foods. The RDAs do *not* address individual biological variation. For one person, 80 mg. of vitamin C might be optimal—for another, 1000 mg. per day works better. Our nutritional needs are as individual as our fingerprints.

Countless patients over the years have told me how much better they feel when taking a balanced vitamin-mineral formula with additional nutrients when indicated. A reduction in winter colds is a very common benefit of such a regimen.

Vitamin C, an antioxidant (taken in doses ranging from 500 to 3000 mg. per day, depending on one's situation), is particularly good for enhancing the immune response, and multiple studies have shown other benefits as well.[68] The other antioxidant vitamins (A and E, coenzyme Q, selenium, and beta carotene) have also been shown to be important for enhancing our body's immune system's function and for warding off infections and cancer.[69] Zinc, which works along the same metabolic pathways as the other antioxidants, is also important for immune response and has been found to be low in many women.[70] Magnesium,[71] other trace minerals, garlic, and onion[72] have also been found to be important in immune system functioning. There may well be an increased requirement for magnesium in those women who are trained endurance athletes or who are otherwise quite physically active.[73]

Until the planet is healed, the soil is replenished, and McDonald's serves fast vegetarian food, many women will need supplements for optimal functioning. I stress "optimal functioning"—a woman is *not* apt to get an outright vitamin deficiency if she doesn't take supplements. But unless she's consistently eating very well, she may not feel her best either.

I recommend a "preconception" supplement to all women who are thinking of getting pregnant (unless their diets are excellent), so that their bodies have optimal levels of nutrients on board at the time of conception. Studies have shown that folic acid in particular can decrease the incidence of neural tube defects such as spina bifida.[74] Vitamin B_6 (which should always be taken with the whole B complex) has been shown to decrease nausea and vomiting associated with pregnancy.[75]

For those women with concerns about osteoporosis who are still eating a high-fat, high-protein diet and for whatever reason aren't going to change, I recommend a multimineral supplement with at least as much magnesium as calcium—800 to 1000 mg. per day is optimal, assuming that another 200 to 300 mg. will come from food. Note that merely taking a supplement into your body doesn't guarantee that it will get absorbed and utilized properly. The gut only absorbs what the body needs that day. Find a supplement that is free of fillers, binders, and artificial ingredients that can block absorption. Chelated minerals work best.

I'd recommend that you consult a nutritionist or other health professional familiar with nutritional supplements and micronutrients, or write to a few companies for information, before you make a choice. Nutritional medicine is a specialty in and of itself with many excellent practitioners who can help guide you. (See Resources.)

Each individual may require specific supplemental foods and nutrients in their diets. Almost all nutritionists, dietitians, and practitioners of nutritional medicine agree that a diet of whole foods, not just a handful of supplements each day, is the keystone of any nutritional program.

CAN DIET HELP IRRITABLE BOWEL SYNDROME AND OTHER DIGESTIVE PROBLEMS? Many women have taken numerous courses of antibiotics for acne, urinary tract infections, and upper respiratory infections. Chronic use of antibiotics kills the normal bowel flora that are necessary for a healthy functioning colon—a place in the body in which essential bacteria play an important role in nutrient absorption and manufacture. In addition, chronic use of aspirin and other nonsteroidal anti-inflammatory medicines (ibuprofen and acetominophen) has also been shown to affect both the stomach's and the intestines' physiological function. (One half to two thirds of patients who use nonsteroidal anti-inflammatory medicine chronically show evidence of inflammation of the small intestine.)[76]

Because of our national penchant to overuse antibiotics and aspirin (and other nonsteroidal anti-inflammatory medicines), and a refined-food diet and high-stress lifestyle, many women have digestive difficulties, such as chronic constipation, excess gas, frequent diarrhea, and lower abdominal distress. All of these conditions may result from an imbalance in normal intestinal bacteria, intestinal parasites of various kinds, overgrowth of intestinal yeast, and an increase in intestinal permeability (leaky gut syndrome). These conditions are collectively known as *intestinal dysbiosis*. Intestinal dysbiosis is often related to and may result in chronic vaginitis, migraines, arthritis, autoimmune diseases, and food allergy.[77]

At Women to Women we diagnose this condition either clinically, from symptoms such as chronic gas or diarrhea, or by sending stool cultures to a lab that specializes in this testing. Intestinal parasites are often diagnosed as well.[78] A variety of supplements, such as acidophilus and bifido bacteria, are then used to help restore normal bowel flora and get the yeast under control. A yeast-free diet is also prescribed for some (see Appendix). A mostly vegetarian whole food diet also helps.

HOW DO I KNOW IF I HAVE FOOD ALLERGIES? Intestinal dysbiosis is often accompanied by food allergies.[79] In our center we use a blood test known as a RAST panel to diagnose this condition. This test should be ordered by a physician familiar with this type of testing and should be performed by a lab that specializes in it. A special diet is then prescribed based on the results. Because food allergy is most often a problem found in women who've had very stressful childhoods (rape, incest, or abuse) and who are continuing to live in dysfunctional jobs or relationships, we emphasize to these women that they will not get well simply from dietary change alone. There is a dramatic synergy between lifestyle choices, stress, and the parts of the immune system that maintain bowel and vaginal health.[80] Supporting their bodies nutritionally while they learn to support themselves emotionally and psychologically helps many women enormously. Studies have shown that this normalizes immune system response. I refer to this step as "replenishing the soil."

DO I HAVE TO GIVE UP COFFEE? Caffeine is a very popular drug worldwide, perhaps *the* most popular. The average American drinks some thirty-two gallons of caffeinated soft drinks and twenty-eight gallons of coffee a year, and more than a thousand proprietary drugs list caffeine as an ingredient. Ninety-five percent of pregnant women consume caffeine during their pregnancies.[81] I enjoy mostly decaffeinated coffee myself and use about three or four cups of caffeinated coffee per week.

Caffeine stimulates the central nervous system and affects the heart, skeletal muscles, and kidneys and also the adrenals. It is associated with increased mental acuity, initially. However, it may also result in rebound confusion once the effect has subsided. In some women caffeine is a factor in breast pain and cysts. An occasional woman is so sensitive to it that one piece of chocolate will cause breast tenderness premenstrually during the month in which she eats that chocolate.

Sleep disorders often disappear when people stop using caffeine—and so does urinary frequency. Some studies have shown that the effects of caffeine on females may vary according to the level of estrogen in their system.[82] Even decaffeinated coffee can be a breast and bladder irritant for some.

Here's a test to see if you're addicted to caffeine: Go without it for three days. If you get a headache—you are addicted. If you don't, it probably doesn't affect you much. Withdrawal from caffeine takes only two or three days. The headache and the fatigue that accompany this withdrawal, however, can be quite debilitating. I recommend that women plan to withdraw over a weekend, or whenever they have time to rest and nurture themselves in other ways. During caffeine withdrawal, drink plenty of water and drink 3–4 cups of camomile tea per day. This tea is considered a "nervine" (nerve tonic) and helps maintain alertness. Many of my patients note that their tolerance to caffeine decreases over the years. Those who have stopped caffeine and then try it again often notice that the drug affects them quite dramatically.

Eliminating caffeine may be a step in the right direction for you. Certainly you will want to do this if you're planning a pregnancy.

I KNOW I SHOULD STOP SMOKING ... I don't lecture smokers because they generally want to quit anyway. Sometimes a few facts help them to make the decision:

- Right now, tobacco companies have targeted adolescent girls as their number-one market for cigarettes because this group has been found to have the lowest self-esteem and is therefore the most likely to start smoking as a result of peer pressure. (Thank you, tobacco companies, and thank you, U.S. government, for all the tobacco subsidies.)
- 41.2 percent of white high school students smoke or use other tobacco products.
- Tobacco kills more *nonsmokers* each year than AIDS, illicit drugs, and teenage drinking.
- Tobacco costs the American public over $100 billion each year.[83]

- One out of every six deaths in the United States is related to tobacco.
- More Americans die each year from tobacco than from fires, car accidents, illegal drugs, murders, and AIDS combined.
- Tobacco kills more people in two days than crack and cocaine kill in a year.[84]
- Tobacco companies know that once hooked, females are less likely to quit than males. (More nurses *start* smoking in nursing school than any other profession.)
- Cigarettes are more addictive than heroin because taking smoke into the lungs immediately produces a profound drug effect in the brain. It's like mainlining the most addictive substance in the world. Some kids are "hooked" after only one cigarette.
- More than four thousand chemicals, including two hundred known poisons such as DDT, arsenic, formaldehyde and carbon monoxide, are housed in tobacco.

Smoking and specific women's health problems have been so well-documented now that the smokers among us simply "shut down" when they hear about them. The power of addiction and denial is nowhere more striking than in the case of a pregnant patient who, despite a history of infertility, continues to smoke throughout her pregnancy. Consider the following data:

- Smokers have a miscarriage rate that is twice as high as nonsmokers. These miscarriages are of genetically normal fetuses.
- Mothers who smoke have a twofold increase in infants who die of sudden infant death syndrome (SIDS).[85]
- Smoking in pregnancy is the number-one cause of low-birthweight babies, who have a much higher death rate than normal-weight babies.
- The children of smoking parents have many more respiratory illnesses (like asthma) per year than those of nonsmokers.
- Smokers are at increased risk for cervical cancer, vulvar cancer, and abnormal Pap smears, possibly because smoking depletes vitamins C and A and beta carotene, antioxidants that are

somewhat protective against cancer.[86] Smoking literally poisons the ovaries.

- Smoking ages the skin more quickly than normal.
- Lung cancer has now passed breast cancer as the number-one cancer killer of women. (You *have* come a long way, baby!)
- Smokers are at increased risk for osteoporosis, premature aging, and heart disease.

Dr. Andrew Weil points out that there are tobacco leaves carved on the pillars of the Capitol building in Washington, D.C.—testimony to the entwined interests of the government and the tobacco companies. Since the handwriting is on the wall for smoking in the United States, however, tobacco growers are now targeting the almost limitless market overseas in such places as China.

How to Quit Smoking
- Know that every attempt at quitting increases your chances of success next time. Give yourself credit for trying.
- For now, when you smoke, try to become very conscious of your smoking. Go outside, breathe in deeply, and pay attention to your lungs.
- Ask your lungs for permission to smoke. Check in with this part of your body and see how it feels.
- When you smoke, just smoke. Try to get as much pleasure from the cigarette as possible. The idea here, as with food, is to change your consciousness around smoking. Doing so will stop the "robot" approach that is the basis for this habit.
- Weight gain is *not* an inevitable part of smoking cessation. The only reason women gain weight is that they are substituting one addiction for another. (The dictum to be thin is so great that many smokers would rather risk lung cancer and death than risk being overweight. A few very honest smokers have told me this.)
- Get support—join a Smokers Anonymous or other group of people going through the same thing.
- Acupuncture and traditional Chinese medicine are known to be of benefit in helping with withdrawal from cigarettes and

NOURISHING OURSELVES WITH FOOD

other addictive substances. In New York City, the March of Dimes and Columbia-Presbyterian Hospital advocate acupuncture-based treatment for addicted clients. One three-year study involving 2,282 cases demonstrated that acupuncture had a 90 percent success rate in a nicotine detoxification program.[87]

CAN I DRINK ALCOHOL? Excess alcohol consumption is associated with increased risk of breast cancer, menstrual irregularities, osteoporosis, and birth defects. As with cigarettes, I ask women who drink alcohol regularly to become conscious of why and how they are using alcohol. If they feel the need to have two drinks every single night "to relax" (whether at home or "out"), I seriously question that behavior. Meditation, listening to music, and taking a long bath are good alternatives.

I point out that two drinks of alcohol per night effectively wipe out rapid eye movement (REM) sleep, the type of sleep associated with dreaming. Dreaming is part of your inner guidance system. Why wipe it out with alcohol?

The amount of alcohol a woman takes in has very little to do with whether she has a problem with alcohol. What determines an alcoholic is her *relationship* to alcohol. One of my patients realized that she felt much more comfortable when she had her bottle of sherry filled by her bedside. She rarely drank it, but she realized that if it weren't there, she'd feel agitated. For that reason, she checked out a few Alcoholics Anonymous meetings and found that she did indeed have a tendency toward alcoholism.

Many women hold the "cocktail hour" as a sacred ritual. When I suggest that they drink spring water or sparkling cider as an alternative, in order to see what effect the alcohol is having on them, the reaction I get gives me a few clues about their relationship to alcohol. One woman said, "But my husband and I look forward to this hour. We have such fun we often forget to eat dinner."(!) Another said that she couldn't substitute a nonalcoholic drink for herself because if she did, "Everyone else would start to look stupid." (Hmmmm.)

Please be good to yourself. Examine your relationship to alcohol and make adjustments if necessary. If you feel you *can't* go without your evening wine or cocktail, you have a problem.

HOW CAN I HELP MY CHILDREN EAT WELL? I was six weeks pregnant with my first daughter when I began to change to a grain-based diet. My second daughter was brought up on whole food from conception onward. Daily I hear the woes of women who say they can't change their diets because no one in their family will eat the food. The process has to be gradual.

Don't ask your family for permission to improve your health—and possibly theirs. Do share with them what you're doing and why.

Enlist their cooperation as much as possible. Almost everyone likes some healthy foods. Find out what your family's favorites are.

Don't push an agenda. If you encounter resistance, just laugh and continue your own program. The stepson of one of my colleagues used to make fun of her food choices when he was an adolescent. He and his friends poked fun at the tofu and rice in the refrigerator and boasted about how delicious their hot dogs were, brandishing them about like trophies. Now, living in an apartment on his own, he has become very interested in his health. He has noticed how much better he feels when he cooks and eats well. He comes to my colleague for cooking and nutritional advice. He and his friends have become great vegetarian cooks.

Respect your family's choices and timing. Back in 1980, my husband was not very thrilled with my brown rice and tofu meals at first. Now he wouldn't eat any other way and boasts of a cholesterol of 130! He has also become a good vegetarian cook. My oldest brother, a former "meat and potatoes kind of guy," has also recently made the switch and likes grains and bean cooking better than any other cuisine.

As my younger daughter grows older, she is increasingly drawn to animal food. She likes hot dogs but keeps them to a minimum. She dislikes all red meat, however. This year she announced that she didn't like a lot of our food. So together we made a list of low-fat, nonvegetarian foods she enjoys. This includes organic chicken, low-fat cookies and crackers (even some with hydrogenated fats), and occasional low-fat yogurt. She is old enough now to be out in the world and to discover what her own tastes are. I can no longer control her diet, so I have compromised with the best quality, lowest-fat choices I can find that she enjoys. When she's not at home, she eats all the things that most American kids her age eat—both good and bad. I've had to learn that I have no control over this and though tempted to nag, realize I am powerless over her choices and behavior. The sooner mothers learn this, the better.

Become informed. When we started to eat a macrobiotic diet and eliminated dairy food, we had to contend with the usual comments of the uninformed. My sister told a pediatrician friend that my children didn't drink milk. Her response was, "They'll die." This is not a scientific response. It is pure emotion, and a typical response.

My children were breast-fed until almost age two. Human milk, a living, dynamic food, is designed for optimal growth and development of baby humans. Cow's milk, very different in composition from human milk, is designed to produce rapid growth and the development of cattle. Children are bigger today than they used to be. Cow's milk produces rapid growth in children, the same as it does in cattle. This is one of the reasons why the American children of relatively small immigrants are so much bigger than their parents. In this country we associate bigger with better.[88]

Since you will find so little cultural support for removing milk from the diet of your children, it is helpful to be well-armed with information. Dr. Frank Oski, chief of pediatrics at Johns Hopkins Medical School, has published a great little book entitled, *Don't Drink Your Milk*,[89] which documents the link between dairy food and allergy, eczema, bed wetting, and ear infections in children. Countless children are needlessly treated with antibiotics for repeated ear infections that would go away if they were taken off dairy food. As a pediatrician, Dr. Oski's honesty about the adverse health effects of dairy food is a much appreciated contribution.

Ask for help and cooperation. My children are involved with the food, with shopping, and with food preparations. Meal decisions and preparation help are a must from those with whom you are sharing meals. Any child of either gender over the age of ten can easily learn the basics of cooking. So can any man of any age.

Our family agreement is that our children can have some junk food such as french fries in moderation when we're traveling or eating out. We enjoy these, too. Making them "forbidden" would simply increase the desire for them. We limit ice cream to one serving per week. Our children don't request it every week, especially in the winter. (When I was their age, I ate ice cream almost nightly, so I see this as an improvement.)

Be flexible. Respect the inner wisdom of each family member. Any mother would be foolish to think that she can control all of her children's dietary choices. Candy, ice cream, and pizza are staple foods in our culture. Your children will probably eat them. This won't be a problem if they've been exposed to healthy food regularly so that their bodies know the difference. My daughters have their own inner guidance to make nutritional choices that are best for them, especially since they've been exposed to some healthy choices. Since that is the philosophical approach I use at the office, why should I expect less of my children, just because I'm their mother?

Before they reached the age of four, obviously I had much more control over what foods they ate than I do now. When they were little I noticed that when they ate ice cream or candy, for example, they'd often have diarrhea or a fever within hours afterward. Other mothers whose children eat whole-food diets report the same experience. Their systems literally "detoxed" or "discharged" the refined food. Even now, I view their illnesses, especially colds, as their bodies' way of fasting, resting, and getting rid of excess. I did the best job I could of creating a firm nutritional foundation for my children. When they think back on "mother's home cooking," they will remember brown rice and collard greens, not roast beef and Yorkshire pudding. This foundation serves them well. When my oldest daughter recently returned from a weeklong school outing, all she wanted was brown rice. She was very tired of the Standard

American Diet. When I've been on the road, I also crave brown rice and freshly steamed greens.

Expect dietary imperfection. My daughters' and my diets are not "perfect." I don't carry brown rice and vegetables with me on the road. Some people do, and it works well for them. Each of us must find her own way, depending upon her background, state of health, and desire for change. A mostly vegetarian, low-protein, low-fat, high-fiber, high-quality diet works for me and for many of my patients—with a good brownie added now and then.

Getting Started

Now you are ready to take this information and do something with it. You can learn to nurture yourself fully while using food to help heal a health problem or for general health maintenance and improvement. Here's a prerequisite for change: Change your relationship with food to nourish and please *you*. When you begin with this attitude in place, your success will be assured. Food will be your ally, a comfort, a health-enhancer, and a delicious way to nourish yourself. Sooner or later, you have to become your own mother— to feed and nourish yourself the way you've always hoped that someone else would do it for you.

No breakthrough in cancer or heart disease treatment can ever approach the success of the diet that will prevent the problem in the first place. Mental, emotional, and physical improvements often accompany dietary improvements. An executive in one of our local firms recently wrote me the following: "As a new student of the macrobiotic philosophy, I have begun to experience dramatic changes within me as a result of the diet and my reorientation to life. Besides the physical changes (weight loss, increase in energy, and general sense of well-being), I have experienced what I can only describe as a 'spiritual connectedness' and motivation to help heal the soul sickness of the earth. This represents a dramatic and somewhat 'strange' shift for me. I've worked for ten years in corporate communications. Although at times I feel a bit mad admitting this focus, I feel compelled to do so.

"I am writing to ask your advice on my idea: I am interested in using the communication skills I have developed over the last ten years to increase awareness of environmental threats to human survival and introduce/reinforce solutions to preserve quality life."

My response to this woman's letter was to support her in her newly forming life's purpose and to share with her my belief that her path would open up for her spontaneously, now that she'd awakened her intuition through dietary change. This woman's experience is not unusual.

When we change in one area of our lives, possibilities always open up in other areas. Sometimes the result is as simple as feeling better, so that the work we're already doing becomes easier. One of my patients who runs a successful art gallery said after noticing this improvement, "Why was I never told to stop caffeine or refined sugar before? I've been to so many doctors, and I've had these headaches for years. Now finally they're gone. Thanks."

Start Where You Are

If you were sitting on the couch in my office for a consultation, together we would both decide on a plan for dietary improvement that would take into account what your life is like and what feels comfortable for you. If you're currently married to an alcoholic whom you're thinking of leaving, diving headlong into whole-food cooking may not be the best use for your energy right now. Al-Anon or another source of support might be a better choice. If you're a single mother of a one- and a three-year-old, I would suggest that you do whatever is necessary to survive the next several years. Feeling guilty about using fast foods is not something I'd encourage in your case.

Make a Choice and Stick with It

Commit to one month of whole grains, beans, and vegetables as your staple foods, while eliminating meat, dairy products, caffeine, and as many refined foods as you can. (When I say eliminate dairy food, I don't suggest that you try to figure out if the muffin you ordered for breakfast has a bit of milk added to the batter. I'm talking here about the dairy food you can see: cream sauces, butter, cheese, cottage cheese, yogurt, ice cream, cream-based soups, and milk.) Eggs are not dairy food—they don't come from cows. (You'd be surprised at how many people think eggs are dairy food—this comes from the old brainwashing of the four basic food groups, with eggs and dairy in the same category.) But if you're trying to clear up a health problem, I'd recommend eliminating eggs as well.

This one-month period is an experiment to see how your body responds to the food. I call it Cleansing Your Dietary Intuition. This program should not be seen as deprivation or punishment. If it feels like a punishment and not a growth opportunity, don't do it—you're not ready.

If grains and beans are too much of a change for you, then start by lowering your dietary fat content to 20 to 40 grams per day if you need to lose weight, or to 30 to 50 grams per day if you don't. Buy a fat gram counter, and become aware of how much fat you're eating. These are now readily available in book stores and even at the check-out counters of many grocery stores. I usually recommend the *T-Factor Diet* and/or *The T-Factor Fat Gram Counter* by Martin Katahn and Jamie Popo-Cordie.[90] If you must eat dairy food, remember to make it low fat and consider limiting it to once or twice per day maximum.

You can experiment with the level of fat that works best for you. Start by determining how much fat is in your diet to begin with. Then cut it to 35 to 40 grams per day if you want to decrease your weight. Stay with this for a few weeks. See how this feels. Some women feel better on 20 grams per day, with occasional increases as needed. Others need 60 to 70 per day. Don't go below 20 grams per day for longer than two to three months, unless you make sure you're getting your essential fatty acid requirement met through supplements. When you're ready, you can add an occasional grain or bean dish to your menu.

Go to Cooking Classes

I recommend cooking classes because most Americans simply are not familiar with many of the staple foods that make up a healthy vegetarian diet, and they simply don't know the basics of grain and bean preparation. These are difficult to learn from a book.

Macrobiotic centers are located in almost every major city. They all offer whole-food cooking classes and are a good start, even if you don't intend to follow an entirely macrobiotic approach. (Far too many vegetarian cookbooks and cooks rely on cream sauces, cheese, and other dairy-rich recipes—avoid them.)

Jeff Woodward, author of *The Healing Power of Food: A Gourmet Cookbook for Lives in Transition*,[91] is a nationally known cook and lecturer on gourmet whole foods cooking. He comes to Maine about four times a year and offers classes on integrating whole foods into our fast-paced lifestyle. Whenever he's in town, I recommend his work to my patients, who find his approach practical, delicious, and fun. One woman said, "My husband and I were truly inspired by what Jeff had to say. I'm so grateful for what I learned. And the food was so good. It feels like a whole new world has opened up for me."

Woodward's classes are a great opportunity for educating not only yourself but also the men in your life. You can arrange a class in your area. For further information or to order *The Healing Power of Food* call or write:

Jeff Woodward,
Traditional Cooking Arts
5336 York Ave. South
Minneapolis, MN 55410
(612) 929-2207

Annemarie Colbin, founder of the Natural Gourmet Cookery School in New York, and author of the classic *Food and Healing*,[92] has a great cooking class on videotape called *The Basics of Healthy Cooking*. From this you can learn whole-grain and bean cooking without leaving your home. Colbin's *Book of Whole Meals* was my first whole-foods cookbook. This book is unique in that it contains a shopping list of staple foods at the beginning so that you can easily stock your kitchen with the necessary supplies. When I was first learning, I had never heard of such foods as kuzu, a thickener that is healthier than cornstarch; miso, a delicious cultured soy product; or the various condiments such as gomasio (sesame salt). *The Book of Whole Meals* is set up to take you through meal preparation in such a way that the entire meal is ready at the same time.

The Natural Gourmet Cookery School, in addition to offering a full range of classes, also offers a natural catering and meal service, as well as a chef training school. (I predict that the demand for chefs trained in whole-food cookery will increase dramatically in the 1990s.) For more information or to order books or a tape:

The Natural Gourmet Cookery School
48 West 21st Street, Suite 202
New York, NY 10010
(212) 645-5170

Rick Perry, chief cook at the Hurricane Island Outward Bound School in Maine, serves whole-food meals to the students all summer. He notes that after a week or two of this food, students notice the difference. He tells the story of one rather tough boy from New York City who at first couldn't understand why he had so much energy and felt so good. The bracing air and atmosphere on Hurricane Island notwithstanding, the boy said to Perry, "I guess it must be the food." Perry's book, *Hurricane Kitchen,* is a wealth of information and recipes for how to cook whole foods for large groups of people.[93] (The yeast gravy recipe is worth the price of the book.) The recipes are "transitional," meaning that they work very well for those who are just starting vegetarian eating but haven't necessarily made the leap yet. The food is delicious, and it's also cheap—much cheaper than a meat-based diet, particularly for large groups.

I also recommend *The Self-Healing Cookbook* by Kristina Turner.[94] This book moves you gradually through different stages toward full vegetarian eating. It also deals very nicely with the emotional aspects of eating and food.

Cook with Good Cookware

Many households have substandard cooking equipment. I, like so many other women and men, used to devalue the art of food preparation by being unconscious about the implements associated with it. Do you have a mismatched set of pots with no lids, hanging around jumbled in your kitchen cabinet? Or is your cookware serviceable and a pleasure to use? Don't you think that you deserve to have the proper instruments for carrying out something so basic as nourishing yourself and others? After all, these items are for daily use. The same goes for good quality knives.

I don't recommend aluminum pots and pans. There is some evidence that aluminum accumulation in the brain may be an etiological factor in Alzheimer's disease and may play a role in other degenerative diseases. When water is heated in an aluminum pot, there is a seventy-five-fold increase in the aluminum level in the heated water. This level greatly exceeds what is considered safe for tap water drinking.[95] So stay away from aluminum cookware in your own kitchen at least.

Microwaves used chronically are also a concern of mine because these change the basic energy of the food. Microwaved infant formula, in one study, was found to change the amino acid structure of the formula and produced an amino acid called d-proline. These changes don't occur when milk is heated in a conventional way. D-proline has been shown to be toxic to the kidneys, brain, nerves, and liver.[96] If this type of amino acid change has been demonstrated in microwaved infant formula, what does microwave cooking do to the essential molecular structure of other foods—a molecular structure to which it took our bodies millennia to adjust?

Food and Consciousness

Guilt is one of the worst foods for the intestines.
                              —Bill Tims, macrobiotic counselor

If you were sitting on a beach in Hawaii reading novels, you could eat almost anything you wanted and suffer few ill effects—even from foods that usually give you problems (provided, of course, that you like Hawaii and the beach). On the other hand, when you're under stress, hurried, or unhappy, digestion and food assimilation are adversely affected. This link is important to understand.

The effects of diet are definitely influenced by states of consciousness. Digestion, absorption, and assimilation of our food is also dependent upon our state of consciousness. So if you're eating brown rice and vegetables out of guilt or as a way to beat yourself up—chances are they won't have nearly the beneficial effects that they're capable of providing.

A now-famous study on heart and blood vessel disease was

conducted at Ohio State University on rabbits. These rabbits were all genetically bred to develop atherosclerosis (hardening of the arteries) and coronary artery disease. The investigators fed the rabbits a high-fat diet to speed up the disease process. At the end of the study, when the rabbits were sacrificed, the researchers found that more than 15 percent of the rabbits had almost no coronary artery disease—their arteries were clean. After much head-scratching, they discovered that the bunnies with the clean arteries were the ones whose cages were at waist level. The female graduate student who fed the rabbits used to take these ones out of their cages and pet and play with them for a while before their feeding.[97] This study has been repeated several times, mostly because no one could believe it initially, but the results were the same. Studies like this fly in the face of what we normally believe is going on. I tell my patients that if they're going to eat prime rib, get a massage—or pray over it first.

People with multiple personality disorder can be very allergic to a food while they are in one personality; that same food doesn't affect them a bit when they are in another personality—in the exact same body. Clearly, more is going on with food and nourishment than simply fat, carbohydrates, proteins, vitamins, and calories. When all is said and done, diet is only one factor in creating health, albeit a very powerful one. According to numerous investigators, dietary patterns that are associated with low cancer and heart disease risk are usually present in those individuals who have other lifestyle factors that are associated with a low risk of cancer. These include less consumption of alcohol and fast food, and more exercise.

I encourage you to experiment with whole, unprocessed food. Understand that your consciousness around a food can change that food's effect on your body. For me, the pleasure of eating out at a restaurant with my family where I can relax and be served, occasionally outweighs the damage of hydrogenated fat in the salad dressing or on the fish. Melvin Morse's study of long-term survivors of near-death experiences showed that they eat better than controls and in general take better care of themselves. They do not do this to avoid dying but because, as a result of their near-death experience, they value their lives more than ever before. Eating well is a way of valuing and nourishing themselves.[98]

George Burns once said, "If I had known I was going to live so long, I'd have taken better care of myself." Part of George Burns's longevity secret is his sense of humor. Don't lose yours—and don't eat without it! Keep food in perspective.

EIGHTEEN

The Power of Movement

Our body creates our soul, as much as our soul creates our body.
—David Spangler[1]

*P*hysical exercise or regular movement of some kind is a vital part of creating health. Our bodies were designed to move, stretch, and run. I exercise because I like the way it feels to have a strong body—including a strong heart. For the first time in years, I have the time to do it without rushing since my children are older. My exercise time is part of my commitment to myself. It would be easy to put off exercising until the house is clean, more writing is done, or I've gone through the mail. Yet I *still* put on my shorts and get going most of the time. The endless household and work duties will always be there, even after I'm dead. If my exercise actually helps me live longer, I'm *saving* time by exercising.

If we wait to take care of ourselves until everything else is done, there will never be time for exercise. If we don't *create* exercise time, we'll never have it. For my part, I enjoy *doing* it. I don't exercise to lose weight, and though I have a family history of heart disease and genetically low HDL (the good cholesterol), I also don't exercise because I'm afraid of heart disease. The old feminist adage "how you do it is what you get" applies to exercise just as it does to any other area of life.

Our Cultural Inheritance

Many women have to heal their early perceptions of themselves and their physical capabilities before they can become comfortable with physical activities. Schools and the culture tend to confuse sports skills with fitness. Being good at batting a ball and being physically fit are not necessarily related. Many girls end up feeling bad about their physical prowess simply because they're not "good" at sports. The only reason many girls don't have the skills is that no one ever taught them. One of my friends who was a pro baseball player told me that when boys are first learning to throw, they also throw "just like a girl." Boys learn to "throw like a boy" from practicing over and over again with those who are more skilled than they. It's part of their cultural heritage.

Are you someone who was never picked for the school softball team? Did you feel you had to quit playing sports with the boys when you started to grow breasts? Check to see if your history and any messages you received as a girl are preventing you from enjoying physical activity now. If they are, bring them to consciousness so you can experience them fully, and then let them go. Brian Swimme, physicist and author of *The Universe Is a Green Dragon*, said it best: "To exercise actually means to bring into action. When we exercise, we bring into action our ancestral memories. Our bodies remember that we lived in trees and forests. We need to crawl and climb and run if we are to develop our intellectual, emotional, and spiritual capacities. . . . We tend to think of exercise as losing weight, as trimming off the fat. But to exercise is to enable the body to remember its past, so that it can stretch out with all its intertwined powers of being and thought and reflection."[2]

Many of the bodily changes we associate with aging have nothing to do with aging per se. Decreased muscle mass and increased fat may be normal in this culture, but these conditions are not necessarily natural—and we needn't expect them. They are caused by inactivity, accompanied by a mindset that expects us to grow weaker as we age. As we have seen, the physical condition of sixty-year-old Tara Humara runners was *better* than that of the twenty-year-olds.

Unfortunately, our own "tribe" collectively believes that we are supposed to fall apart when we age. We have *no* culturally supported tradition that teaches us that we can improve with age. Though countless exceptions to this rule exist, we still suffer under the collective delusion about what happens to our bodies with age.

Benefits of Exercise

Joanne Cannon, a wellness educator, defines physical prowess as "the ability to meet the physical demands of one's day, plus one emergency." I like that definition because it is so individualized. Feeling strong and capable is an essential ingredient to building health. Studies show that women who are moderately physically active enjoy the following benefits more than sedentary women:[3]

- Lower cancer rates and better immune system function (more white blood cells and increased levels of immunoglobulins)[4]
- A life expectancy that is on average seven years longer[5]
- Less depression and anxiety, and better mental efficiency and speed (higher IQ scores with exercise in some studies)[6]
- More relaxation, more assertiveness, more spontaneity and enthusiasm; a better attitude about their bodies and better self-acceptance[7]
- Stronger bones, increased bone thickness, increased bone mass, and increased ability of the bone to resist mechanical stress and fracture[8]
- More restful sleep[9]
- Higher self-esteem[10]

Another benefit of physical exercise is that it increases insulin sensitivity and can therefore prevent noninsulin-dependent diabetes.[11] It is also energizing. If you're always tired, it may be because you don't move enough. (But sometimes it's because you need to rest. You'll have to check this out for yourself.) For women with PMS, exercise often alleviates symptoms.[12] And pregnant women who exercise moderately have decreased constipation, hemorrhoids, varicose vein complications, and morning sickness.[13]

Even women who are disabled or confined to a wheelchair can benefit from strengthening their upper bodies and increasing their cardiovascular fitness. Adding regular exercise to any dietary regimen that we are on improves its effectiveness. So if you follow a low-fat diet, adding exercise will help it along. You'll lose excess fat and feel better sooner than if you didn't exercise.

Exercise and Intuition

The mind pervades the body. Moving my body rhythmically and repetitively helps me tap into my intuition, and more of my mind becomes available to me—the mind in my legs, in my heart, and in my biceps. Exercising feels like a necessary process for fully digesting my thoughts. Raising my heartbeat brings into play *more* of myself. My body wakes up—and so does my mind. During my workouts insights arise spontaneously.

Studies have shown that repetitive movement increases alpha waves in the brain—and alpha state is associated with enhanced intuition. Exercising hard is the perfect balance for the mental activity so often required in modern life.

People have very different approaches to exercise and physical activity. Each of us has an innate sense of what feels right for our bodies. As a scholar in a family of "jocks," I've had to find my own truth about what works best for me.[14] You will need to find yours, too. Your truth will not necessarily be what any outside authority tells you is "the right way to do it." And different approaches to exercise work best at different times in people's lives. For some, a twenty-minute walk three times a week is all that is necessary. For others, aerobics, weight training, or dance feels the best. Above all, exercise and body movement should be joyful and fun.

Ways to Move the Body

Aerobic Exercise and Target Heart Rate

Back in the 1960s, the concept of aerobic exercise was a revolutionary breakthrough in exercise physiology. Exercising aerobically keeps the heart, lungs, and entire cardiovascular system in good shape. It also burns off excess fat. Aerobic activity is exercise in which the heart rate is elevated for 15 to 20 minutes into what is called "the target zone."

To calculate your target heart rate:

1. Subtract your age from 220.
2. Subtract your resting heart rate (beats per minute) from this figure.
3. Multiply this figure by your "exercise quotient." This is 0.6 for a beginner or 0.8 for an advanced exerciser.
4. Add your resting heart rate to the figure from Step 3. This number is your target heart rate in beats per minute. You can divide by 6 to find out your heart rate for a ten-second interval.

Example: Your age is thirty-two. Your resting heart rate is 60, and you are a beginner. Hence: $220 - 32 = 198. 198 - 60 = 138. 138 \times 0.6 = 82.8. 82.8 + 60 = 142.8$. Your target heart rate is 143 beats per minute, or 13 beats for a ten-second interval.

Most experts agree that twenty minutes of aerobic-type exercise three times a week is adequate for cardiovascular fitness.

Aerobic Weight Training

Aerobic exercise *plus* weight training is more effective than aerobics alone because the weight training increases the amount of muscle in the body relative to fat and does so much more effectively than aerobics alone.[15] This is a relatively new understanding.

Studies show that as we age, we create an average of one and a half pounds of fat per year. We also lose a half pound of muscle each year if we don't exercise regularly. Muscle loss results in fat gain. Weight training prevents the muscle loss that too often accompanies aging. Aerobic weight training produces more muscle gain on average than aerobics alone. It also shapes muscles resulting in a healthier appearance. The increase in muscle strength that comes with weight training is very beneficial to women, who are often weak in their upper bodies. (Older women break their hips not only because of osteoporosis but because of muscle weakness and decreased strength, which makes them more susceptible to falling.)

Aerobic exercise combined with weight training results in more fat loss and produces more muscle gain compared to aerobics alone. The reason this is so important is that one pound of muscle requires

30 to 50 calories a day just to stay alive. One pound of fat requires fewer calories for maintenance. People with more muscle have higher metabolic rates. This is one reason that overweight women with lots of body fat often maintain their weight even when eating relatively little. To change their metabolic rate, they need to increase their physical activity. This results in a change in their "set point"— the point at which our body weight stays the same when we eat freely according to our appetite.

It is well-known that bone-mineral content may increase with physical activity.[16] Putting "vertical vectors of force" on bones through a weight-bearing exercise such as walking, jogging, biking, weight training, or stairclimbing sets up a minielectrical current in the bone known as a piezoelectric effect. This current actually draws in calcium and other minerals we need for bone density and strength. Twenty minutes of weight-bearing exercise daily, or thirty minutes three times a week, is ideal for this purpose.

Martial Arts

Martial arts training such as aikido or tai chi combines the body, mind, and spirit very consciously. Studies of individuals who do tai chi regularly, for example, have found that tai chi modifies their biological function via their nervous and hormonal systems, more than controls it. It has been shown to be effective in the treatment of heart disease, hypertension, insomnia, asthma, and osteoporosis. It decreases depression, tension, anger, fatigue, confusion, and anxiety.[17]

When I was in college, I got a green belt in jujitsu. Though that's not much of an accomplishment, I did have to spar with a couple of big guys from Cleveland Heights in order to earn it. From that, I learned that I have the strength and the will to fight someone in self-defense if I need to. Studies of men who rape show that they tend to go after women who seem the most vulnerable. The self-confidence and resulting self-confident stance that comes from knowing you can fight for yourself is conveyed in the energy field around you and is one way to decrease your chances of being raped. Martial arts can also help you discover your voice.[18]

Gentle Approaches to the Body

The effects of gravity over time and "buckling under" to life's stresses quite literally "wear us down." Our muscles and our alignment deteriorate over time unless we become aware of this and do something to counteract it. Yoga, Feldenkrais, Alexander work, and other gentle body-realigning techniques are a wonderful way to relax, stretch, and gently stimulate the muscles and internal organs. They also help maintain the body in proper alignment to gravity and keep the spine and joints supple.

Exercise and Addiction

Just about anything can be used addictively, and exercise is no exception. Some people have actually gone to rehab for running addiction. When we use exercise to run away from the stress in our lives, it is no different from the addictive use of Valium. (It may be a healthier choice initially, but it is still an addiction.)

Our society's attitude toward exercise as a fix is illustrated perfectly by an article that appeared in *Longevity* magazine in May 1991 (just before "swimsuit season"). The article was entitled "The Quickest Fixes: Emergency Diet/Shape-up Strategies from 8 Famous Bodies."[19] In the top left-hand corner was the line "30 Days to Summer." (This serves to "hook" you into the crisis-intervention mode for cellulite management.)

Celebrities and their nearly impossible routines were featured. When I read this article, I couldn't believe what I was reading. How many of us have personal trainers—or have the time to work out even an hour a day? Presenting this information on celebrity women to ordinary mortals and expecting us to meet their standards is ridiculous. Celebrity women make careers out of having perfect bodies, and their bodies pay a price for it. It's part of their work. They don't accomplish this in addition to raising a family and holding down another job. You don't have to be a drug and alcohol counselor to see the language and the process of addiction in this article—and hundreds more like it. Celebrity women fall prey to the same addictive tendencies as the rest of the culture—"I just do it harder," said Jane Fonda in the *Longevity* article, when asked what kind of exercise she does when she needs to shed a few pounds fast.

They just have more money for child care—and more time for exercise!

Unfortunately, many women do use exercise as a fix to run away from stress or as a way to keep their weight down. Though exercise does accomplish both of these goals, you'll never establish a healthy relationship with exercise and your body if you do the exercise strictly for stress and/or weight control.

Exercise, Amenorrhea, and Bone Loss

Studies have repeatedly shown that female athletes whose menstrual cycles have stopped suffer from premature bone loss.[20] In the past, I feared that this data would be used to scare women away from choosing to use their bodies as fully and powerfully as men. (Having a baby uses your body as fully and powerfully as any athletic event I can think of.)

Follow-up studies have shown that the reason many women athletes stop having periods is the same reason that many women go on stringent diets or become anorectic: They don't eat enough, and their total body fat becomes very low. This results in loss of periods (amenorrhea) and early osteoporosis.[21] In one study, when women who had developed amenorrhea from exercise ate 500 to 700 calories more per day, their periods returned. (Most competitive women runners won't do this.)

A study done by Dr. Nancy Lane indicates that women marathon runners who exercise to the point of becoming amenorrheic have bone density comparable to that of fifty-year-old women. There is no definite point at which running may begin to have deleterious effects on a woman's body, although in competitive runners it appears to begin at about 50 miles of training per week.

Not all women are at risk for losing their periods from extreme amounts of exercise. In Dr. Lane's study, amenorrhea from excess exercise was primarily a problem of young, childless women. After a woman has had children, she is less likely to develop this problem because childbearing appears to make her hormonal system difficult to suppress via extreme exercise. Her monthly cycling becomes harder to turn off. That's why women runners in their thirties and forties who've had children rarely become amenorrheic.[22] I believe that there's another reason why women who have had children are at less risk for exercise-induced amenorrhea: They are much less likely to maintain ruthless competitiveness, and this is associated with a change in body chemistry. Having a child often changes a woman in very fundamental ways—emotionally, psychologically, physically, spiritually.

Still another reason these women become amenorrheic is that, as studies have shown, leanness *combined* with chronic concern about becoming overweight is associated with disturbed menstrual cycles.[23] Women athletes are just as influenced by the cultural desire to be thin as other women. For that reason, their caloric intake is often lower than it has to be for the level of activity in which they participate. Eating disorders are just as common in athletic women as they are in nonathletic women, but athletic women sometimes use the training as a form of weight control. They exercise heavily—then they don't eat. This is no different from other forms of anorexia.

Since resumption of menses can take some time, progesterone therapy to help restore bone mass is often helpful. Once ovulatory periods have resumed, bone mineral density also begins to improve.[24]

My Exercise Story: Making Peace

I grew up, as I've mentioned, in an atmosphere teeming with physical activity and exercise. Most of it was outgoing and energetic like jogging and skiing. Even on Christmas Day, to my chagrin, my parents and siblings would race out the door to "hit the slopes." Though my mother did yoga and I learned the basic postures in the eighth grade, this was done not as an inner meditation with attention to breathing—it was a humorous competition to see who could actually get their bodies into the postures. We especially liked doing yoga headstands—they looked impressive.

My sister regarded any meditative stretching or muscle toning as a sissy approach. When not on the racing circuit, she was out running up our back hill with ski poles doing "dry land training." Every family vacation was camping or hiking, and most of the hiking had a "race to the summit" feeling and I didn't even pretend to be interested. I enjoyed being out in nature, but not as a competitive event.

My ski-racer sister now does yoga and tai chi regularly, paying attention to her breathing and inner feelings. After years of pushing and multiple injuries, she can no longer look at a Nautilus machine. I, on the other hand, am currently interested in aerobic weight training, though I change my exercise routine regularly depending upon how I'm feeling. Our paths have crossed as both of us have reached a balanced approach to physical activity.

When I was in medical school and residency, I jogged for 20 to 30 minutes three to four times a week and did a bit of yoga for balance. Unfortunately, I was chasing the elusive "runner's high" in those days. Looking back on those years, what I remember most is how wonderful it felt to be out in the sunshine and fresh air after all those hours of being confined inside a hospital. I looked forward to my runs for that reason, but I also wanted to get my 30 aerobics points for the week. To accomplish this, I ran in place even at stoplights. I wish I had been even *more* aware of the air and the light—and less aware of how far I was running or how high my pulse rate was. I didn't know then that running is best done for the enjoyment of the process. I was doing it to get something—not because of enjoying the process (classic addictive behavior).

During my pregnancies I did prenatal yoga. I found, like many pregnant women, that jogging just felt awful. I've never returned to it. After the children were born and while they were little (below age four), I occasionally went for a walk, but that was about it for a few years. (I don't remember much from those years—it's a blur of diapers and fatigue.) When I came home at the end of the day, I couldn't bring myself to go out the door to exercise. The children seemed to need my attention too much. Learning to balance my needs and theirs took awhile. They're only little once, and my instincts told me that being with them as much as I could was crucial.

As the children grew older, though, I bought a NordicTrack and set it up in front of the television. I did 20 minutes of this three times a week or so while watching *Entertainment Tonight* or other such fare or listening to music. During the first few months my children whined, complained, and constantly asked me to get them a drink, tie their shoes, or do something that would focus my attention completely on them. Pointing out to them that they could color or play right in the same room with me and that I wasn't going to leave them to exercise worked. The children understood. When I was clear about my needs, without feeling guilty about them, even young children would cooperate for short periods of time. I also promised them that when I was finished I would play with them, or in some other way give them the attention they needed. This worked well for a number of years.

Our whole approach to fitness and sports needs to be completely revamped if lifetime fitness is our goal. Individual sports or activities that teenagers enjoy long after they've finished school need to be added to every school's physical fitness curriculum. Though tennis, yoga, dance, and martial arts are often available at the college level, I'd like to see them in elementary schools.

Getting Started

STEP ONE: CHOOSE AN EXERCISE PROGRAM. It is just as healthy to discard the concept of the "ideal" amount of exercise as it is to discard the concept of the "ideal" weight. When people ask me what exercise program is best, I reply, "The one that you'll actually do." My patients participate in a very wide variety of activities, ranging from yoga, tai chi, and dance to teaching Outward Bound courses.

Try this: Recall a time in childhood when you were outside playing—skipping, jumping rope, or throwing a ball just for fun. Or perhaps you remember dancing—twirling around till you fell on the ground dizzy. Play with this memory in your mind for a while, and feel how it felt. Smell how it smelled. Feel the sun or wind on your face. Feel how good it felt to move your body with joy and energy, stretching it to its full capacity.

When you are ready, bring yourself back into the present. Begin moving your body the way you used to. See how it feels now. Be *in* your body. Enjoy it, appreciate it—experiment with moving it. Did any type of movement come to mind as something that felt really good? What was it? How could you incorporate that into your life now?

STEP TWO: MAKE A COMMITMENT TO MOVE YOUR BODY. Commit to moving your body in some way or in some form three times a week for 20 to 30 minutes. Combining exercise with a low-fat diet is an ideal combination for weight loss and increased energy.

Make exercise as simple as possible for yourself. For me, that means coming home from work and putting on my T-shirt and shorts. My exercise equipment is right in the family room in front of the television. I don't have to do any elaborate setup. The house is for me to live in, not to look perfect in case company comes. We move it when we have guests, then get it out again.

Commit to doing an exercise program for one month. Within that time your body will probably come to look forward to exercise.

If you drop out for a while, let yourself know that you will get back to it when you can. Don't spend a minute beating yourself up.

STEP THREE: WATCH OUT FOR SELF-SABOTAGE. One of the most common reasons that women stop exercising is that they do too much too soon (addictive behavior). Having been out of shape for three years, they vow that they'll run three miles a day for a week and get in shape fast. A much better approach is to *do less* each day than you are capable of—at least for a while. This will give your body the message that it can trust you to take care of it and not push it to exhaustion. Your body will get the idea that exercise is fun! Dogs love to go for their walks—and we would be just as enthusiastic if we followed our instincts as well as animals do.

If you *never* push yourself, on the other hand, and always do *less* than is expected or needed, consider giving yourself a little push. It's good to know your body is capable of the long haul when necessary. Don't ever use exercise as a way to beat your body into submission or to punish it for not looking perfect. (Anne Wilson Schaef says that she thinks addiction to self-abuse is probably the most common addiction in our culture, and I would agree.)

Be aware of using exercise as a way to run away from your feelings or as a way to decrease stress. Though exercise can "blow off steam," if it's used primarily for this purpose it can become a "fix" anytime you feel stressed. You'll use exercise to "medicate" your emotional pain. It's much better to deal with the source of the stress than to use exercise as a fix.

If you hate your exercise program and have to manipulate or force yourself into doing it, you'll just build up resistance at some level. You'll eventually quit or manage to get injured, or you'll make the exercise program into an external authority controlling you— and you'll sabatoge yourself to get out of doing it.

STEP FOUR: ENJOY YOURSELF. One of my patients, an art teacher in her forties, started going to a gym for weightlifting. She's having a great time pumping iron. Newly divorced and on her own, her muscle-strengthening reflects the strengthening she's doing in other areas of her life as well. She looks and feels wonderful—and powerful. Exercise releases naturally occurring substances called endorphins, which are related to morphine and the other opiates. For this reason exercise does naturally produce a feeling of well-being.

Give physical activity a try. If, as David Spangler says, "our body creates our soul as much as our soul creates our body," maybe your soul could use a better set of biceps!

NINETEEN

Healing Ourselves, Healing Our World

If you bring forth what is within you,
What you bring forth will save you.
If you do not bring forth what is within you,
What you do not bring forth will destroy you.

Jesus, in The Gospel According to Thomas

All of us must acknowledge our female heritage and bear witness to it if we are to heal ourselves. We carry in our own bodies not only our own pain but that of our mothers and grandmothers, however unconsciously. Hatred of the body is very deep in most women—generations deep. Most of us had mothers who were brought up to distrust their own bodies and the processes of their bodies. So had their mothers, grandmothers, and greatgrandmothers before them.

From time to time I have a very vivid experience of entering a place inside myself that I call "the pain of women." The first time it happened, at an intensive with Anne Wilson Schaef, I felt my consciousness going backward in time, as layers and layers and centuries and centuries of denial peeled away. My entry into this process was when Anne said to me, "You're so tired" and then suggested I lie down on a mat to see "what comes up." Having a woman, a mentor, acknowledge my tiredness instead of demanding more sacrifice was one of the most profound experiences of my life. At first, as she sat with me and told me to stay with myself, I felt how strongly my body resisted feeling what I was feeling. I experienced how good I was at pushing down my tears and getting on with whatever I had to do. But eventually, as Anne suggested that I simply stay with myself, I felt my consciousness go backward through all the times when I had never rested: when I'd had my children, during residency, during medical school, during college, during high school. Backward, backward—through my childhood—"Don't ask for a lighter pack, ask for a stronger back," I heard my mother say. And I wept for myself and for that part of me that so needed rest. When I had finished crying all the tears that I had never cried for myself, I began to weep for my mother—for all the times that she had not been allowed to feel or to rest, for all the times that she was up all night with a sick child, for the endless grief of losing two children.

And when that was over, I felt my grandmother's grief, raised by her twelve-year-old sister after her own mother had died in childbirth. When that was complete, I went backward further still—until I was wailing for all women, for all the pain, for all the labors unattended, for all the injustice, for so many thousands of years. What had started as very personal became universal: not my pain, but *the* pain.

When it was over, several hours later, I knew exactly why I was on earth and what my mission was: to work toward healing this collective pain. I knew in a flash that there are no mistakes, that I had been destined to become an obstetrician/gynecologist, and that no other path would have served as well. I knew why I had cried so many years before in medical school, when I had first witnessed the birth of a baby: I had tapped into the same "field." Seeing the birth had brought up emotions for me that I had no words for back in 1973. I only knew that I had been moved beyond all reason by this birth and that there was no other field of medicine for me except the care of women. But I pushed those emotions down then, instead of experiencing them fully, as I did on so many other occasions. Two days after this experience I got my period, confirmation for me that our deepest material often comes to consciousness premenstrually—the time when the veil between the worlds is thinner.

About a week later, I was relating my experience of this deep process to my mother over the phone. When I had finished, she was silent for a long time. Then she said, "I was sexually abused. I remember the room, I remember the smell of his pipe. I can see it as though it were happening now. It was old Bill, the man who rented a room from my mother. He told me never to tell anyone. I felt dirty. I was eight years old."

My mother, at sixty-three, had not remembered this part of her history before that moment. Somehow I had broken into the family memory bank with my process—and the contents were easier for her to get to as well. A few months prior to this, she had been having a recurrent dream in which there were horrid growths on her body. She'd awaken in terror. She now knew that these dreams were related to her long-suppressed abuse; the growths on her skin were symbolic of material coming up to consciousness "just under the surface"—ugly material, horrid material.

Mom was alone in her cabin when I called and she remembered her abuse. I asked her if she would be all right after we hung up. She said she would but that she'd call back if she needed support. I suggested that she be willing to stay with "that which was not acceptable." She prayed for guidance and let herself experience the sickening feelings that had surfaced with the sexual abuse memory. She then went to bed. Her loft window was open—it was a warm autumn night—and she later told me that three blue lights came in the window, followed by a large gleaming sphere of white light. The next thing she knew, it was morning. She awakened feeling profoundly at peace, knowing that she had had an experience of grace.

Our Mothers: Our Cells

Our memories are stored up in our bodies. Incest memories surface after a uterine biopsy, and sadness arises after pelvic surgery, all for a reason. We carry our personal history in our tissue, like data banks. But we carry much more than what is simply personal. On some level, we carry everyone and everything—the collective—all there within and around our very cells.

It's known that mitochondrial DNA, the DNA that carries out the daily activities of the cytoplasm of the cell, is inherited strictly through the maternal line. The entire human race can be traced back to a group of females in Africa.[1] This fact lends biological credence to my experiences and those of my patients who've entered into realms of experience that don't fit logical thinking. Sometimes body symptoms are the doorway not only into our own individual pain but into the collective pain of others.

An old Sufi saying captures the essence of what this means and what each of us must do with it:

> *Overcome any bitterness that may have come to you because you were not up to the magnitude of the pain that was entrusted to you. Like the mother of the world who carries the pain of the world in her heart, each one of us is part of her heart and therefore endowed with a certain measure of cosmic pain. You are sharing in the totality of that pain.*
>
> *You are called upon to meet it in joy instead of self-pity. The secret is to offer your heart as a vehicle to transform cosmic suffering into joy.*

Stephen Levine taught me that the work we do to let go of our suffering diminishes the suffering of the whole universe. When we have room for our own pain, we have room for the pain of others and we actually help "carry" the suffering of others. Only then can it be transformed into joy.

A Ritual of Reclaiming: Brenda's Story

Several years ago, my closest friend from childhood decided that she'd like to have her IUD removed in order to get pregnant. She'd been using IUDs for contraception for almost eighteen years with no problem, but now, at the age of forty, she had met a man with whom she wanted to share her life and have children. Because this decision was a major turning point in her life, she wanted someone close to her to share it. So she asked me to remove the IUD while she was here visiting in Maine.

We decided to do a simple ceremony prior to the procedure—to bring intent and consciousness to the process of removing the IUD and inviting in a child. So on a glorious Sunday afternoon in autumn, with the trees ablaze with color, we went over to Women to Women, set up a circle of cloth on the carpet in my office, picked a geranium from an office plant, and gathered a few sea shells to place in our circle. We filled a shell with water, lit some candles, and then, sitting around our small circle, we acknowledged the forces of nature, God, and the mysteries of life, and we invited them to be present with us.

We called Brenda's fiancé on the phone (he was at work in another state at the time). I asked each of them to speak about their fears and hopes for a child, which they did. The fiancé had already had a child many years before, but he was eager for a chance to participate more fully in the process this time. His support and love for Brenda were very evident and clear as he spoke; he had no doubts about his willingness to participate in parenthood. His commitment to support her was strong and inspiring. Their relationship felt like the very embodiment of the masculine at its best when it is in full support of the feminine.

Brenda herself, though eager to have a baby, voiced a concern that she wouldn't know how to give birth. Despite her fear, she was ready to proceed with the IUD removal. We said good-bye to her fiancé, promising to call back as soon as we had completed the procedure.

Now we moved into one of my exam rooms, and I placed a small amount of local anesthetic in the cervix. Once Brenda felt ready, I asked her to cough while I pulled out the IUD. (Coughing while something is going into or coming out of the cervix often interferes with pain pathways and thus makes the procedure more comfortable.)

I told her that she would feel the visceral sense of her uterus as the IUD was pulled out and that this would be a good time for her to tune in to the information stored in there. I told her that the body holds memories and that these sometimes come to the surface during an office procedure such as an endometrial biopsy or an IUD removal. I explained that I would be taking some time after the procedure to "put her energy field back together" by placing my hands over the uterus. Her job was to simply pay attention to any thoughts or feelings that came up.

The IUD came out with no difficulty. I then took Brenda's heels out of the stirrups, had her lie flat, and then ran my hands over her body from head to toe several times, doing therapeutic touch. When finished, I laid my hands over her lower abdomen. She began to cry and laugh at the same time as her body released the tension and the emotional charge associated with this sort of procedure. I encouraged her to do whatever she had to do for herself. And I reminded her to simply stay with whatever was coming up.

After crying for a bit, Brenda closed her eyes and then began to laugh. She spoke of being in a forest, with light shining down through the tall trees. She described herself as being young, too young. Then she became frightened again. At this time, I didn't know exactly what was going on, but I simply remained with my hands over her lower abdomen. She told me that having my hands there felt good and she wanted me to keep them there.

She continued to recount being a young girl, alone in the woods. She was pregnant there, without the support of anyone. Her body began to go through what looked like labor. She kept saying, "It's too soon. I don't know how to do this." She began to go through contractions and then pushing. (I've sat with enough women in labor to know what a laboring woman's body goes through.) After about ten minutes she looked down at what sounded like a thirty-week-size stillborn when she described it. And she asked me, "What is that white ropelike thing going into my vagina?" She was describing the umbilical cord. I told her what it was and said that she'd have to deliver the placenta. Her body then went into another contraction and went through the motions of pushing out a placenta. Brenda had never seen a thirty-week premature baby, a placenta, or a white translucent umbilical cord, but she was able to describe them perfectly—but with the curiosity of a young girl who didn't know exactly what was happening to her, not a worldly forty-year-old.

At this point, the "energetic" labor and delivery complete, Brenda began to laugh and also to chant "O-ne-an-ta, O-ne-an-ta." It sounded like a Native American language. During this time she said, "I know the whole language." I wish I had had a tape recorder—we might have figured out what language it was.

We stayed in the exam room a while longer while Brenda returned to the twentieth century and stretched her legs. Both of us were amazed by what had just happened. I reminded her that her body did in fact know how to give birth—she had just gone through it, though not on what we'd conventionally call a physical level. Nevertheless, her body now "knew" or "remembered" what labor and delivery were like, and her fear of the process was gone. We returned to my office, sang a lullaby together, and blew out the candles. When she was ready, she called her fiancé and related the experience.

Brenda had tapped in to the collective unconscious, had gained access to some ancient memory that still lived on in her cells. It was an extraordinary experience. I believe that in taking out her IUD and allowing her process to unfold, we were able to heal something deep, on a level that is available to all of us but that we rarely allow ourselves to touch.

Martha, when she had her stomach pain described in Chapter 2, did the same thing. *Our bodies contain information that is beyond our intellectual mind's capacity to understand. We are much more than we think we are.*

Conquering Our Fear of Our Shaman Past

In the Middle Ages, 9 million women were burned as witches. This witch craze, fueled by the Catholic Church, lasted for hundreds of years and has been well documented by others.[2] It's not uncommon for women who are reclaiming their power or speaking their personal truths to have terrifying dreams of being burned. I have heard this countless times in my work. The burning times have been suppressed for centuries but are now surfacing in our consciousness.

When a woman enters into the work of healing her body and speaking her truth, she must break through the collective field of fear and pain that is all around us and has been for the past five thousand years of dominator society. It is a field filled with the fear of rape, of beating, of abandonment.

Rupert Sheldrake, a British biologist, posits that all the knowledge of the earth's past exists all around us as electromagnetic fields of information, or "morphogenic fields."[3] When an athlete first breaks a world record, Sheldrake notes, he or she often has to work for years to do it and is often told that it can't be done—that it is not humanly possible. It was once felt, for example, that no one would ever be able to run a mile in under four minutes. Yet once a record is broken, suddenly athletes all over the world begin breaking it. Sheldrake explains that the morphogenic field around this world record is changed by the first person who breaks it, thus making it easier for others to equal that performance by tapping into the new morphogenic field.

Women all over the planet are finding the courage to break through the collective morphogenic field of shame, fear, and pain. One of my patients recently went home to tell her father what it was like to grow up in a household in which he had sexually abused her sisters and herself for years. She stood there and told all of it, not to change him but to break the years of silence. She later told me, "I am ready to go on national television with my father's name. He not only ruined my girlhood, but also has abused almost every girl in my neighborhood!" Another one of my patients recently had a mastectomy. When she is casually asked how she is doing, she graciously says, even to a male businessman who doesn't know about it, "I am healing very beautifully from my mastectomy. You do know I had one, don't you?" Both of these women are breaking the silence—releasing the secrets that keep all of us trapped. They are saying, "No more!" All over the world, women like this are changing the morphogenic field of fear and silence.

Breaking the silence takes courage. I know of no woman who has tapped her inner source of power without going through an almost palpable veil of fear, often feeling as though her very life would be threatened by telling the truth. The journalist Vivian Gornick says, "For a woman, coming off fear is like an addict coming off drugs." I don't know any way around this fear except to go through it with the help of others who've also experienced it and come out on the other side. Millions of women healers and wise women, and the men who have supported them, have been killed for telling the truth. It is little wonder, given the collective history of women, that we are afraid. When we deny this fear or discount its presence in others, we only give it more power. Experiencing the fear we collectively hold is a very important step toward healing—we need not judge it in others or in ourselves.

But as each of us acknowledges and moves through her fear, it becomes that much easier for the next woman to heal, just as when a world record is broken. We are changing the morphogenic field together, as thousands of women break through their fields of fear at the same time. The first women who told the truth about their incest were accused of making it up. Now, when a woman remembers and speaks, support, books, and meetings are available for her. She's no longer alone.

I often think of myself as standing on the shoulders of all the strong women who came before me and being supported by them, women who had the courage to speak their truths even in the face of great opposition. I reassure myself with the thought, "They can't burn me this time. There are too many of us this time. This time I am safe."

Our Dreams: Earth's Dreams

Women are rising like yeast all over the planet.
                                        —Sonia Johnson

As we heal, through feeling our grief and our joy, the Earth heals. Part of the rise of the feminine that I see happening all over the country (and the world) is the strengthening of ties between women. Gwendolyn, one of the women we met earlier, said that as a result of her healing, "What has come into my life are beautiful female relationships. This never happened before because I put so much energy into men. Now a sisterhood is starting to happen. When you take the time to tune in to yourself and your needs, the sisterhood starts happening."

I couldn't do the work I do without the support of my sisters throughout the country. My women friends and colleagues sustain me. I feel supported and blessed. Brian Swimme once wrote that we humans are the space where the Earth dreams. Our personal dreams aren't ours alone—they are the Earth dreaming through us. Our heart's desire is the desire of the Earth—it is what She is asking you to do. The addictive system has told us that "if it doesn't hurt, it is not worth doing—no pain, no gain." But often just the opposite is true. If what you are doing gives you no joy, no pleasure, no sense of purpose, no sense of fulfillment—it is *not* worth doing. Your state of health is the barometer of this. Your cells know what you need to do—*listen!*

Every cell in your body reponds to your inner dreams. They are necessary for your health and for that of our planet. The dreams the Earth dreams through you are different from the ones She dreams through me. But I need to hear your dreams, and you need to hear mine—otherwise we don't have the whole story. The addictive system has had a vested interest in keeping us from hearing each other for centuries. But our time has come. Let's listen to each other.

Personal Healing Is Planetary Healing

For all of written history, the Earth and the natural world have been viewed as feminine, with "virgin resources" to be "exploited." What happens to individual women and what happens to our planet are linked. Our personal degradation of nature, women, and the feminine must now cease—if it does not, nothing else will matter.

Science as it is currently practiced will not save us. It lacks the voice of intuition, the feminine voice, the voice that speaks from our bodies. We require balance now. We require embodied wisdom that is filtered through *all of us*—including what the mind of our bodies and our inner guidance is telling us.

A crowd of women were shown on a recent cover of *Ms.* magazine with the headline RAGE + WOMEN = POWER.[4] This message made me uncomfortable, until I saw the potential embedded in it. The anger and rage of silenced women, when used as fuel for change, is indeed power. But it must be power from within, power that is fully grounded and centered—not rage directed *against* someone or something. Rage *transformed* is power. Rage transformed is *strength*.

Anne Wilson Schaef writes "As women we have been limited as to what we can do, say, think, and feel. We may hate to admit it, yet deep down, we know that there are many forces that limit our lives over which we have no control. Only a person with no feelings would not feel the smolder of rage at times. We thought we had only two options: to go along with authority and thus support it, or to fight it and thus support it. Either way we lose. There is a third option. We can be ourselves. We can see what is important for us and do it. And—we may have to go through our anger before we can exercise this option."[5]

To name your work "political," especially when it comes to your body and to things that are "womanly," is an act of power. If you are a mother, believe me, your work is political. If you are a nurse, a childcare worker, or *anything* else—your work is political. If you're healing a fibroid tumor or remembering your incest, you are doing political work.

How refreshing to see our body's healing as political. Let us give it the importance that it deserves! Gloria Steinem once said, "Any woman who is up off her ass is part of the women's movement." I like that a lot—it leaves room for a wide range of interpretations. We have many choices. No one but you gets to define your healing or your politics for you. Do you need to take six weeks off from work to heal from pelvic surgery? Think of it as political. And then when you've learned from it, see if you can channel future energy outward from your body into work that is positive and life-affirming.

In the epilogue to her book on her recovery from breast cancer, *Burst of Light,* poet Audre Lorde writes, "I had to examine in my dreams as well as in my immune function tests the devastating effects of overextension. Overextending myself is not stretching myself. I had to accept how difficult it is to monitor the difference. Caring for myself is not self-indulgence, it is self-preservation, and that is an act of political warfare."[6]

In a political system that has not represented womanly values, each woman must represent herself and become a lobbyist for her own needs. Caring for yourself as well as you possibly can, *whether or not* you have a socially acceptable illness, is *indeed* an act of political warfare.

Physician, Heal Thyself—Revisited

My inner guidance came to me through the mind of my uterus while I was in the process of writing this book. I was diagnosed with a fibroid tumor that made my uterus about thirteen-weeks' size. I had no symptoms. I had been eating an essentially dairy-free, low-fat diet for years. At first I was saddened and didn't want anyone to know about it. I grieved for the loss of my "normal" uterus. When Annie Rafter[7] did my pelvic exam and told me about the fibroid, the first thought that flashed through my mind was, "I better get this book finished this year, because I'm sure this growth is related to it."

I felt intuitively that it had started to grow in the early stages of my writing process, two years before. I also thought, "Damn, I've been hanging around too many women with fibroids. Maybe I caught one."[8]

I felt as though I had done something wrong, as though I had somehow failed. I was reminded that our emotions don't always match our level of intellectual development. I was humbled. Later that night, as I lay in my bed, I put my hands over my lower abdomen and said to my uterus, "Okay, now I have to take my own medicine and tune in to what you're telling me." My uterus gave me the following message: "This fibroid is a reminder that you need to learn how to move energy through your body more efficiently. If you take care of yourself now and pay attention, you'll avoid more serious problems in the future. This is also a wonderful opportunity to teach other women by example. Remember, the work you're doing with others applies to you. You've always believed that it is possible to dematerialize fibroids. Here's your chance." I meditated on creativity and what was needing to be birthed through me.

The next day, I began a regimen of castor oil packs, and I started a course of acupuncture, something I'd been wanting to do as a general preventive measure for a long time. My acupuncturist told me that my kidney and triple warmer meridians were very low and had been for some time. This was related to overwork and stress. I was reminded of a chronic energy pattern called, in Oriental medicine, "stuck blood" or "stuck *chi*," on the right side of my body. My previous migraine headaches had been on my right side; Caroline Myss had once diagnosed energy leaking out of my right hip, manifesting as a hip problem on the right; my breast abscess had been on the right; and now I had a fibroid on the right side of my uterus. All were on the right side of my body—the "masculine" or yang side—and all were related in an energy sense. What that meant to me was that it had been important to develop a strong foundation for my work and to take it out into the world—this was my "masculine" task. Up until the past few years, I've been afraid of doing so because of my perception that the world wasn't ready to hear it and that it would be dangerous for me. Hence, the repeated "wounds" on my right side. The fibroid was simply the latest manifestation—and a timely one at that, given my life's work with women. And despite my on-going recovery from relationship ad-diction, I still realized how much I wanted the approval of others and I finally understood how powerless I am over what people will think of me. It became clear that the fibroid was about more than the book and the depleted acupuncture meridians. After several months of acupuncture and castor oil packs, it seemed to get larger, not smaller. My learning had to go much deeper. What did I need to learn? I asked a trusted friend to bring her Motherpeace cards to the office so that I could use her skill with these to tune in to the fibroid further. She had me shuffle the cards, spread them out, and then ask a question. The question I asked was, "What is the highest purpose that my fibroid is teaching me?" With the thought clearly in mind, I picked a card for guidance. The card I picked signifies "bondage." It shows a person with chains around her hands, neck, and legs. From reading about this image further and meditating on its meaning, I realized that my entire relationship with my office and with my profession needed to change—that I was in bondage to an obsolete form. While my heart wanted to write, lecture, and teach women a whole new way of being in relationship with their bodies, my intellectual sense of "responsibility" dictated that I continue to practice medicine in the way I had been trained: see patients, do surgery, and do my share of emergency calls like every-body else (my relationship addiction in yet another guise!). The fibroid was a manifestation of my responsibility addiction to the old form, resulting in a block to the new creative forms that now needed expression. I realized that I needed more freedom. I needed to change my practice to teach more of the material in this book. I needed to be responsible to my deepest dreams and my innermost wisdom.

Women's health will never change substantially unless large groups of women begin to reclaim the wisdom of their bodies collectively. For me to do this meant letting go of being "the doctor" to the hundreds of women I'd enjoyed working with so much over the years. I didn't want to leave the practice of medicine—I wanted to transform it. I knew that I could no longer do primary care with all of its cultural assumptions, assumptions that were chaining me to limits that I could no longer tolerate.

The fibroid was symbolic of the endless piles of charts on my desk and the number of phone calls demanding my attention. I needed to let go of these and reinvent the practice of medicine in a whole new way. I realized at a deeper level than ever before that one-on-one health care, though valuable, tends to isolate each woman's problem and doesn't allow physicians the time necessary to educate her fully about all the issues that can affect her body and how she has the power to transform them. So I began to move toward teaching women in groups how to create health on a daily basis.

I wrote a letter to my patients that said, "I am not leaving the practice of medicine. I am redefining it and expanding into new areas that are critical to truly improving women's health over the long term." I told them that disease-screening—which my training had prepared me for—and creating health, where my heart was taking me, were two different things. I had to concentrate on a new form now. In my letter to my patients I asked them to consider the following questions. I ask you to do the same.

- What would it be like if you reclaimed the wisdom of your body and learned how to trust its messages?
- What would your life be like if you no longer feared germs or cancer?
- How would your life be different if your body were your friend and ally?
- How would your life be different if you learned how to love and respect your body as though it were your own precious creation, as valuable as a beloved friend or child? How would you treat yourself differently?
- What would it be like to know, in the deepest part of you, that every part of your anatomy and each process of your female body contained wisdom and power?

These are the questions I am living and teaching as my new creating-health practice evolves. My fibroid served me well as a kick in the pants from my body and soul. It brought me to a crucial next step that I might not otherwise have taken (at least, not so soon). I am grateful for it and the political significance it has had in my own life. Several months before this book was completed, I no longer cared whether my fibroid stayed or went. Then, as I completed the final stages of my writing and began teaching more and more groups of women, the fibroid gradually started to shrink. It may not go away completely. I suspect it may instead remain in my body as a barometer whose size alerts me to whether I'm being true to myself and to the work I love the most.

Making the World Safe for Women: Start with Yourself

If we are ever to create safety in the outside world for ourselves, we must first create safety for ourselves *right in our own bodies.* If, as we undress for bed, we look in the mirror and beat ourselves up for our breast size or our cellulite, we are not walking our walk. *We are not safe with ourselves.* If we can't create a safe space *within ourselves* for our own bodies—their shape, their size, their natural functions, and their weight; if we are forever putting down our bodies, starving them, and giving them adverse messages, how can we ever expect anyone else to create health for us on the outside? Even if they did, we'd still be carting around our own internal terrorist!

The truth is that we can change only ourselves, not anyone or anything else. This is good news—it means we don't have to wait for someone else to do it for us. A friend of mine gave her daughter a T-shirt that says, "What if the knight in shining armor never comes?" What a thought! What a relief, in fact! After centuries of being told that someone else could, should, and would take care of us, we now have a chance to learn how to take care of ourselves—together. The Boston Women's Fund brochure says on the cover, "The people we've been waiting for are us." Aren't you energized just reading that? We can start saving ourselves *now.* We can start living our lives *now.*

When we change ourselves *inside* by allowing ourselves to experience and own our long-suppressed emotions and woundings *as well as* our hopes and dreams for ourselves, our families, and our planet, the conditions of our lives change on the *outside.* Working for social changes must go hand in hand with the willingness to heal within ourselves all the internalized messages of blame, self-doubt, and self-hatred that are encoded in our very cells. Otherwise, our actions originate out of unhealthy places within us and often re-create polarization and pain. Being led by the spirit means living in tune with our inner guidance. Listen quietly. What do you need to do next? Perhaps just being still for a moment is the best way to heal or to serve. Perhaps there's nothing you need to *do* right now. There is no one "right way" to heal your body. The same goes for any area of life. You must find the way yourself. Emerson once wrote, "The essence of heroism is self-trust." Self-trust is more than the essence of heroism. It is also the basis for trusting our intuition and the healing voice of our cells. Sorting out the genuine messages from our innermost selves (and cells) is no small task. It is indeed the work of heroes.

It takes courage to learn to respect yourself and your body, regardless of how wounded you've been, regardless of your current weight, regardless of who you married or what your sexual prefer-ence is. The women whose stories I've shared with you are ordinary women; they are healing women. Their stories are the stories of planetary wounding and healing. These women are my heroes.

Self-healing is a highly personal and individual process. Self-healing requires personal disarmament, refusing to be at war any longer with a part of your body that's trying to tell you something. Let the arms race end with you. One of my patients, a fifteen-year member of Alcoholics Anonymous, summed this up beautifully: "Each morning I pray for willingness to do whatever it is I must do. *And I also pray to remain teachable.* There have been times in my life when no one could teach me anything. I thought I knew it all. I never want to be there again."

Commit to living your dreams—one day at a time. This is the process that is required to heal our families, our communities, and our planet. May you go forth now, to take a nap, to embrace a child, to feel the sun on your face, or to eat a good meal slowly, knowing deep within you that the next step for healing and living joyfully is already there, waiting for you to listen to it, waiting to be born into the world—through you, dear woman.

Women to Women Guidelines for a Healthy Approach to Food

EATING RECOMMENDATIONS*
(GENERAL GUIDELINES FOR A HEALTHY
APPROACH TO FOOD)

1. Learning to pay attention to when you are really hungry is oftentimes the most difficult single thing you need to learn about yourself. The best way to do it is to use some type of scale for yourself: for example, 1 being extremely hungry and 8 being full, with 4 being comfortably satisfied. This seems to work well for many people. If you are at 1 or 2, I recommend you sit down and have a meal. If you are 3 to 8, wait to eat until you are truly hungry—1 or 2 on your scale.

2. Eat only when sitting down, preferably at the dining-room table or some other area in which you feel comfortable eating.

3. No reading, writing, or watching TV while eating. What this does is allow you to notice your behavior while eating. The questions to ask yourself are: Are you eating quickly? Are you eating slowly? Are you chewing your food? You want to start paying attention to these things.

4. During any situation in which you find yourself reaching for food, try to take a moment aside and sit down and close your eyes and evaluate what is happening in your body. Most often, what is happening in your body can be translated into an emotion. It could oftentimes prevent overeating or a binge if you acknowledge and deal with this emotion.

5. Keep a diary of the foods you are eating. [You may wish to follow the Sample Healthy Diet on pp. 658–59.] Chart the foods as you eat them, not at the end of the day, as we often forget some of the things we have eaten.

* *Source:* Marcelle Pick, RNC, Women to Women, Yarmouth, ME.

SAMPLE HEALTHY DIET*

	Day 1	Day 2	Day 3	Day 4	Day 5	Day 6	Day 7
BREAKFAST	Sour FRUIT (grapefruit or strawberries); herbal tea	VEGGIES (sautéed, raw, or steamed, leftovers); salad or hash browns w/olive oil	Whole-grain variety CEREAL, hot or cold; w/soy, nut, or grain milk (granola-oatmeal)	Tofu and veggie SCRAMBLE, spices; water or decaf, or free choice	Sweet FRUIT (orange, apple, banana); fruit juice	Whole-grain bagel, toast or naturally sweet muffin	1 organic egg (omelette or scramble) and veggies (lots), or no breakfast
How do I feel							
SNACKS	Raw almonds (couple of handfuls, chewed well)	Pear	Orange	Burritos, corn chips (couple of handfuls)	Whole-grain nonyeasted crackers, or free choice	Raw and steamed veggies, w/ or w/out natural dip/cashew butter (1 tbsp.)	Natural fruit juice spritzer
How do I feel							
LUNCH	Veggie or bean SOUP (fresh, pkgd, or canned); whole-wheat/salad; water	Natural deli SANDWICH on whole-grain bun (hummus, tofu salad, soy cheese); water	Fish SALAD w/veggies and tofu mayo or natural dressing; water	Almond butter in celery salad w/Paul Newman dressing; w/added herbs; water	Brown rice or whole-grain and veggie SALAD w/natural dressing or olive oil and lemon; water	Natural pizza (fresh or frozen), soy cheese, veggie, salad; water	Veggie BURGER, whole wheat bun; natural chips; salad; water

How do I feel							
MUNCHIES	Rice Dream (½ cup); or natural ice cream	Natural cookies (whole-wheat, naturally sweetened), or Westbrae Snaps (2–3)	Organic popcorn w/low # cold-pressed oil & sea salt	Grapes or apple	Oven-roasted sunflower seeds	Dried FRUIT (dates, raisins, currants, apricots)	Free choice or leftovers
DESSERT	(carob chip, fudge twirl, lemon)						
How do I feel							
DINNER (starch & veggies)	Broiled or pan sautéed FISH; herbs; veggies; salad (opt.), natural beer (opt.); water	Whole-wheat or corn pancakes; or veggie crêpes; or veggie chili & salad; water	Whole-wheat PASTA w/Ragu homestyle nonmeat sauce; mixed veggie salad; water	Long-grain organic brown rice and veggie STIRFRY; tofu, fish, organic chicken (opt.); water	Mexican bean TACO, or tostada, or enchilada, w/whole-corn tortilla; salad; water	Free choice, or simply varied veggies w/tofu; tempeh; water	Whole-grain PASTA (wheat or buckwheat); or stirfry w/lots of veggies; water
How do I feel							
BEVERAGES	Pure filtered water, or natural soda	Pure filtered water, or Poland Spring	Pure filtered water, or free choice	Pure filtered water, or herbal ice tea	Pure filtered water, or coffee substitute	Pure filtered water, or natural wine	Pure filtered water, or carob tea
How do I feel							
GENERAL OBSERVATIONS							

*Source: Marcelle Pick, RNC, Women to Women, Yarmouth, ME.

6. Try not to be judgmental of yourself. All the things you are trying to do are working toward changing your behavior. It does take patience on your part, and it takes time. In other words, be gentle with yourself.

7. At the end of each meal, jot down in your daily food journal [see Sample Healthy Diet] how you feel physically after you have eaten. Do you feel bloated? Do you feel full? Do you feel hungry? Do you feel deprived? If you do, ask yourself why.

8. A very important element is to notice how often you are comfortably wanting to eat. Some people like three meals a day; some people like two meals a day; and others feel much more comfortable having snacks throughout the day. Listen to what your body is trying to tell you, and then accommodate your eating accordingly. This may also vary depending on the day of the month, especially for women when they are still menstruating.

YEAST-FREE DIET*
GUIDELINES

The following foods contain yeast or mold and should be avoided during the yeast-free diet:

1. Baker's yeast is added to most breads, biscuits, buns, rolls, pretzels, crackers, and pastries. Yeast-free products such as RyKrisp, Wasa lite rye, taco shells, rice cakes, Kavli Norwegian quick breads, and muffins may be substituted.

2. Yeast is present in all fermented beverages: in alcoholic beverages, medications containing alcohol, root beer and ginger ale, and vanilla. Dry cereals, coffee substitutes, and milk drinks to which *malt* has been added should also be avoided.

3. Dried fruits, commercially produced fruit juice (canned and frozen), canned tomatoes, tomato juice, and all teas (except herbal) contain yeast or molds.

4. Cheese of all kinds, including cottage cheese, buttermilk, and sour cream, contain yeast. Skim milk and plain yogurt and butter can be used for some people, but we suggest you try to stay away from them.

5. Mushrooms and truffles are yeastlike foods.

6. All fermented condiments or condiments containing vinegar should be avoided. Soy sauce, tamari, miso, tempeh, sauerkraut, olives, and pickles, as well as catsup, mayonnaise, salad dressings, barbecue sauce, prepared mustard, and horseradish fall into this category. Homemade vinegar-free mayonnaise and salad dressings may be substituted.

7. Wash fruits and vegetables to eliminate the yeast on their surfaces, and avoid overripe produce.

8. Medications derived from mold or yeast should be avoided: penicillin, mycin, chloromycetin, tetracyclines, vitamin B capsules or tablets made from yeast,

* *Source:* Women to Women, Yarmouth, ME.

multivitamins with B vitamins made from yeast, Zylax (and other Lilly products containing B_{12}), Laxo-Funk, PHoscaron—D, and ViLitron Drops, Mead Johnson's vitamins (which contain B_{12}), Squibb vitamins with yeast sources noted on label, Parke Davis Vibex, Merck, Sharpe and Dohme's vitamins containing B_{12}, Lederle vitamins, Endo vitamins including Manibee and S.C.T. and Massengill vitamins.

Abbott vitamins, Mead Johnson and Merck, Sharpe and Dohme vitamins which do contain B_{12}, Robin's Allbee with C, Upjohn and Hoffmann-LaRoche vitamin products, Endo vitamins except for Manibee and S.C.T. and Parke Davis vitamins except Vibrex were yeast-free as of 1957.

A diet that eliminates most sources of yeast consists of the following foods:

1. Fresh vegetables, raw and cooked (large amounts)
2. Fish, fowl, and lean meat
3. Fresh fruits, raw or cooked
4. Whole grains
5. Raw nuts and seeds
6. Legumes
7. Skim milk, plain yogurt, and butter
8. Cold pressed vegetable oils

Within these guidelines, some alternatives for breakfast include:

1. Eggs, poached or soft boiled
2. Hot cereal (oatmeal, buckwheat, millet, or brown rice)
3. Granola (unsweetened)
4. Essenc bread or Dimpflmeier's Sour Rye
5. Baked or steamed potatoes

For lunch, salads and cooked vegetables are the focus:

1. Vegetable salad
2. Steamed vegetables
3. Baked squash, onions, parsnips, sweet potato, etc.
4. Vegetable soup
5. Sandwiches on yeast-free bread (like tuna with yeast-free mayo)
6. Baked, broiled, or steamed fish, fowl, or lean meat
7. Butter (in moderation)
8. Salad dressings of oil, fresh lemon, dry mustard, minced garlic, herbs, and salt

Dinner options are the same as for lunch.

Snack foods might include:

1. Fresh fruit
2. Vegetables
3. Nuts and seeds
4. Plain yogurt, with chopped fresh fruit
5. Rice cakes, Wasa lite rye, RyKrisp, Kavli crispbread

Beverages suitable during this yeast-free period are:

1. Spring water
2. Salt-free seltzer water, with freshly squeezed lemon, lime/orange
3. Home-squeezed fruit juices or vegetable juices
4. Herb teas without the ingredient Matte
5. Homemade soda (½ fruit juice, ½ seltzer)
6. Broth made from vegetables

YEAST AND MOLD AVOIDANCE CHECKLIST* (SIMPLIFIED VERSION)

You may eat whatever items have checkmarks by them, unless you are avoiding them for other reasons. Keep a food and symptom diary. Always read labels carefully.

Dairy Products
- √ butter
- NO cheeses
- √ eggs
- NO ice cream
- √ margarine
- √ milk (cow)
- √ milk (goat)
- √ yogurt (plain)

Meats and Poultry
(Watch out for fried and breaded meats, hot dogs and cold cuts.)
- √ beef
- √ chicken
- √ duck
- √ lamb
- √ liver (beef)
- √ pork
- √ turkey
- √ veal

Fish
- √ bass
- √ bluefish
- √ carp
- √ clams
- √ codfish
- √ crab
- √ flounder
- √ haddock
- √ halibut
- √ herring
- √ lobster
- √ mackerel
- √ oyster
- √ pike
- √ perch
- √ swordfish
- √ salmon
- √ sardines
- √ scallops
- √ shrimp
- √ smelt
- √ trout
- √ tuna
- √ whitefish

Cereal and Grains
- √ barley
- √ buckwheat
- NO cane sugar
- √ corn
- NO malt
- √ oat
- √ rice
- √ rye
- √ wheat
- √ millet
- √ pasta
- √ rice cakes

* *Source:* Women to Women, Yarmouth, ME.

√ brown rice
   crackers
√ corn tortillas
√ Nutri-Grain
   cereals
√ shredded wheat
√ puffed rice, corn
   and wheat

Nuts
√ almonds
√ brazil nuts
√ cashews
√ coconut
√ filbert nuts
NO peanuts
√ pecans
√ pistachios
√ walnuts
√ tahini
√ cashew butter
√ almond butter

Fruits
√ apple
√ avocado
√ banana
√ blackberry
√ blueberry
√ cantaloupe
√ cherry
NO date
NO fig
NO grape
√ grapefruit
√ honeydew melon
√ lemon
√ lime
√ nectarine
√ orange
√ peach
√ pear
√ pineapple
√ plum
NO prune

√ raspberry
NO raisin
√ strawberry
√ tangerine
√ watermelon

Vegetables
(fresh and frozen)
√ artichoke
√ asparagus
√ beet
√ broccoli
√ brussels sprouts
√ cabbage
√ carrot
√ cauliflower
√ celery
√ corn
√ cucumber
√ eggplant
√ endive
√ green pepper
√ kidney beans
√ kohlrabi
√ leek
√ lentils
√ lettuce
√ lima beans
NO mushroom
NO olive
√ onion
√ parsley
√ parsnips
√ peas (green)
√ pimento
√ potato (sweet or
   white)
√ pumpkin
√ radish
√ red pepper
√ rhubarb
√ soy beans
√ spinach
√ squash

√ string beans
√ tomato
√ turnip
√ chick peas
   (garbanzos)
√ navy beans

Miscellaneous
NO baker's yeast
NO brewer's yeast
NO cake
NO candy
√ carob
NO chewing gum
NO chocolate
NO cookies
√ gelatin
NO honey
NO maple syrup
NO sugar
NO any other sweets

Condiments and Spices
√ allspice
√ bay leaf
√ caraway seed
√ cinnamon
√ clove
√ dill
√ fenugreek
√ ginger
√ garlic
NO ketchup
√ licorice
√ mace
√ marjoram
NO mayonnaise
√ mint
NO mustard
√ nutmeg
√ oils
√ oregano
√ paprika
√ peppermint
√ poppy seeds

√	sage	**Beverages**		√	tap water
NO	salad dressings	NO	alcohol	NO	tea
√	sesame seeds	NO	chocolate drinks	√	seltzer
√	shortenings	NO	coffee (regular)	NO	Pero, Postum,
√	sunflower seeds	√	coffee (Swiss,		Cafix, Bambu
√	thyme		water-process,	√	fresh-squeezed
NO	vanilla		Decaff)		juices
NO	vinegar	NO	fruit juice	√	herbal teas
√	white pepper	√	milk	√	Pau d'Arco
√	dry mustard	NO	soda	√	Dacopa
		√	spring water		

DIETARY GUIDELINES FOR THOSE WHOSE EXCESSIVE SUGAR CRAVINGS OR WHOSE COMPULSIVE EATING IS OUT OF CONTROL*

This is meant to be a flexible plan that can be modified for individual needs. Portion sizes are suggestions only. You may need more or less food than others. Additional information is necessary if you have weight problems or allergies. *If you have food allergies, you may have to avoid some of the listed foods.* People who do not have specific medical problems may also follow this diet guide.

Important Instructions to Read Prior to Starting the Diet

Not everyone has the same nutritional requirements, and what might be healthful for some people may give you an allergic reaction. The most common sensitivities are to wheat, milk, and dairy products, yeast, corn, eggs, beef, and citrus. Your health practitioner will help you detect any suspicious foods that may cause symptoms. Personal experimentation is required in these programs to achieve the ultimate goal of maintaining a lifetime of healthful and wholesome eating habits.

It is essential to *read labels* on all products until you are familiar with the ingredients. The order of ingredients determines the amount of that substance in the product (first on the list is the highest amount, and last is the lowest). Do not use products that contain artificial flavors, colors, sweeteners, or preservatives.

Remember: The safest and most reliable grocery store is a *health food store.* However, even these stores carry products that are not entirely healthy and might contain substances that you do not tolerate. So again, reading labels while shopping is important.

Try to *avoid salt* in your diet. You may use tamari (soy sauce) as an alternative, but this also contains a great deal of salt and should be diluted and used sparingly. *Do not use soy sauce if you have a yeast allergy.* Use other herbs and spices, including onion and garlic. Try lemon for accent to reduce your desire for salt—this craving is a learned habit.

* *Source:* Women to Women, Yarmouth, ME.

For beverages, try *unsweetened fruit juices*, diluted with at least an equal amount of filtered or spring water, herbal teas, vegetable juices, and grain cereal beverages (like Cafix and Postum).

Make fresh salad dressings with herbs, spices, yogurt, lemon juice, or oil and vinegar. Use only extra-virgin olive oil or unrefined flaxseed oil. *Do not use vinegar if you are yeast sensitive.* Dressings should not contain sweeteners. Many dressings are available with no salt added and can be found in health food stores. Unsweetened catsup and mayonnaise, with no additives or sweeteners, are also available in health food stores.

Totally Avoid: Sugar; white or refined flour products (pastries, white breads, and all foods of a related nature); caffeine (diet sodas, coffee, tea, chocolate drinks); alcoholic beverages; white rice; all products made with barley malt, honey, maple syrup, concentrated fruit juice, molasses, or artificial sweeteners; *all* margarine and partially hydrogenated vegetable oils; dried fruits. Avoid artificial flavors, colors and preservatives. *As your condition improves*, some natural sweeteners and dried fruits may be added back to your diet in moderation, but check with your health practitioner first.

If you are on a *yeast-free diet, avoid all bread, cheese, pickles, vinegar, sau-erkraut, soy sauce, sprouts, berries, melons, and alcohol.* Please note: Not all foods on this diet are recommended to people with various food allergies, so be careful when selecting your meals and snacks. If you are in doubt about any particular food, please consult your health practitioner.

SUGGESTED FOOD GROUP CHOICES

Select a variety of natural, unprocessed foods from the following lists. (See page 660 for restrictions if you are yeast sensitive.)

Proteins

½–¾ cup peas and beans, such as lentils, chickpeas, pinto beans, kidney beans, split peas, navy beans, aduki beans, black beans, lima beans; see recipe books for varieties of preparation

3–4 oz. soy protein (tofu or tempeh; do not use tempeh if you are yeast sensitive)

½ cup low-fat, plain, or herb cottage cheese (no fruit flavors, as they contain sugar)

1 cup plain low-fat yogurt

1–2 eggs, hard-boiled, soft-boiled, or poached

1–2 oz. nuts or seeds

1–2 Tbsp. nut butter, such as almond or hazelnut

3–4 oz. fish (salmon is best)

3–4 oz. chicken or lean meat (These may be used sparingly if you choose to include them in your food selections. However, we encourage you to try a more vegetarian diet without dairy.)

Grains and Starchy Vegetables

1–2 slices of 100 percent whole-wheat or whole-grain bread. Whole-wheat tortillas, chapati, or matzoh are made without yeast, as are Wasa lite rye crackers and puffed rice cakes

½–1 cup cooked oatmeal (not instant) or other grain cereal such as Cream of Rye or brown rice

½–1 cup brown rice, millet, barley, buckwheat (kasha, or groats), rye, quinoa, teff, or whole-grain pasta, such as soba (buckwheat) or whole-wheat noodles

1–2 cup popcorn (air popped, no salt)

Starchy vegetables (potatoes, sweet potatoes, yams, winter squash, turnips)

Vegetables

alfalfa sprouts
asparagus
avocado
beets
broccoli
brussels sprouts
cabbage—red or green
cauliflower
carrots
celery
collard greens
corn
cucumbers
eggplant

kale
green or red pepper
lettuce (all kinds)
lima beans
mung bean sprouts
okra
onions
mustard greens
parsley
peas
potatoes
radishes
spinach
string beans

summer squash
sweet potatoes/yams
tomatoes
turnips and turnip greens
winter squash (acorn, butternut, hubbard, etc.)
zucchini

These are suggestions only; all other vegetables are acceptable. Choose fresh rather than canned or frozen. Try to have a variety of green and orange or yellow vegetables daily.

Fruits

apples
apricots
avocado
banana
blackberries
blueberries
strawberries

raspberries
cherries
½ grapefruit
kiwi fruit
½ cantaloupe
honeydew or other melon
orange

papaya
peach
pear
pineapple
plum

A portion of fruit is approximately ½–1 cup.

Snacks

About Snacks: Choose all your snacks from the other food lists, and select a wide variety during the day. You can interchange meals and snacks with regard to timing and portion size, but it is important that you remember not to overeat at any one time as well as during the whole day. As always, use common sense.

Snack Choices

- *½ portion of a protein choice:* plain yogurt; some leftover lentil soup; a few almonds, hazelnuts, or walnuts; sunflower or pumpkin seeds (unsalted nuts and seeds); a small piece of fish; a tofu burger; hummos (a chickpea/sesame/lemon/garlic purée used as a dip); or low-fat cottage cheese
- *½ portion of whole-grain or starchy vegetable* such as a baked potato; whole-grain bread with almond butter or any of the listed proteins or tofu salad; whole-grain bread or puffed rice cakes with mashed banana or unsweetened apple butter or low-fat cottage cheese; leftover brown rice with tofu and/or vegetables; oatmeal with fruit
- *fruit* (Be careful about the quantity of fruit in a day if you are yeast sensitive; you may tolerate only 1–2 fruits per day.)

SUGGESTED MEAL PLAN AND SCHEDULE

OPTIONAL: Upon rising, 1 fruit, or unsweetened fruit juice diluted with at least an equal amount of filtered or spring water. If you have candidiasis, you may do better limiting the amount of fruit to 1–2 pieces per day.

If you have food allergies, individual consultation is necessary. If you have candidiasis, avoid any food containing yeast or fermentation products, or those that might be moldy; this includes leftovers kept too long, in addition to the previous listings.

Breakfast:
1 serving of protein
1 fruit (if not already eaten earlier)
1 grain (hot cereals such as oatmeal or multigrain usually contain adequate protein but may be mixed with seeds or nuts. Another option is 100% whole-grain bread with poached or boiled eggs, or yogurt with fresh fruit and oat bran or seeds, such as sunflower or flax seeds. Take morning nutritional supplements after breakfast.)

Midmorning snack: Snacks are optional if you do not have hypoglycemia.

Lunch:
1 serving of protein
1 grain or starchy vegetable (such as squash or potato)
Fresh salad with dressing or fresh lemon juice and/or lightly steamed vegetables. Avoid vinegar if you are yeast sensitive. If you are unsure about ingredients in a restaurant, ask for oil and lemon or vinegar
Midday supplements, if recommended.

Midafternoon snack: From the snack list, but choose a different selection from midmorning.

Optional:
Before dinner, 4 oz of unsweetened fruit juice, diluted as above, or vegetable juice or 1 whole fruit.

Dinner:
1 serving of protein
1 grain
Fresh salad and/or cooked vegetables
1 fruit (if not eaten prior to dinner)
Take evening supplements as recommended

Evening snack: Very helpful if you have hypoglycemia; otherwise optional.

Talk to your health practitioner about the frequency of meals and snacks. It is best to maintain the frequency of meals and snacks and adjust the portion size to achieve the appropriate caloric intake. If you have a weight problem, be sure to discuss your needs. If the recommended portions are not adequate, they can be modified depending on metabolic rate and activity levels. Remember that no one diet can cover all individual needs. Use common sense and professional advice to make sensible choices, and try to have as much variety in your diet as possible.

MEAL PLAN FOR SELF-NURTURANCE
(FOR THOSE WHOSE COMPULSIVE EATING IS OUT OF CONTROL OR WHO WANT A SOUND PLAN FOR FOOD RECOVERY)

Guidelines

1. This program of eating is designed for those people who have identified themselves as having difficulty with food. They must abstain from all whole flours and sugar. Total abstinence from foods not allowed in this food plan is an absolute necessity.

2. This plan takes into account basic health needs, bodily readjustments, and sound nutrition. There are only three meals with an after-dinner adjustment to reduce metabolic problems that often occur.

3. While on this meal plan, it will be necessary for you to weigh and measure all food until you get comfortable with the portion size. Invest in nested measuring cups, a liquid measuring cup, measuring spoons, and a good scale.

4. Look for sugar on package labels. Sugar must be listed fifth or lower on salad dressings and should not be in soft drinks, cereals, seasonings, or sauces. Dextrose, sucrose, fructose, corn syrup, corn sweetener, honey, syrup, molasses—all are sugars to avoid. Acceptable sugar substitutes are saccharine, Sweet n' Low, Nutra-Sweet.

Multiple Allergies

Complex combinations

SAMPLE TRANSITION MENU*

(These meals have been created without corn, dairy, wheat, peanuts, citrus, caffeine, soy, eggs, yeast, or red meat, for those with food allergies.)

	Monday	Tuesday	Wednesday	Thursday	Friday	Saturday	Sunday
Breakfast	Homemade mixed grain cereal	Oatmeal	Homemade mixed grain cereal	Millet porridge	Homemade mixed grain cereal	Rice cream cereal	Homemade pancakes from non-allergen grains, topped with apple butter

You may use any milk substitute you can tolerate: soy milk, almond milk, coconut milk, rice milk (amazake). Use cooked potato or sweet potato for additional calories if necessary. Nuts, seeds, fruits are cereal topping options.

	Monday	Tuesday	Wednesday	Thursday	Friday	Saturday	Sunday
Lunch	Millet salad or croquettes Cold fish plate Watercress	Vegetable barley soup Chicken salad Rice cakes	Bean/avocado on rice cakes Boiled vegetable salad	Tuna fish salad RyKrisp Cold sliced beets with olive oil dressing	Roast turkey Mashed potato Broccoli	Wild rice salad Steamed kale Rice cakes with tahini	Hummos with vegetables Rice cakes Green beans Brown rice
Dinner	Grilled fish New potatoes Green salad Broccoli	Brown rice Dal (lentils) Steamed greens Sugar snap peas	Artichoke with warm garlic oil Quinoa noodles with salmon or shrimp Kale salad	Corn on cob Organic turkey burger Baked sweet potato brussels sprouts	Chickpea patties Basmati or brown rice Red cabbage salad Steamed greens	Stir-fried vegetables with scallops Brown rice Green salad	Aduki bean soup Baked chicken Watercress salad Steamed carrots

Dessert

Good dessert choices include fresh or cooked fruits, muffins, rice cakes with spreads, and mochi. Do not use concentrated sweeteners such as honey, barley malt, rice syrup, any form of sugar, maple syrup, fructose, or corn syrup.

Source: Women to Women, Yarmouth, ME.

5. Look for sugar in your medications. Some sugar-free cough medications available are: Cerose DM (Ives), Codimal (Central), Conar Suspension (Beecham), and Sorbutuss (Dalin).

6. *Low calorie* or *lite* on a product label does not necessarily mean sugar free; read the product content list. A manufacturer may adjust calorie content by changing the fat content and not change or omit sugar products.

7. Flour and cornstarch are items to avoid. Modified food starch as found in some dressings may be used with discretion. Arrowroot is acceptable as a thickener.

8. Fresh, frozen, or canned products are acceptable as long as no sugar is added to them.

9. For those with elevated cholesterol, limit egg intake to three times per week total. This meal plan should help alleviate elevated triglycerides, problems caused by excess carbohydrate and alcohol calories.

10. For abstainers with high blood pressure who are prescribed a low-sodium diet, remember—fresh is best, and frozen foods (meats and vegetables) are a good alternative. Always read the label for salt content as well as sugar. Also, cooked cereals that are "instant" have a higher sodium content than "regular" cooking varieties.

11. Tomato juice or vegetable cocktail juice made without sugar may be used as a vegetable substitute; 1 cup juice equals 1 cup vegetable.

12. If fresh fruit is not available, fruit may be canned or frozen in water or natural juices with no added sugar (pour off the juice). Juices may be used; see fruit choices for serving sizes (they vary).

13. Soy sauce whose label lists sugar fifth or lower is acceptable. Lite soy sauce is lower in sodium, not sugar. Tamari sauce is an acceptable seasoning sauce, similar to soy sauce.

14. For food preparation, regular mustard, low-calorie mayonnaise and sugar-free catsup are approved. Whipped dressings should not be used. Up to ½ cup of tomato sauce and one tablespoon of lemon juice may be used in food preparation.

15. Salad dressing should be limited to 2 ounces per day.

16. Caffeine products—coffee, tea, cola, and chocolate—should be avoided because caffeine is an appetite stimulant.

17. You may use part of your nondairy milk allowance as decaffeinated coffee lightener. One percent milk may be used in this plan.

18. If constipation is a problem, eight 8-ounce glasses (64 ounces) of water per day along with the cereal, the fresh fruit, and the vegetables in your meat plan will help. Exercise will also help.

19. Once you are within five pounds of your goal, you may introduce items allowed on the maintenance plan. Again, it will be necessary to weigh and measure these items until you become used to the portions allowed.

Protein Choices
Eggs—breakfast, 1 large; lunch or dinner, 2 large
Dried beans—1 c. cooked*
Vegetarian protein—4 oz. (tofu, tempeh)

Nondairy Milk (½ protein)
Soy cheese—2 oz.

Cereal and Grain Choices
Mixed grain—1 tbsp. corn germ, 2 tbsp. oat bran
1 c. Ralston Sunflakes (rice and corn)
1 c. New Morning Oatios
1 c. any fruit juice-sweetened cereal
½ c. cooked oatmeal
½ c. cooked brown rice
½ c. cooked barley
½ c. cooked kasha or buckwheat
½ c. cooked soy cereal
½ c. any cooked nonwheat, sugar-free cereal (½ c. dry cereal, ⅔ c. water)
For any wheat-free, sugar-free, ready-to-eat cereals, follow serving portion listed on side panel of cereal.

Starchy Vegetable Choices
(two per week)
Dried beans*: lima, navy, white, pinto, etc.—½ c. (cooked)
Corn: kernel—(1 c.)
Corn: ear—(5"–6")
Parsnips—1 c.
Peas, dried—1 c.
Peas, green—1 c.
Potato: Fresh sweet yam—½ medium
Potato: mashed yam—½ c.
Potato: white, baked—1 small
Potato: white, mashed—1 c.
Pumpkin—1 c.
Squash: winter acorn, hubbard, butternut, spaghetti—1 c.
Rice—½ c. cooked

Fruit and Juice Choices
Apple—4" diameter   Apricots—3 medium
Apple juice—⅔ c.   Banana†—1 small
Applesauce (natural)—1 cup

* One cup of cooked dried beans and rice also equal one protein choice.
† These fruits are calorie dense.

Berries: boysenberries,
    blackberries, blueberries,
    raspberries—1 c.
Cantaloupe—½ (6″ diameter)
Cranberries—1 c.
Cranberry juice—1 c. (low-calorie)
Grapefruit—½ large
Grapefruit juice—1 cup
Grapes—1 cup
Honeydew, casaba, or crenshaw
    melon†—¼ (7″ diameter)
Kiwi—2
Lemons and limes—2
Mandarin oranges—1 c.
Mango—1 small
Nectarine—1 medium

Orange—1 large
Orange juice—1 c.
Papaya—1 c.
Peach—1 large (3 halves, canned)
Pear—1 large (3 halves, canned)
Persimmon (native)—2 medium
Pineapple—1 c. or ¼ pineapple
Plums—3 medium
Prunes; stewed or in juice—3
    medium
Prune juice—½ c.
Rhubarb—1 cup
Strawberries—1 c.
Tangerine—2
Watermelon—2 c.

Vegetable Choices
(full cup)

Artichoke (not marinated in oil)
Asparagus
Bamboo shoots
Beans, yellow or green
Bean sprouts
Beets
Bok choy
Broccoli
Brussels sprouts
Cabbage
Carrots
Cauliflower
Celery
Chicory
Chinese Cabbage
Cucumber
Eggplant
Endive
Escarole
Greens: beets, chard, collard, dan-
    delion, kale, mustard, spinach,
    turnip

Lettuce
Mushrooms
Okra
Onions
Parsley
Peppers, red or green
Pickles‡ (not sweet)
Radishes
Rhubarb
Romaine
Rutabagas
Sauerkraut‡
Snow pea pods
Summer squash, yellow
Tomatoes
Tomato juice‡
Turnips
Vegetable juice‡
Water chestnuts
Watercress
Zucchini

† These fruits are calorie dense.
‡ These choices are high in sodium and should not be used on a sodium-restricted
   meal plan.

Fat Choices
Approved salad dressings—2 oz./day
Polyunsaturated oil—2 tsp./week (corn, safflower or sunflower oil), or ⅓ tsp./ day

Condiments
Any sugar-free, wheat-free spice or sauce, including but not limited to mustard, tamari sauce, salsa, and Kikkoman Lite Soy Sauce.
Limit spice and condiment use to the levels recommended in recipes, or no more than 1 teaspoon per day of any one spice and no more than 1 ounce per meal of any one sauce.

MENU OUTLINE

Breakfast
1 selection from nondairy milk choices
1 selection from protein choices
1 selection from cereal and grain choices
1 selection from fruit choices
Calorie-free beverage*

Lunch
1 selection from protein choices
1 selection from vegetable choices
1 c. of salad or vegetable or 3 raw vegetables
1 oz. low or no-cal dressing
Calorie-free beverage*

Dinner
1 selection from protein choices
1 selection from vegetable choices
2 c. salad
Up to 1 oz. low or no-cal salad dressing
Starchy vegetable (2 times per week)
Calorie-free beverage*

Metabolic Adjustment (4 hours before or after evening meal)
1 selection from cereal and grain choices
1 selection from nondairy milk choices
1 selection from fruit choices

A clear soup can be added for lunch or dinner each day.

* Caution: NutraSweet products have become binge foods for some people.

Resources

Christiane Northrup, M.D., F.A.C.O.G.
Women to Women
One Pleasant Street
Yarmouth, ME 04096
(207) 846-6163

GENERAL READING LIST

Medical Education/Society As an Addictive System

Berry, Carmen Renee, *When Helping You Is Hurting Me,* New York: Harper and Row, 1988.

Fassel, Diane, *Working Ourselves to Death.* Harper San Francisco, 1990.

Gabbard, Glen O. and Roy W. Menninger, "The Psychology of Postponement in the Medical Marriage," *Journal of the American Medical Association,* vol. 261, no. 16 (Apr. 28, 1989), pp. 2378–81.

McKegney, Catherine P., "Medical Education: A Neglectful and Abusive Family System," *Family Medicine,* vol. 21, no. 6 (Nov.–Dec. 1989), pp. 452–57.

Richman, Flaherty, Rospenda, and Christensen, "Mental Health Consequences and Correlates of Reported Medical Student Abuse," *Journal of the American Medical Association,* vol. 267, no. 5 (Feb. 5, 1992).

Schaef, Anne Wilson, *When Society Becomes an Addict.* Harper San Francisco, 1986.

———. *The Addictive Organization.* Harper San Francisco, 1988.

———. *Beyond Therapy, Beyond Science.* Harper San Francisco, 1992.

Travis, John and Meryn Callander, *Wellness for Helping Professionals: Creating Compassionate Cultures.* Wellness Associates Publishing, Box 5433-P, Mill Valley, CA 94942.

Gender and Sexual Abuse: Medical and Psychological Consequences: Feminist Perspectives

Bachmann, Moeller, "Childhood Sexual Abuse and the Consequences in Adult Women," *Obstetrics and Gynecology,* vol. 71, no. 4 (Apr. 1988), pp. 631–42.

Ehrenreich, Barbara and Deirdre English, *For Her Own Good: 150 Years of the Experts' Advice to Women.* Garden City, NY: Anchor Books, 1989.

Eisler, Riane, *The Chalice and the Blade: Our History, Our Future.* Harper San Francisco, 1987.

Epperson, Sharon, "Studies Link Subtle Sex Bias in Schools with Women's Behavior in the Workplace," *The Wall Street Journal* (Sept. 16, 1988). See also the American Association of University Women 1991 study on this subject.

Gise and Paddison, "Rape, Sexual Abuse, and Its Victims," *Psychiatric Clinics of North America,* vol. 11, no. 4 (Dec. 1988), pp. 629–48.

Green, Arthur, "Child Maltreatment and Its Victims: A Comparison of Physical and Sexual Abuse: The Violent Patient," *Psychiatric Clinics of North America,* vol. 11, no. 4 (Dec. 1988), pp. 591–610.

Hesse, Lori, "Crimes of Gender," *World Watch* (Mar.–Apr. 1989), pp. 12–21.

Hilberman, "The Impact of Rape," in M.T. Notman and C.C. Nadelson, eds., *The Woman Patient: Medical and Psychological Interfaces, Vol. 1: Sexual and Reproductive Aspects of Women's Health Care,* New York: Plenum Press, 1978.

Reiter, Robert and J. Gambone, "Nongynecologic Somatic Pathology in Women with Chronic Pelvic Pain and Negative Laparoscopy," *Journal of Reproductive Medicine,* vol. 36, no. 4 (Apr. 1991), pp. 253–59.

Women and Depression Task Force of the American Psychiatric Association, report of the August 1989 Meeting, *Brain/Mind Bulletin* (1989), p. 3.

Healing from Sexual Abuse

Bass, Ellen, and Laura Davis, *The Courage to Heal: A Guide for Women Survivors of Child Sexual Abuse,* New York: Harper Perennial, 1989.
Audiocassettes of this book read by the authors are available through Caedmon Self-Help Soundbooks. This pioneering book and tape series are landmark healing tools for women survivors of child sexual abuse. The healing process is explained and developed fully.

Blume, E. Sue, *Secret Survivors: Uncovering Incest and Its Aftereffects in Women,* New York: Ballantine, 1989. Includes a very helpful Incest Survivors Check List.

Russell, Diana, *The Secret Trauma,* New York: Basic Books, 1986.

The Healing Woman
P.O. Box 3038
Moss Beach, CA 94038
(415) 728-0339

The Healing Woman is a national monthly newsletter designed to help women in their recovery from the devastating effects of childhood sexual abuse.

Ecological/Partnership/Feminist Perspectives

Gray, Elizabeth Dodson, *Patriarchy as a Conceptual Trap*, Wellesley, MA: Roundtable Press, 1981.

Hubbard, Ruth, *The Politics of Women's Biology*, New Brunswick, NJ: Rutgers University Press, 1990.

Johnson, K. and Tom Ferguson, *Trusting Ourselves: The Sourcebook on Psychology for Women*, New York: Atlantic Monthly Press, 1990.

Johnson, Sonia, *From Housewife to Heretic*, Garden City, NY: Doubleday, 1981.

———. *Going Out of Our Minds: The Metaphysics of Liberation*, Freedom, CA: Crossing Press, 1987.

———. *Wildfire: Igniting the She/volution*, Estancia, NM: Wildfire Books, 1989.

———. *The Ship That Sailed into the Living Room*, Estancia, NM: Wildfire Books, 1991.

Schaef, Anne Wilson, *Women's Reality*, New York: Harper and Row, 1982.

Wolf, Naomi, *Fire with Fire: The New Female Power and How It Will Change the 21st Century*, New York: Random House, 1993.

Energy Medicine: The Science of the Mind/Body Connection

Alternative Medicine: The Definitive Guide, compiled by the Burton Goldberg Group, Future Medicine Publishing, Inc., Puyallup, Washington, 1993.

Anderson, Robert, *Wellness Medicine*, Lynnwood, WA: American Health Press, 1987.

Becker, Robert, *The Body Electric*, New York: William Morrow, 1985.

Brain/Mind Bulletin/New Sense, a newsletter about leading edge thinking in science, technology, mind/body connection, medicine, and the like. P.O. Box 42211, Los Angeles, CA 90042.

Breslow, Rachelle, *Who Said So: A Woman's Journey of Self-Discovery and Triumph over Multiple Sclerosis*, Berkeley, CA: Celestial Arts, 1991.

Chopra, Deepak, *Quantum Healing*, New York: Bantam, 1989.

Cousins, Norman, *Head First: The Biology of Hope*, New York: Dutton, 1989.

Dossey, Larry, *Meaning and Medicine*, New York: Bantam, 1991.

———. *Space, Time, and Medicine*, Boston: Shambhala, 1982.

———. *Beyond Illness, Discovering the Experience of Health*, Boston: Shambhala, 1984.

Gerber, Richard, *Vibrational Medicine*, Santa Fe, NM: Bear and Co., 1988.

Levine, Barbara, *Your Body Believes Every Word You Say*, Aslan Publishing, 310 Blue Ridge Drive, Boulder Creek, CA 95006; 1991. This book illustrates beautifully the way our bodies manifest our beliefs physically.

Morse, Melvin, *Transformed by the Light*, New York: Random House/Villard Books, 1992. Fascinating research on the lives of those who have survived near-death experiences.

Murphy, Michael, *The Future of the Body: Explorations into the Further Evolution of Human Nature*, Los Angeles: Jeremy Tarcher, 1992.

Myss, Caroline, *The Human Energy System* videocassette lecture. To order, write to Caroline Myss, 1210 Hirsch St., Melrose Park, IL 60160.

Psychoneuroimmunology: The Scientific Basis for Holism in Medicine, Raleigh, NC: American Holistic Medical Association, 1990.

Sagan, Leonard, *The Health of Nations: True Causes of Sickness and Well-being*, New York: Basic Books, 1987.

Shealy, Norman, and Caroline Myss, *The Creation of Health*, Walpole, NH: Stillpoint Publications, 1987.

Healing

Langer, Ellen J. *Mindfulness*, Reading, MA: Addison-Wesley, 1989.

Levine, Stephen, *Healing Into Life and Death*, New York: Doubleday, 1987.

Matthew, Marti Lynn, *Pain: The Challenge and the Gift*, Walpole, NH: Stillpoint, 1991.

EXERCISE

Melpomene Foundation
(612) 642-1951
Organization that promotes education and research into women's health and fitness issues, including exercise and pregnancy, amenorrhea, menopause, larger women, and aging.

REFERRAL SOURCES FOR HOLISTIC TREATMENTS

The Health Resource Newsletter
209 Katherine Drive
Conway, AR 72032
(501) 329-5272
FAX (501) 329-8700
The Health Resource was founded by Janice Guthrie as a result of her personal experience of illness and her desire to become an active partner in her care and treatment. This medical information service provides you with an individualized comprehensive research report on your specific medical problem. Information on conventional and alternative treatments is offered as well as information on research, specialists, books, and resource organizations. To order a report, call, write, or fax.

World Research Foundation
15300 Ventura Blvd.
Suite 405
Sherman Oaks, CA 91403
(818) 907-5483

Publishes information from around the world on health subjects and alternative approaches to conventional medicine. Excellent book reviews.

HOLISTIC HEALTH CARE ORGANIZATIONS

Institute for Noetic Sciences
475 Gate Five Road
Suite 300
Sausalito, CA 94965
(415) 331-5650

Citizens for Health
P.O. Box 1195
Tacoma, WA 98401
(800) 354-2211

Publishes a newsletter, supports research, and holds educational conferences on the mind/body/spirit continuum. Also serves as a networking organization.

Association of Holistic Healing Centers
109 Holly Crescent, Suite 201
Virginia Beach, VA 23451
(804) 422-9022

Mission Statement: The AHHC is dedicated to providing opportunities for individuals, groups, and centers actively involved in the healing arts to join together for holistic community and synergy. The focus of the organization is threefold: (1) to provide its membership with quarterly newsletters, seminars, and educational tours to healing centers for the purpose of sharing new ideas, research, and clinical experiences of healing interventions; (2) to sponsor conferences, workshops, and retreats in which educators and healers can in turn manifest their creative skills and minister to those in need of spiritual, mental, emotional, and physical healing; and (3) to support the evolutions of prototype centers.

National Wellness Coalition
Contact: Janet Smith
P.O. Box 3778
Washington, DC 20007-0278
(202) 333-1638

Mission Statement: The National Wellness Coalition addresses the root causes of illness in our society, providing us with new ways of caring for each other and ourselves—in our places of work, our communities, our families, and our own lives. By making wellness, rather than issues of financing, the primary focus of policy efforts, we practice true cost effectiveness.

This Washington based organization's goal is to develop a national wellness policy agenda—a blueprint for shifting the focus of our healthcare system and our society from illness and crisis intervention to wellness by the year 2000.

Shealy Institute
1328 East Evergreen St.
Springfield, MO 65648
(417) 865-5940

Founded by Dr. Norman Shealy, the founder of the American Holistic Medical Association, the Shealy Institute runs both in-patient and out-patient programs for treating chronic pain and stress-related illnesses. As a neurosurgeon, Dr. Shealy's programs combine the best of conventional medicine with effective alternatives to drugs and surgery.

American Association of
   Naturopathic Physicians
P.O. Box 20386
Seattle, WA 98102
(206) 323-7610

American Holistic Medical
   Association
4101 Lake Boone Trail, Suite 201
Raleigh, NC 27607
(919) 787-5181

American Holistic Nurses
   Association
4101 Lake Boone Trail, Suite 201
Raleigh, NC 27607
(919) 787-5181

Holistic Dental Association
974 North 21st Street
Newark, OH 43055-2922
(614) 366-3309

Homeopathic Academy of
   Naturopathic Physicians
14653 South Graves Road
Mulino, OR 97042
(503) 873-4542

International Foundation for
   Homeopathy
2366 Eastlake Ave. East, #30
Seattle, WA 98102
(206) 324-8230

International Society for the Study
   of Subtle Energies and Energy
   Medicine
356 Goldco Circle
Golden, CO 80403
(303) 278-2228

National Center for Homeopathy
801 North Fairfax Street, Suite 306
Alexandria, VA 22314
(703) 548-7790

Physicians Association for
   Anthroposophical Medicine
P.O. Box 269
Kimberson, PA 19442

Recovery/Spirituality/Living in Process

Wilson Schaef Associates
P.O. Box 18686
Boulder, CO 80308
(303) 444-5735

Schaef facilitates Living in Process seminars throughout the world and maintains a list of process facilitators throughout the United States and in some locations abroad. Her home base for these seminars is at Boulder Hot Springs in Montana. Call or write for a current brochure. Tapes and books also available. Referrals to process facilitators in your area are available.

Books

The Courage to Change: One Day at a Time in Al-Anon, New York: Al-Anon Family Group Headquarters, Inc., 1992.

One Day at a Time in Al-Anon, New York: Al-Anon Family Group Headquarters, Inc., 1973.

For information and catalogs of literature write:

Al-Anon Family Group Headquarters, Inc.
P.O. Box 862
Midtown Station
New York, NY 10018-0862
(212) 302-7240

MENSTRUAL CYCLE

Organization

Menstrual Health Foundation
104 Petaluma Ave.
Sebastopol, CA 95472
(707) 829-2744

Dedicated to empowering women in the area of the "Menstrual Matrix," the years between menarche and menopause. Wonderful publications and products to help all women celebrate their cycles. Especially lovely materials for introducing the menstrual cycle to young women.

Natural Hormones

Women's International Pharmacy
5708 Monona Dr.
Madison, WI 53719-3152
(800) 279-5708
(608) 221-7819

This pharmacy specializes in individualized natural hormonal treatment for women. Estriol, DHEA, natural progesterone available by prescription. Maintains referral list of health professionals who prescribe their products. Carries patented time release progesterone developed by Delk and Hargrove.

Madison Pharmacy Associates
429 Gammon Place
Madison, WI 53719
Pharmacy line: (800) 558-7046
PMS Access, a national hotline for PMS information: (800) 222-4767

Excellent source for natural progesterone products, including progestrol capsules and PMS information. Supplements specific to PMS are also available. Also makes Procycle, a supplement for PMS. Clinic and support group referrals are available for a fee.

Professional and Technical Services
333 Northeast Sandy Boulevard
Portland, OR 97232
(503) 231-7244
(800) 648-8211

Manufactures natural progesterone skin cream and oil (ProGest) and other products. This company provides extensive supporting information about its products and their use. It sponsors research addressing the role of natural progesterone in preventing and reversing osteoporosis.

EsGen Cream, a transdermal estrogen cream, is applied to the skin. It comes from all-natural plant sources. Comes with full instructions and is a nice alternative to systemic ERT for some women. Must be used with a source of natural progesterone such as ProGest. Available through Professional and Technical Services. For use when under health care professional guidance.

Dixie PMS Center
2161 Newmarket Parkway
Suite 222
Marietta, GA 30067
(800) 767-9232

Serves as a hot-line for women who desire natural approaches to their health care. It maintains a referral network for health care practitioners who use natural methods such as natural progesterone.

Progesterone

Lee, John R., *Progesterone: The Multiple Roles of a Remarkable Hormone,* Sebastopol, CA: BLL Publishing (P.O. Box 02068), 1993.

Books

Cameron, Anne, *Daughters of Copper Woman,* Erie, KS: Inland Publishers, 1988.

George, Demetra, *Mysteries of the Dark Moon: The Healing Power of the Dark Goddess,* Harper San Francisco, 1992.

Lark, Susan, *PMS Self-Help Book,* Santa Monica, CA: Forman Publishing, 1984.

Shuttle, Penelope, and Peter Redgrove, *The Wise Wound,* New York: Grove Press, 1988.

Taylor, Dena, *The Red Flower: Rethinking Menstruation,* Freedom, CA: The Crossing Press, 1988.

Seasonal Affective Disorder/Light Therapy

Women with PMS often have SAD and are helped by light therapy. Light can also help ovulatory and other menstrual cycle disturbances.

Liberman, Jacob, *Light: Medicine of the Future,* Santa Fe, NM: Bear and Co., 1991.

Goodrich, Janet, *Natural Vision Improvement,* Berkeley, CA: Celestial Arts, 1986.

The SunBox Company
19217 Orbit Drive
Gaithersburg, MD 20879
(800) 548-3968

Provides excellent quality lighting units, full-spectrum bulbs, and accurate information on the therapeutic use of light.

Vagina/Cervix

Human Papilloma Virus Information, American Social Health Association publishes HPV News, P.O. Box 13827, Research Triangle Park, NC 27709.

Provides educational support from leading HPV experts around the country. Membership is $25.00 per year. Publications, advocacy, local support groups, research. Provides accurate medical information and emotional support for those affected by HPV and genital warts.

Endometriosis

Laversen, Niels H., M.D., Ph.D. and Constance DeSwann. *The Endometriosis Answer Book: New Hope, New Help.* New York: Rawson Associates, 1988.

Endometriosis Treatment Program
St. Charles Medical Center
2500 N.E. Neff Road
Bend, OR 97701
(800) 446-2177

Based on the pioneering surgical treatment of endometriosis developed by Dr. David Redwine. Has treated women from throughout the United States and Canada for their endometriosis pain upon referral from their physicians. Nancy Peterson, the spokeswoman for the program, travels extensively throughout the United States giving educational talks on endometriosis. A very informative newsletter is also available.

The Endometriosis Alliance of Greater New York
Old Chelsea Station
P.O. Box 634
New York, NY 10113-0634

A networking and educational organization for those with endometriosis.

Castor Oil Packs

Known also as the palma Christi, castor oil packs are wonderful for healing menstrual problems, urinary tract infections, joint aches and pains, and abdominal distress. Applied to the upper chest, they also can relieve a cough. The usual treatment frequency is one hour for three to five times a week. (Don't use them during the heaviest days of the menstrual period.) Used once per week, they are also good preventive medicine. They have been shown to increase immune system functioning.

A castor oil pack consists of wool flannel saturated with castor oil applied directly to the skin. A plastic bag is put over this to keep the oil where it belongs, and a heat source is applied. We highly recommend a hot water bottle or a Fomentek bag for this purpose. Though a heating pad can be used, a nonelectrical source of heat is preferred. Once a castor oil pack is made up, it can be stored for months in a plastic bag and reused over and over, simply adding more oil as necessary.

Castor oil, flannel, and Fomentek bags are available from Women to Women (full instructions included). Castor oil and flannel can also be ordered from Home Health Products, Virginia Beach, VA; (800) 468-7313

Melaleuca Oil

Melaleuca oil is a type of tea tree oil that is very good for preventing herpes outbreaks. Apply to the affected area immediately, at the first sign of tingling. The outbreak will usually be prevented. Available from Women to Women or from the Melaleuca Co., 3910 So. Yellowstone Highway, Idaho Falls, ID, 83402-6003; telephone: (208) 522-0700.

Sexuality

Chia, Mantak, and Maneewan Chia, *Cultivating Female Sexual Energy*, Huntington, NY: Healing Tao Books, 1986.

Muir, Charles, and Caroline Muir, *Tantra: The Art of Conscious Loving*, San Francisco: Mercury House, 1989.

Sevely, Josephine Lowndes, *Eve's Secrets: A New Theory of Female Sexuality*, New York: Random House, 1987.

NATURAL FAMILY PLANNING

Books

Billings, E.L., J. J. Billings, and M. Catarinich, *The Atlas of the Ovulation Method*, 5th ed., Ovulation Method Research and Reference Center of Australia, 1989. Telephone: in Maryland, (301) 897-9323.

Hilgers, T.W., *The Medical Applications of Natural Family Planning: A Contemporary Approach to Women's Health Care*, Omaha, NE: Pope Paul VI Institute Press, 1991. Telephone: (402) 390-6600.

Wilson, M.A., *The Ovulation Method of Birth Regulation,* New York: Van Nostrand Reinhold, 1981. Telephone: (301) 627-3346. A how-to manual, with examples of women's charts from all over the world. Written by a pioneer in teaching the Ovulation Method internationally.

Organizations
American Academy of Natural Family Planning, (314) 569-6495. Uses Creighton Model Ovulation Method, USA and Canada.

Pope Paul VI Institute for the Study of Human Reproduction
6901 Mercy Road
Omaha, NE 68106
(402) 390-6600

Provides referrals of physicians who have been trained as natural family planning medical consultants. Conducts a comprehensive natural family planning medical consultant training course for physicians annually in Omaha. Most physicians trained through this course are family physicians or obstetricians/gynecologists. Uses the Creighton Model Ovulation Method, USA and Canada.

Billings Ovulation Method Association, USA
P.O. Box 30329
Bethesda, MD 20824-0239
(301) 897-9323
(Ovulation Method: USA)

Family of the Americas Foundation
P.O. Box 1170
Dunkirk, MD 20754-1170
(301) 627-3346
(Ovulation Method: International and USA)

Couple to Couple League
P.O. Box 111184
Cincinnati, OH 45211-1184
(513) 661-7612
(Symptothermal Method: USA and International)

Institute for Reproductive Health at Georgetown University
3 PHC
3800 Reservoir Road NS
Washington, DC 20007
(202) 687-1392
(Ovulation Method and Symptothermal Method: International)

PREGNANCY AND BIRTHING

LaLeche League International
9616 Minneapolis Avenue
Franklin Park, IL 60131
(708) 455-7730
Leaders and pioneers in promoting and supporting the womanly art of breast-feeding.

International Childbirth Education Association
P.O. Box 20048
Minneapolis, MN 55420
(612) 854-8660
Information and resource center for birth information of all kinds. They supply an excellent catalog of relevant books and other information.

Books

Baker, Jeanine Parvati, *Conscious Conception: Elemental Journey Through the Labyrinth of Sexuality,* North Atlantic, 1986.

Chamberlain, David, *Babies Remember Their Births,* New York: Ballantine, 1989.

McGarey, Gladys, *Born to Live,* Phoenix, AZ: Gabriel Press, 1980.

Noble, Elizabeth, *Channel for a New Life.* Videotape of an extraordinary normal birth. Particularly valuable to hear the "deep process" sounds made by the mother during this birth. Available from Elizabeth Noble, 448 Pleasant Lake Ave., Harwich, MA 02645.

Odent, Michel, *Birth Reborn,* New York: Pantheon Books, 1984.

Peterson, Gayle, and Lewis Mehl, *Birthing Normally,* Berkeley, CA: Mindbody Press, 1981.

Verney, Thomas, *The Secret Life of the Unborn Child,* New York: Delacorte Press, 1982.

Circumcision Information

National Organization of Circumcision Information and Resource Centers
P.O. Box 2512
San Anselmo, CA 94979-2512
(415) 488-9883

Circumcision Resource Center
P.O. Box 232
Boston, MA 02133
(617) 523-0088

Article

Spock, Benjamin, "Circumcision: It's Not Necessary," *Redbook,* April 1989, p. 53.

HYSTERECTOMY

Cutler, Winnifred, *Hysterectomy Before and After,* New York: HarperCollins, 1990.

Goldfarb, Harold, *The No-Hysterectomy Option: Your Body-Your Choice,* New York: Wiley, 1990.

Harris, Dean, *Recovering from a Hysterectomy,* New York: HarperPaperbacks, 1992.

HERS Foundation
422 Bryn Mawr Ave.
Bala-Cynwyd, PA 19004
(215) 667-7757

Hysterectomy Educational Resources and Services
A national referral service for women who need information about how to avoid hysterectomy. Maintains a network of empathetic physicians.

MENOPAUSE

Books

Borton, Joan, *Drawing from the Women's Well* (1992), LuraMedia, 7060 Miramar Road, Suite 104, San Diego, CA 92121; (619) 578-1948.

Clow, Barbara Hand, *The Liquid Light of Sex: Understanding Your Key Life Passages,* Santa Fe, NM: Bear and Co., 1991.

Greenwood, Sadja, M.D., *Menopause, Naturally: Preparing for the Second Half of Life,* Volcano, CA: Volcano Press, 1989.

McCain, Marian Van Eck, *Transformation through Menopause,* Amherst, MA: Bergen and Garvey, 1991.

Sheehy, Gail, *Menopause: The Silent Passage,* New York: Pocket Books, 1993.

A Friend Indeed: Newsletter for Women in the Prime of Life
Box 515, Place du Parc Station
Montreal, Quebec
Canada H2W 2P1
(514) 843-5730

This monthly newsletter explores the standard scientific approach to menopause as well as alternatives to hormones. Topics such as premature menopause, atrophic vaginal changes, women's emotions, and the taboo of menopause are covered.

Menopause News
2074 Union Street
San Francisco, CA 94123
Telephone inquiries: (800) 241-MENO

This newsletter provides the most balanced information on natural approaches to menopause that I have yet read. I have learned a great deal from the information contained in each issue and highly recommend it.

ERT Alternatives

For natural estrogen (estradiol, 0.5 mg.) combined with natural progesterone (100 mg.) as an excellent ERT source. (It is also available at lower doses.) Women on this preparation do not get periods, as it maintains an inactive endometrium with none of the side effects of progestin. Available by prescription from

Delk Pharmacy
1602 Hatcher Lane
Columbia, TN 38401
(615) 388-3952.

Pharmacist Joseph Delk and Dr. Joel Hargrove have developed and tested this form of hormonal replacement for many years. It is available by prescription from the Delk Pharmacy, which will mail it anywhere in the United States.

BREASTS

Love, Susan, *The Breast Book*, Reading, MA: Addison-Wesley, 1990.

The Bosom Buddy Club
Joan Dawson
1057 Columbia Place
Boulder, CO 80303
(303) 494-8252

A support group for women who are considering or who have had a prophylactic mastectomy.

For Those with a Positive Family History of Breast Cancer

To determine your statistical risk for breast cancer if you have a family history, you can become part of Strang's National High Risk Registry, located throughout the country. The program is free, and your risk will be accurately assessed. For more information, write to:

Strang Cancer Prevention Center
National High Risk Registry
428 East 72nd St.
New York, NY 10021
(212) 794-4900

NUTRITION AND HEALTH

Books

Adams, Carol, *The Sexual Politics of Meat: A Feminist-Vegetarian Critical Theory*, New York: Continuum, 1990.
Colbin, Annemarie, *Food and Healing*, New York: Ballantine, 1988.
Manahan, William, *Eat for Health*, Tiburon, CA: H.J. Kramer, 1989.

Nutrition Action Health Letter
Center for Science in the Public Interest
Suite 300
1875 Connecticut Avenue, N.W.
Washington, DC 20009-5728
Priestley, Joan, *Essential Supplements for Women* (1991), Thorsons, 77–85 Fulham
  Palace Rd., Hammersmith, London, W68JB, England.
Robbins, John, *Diet for a New America,* Walpole, NH: Stillpoint.
Roth, Geneen, *When Food Is Love,* New York: Dutton, 1990.
Turner, Kristina, *The Self-Healing Cookbook,* Grass Valley, CA: Earthtones Press,
  1990.
Weil, Andrew, *Natural Health, Natural Medicine,* Boston: Houghton Mifflin,
  1990.

Organizations

The Vegetarian Resource Group
P.O. Box 1463
Baltimore, MD 21203
(301) 366-VEGE

This group has developed a packet of 30 quantity recipes for institutions. They work with food services in hospitals, universities, and schools to incorporate vegetarian foods into the menus.

Mountain Ark Trading Company
120 South East Ave.
Fayetteville, AR 72701
(800) 643-8909

This mail-order company supplies almost everything the vegetarian cook could want: high quality knives, cookware, organic beans, rice, vegetables, snacks, and lots more. Their catalog provides a short course in whole foods and their uses.

Macrobiotics

Kushi Institute of the Berkshires
Box 7
Becket, MA 01223
(413) 623-5742

Maine Seaweed Company
P.O. Box 57
Steuben, ME 04680
(207) 546-2875

Run by Larch Hansen, this company harvests Maine coast sea vegetables and trains apprentices to harvest, so that ecologically sound harvest practices can be established throughout the coast of Maine. Larch has worked with the same plant beds for sixteen years, in such a way that they can regenerate year after year. He has also set a standard for sea vegetable quality. Publications: *Thoughts of a Seaweed Harvester*, $3.00; *Edible Sea Vegetables of the New England Coast* (a forager's guide with recipes and anecdotes), $2.00.

Physicians Committee for Responsible Medicine
P.O. Box 6322
Washington, DC 20015
(202) 686-2210

Cooking Classes

Annemarie Colbin
The Natural Gourmet Cookery School
48 West 21st St., Suite 202
New York, NY 10010
(212) 645-5170

Trains whole food chefs, teaches cooking classes, and sells cookware, cookbooks, and a cooking class video. Colbin is also the author of some excellent cookbooks.

Jeff Woodward
Traditional Cooking Arts
5336 York Ave. South
Minneapolis, MN 55410
(612) 929-2207

Woodward is the author of *The Healing Power of Food*, which he distributes. He travels to various locations throughout the country to teach cooking classes. They can be arranged in your area. He also sells excellent cookware, cookbooks, and cooking supplies.

Notes

Chapter 1: The Patriarchal Myth and the Addictive System

1. Jamake Highwater, *Myth and Sexuality* (New York: Penguin, 1988), pp. 8–9.
2. Anne Wilson Schaef, *The Addictive Organization* (Harper San Francisco, 1988), p. 58.
3. David Sadker and Myra Sadker. Sharon Epperson, "Studies Link Subtle Sex Bias in Schools with Women's Behavior in the Workplace," *The Wall Street Journal* (Sept. 16, 1988). See also American Association of University Women. 1991. *Shortchanging Girls, Shortchanging America*. Washington, D.C.: AAUW. American Assoc. of University Women, 1992. *How Schools Shortchange Girls*. Washington, D.C.: AAUW Educational Foundation and National Education Foundation.
4. Simone de Beauvoir, *The Second Sex* (New York: Alfred A. Knopf, 1953).
5. Anne Wilson Schaef, *Women's Reality: An Emerging Female System in a White Male Society* (Minneapolis, MN, 1985).
6. Anne Wilson Schaef and Diane Fassel, *The Addictive Organization* (Harper San Francisco, 1988).
7. Sonia Johnson, *Going Out of Our Minds: The Metaphysics of Liberation* (Freedom, CA: Crossing Press, 1987), p. 267.
8. Data from Oxfam America, 115 Broadway, Boston, Massachusetts 02116.
9. B. Grad et al., "An Unorthodox Method of Treatment on Wound Healing in Mice," *International Journal of Parapsychology*, vol. 3, pp. 5–24. This well-designed study showed that wound healing in mice was speeded up significantly (p. < .01) when a self-styled healer passed hands over the animal's cage.
10. Randolph C. Byrd, "Positive Therapeutic Effects of Intercessory Prayer in a Coronary Care Unit Population," *Southern Medical Journal*, vol. 81, no. 7 (July 1933), pp. 826–29.
11. Quoted in *Health*, vol. 6, no. 2 (Apr. 1992). Data on doctors from "Unhealthy

Doctors," report issued by School of Medicine, University of California at Los Angeles.

12. Stephen Hall, "Cheating Fate," *Health* (Apr. 1992), p. 38. Every doctor has seen at least a few cases of "spontaneous remission," and every year these cases are reported in the medical literature. Far too often, instead of being studied, they are ignored. Their existence flies in the face of the medical belief system.

13. Thomas E. Andreoli et al., *Cecil: Essentials of Medicine,* 2d ed. (Philadelphia: W.B. Saunders and Co., 1990), pp. 422–23.

14. J. M. Thorp and W. A. Bowes, "Episiotomy: Can Its Routine Use Be Defended?" part 1, *American Journal of Obstetrics and Gynecology,* vol. 160, no. 5 (May 1989), pp. 1027–30; and S. B. Thacker and H. D. Banta, "Benefits and Risks of Episiotomy: An Interpretive Review of the English Literature, 1860–1980," *Obstetric and Gynecological Survey,* vol. 36 (1983), pp. 322–38.

15. Anne Wilson Schaef, *When Society Becomes an Addict,* Harper San Francisco, 1987, p. 72.

16. Clarissa Pinkola Estes, *Women Who Run With the Wolves: Myths and Stories of the Wild Woman Archetype* (New York: Ballantine, 1992), p. 33.

17. My understanding of the addictive system began when I first learned about codependence. But I later learned that the concept of codependence requires further clarification if it is to be useful in helping people. Codependence is a murky term that keeps people stuck because it describes behavior only in reference to another individual. For example, "If it weren't for my husband's drinking, my life would be fine." Calling someone codependent doesn't name the behavior as the problem of the individual herself. *Relationship addiction* is a much more accurate term because it refers to self-destructive behavior that only the individual herself can change. See Anne Wilson Schaef, *Escape from Intimacy: Untangling the "Love" Addictions: Sex, Romance, and Relationships* (Harper San Francisco, 1990). We can be sure that a relationship that we can preserve only by putting our own needs last or pretending that we don't have any needs is not healthy for us in the first place. This type of unhealthy relationship is an addictive relationship.

18. Schaef, *When Society Becomes an Addict,* p. 72.

19. Patricia Reis, "The Women's Spirituality Movement: Ideas Generated and Questions Asked." Presentation to feminist seminar, Proprioceptive Writing Center, Maine (Dec. 3, 1990).

Chapter 2: Feminine Intelligence and a New Mode of Healing

1. Stephanie Field et al., *Science News,* vol. 127, no. 301; reported in *Brain/Mind Bulletin* (Dec. 9, 1985).

2. Marshall H. Klaus and John H. Kennel, *Parent/Infant Bonding,* 2d ed. (St. Louis: C. V. Mosby Co., 1982).

3. L. F. Berman and S. L. Syme, "Social Networks, Host Resistance, and Mortality: A Nine-Year Follow-up of Alameda County Residents," *American Journal of Epidemiology,* vol. 109 (1978), pp. 186–204.

4. Jeanne Achterberg, *Imagery in Healing: Shamanism and Modern Medicine* (Boston: Shambhala, 1985).

5. Anne Moir and David Jessel, *Brain Sex* (New York: Carol Publishing Co., a Lyle Stuart Book, 1991), p. 195.

6. Robert Bly and Deborah Tannen, "Where Are Women and Men Today," *New Age* (Jan.-Feb. 1992), p. 32.

7. S. J. Schleifer et al., "Depression and Immunity: Lymphocyte Function in Ambulatory Depressed Patients, Hospitalized Schizophrenic Patients, and Patients Hospitalized for Herniorrhaphy," *Archives of General Psychiatry,* vol. 42 (1985), pp. 129–33.

8. J. K. Kiecolt-Glaser et al., "Stress, Loneliness, and Changes in Herpes Virus Latency," *Journal of Behavioral Medicine,* vol. 8, no. 3 (1985), pp. 249–60.

9. The following autoimmune diseases affect women much more frequently than men. Systemic lupus erythematosus—90 percent of sufferers are women. Myasthenia gravis—85 percent are women. Autoimmune thyroid disease—80 percent are women. Rheumatoid arthritis—75 percent are women. Multiple sclerosis—70 percent are women.

10. S. F. Maier et al., "Opiate Antagonists and Long Term Analgesic Reaction Induced by Inescapable Shock in Rats," *Journal of Comparative Physiology and Psychology,* vol. 4 (Dec. 1980), pp. 1177–83; M. L. Laudenslager, "Coping and Immunosuppression: Inescapable But Not Escapable Shock Suppresses Lymphocyte Proliferation," *Science* (Aug. 1983), pp. 568–70; Steven E. Locke et al., "Life Change Stress, Psychiatric Symptoms and Natural Killer Cell Activity," *Psychosomatic Medicine,* vol. 46, no. 5 (1984), pp. 441–53; B. S. Linn et al., "Degree of Depression and Immune Responsiveness," *Psychosomatic Medicine,* vol. 44 (1982), p. 128.

11. R. J. Weber and C. B. Pert, "Opiatergic Modulation of the Immune System," in E. E. Muller and Andrea R. Genazzani, eds., *Central and Peripheral Endorphins* (New York: Raven Press, 1984), p. 35.

12. R. L. Roessler et al., "Ego Strength, Life Changes, and Antibody Titers," paper presented at the annual meeting of the American Psychosomatic Society, Dallas, Texas (Mar. 25, 1979).

13. Ellen Langer, *Mindfulness* (Reading, MA: Addison-Wesley, 1989), pp. 100–13.

14. Maude Guerin, "Psychosocial Lecture Notes," department of obstetrics and gynecology, Michigan State University School of Medicine, Lansing, MI (1991).

15. Elisabeth Kübler-Ross, *On Death and Dying* (New York: Macmillan, 1969).

Chapter 3: Inner Guidance

1. Stephen Sullivan, "Inhibition of Salivary and Lacrimal Secretion by an Enkephalin Analogue," *American Journal of Psychiatry,* vol. 139, no. 3 (Mar. 1982), pp. 385–86.

2. W. H. Frey et al., "Effect of Stimulus on the Composition of Tears," *American Journal of Ophthalmology,* vol. 92, no. 4 (1982), pp. 559–67.

3. Olga and Ambrose Worrall, *The Gift of Healing* (Columbus, OH: Ariel Press,

1985). The work of Olga Worrall, a world-renowned intuitive healer, was studied and documented by physicians at Johns Hopkins School of Medicine. The book is available from Ariel Press, P.O. Box 30975, Columbus, OH 43230. Her work is currently being carried on by Dr. Robert Leichtman. Edgar Cayce is another well-known medical intuitive.

4. Marilyn Ferguson, "Commentary: Waking Up in the Dark," *Brain/Mind and Common Sense* (Apr. 1993), p. 3.

5. Fox quoted in Michael Toms, "Renegade Priest: An Interview with Matthew Fox," *The Sun,* issue 89 (Aug. 1991), p. 10.

Chapter 4: The Female Energy System

1. Graham Bennette, "Psychic and Cellular Aspects of Isolation and Identity Impairment in Cancer," *Annals of the New York Academy of Science,* vol. 131 (1972), pp. 352–63.

2. C. E. Wenner and S. Weinhouse, "Diphosphopyridine Nucleotide Requirements of Oxidations by Mitochondria of Normal and Neoplastic Tissues," *Cancer Research,* vol. 12 (1952), pp. 306–7.

3. I am talking about common patterns here. Some illnesses are mysterious—almost archetypal—and don't fit the personal patterns I describe in this section.

4. D. B. Clayson, *Chemical Carcinogenesis* (London: Churchill Publishers, 1962).

5. Caroline B. Thomas and K. R. Duszynski, "Closeness to Parents and the Family Constellation in a Prospective Study of Five Disease States: Suicide, Mental Illness, Malignant Tumor, Hypertension, Coronary Heart Disease," *Johns Hopkins Medical Journal,* vol. 134 (1974), pp. 251–70.

6. See Norm Shealy and Caroline Myss, *The Creation of Health* (Walpole, NH: Stillpoint Publications, 1988), which goes into much more detail on the human energy system. Dr. Shealy, a neurosurgeon who founded the American Holistic Medical Association, has done extensive research on energy medicine with Caroline Myss. A world-renowned medical intuitive, Myss needs to know only the name and age of an individual to be able to give a full diagnostic reading; the individual can be located anywhere in the world. For several years, she has given energy readings on my own patients, whose physical conditions were correlated with their energy anatomy. Myss's intuitive ability appeared in her life suddenly and very unexpectedly. She had not been previously interested in illness or healing, and for a while after it did appear, she was "angry with God" for saddling her with this gift. In the mid-1980s, Dr. Shealy scientifically tested her ability and accuracy at the Shealy Institute, and she began working and writing with him. Much of the material in this chapter is based on my own work with her.

7. G. A. Bachmann et al., "Childhood Sexual Abuse and Consequences in Adult Women," *Obstetrics and Gynecology,* vol. 71, no. 4 (1988), pp. 631–41.

8. R. C. Reiter et al., "Correlation Between Sexual Abuse and Somatization in Women with Somatic and Nonsomatic Pain," *American Journal of Obstetrics and Gynecology,* vol. 165, no. 1 (1991), p. 104.

9. Scientific studies supporting this premise include M. Tarlau and M. A. Smalheiser, "Personality Patterns in Patients with Malignant Tumors of the Breast and Cervix," in *Psychosomatic Medicine,* vol. 13 (1951), p. 117. In this study of women with cervical cancer, most of the subjects had uniformly negative feelings toward heterosexual relations. Most of them had a higher incidence of premarital sexual experiences, and nearly 75 percent had had multiple marriages ending in divorce or separation.

10. "The differences in body image scores between the body-exterior cancer group and the body-interior cancer group seem to reflect basic differences in personality orientation." Fisher and Cleveland, "Relationship of Body Image to Site of Cancer," *Psychosomatic Medicine,* vol. 18, no. 4 (1956), p. 309.

11. Tarlau and Smalheiser, (see note 9).

12. J. I. Wheeler and B. M. Caldwell, "Psychological Evaluation of Women with Cancer of the Breast and Cervix," *Psychosomatic Medicine,* vol. 17, no. 4 (1955), pp. 256–60; M. Reznikoff, "Psychological Factors in Breast Cancer: A Preliminary Study of Some Personality Trends in Patients with Cancer of the Breast," *Psychosomatic Medicine,* vol. 17 (1955), p. 96; and A. H. Labrum, "Psychological Factors in Gynecologic Cancer," *Primary Care,* vol. 3, no. 4 (1976), pp. 811–24.

Chapter 5: The Menstrual Cycle

1. E. Hartman, "Dreaming Sleep (The D State) and the Menstrual Cycle," *Journal of Nervous and Mental Disease,* vol. 143 (1966), pp. 406–16; and E. M. Swanson and D. Foulkes, "Dream Content and the Menstrual Cycle," *Journal of Nervous and Mental Disease,* vol. 145, no. 5 (1968), pp. 358–63.

2. F. A. Brown, "The Clocks: Timing Biological Rhythms," *American Scientist,* vol. 60 (1972), pp. 756–66; M. Gauguelin, "Wrangle Continues over Pseudoscientific Nature of Astrology," *New Scientist* (Feb. 25, 1978); W. Menaker, "Lunar Periodicity in Human Reproduction: A Likely Unit of Biological Time," *American Journal of Obstetrics and Gynecology,* vol. 77, no. 4 (1959), pp. 905–14; and E. M. Dewan, "On the Possibility of the Perfect Rhythm Method of Birth Control by Periodic Light Stimulation," *American Journal of Obstetrics and Gynecology,* vol. 99, no. 7 (1967), pp. 1016–19.

3. R. P. Michael, R. W. Bonsall, and P. Warner, "Human Vaginal Secretion and Volatile Fatty Acid Content," *Science,* vol. 186 (1974), pp. 1217–19.

4. Demetra George, *Mysteries of the Dark Moon: The Healing Power of the Dark Goddess* (Harper San Francisco, 1992), pp. 70–71.

5. Menaker, "Lunar Periodicity" (see note 2).

6. Lunar data adapted from Caroline Myss.

7. Hartman, "Dreaming Sleep," and Swanson and Foulkes, "Dream Content" (see note 1).

8. Therese Benedek and Boris Rubenstein, "Correlations Between Ovarian Activity and Psychodynamic Processes: The Ovulatory Phase," *Psychosomatic Medicine,* vol. 1, no. 2 (1939), pp. 245–70.

9. Bernard C. Gindes, "Cultural Hypnosis of the Menstrual Cycle," *New Concepts of Hypnosis* (London: George Allen Press, 1953).

10. Diane Ruble, "Premenstrual Symptoms: A Reinterpretation," *Science,* vol. 197 (July 15, 1977), pp. 291–92.

11. For further information, see Riane Eisler, *The Chalice and the Blade: Our History, Our Future* (Harper San Francisco, 1988); and Marija Gimbutas, *Goddesses and Gods of Old Europe, 7000 to 3500 B.C.* (Berkeley and Los Angeles: University of California Press, 1982). The degradation of women's wisdom took place gradually. By the time European settlers arrived in what would become the United States, native tribes were mixed in their approach to women. Some degraded them and their bodily processes, setting them apart in shame, while others revered women's wisdom.

12. Credit for the term *offices of womanhood* goes to Tamara Slayton. See also Brooke Medicine Eagle, "Women's Moontime: A Call to Power," *Shaman's Drum,* vol. 4 (Spring 1986) p. 21.

13. Brown and W. M. O'Neil, cited in P. Shuttle and P. Redgrove, *The Wise Wound* (New York: Grove, 1986).

14. Quoted by Dr. Ronald Norris at lecture on PMS, Rockland, ME (Nov. 1982).

15. R. Loudall, P. Snow, and J. Johnson, "Myths about Menstruation: Victims of Our Folklore," *International Journal of Women's Studies,* vol. 1 (1984), p. 70; W. M. O'Neil, *Time and the Calendars* (Manchester University Press, 1976); P. L. Brown, *Megaliths, Myths and Men: An Introduction to Astro-Archeology* (Blandford Press, 1976).

16. Dr. John Goodrich, lecture on adolescent gynecology, Maine Medical Center, Portland, Maine (July 29, 1992).

17. Quoted from a Tampax box insert, given to me by Gina Orlando.

18. Michael, Bonsall, and Warner, "Human Vaginal Secretion" (see note 3).

19. M. K. McClintock, "Menstrual Synchrony and Suppression," *Nature,* vol. 299 (1971), pp. 244–45.

20. M. C. P. Rees, A. Anderson, et al., "Prostaglandins in Menstrual Fluid in Menorrhagia and Dysmenorrhea," *British Journal of Obstetrics and Gynaecology,* vol. 91 (1984), p. 673.

21. G. E. Abraham, "Primary Dysmenorrhea," *Clinical Obstetrical Gynecology,* vol. 21, no. 1 (1978), pp. 139–45.

22. F. Facchinetti et al., "Magnesium Prophylaxis of Menstrual Migraine," *Headache,* vol. 31 (1991), pp. 298–304; Facchinetti, "Oral Magnesium."

23. E. B. Butler and E. McKnight, "Vitamin E in the Treatment of Primary Dysmenorrhea," *Lancet,* vol. 1 (1955), pp. 844–47.

24. During the menstrual cycle, excess epinephrine released via stress (known as autonomic overdrive) may disrupt the natural autonomic nervous system balance. E. W. Winenman, "Autonomic Balance Changes During the Human Menstrual Cycle," *Psychophysiology,* vol. 8, no. 1 (1971), pp. 1–6.

25. There is no uniformly agreeable definition of PMS in the medical literature, so

many of the studies on the incidence of this disorder disagree. Regardless of medical definition, the experience of thousands of women around their menstrual cycle is one of emotional and physical suffering. R. L. Reid and S. S. Yen, "Premenstrual Syndrome," *American Journal of Obstetrics and Gynecology,* vol. 139 (1981), p. 86.

26. Ronald Norris, "Progesterone for Premenstrual Tension," *Journal of Reproductive Medicine,* vol. 28, no. 8 (Aug. 1983), pp. 509–15.

27. D. L. Jakubowicz, E. Godard, and J. Dewhurst, "The Treatment of Premenstrual Tension with Mefenamic Aid: Analysis of Prostaglandin Concentration," *British Journal of Obstetrics and Gynaecology,* vol. 91 (1984), p. 78.

28. In one study, PMS patients consumed five times more dairy products than controls without PMS. The excess calcium intake from the dairy products may hinder magnesium absorption. G. S. Goci, and G. E. Abraham, "Effect of Nutritional Supplement . . . on Symptoms of Premenstrual Tension," *Journal of Reproductive Medicine,* vol. 83 (1982), pp. 527–31.

29. A. M. Rossignol, "Caffeine-Containing Beverages and Premenstrual Syndrome in Young Women," *American Journal of Public Health,* vol. 75, no. 11 (1985), pp. 1335–37.

30. B. L. Snider and D. F. Dietman, "Pyridoxine Therapy for Premenstrual Acne Flare," *Archives of Dermatology,* vol. 110 (July 1974); G. E. Abraham and J. T. Hargrove, "Effect of Vitamin B on Premenstrual Tension Syndrome: A Double Blind Crossover Study," *Infertility,* vol. 3 (1980), p. 155; M. S. Biskind, "Nutritional Deficiency in the Etiology of Menorrhagia, Cystic Mastitis, Premenstrual Syndrome, and Treatment with Vitamin B Complex," *Journal of Clinical Endocrinology and Metabolism,* vol. 3 (1943), pp. 227–334; and R. W. Engel, "The Relation of B Complex Vitamins and Dietary Fat to the Lipotropic Action of Choline," *Journal of Biological Chemistry,* vol. 37 (1941), p. 140.

31. D. G. Williams, "The Forgotten Hormone," *Alternatives,* vol. 4, no. 6 (1991), p. 11.

32. B. L. Denrefer et al., "Progesterone and Adenosine 3, 5′Monophosphate Formation by Isolated Corpora Lutea of Different Ages: Influence of Human Chorionic Gonadotropin and Prostaglandins," *Journal of Clinical Endocrinology and Metabolism,* vol. 3 (1943), pp. 227–34.

33. B. R. Goldin et al., "Estrogen Excretion Patterns and Plasma Levels in Vegetarian and Omnivorous Women," *New England Journal of Medicine,* vol. 307 (1982), pp. 1542–47; B. R. Goldin et al., "Effect of Diet on Excretion of Estrogens in Pre- and Post-Menopausal Women," *Cancer Research,* vol. 41 (1981), pp. 3771–73.

34. G. E. Abraham, "Nutritional Factors in the Etiology of the Premenstrual Tension Syndromes," *Journal of Reproductive Medicine,* vol. 28 (1983), p. 446; M. Lubran, and G. Abraham, "Serum and Red Cell Magnesium Levels in Patients with Premenstrual Tension," *American Journal of Clinical Nutrition,* vol. 34 (1982), p. 2364; G. E. Abraham and J. T. Hargrove, "Effect of Vitamin B on Premenstrual Tension Syndrome: A Double Blind Crossover Study," *Infer-*

tility, vol. 3 (1980), p. 155; F. Facchinetti et al., "Oral Magnesium Successfully Relieves Premenstrual Mood Changes," *Obstetrics and Gynecology,* vol. 78, no. 2 (Aug. 1991), pp. 177–81; and Snider and Dietman, "Pyridoxine Therapy."

35. R. S. Landau et al., "The Effect of Alpha Tocopherol in Premenstrual Symptomatology: A Double-Blind Trial," *Journal of the American College of Nutrition,* vol. 2 (1983), pp. 115–23; M. R. Werbach, *Nutritional Influences on Illness* (Tarzana, CA: Third Line Press, 1988).

36. L. M. Abraham, "Serum and Red Cell Magnesium Levels" (see note 34); F. Facchinetti, "Oral Magnesium" (see note 22).

37. B. L. Parry et al., "Morning vs. Evening Bright Light Treatment of Late Luteal Phase Dysphoric Disorder," *American Journal of Psychiatry,* vol. 146 (1991), p. 9.

38. J. Ott, *Health and Light* (New York: Pocket Books, 1978); Z. Kime, *Sunlight Could Save Your Life* (Penryn, CA: World Health Publications, 1980); available by writing: World Health Publications, P.O. Box 400, Penryn, CA 95663.

39. Kim Dirke et al., "The Influence of Dieting on the Menstrual Cycle of Healthy Young Women," *Journal of Clinical Endocrinology and Metabolism,* vol. 60, no. 6 (1985), pp. 1174–79.

40. I. Goodale, A. Domar, and H. Benson, "Alleviation of Premenstrual Syndrome Symptoms with the Relaxation Response," *Obstetrics and Gynecology,* vol. 75, no. 4 (Apr. 1990), pp. 649–89.

41. J. Prior et al., "Conditioning Exercise Decreases Premenstrual Symptoms: A Prospective Controlled Six-Month Trial," *Fertility and Sterility,* vol. 47 (1987), pp. 402–9.

42. Parry, "Morning vs. Evening" (see note 37). For a full discussion of light therapy, see J. Liberman, *Light Medicine of the Future: How We Can Use It to Heal Ourselves Now* (Santa Fe, NM: Bear and Co., 1991).

43. Controlled trials of natural progesterone that have been reported in the gynecological literature *do not* bear out my experience here. I think that this is because diet, exercise, and supplements have not been part of these studies, and also because women in these studies have not been taught how to think about their PMS as a signal that their lives are out of balance.

44. For years, those interested in PMS have batted around the idea of a "menotoxin" present in women around the time of their periods because of this Jekyll-Hyde phenomenon and also because skin breakouts were worse premenstrually.

45. A. Barbarino, L. De Marinis, G. Folli, et al. "Corticotrophin-Releasing Hormone Inhibition of Gonadotropin Secretion During the Menstrual Cycle," *Metabolism,* vol. 38 (1989), pp. 504–6; Nagata, Kota, Seki, and Furuya, "Ovulatory Disturbances: Causative Factors Among Japanese Women Student Nurses in a Dormitory," *Journal of Adolescent Health Care,* vol. 7 (1986), pp. 1–5; and M. R. Soules, R. I. McLachlan, E. K. Marit, et al., "Luteal Phase Deficiency: Characterization of Reproductive Hormones over the Menstrual Cycle," *Journal of Clinical Endocrine Metabolism,* vol. 69 (1989), pp. 804–12.

46. S. Zuckerman, "The Menstrual Cycle," *Lancet* (June 18, 1949), pp. 1031–35.

47. Cystic and adenomatous hyperplasia of the endometrium is very common after periods of amenorrhea or anovulation. It is a benign condition if there is no "atypia" of the cells. A good gynecological pathologist can make a prediction as to how dangerous this condition is, depending upon the nature of the cells present on the specimen.

48. Clomid has an estrogenlike structure. Its presence in the first half of the menstrual cycle causes the hypothalamus to put out increased levels of the hormones LH and FSH, thus stimulating the ovary to produce an egg.

49. Dewan, "Perfect Rhythm Method of Birth Control" (see note 2).

50. J. D. Cohen and H. W. Rubin, "Functional Menorrhagia: Treatment with Bioflavonoids and Vitamin C," *Current Therapeutic Research,* vol. 2 (1960), p. 539.

51. D. M. Lithgow and W. M. Politzer, "Vitamin A in the Treatment of Menorrhagia," *South African Medical Journal,* vol. 51 (1977), p. 191.

52. Kelley et al., "The Relationship between Menstrual Blood Loss and Prostaglandin" *Leukotrienes Medicine,* vol. 16 (1984), p. 69; A. Anderson et al., "Reduction of Menstrual Blood Loss by Prostaglandin-Synthetase Inhibitors," *Lancet,* (1976), p. 774.

53. I was introduced to this concept by Tamara Slayton.

Chapter 6: The Uterus

1. S. Zuckerman, "The Menstrual Cycle," *Lancet,* (June 18, 1949), pp. 1031–35.

2. While doing the research for this book, I was amazed by the lack of data on the uterus itself, separate from childbearing. The silence on this organ speaks volumes.

3. M. E. Davis, "Complete Caesarean Hysterectomy," *American Journal of Obstetrics and Gynecology,* vol. 62 (1951), p. 838; cited in Robert C. Park and Patrick Duff, "Role of Cesarean Hysterectomy in Modern Obstetric Practice," *Clinical Obstetrics and Gynecology,* vol. 23, no. 2 (June 1980), p. 602. Note: Cesarean hysterectomy is never done routinely—it is far too risky. I use these quotations only to illustrate the authors' attitudes toward the uterus.

4. Celso-Ramon Garcia and Winnifred Cutler, "Preservation of the Ovary: A Reevaluation," *Fertility and Sterility,* vol. 42, no. 4 (Oct. 1984), pp. 510–14.

5. Information from Caroline Myss.

6. Dr. Isaac Schiff (Chairman of the Department of Gynecology at Massachusetts General Hospital) at the "Grand Rounds," conference at Maine Medical Center, Portland, ME.

7. Nancy Petersen and B. Hasselbring, "Endometriosis Reconsidered," *Medical Self Care* (May-June 1987).

8. David B. Redwine, "The Distribution of Endometriosis in the Pelvis by Age Groups and Fertility," *Fertility and Sterility,* vol. 47 (Jan. 1987), p. 173.

9. Supporting evidence can be found in Vaughan Bancroft, C. A. Williams, and

M. Elstein, "Minimal/Mild Endometriosis and Infertility: A Review," *British Journal of Obstetrics and Gynaecology*, vol. 96, no. 4, pp. 454–50; The role of minimal or mild endometriosis in the etiology of infertility remains unclear, but an increased prostanoid content and macrophage activity in peritoneal fluid may exert an effect by a variety of mechanisms, including altered tubal motility, sperm function, and early embryo wastage. Ovarian function may be altered in a variety of ways, including many subtle abnormalities detectable only by detailed investigation. Autoimmune phenomena may also be contributory.

10. John Sampson, "Peritoneal Endometriosis Due to the Menstrual Dissemination of Endometrial Tissue into the Peritoneal Cavity," *American Journal of Obstetrics and Gynecology*, 1984.

11. This theory is based on the work of Dr. David Redwine, who along with Nancy Petersen, a registered nurse, is the founder of the St. Charles Medical Center endometriosis treatment program in Bend, OR.

12. Petersen and Hasselbring, "Endometriosis Reconsidered." See also David Redwine, "Age-Related Evolution in Color Appearance of Endometriosis," *Fertility and Sterility*, vol. 48, no. 6 (Dec. 1987), pp. 1062–63; and David Redwine, "Is Microscopic Peritoneal Endometriosis Invisible," *Fertility and Sterility*, vol. 50, no. 4 (Oct. 1988), pp. 665–66.

13. Norbert Gleicher, "Is Endometriosis an Autoimmune Disease?" *Obstetrics and Gynecology*, vol. 70, no. 1 (July 1987); E. Surrey and J. Halme, "Effect of Peritoneal Fluid from Endometriosis Patients on Endometrial Stromal Cell Proliferation in Vitro," *Obstetrics and Gynecology*, vol. 76, no. 5, part 1 (Nov. 1990), pp. 792–98; S. Kalma et al., "Production of Fibronectin by Peritoneal Macrophages and Concentration of Fibronectin in Peritoneal Fluid from Patients With or Without Endometriosis," *Obstetrics and Gynecology*, vol. 72 (July 1988), pp. 13–19; J. Halme, S. Becker, and S. Haskill, "Altered Maturation and Function of Peritoneal Macrophages: Possible Role in Pathogenesis of Endometriosis," *American Journal of Obstetrics and Gynecology*, vol. 156 (1987), p. 783; J. Halme, M. G. Hammond, J. F. Hulka, et al., "Retrograde Menstruation in Healthy Women and in Patients with Endometriosis," *Obstetrics and Gynecology*, vol. 64 (1984), pp. 13–18.

14. Conventional insurance is set up to cover only certain treatment modalities and often does not cover relatively inexpensive measures to maintain health. Much has been written about the politics of medical treatment, a topic that is beyond the scope of this book. Though all of us end up paying for very expensive conventional medical treatments such as GnRH agonists, individuals with insurance don't bear this cost *directly* and therefore don't want to pay for modalities that aren't covered by insurance.

15. Francis Hutchins, Jr., "Uterine Fibroids: Current Concepts in Management," *Female Patient*, vol. 15 (Oct. 1990), p. 29.

16. A. D. Feinstein, "Conflict over Childbearing and Tumors of the Female Reproductive System: Symbolism in Disease," *Somatics* (Fall/Winter 1983).

17. R. C. Reiter, P. L. Wagner, and J. C. Gambone, "Routine Hysterectomy for Large Asymptomatic Leiomyomata: A Reappraisal," *Obstetrics and Gynecology*, vol. 79, no. 4 (Apr. 1992), pp. 481–84.

18. An entire body of literature on the healing power of sound is available. Each chakra, for example, is associated with a certain vibration. Healers who use sound may suggest that a person sing certain tones or listen to specially designed music. For more information about this treatment, read: W. David, *The Harmonics of Sound, Color, and Vibration: A System for Self Awareness and Evolution* (Marina Del Rey, CA: DeVorss and Co., 1985); Kay Gardner, *Sounding the Inner Landscape* (Caduceus Publications, 1993).

19. L. Zussman et al., "Sexual Response after Hysterectomy-Oophorectomy: Recent Studies and Reconsideration of Psychogenesis," *American Journal of Obstetrics and Gynecology*, vol. 140, no. 7 (Aug. 1, 1981), pp. 725–29.

20. B. Ranney and S. Abu-Ghazaleh, "The Future Function and Control of Ovarian Tissue Which Is Retained in Vivo During Hysterectomy," *American Journal of Obstetrics and Gynecology*, vol. 128 (1977), p. 626.

21. Urinary incontinence is often very responsive to biofeedback. I always recommend a course of biofeedback in these women before a surgical solution. Kegel's exercises, when properly done, are very effective for helping incontinence. Ninety-nine percent of women don't know how to do them properly. Biofeedback helps a woman learn how to contract her vaginal and pelvic floor muscles, not just her abdominals. See also B. J. Parys et al., "The Effects of Simple Hysterectomy on Vesicourethral Function," *British Journal of Urology*, vol. 64 (1989), pp. 594–99; S. J. Snooks et al., "Perineal Nerve Damage in Genuine Stress Urinary Incontinence," *British Journal of Urology*, vol. 42 (1985), pp. 3–9; C. R. Wake, "The Immediate Effect of Abdominal Hysterectomy on intervesical Pressure and Detrusor Activity," *British Journal of Obstetrics and Gynaecology*, vol. 87 (1980), pp. 901–2; A. G. Hanley, "The Late Urological Complications of Total Hysterectomy," *British Journal of Urology*, vol. 41 (1969), pp. 682–84.

22. J. H. Manchester et al., "Premenopausal Castration and Documented Coronary Atherosclerosis," *American Journal of Cardiology*, vol. 28 (1971), pp. 33–37; A. B. Ritterband et al., "Gonadal Function and the Development of Coronary Heart Disease," *Circulation*, vol. 27 (1963), pp. 237–87.

23. A. J. Friedman et al., "A Randomized Double-Blood Trial of Gonadotropin . . . in the Treatment of Leiomyomata Uteki," *Fertility and Sterility*, vol. 49 (1987), p. 404.

24. Progestin hormone, in the form of Provera or Aygestin, can be taken daily on days 14 to 28 of the menstrual cycle to decrease excess buildup of endometrial tissue inside the uterus. This treatment sometimes works like a D&C and in fact is sometimes called a "medical D&C." I recommend this approach for those women whose heavy bleeding is unaffected by dietary change or for whom dietary change is impractical. It is sometimes used in addition to other therapies, such as acupuncture. Each case is individualized.

25. Alan de Cherney, M.D., chairman of the Department of Obstetrics and Gynecology, Tufts University Medical Center, is a pioneer in this surgery and has trained physicians throughout the country in this technique.

26. Shiatsu massage is a type of massage that uses pressure on acupuncture meridians to stimulate the flow of chi in the body.

27. Because of the size and location of the fibroids, she was not a candidate for endometrial ablation.

28. Hysterectomy Educational Resources and Services (HERS) provides articles, telephone consultations, and referrals to physicians who offer alternatives to surgery. Write: HERS, 422 Bryn Mawr Avenue, Bala Cynwyd, PA 19004.

Chapter 7: The Ovaries

1. R. H. Asch and R. Greenblatt, "Steroidogenesis in the Postmenopausal Ovary," *Clinical Obstetrics and Gynecology*, vol. 4, no. 1 (1977), p. 85.

2. E. R. Novak, B. Goldberg, and G. S. Jones, "Enzyme Histochemistry of the Menopausal Ovary Associated with Normal and Abnormal Endometrium," *American Journal of Obstetrics and Gynecology*, vol. 93 (1965), p. 669; and C. R. Garcia and W. Cutler, "Preservation of the Ovary: A Reevaluation," *Fertility and Sterility*, vol. 42, no. 4 (Oct. 1985), pp. 510–14.

3. K. P. McNatty et al., "The Production of Progesterone, Androgens, and Estrogens by Granulosa Cells, Thecal Tissue, and Stromal Tissue by Human Ovaries in Vitro," *Journal of Clinical Endocrinology and Metabolism*, vol. 49 (1979), p. 687.

4. B. Dennefors et al., "Steroid Production and Responsiveness to Gonadotropin in Isolated Stromal Tissue of Human Postmenopausal Ovaries," *American Journal of Obstetrics and Gynecology*, vol. 136 (1980), p. 997; and G. Mikhail, "Hormone Secretion of Human Ovaries," *Gynecological Investigation*, vol. 1 (1970), p. 5.

5. Mantak Chia and Maneewan Chia, *Cultivating Female Sexual Energy: Healing Love Through the Tao* (Huntington, NY: Healing Tao Books, 1986), available from Healing Tao Books, 2 Creskill Place, Huntington, NY 11743.

6. Frank P. Paloucek and John B. Graham, "The Influence of Psychosocial Factors on the Prognosis in Cancer of the Cervix," *Annals of the New York Academy of Sciences*, vol. 125 (1966), pp. 815–16.

7. Kelly et al., "Psychodynamic Psychological Correlates with Secondary Amenorrhea," *Psychosomatic Medicine*, vol. 16 (1954), p. 129; M. M. Gill, "Functional Disturbances in Menstruation," *Bulletin of the Menninger Clinic*, vol. 7 (1943), p. 12.

8. T. Piotrowski, "Psychogenic Factors in Anovulatory Women," *Fertility and Sterility*, vol. 13 (1962), p. 11; T. Loftus, "Psychogenic Factors in Anovulatory Women; Behavioral and Psychoanalytic Aspects of Anovulatory Amenorrhea," *Fertility and Sterility*, vol. 13 (1962), p. 20.

9. W. Menaker, "Lunar Periodicity in Human Reproduction: A Likely Unit of Biological Time," *American Journal of Obstetrics and Gynecology*, vol. 77, no. 4

(1959), pp. 905–14; E. M. DeWan, "On the Possibility of the Fact of the Rhythm Method of Birth Control by Periodic Light Stimulation," *American Journal of Obstetrics and Gynecology,* vol. 99, no. 7 (1967), pp. 1016–19.

10. Though some might argue that all cysts should therefore be removed when they are first diagnosed and are relatively small, I disagree. Not all cysts grow rapidly, and not all cysts replace all normal ovarian tissue. And of course, some cysts go away on their own.

11. B. S. Centerwall, "Premenopausal Hysterectomy," *American Journal of Obstetrics and Gynecology,* vol. 139 (1981), p. 38; and R. Punnonen and L. Raurama, "The Effect of Long-Term Oral Oestriol Succinate Therapy on the Skin of Castrated Women," *Annals of Gynaecology,* vol. 66 (1977), p. 214.

12. J. G. Annegers et al., "Ovarian Cancer: Reappraisal of Residual Ovaries," *American Journal of Obstetrics and Gynecology,* vol. 97 (1967), p. 124; G. V. Smith, "Ovarian Tumors," *American Journal of Surgery,* vol. 95 (1958), p. 336; V. S. Counsellor et al., "Carcinoma of the Ovary Following Hysterectomy," *American Journal of Obstetrics and Gynecology,* vol. 69 (1955), p. 538; and R. H. Grogan, "Reappraisal of Residual Ovaries," *American Journal of Obstetrics and Gynecology,* vol. 97 (1967), p. 124.

13. Theodore Speroff, "A Risk-Benefit Analysis of Elective Bilateral Oophorectomy: Effect of Changes in Compliance with Estrogen Therapy on Outcome," *American Journal of Obstetrics and Gynecology* (Jan. 1991), pp. 165–74.

14. D. W. Cramer and B. L. Harlow, "Author's Response to Progress in Nutritional Epidemiology of Ovarian Cancer," *American Journal of Epidemiology,* vol. 134, no. 5 (1991), pp. 460–61; D. W. Cramer et al., "Galactose Consumption and Metabolism in Relationship to Risks for Ovarian Cancer," *Lancet,* vol. 2 (1989), pp. 66–71; D. W. Cramer, "Lactose Persistence and Milk Consumption as Determinants of Ovarian Cancer Risk," *American Journal of Epidemiology,* vol. 130 (1989), pp. 904–10; D. W. Cramer et al., "Dietary Animal Fat and Relationship to Ovarian Cancer Risk," *Obstetrics and Gynecology,* vol. 63, no. 6 (1984), pp. 833–38.

15. C. J. Mettlin and M. S. Diver, "A Case-Control Study of Milk-Drinking and Ovarian Cancer Risk," *American Journal of Epidemiology,* vol. 132 (1990), pp. 871–76; C. J. Mettlin, "Invited Commentary: Progress in Nutritional Epidemiology of Ovarian Cancer," *American Journal of Epidemiology,* vol. 134, no. 5 (1991), pp. 457–59.

16. D. W. Cramer, W. R. Welsh, R. E. Scully, and C. A. Wojciechowski, "Ovarian Cancer and Talc: a Case-Control Study," *Cancer,* vol. 50 (1982), pp. 372–76; W. J. Henderson, T. C. Hamilton, and K. Griffiths. "Talc in Normal and Malignant Ovarian Tissue." *Lancet,* vol. 1 (1979), p. 499.

17. G. E. Egli, M. Newton, "The transport of carbon particles in the human female reproductive tract." *Fertility and Sterility,* vol. 12 (1961), pp. 151–55.

18. B. L. Harlow et al., "The Influence of Lactose Consumption on the Association of Oral Contraceptive Pills and Ovarian Cancer Risk," *American Journal of Epidemiology,* vol. 134, no. 5 (1991), pp. 445–61.

19. S. E. Hankinson, et al., "Tubal ligation, hysterectomy, and risk of ovarian cancer: a prospective study," *J.A.M.A.* (Dec. 15, 1993); A. S. Whittemore, R. Harris, J. Intyre, and the Collaborative Ovarian Cancer Group, "Characteristics Relating to Ovarian Cancer Risk: Collaborative Analysis of 12 US Case-Control Studies." "Part II: Invasive Epithelial Ovarian Cancers in White Women," *American Journal of Epidemiology,* vol. 136 (1992), pp. 1184–1203.

20. C. Granai, "Sounding Board: Ovarian Cancer: Unrealistic Expectations," *New England Journal of Medicine,* vol. 327, no. 3 (1993), pp. 197–200.

21. Gilda Radner, a well-known comedienne and wife of actor Gene Wilder, died of familial ovarian cancer. To prevent this from happening to others, Wilder has publicized the genetic risk for those who have this disease in their families, usually in first-degree relatives on the mother's side of the family.

22. J. K. Tobachman et al., "Intra-abdominal Carcinomatosis after Prophylactic Oophorectomy in Ovarian Cancer Prone Families," *Lancet,* vol. 2 (1982), p. 795; and Elvio Silva and Rosemary Jenkins, "Serious Carcinoma in Endometrial Polyps," *Modern Pathology,* vol. 3, no. 2 (1990), pp. 120–22.

Chapter 8: Reclaiming the Erotic

1. Josephine Lowdes Sevely, *Eve's Secrets: A New Theory of Female Sexuality* (New York: Random House, 1987), pp. 89–90.

2. Caroline Muir and Charles Muir, *Tantra: The Art of Conscious Loving* (San Francisco: Mercury House, 1989).

3. The Muirs teach that finding the sacred spot is often difficult for a woman to accomplish alone. Even if she does locate it, it may be very difficult for her to stimulate it herself, which is the only way to access its healing power and its sexual and spiritual potential. Nevertheless, you can try to locate it in the following way: Squat with two fingers inside the vagina, press your fingers upward toward the navel while pressing down on the pubic bone with the other hand. If you can manage to stimulate or massage the area, the spot will swell. You may then be able to feel it between your fingers. For most women, this part of their awakening process requires the loving touch of a partner who respects the vulnerable nature of this spot.

4. Muir and Muir, *Tantra,* p. 74 (see note 2).

5. Naura Hayden, *How to Satisfy a Woman Every Time and Have Her Beg for More* (New York: Biblio-Phile). Though I don't agree with everything in this book, it's a very practical guide for satisfactory heterosexual lovemaking. A good book to give to a male partner, it can be obtained by writing to Biblio-Phile at P.O. Box 5189, New York, NY 10022.

6. Paula Brown Doress and Diana Laskin Siegal, *Ourselves Growing Older* (New York: Simon and Schuster, 1987).

7. H. B. Van de Weil, W. C. Schultz et al., "Sexual Functioning Following Treatment of Cervical Cancer," *European Journal of Gynecologic Oncology* (1988), pp. 275–81.

8. So-called "natural" male sexual needs are also deeply influenced by the culture. Barbara Hand Clow, in *The Liquid Light of Sex* (Santa Fe, NM: Bear and Co., 1991), points out that many men in this culture achieve erection via their third chakra power centers. But erection achieved in this way is a form of power over others, and erections maintained through third chakra energy are the basis of rape, which is not about sexuality at all but about power and dominance. Caroline Myss says that in this culture the size of a man's wallet and the size of his erections are related. When a man is able to clear his lower chakras of negativity, his erections are achieved more through fourth chakra or heart energy. Then the act of intercourse becomes an act of sharing, caring, and love. The orgasm achieved in this way is symbolic of this man's love not only for the woman he's with but for creation itself.

9. "A View from Above: The Dangerous World of Wannabes," *Time* (Nov. 25, 1991), p. 77.

10. "A View from Above" (see note 9).

11. John Stoltenberg, *Refusing to Be a Man: Essays on Sex and Justice* (New York: Penguin, 1990). Data quoted by Stoltenberg are from, "Chicago: 'Out Reach' Is the Name of the Game," *Family Planner*, vol. 8 (Mar.-Apr. 1977), pp. 2–4.

12. Barbara Walker, *The Women's Encyclopedia of Myths and Secrets* (Harper San Francisco, 1983), pp. 1049–51. Scholarly research on the whole issue of the virgin birth has been done. "In ancient times impregnation by a ghost used to be 'the acceptable explanation for pregnancy in most pagan countries where the sexual act was part of the fertility rites,' so Christians thought impregnation by spirits was still credible, whether the alleged father was a dead hero, a devil, an incubus, or even—in some sects—the Holy Ghost again." R. Holmes, *Witchcraft in History* (Secaucus, NJ: Citadel Press, 1974); quoted in Walker, *Encyclopedia*, p. 1050.

13. Elizabeth Cady Stanton, *The Original Feminist Attack on the Bible* (New York: Arno Press, 1974), p. 114; quoted in Walker, *Encyclopedia*, p. 1051 (see note 12).

14. Barbara Walker points out that the Hebrew Gospels designated Mary by the word *mah,* mistakenly translated as "virgin" but really meaning "young woman." See also Esther Harding, *Women's Mysteries, Ancient and Modern* (New York: Rider and Co., 1955).

15. Women's sense of smell is more acute than men's. A smell can evoke an entire stream of memories, either positive or negative. Smell is the longest-remembered sense. A particular smell evokes associated memories more than the senses of vision, hearing, and skin sensation. The olfactory center is located in the brain in an area that is intimately connected with memory function.

16. Part of normal dolphin life is being sexual with each other. Male dolphins often wrap their penis around a female's lower body, playfully—not to procreate but simply to communicate. Male dolphins sometimes do this when they are communicating with humans too. This happened to my sister once—she described her dolphin encounter as an ecstatic experience.

17. Mantak Chia and Maneewan Chia, *Cultivating Female Sexual Energy: Healing Love Through the Tao* (Huntington, NY: Healing Tao Books, 1986); available from Healing Tao Books, 2 Creskill Place, Huntington, NY 11743.

18. For more information on weighted cones, how to use them, and medical studies showing their effectiveness, contact the Dacomed Corporation, 1701 East 79th Street, Minneapolis, MN 55425; tel. (800) 823-1108 or (612) 854-7522.

19. Chia and Chia, *Cultivating* (see note 17).

20. I have replaced the repugnant term *masturbation* with the term *self-love*, or as a friend of mine calls it, "Being your own best friend."

Chapter 9: Vulva, Vagina, and Cervix

1. R. Good, "Attitudes Toward Douching," *Female Patient*, vol. 15 (Oct. 1990), pp. 53–57.

2. See the book by the Body Shop Team, *Mamamoto: A Celebration* (New York: Viking, 1992), p. 78.

3. Barbara Walker, *The Women's Encyclopedia of Myths and Secrets* (Harper San Francisco, 1983), p. 1034.

4. M. Tarlau and M. A. Smalheiser, "Personality Patterns in Patients with Malignant Tumors of the Breast and Cervix," *Psychosomatic Medicine*, vol. 13, p. 117 (1951). Women with cervical cancer characteristically experienced an early rejection; the patients grew up in homes lacking a male figure due to the death or desertion of the father.

5. James H. Stephenson and William Grace, "Life Stress and Cancer of the Cervix," *Psychosomatic Medicine*, vol. 16, no. 4 (1954), pp. 287–94.

6. A. Schmale and H. Iker, "Psychological Setting of Uterine Cervical Cancer," *Annals of the New York Academy of Sciences*, vol. 125 (1966), pp. 807–13.

7. Leopold G. Koss, "Human Papilloma Viruses and Genital Cancer," *Female Patient*, vol. 17 (Feb. 1992), pp. 25–30.

8. J. Buscema, "The Predominance of Human Papilloma Virus—Type 16 in Vulvar Neoplasia," *Obstetrics and Gynecology*, vol. 71, no. 4 (1988), pp. 601–5.

9. R. Kiecolt Glaser, J. K. Glaser, C. E. Speicher, and J. E. Holliday, "Stress, Loneliness, and Changes in Herpes Virus Latency," *Journal of Behavioral Medicine*, vol. 8, no. 3 (1985), pp. 249–60.

10. To diagnose warts that aren't visible, or so-called flat warts, the penis must be bathed in vinegar and then viewed through some sort of magnifying lens. Only then will the flat white warts be obvious to those who know what to look for. Treatment issues for men are exactly the same as for women.

11. For more information about podofilox, you or your doctor can write to Oclassen Pharmaceuticals, Inc., 100 Pelican Way, San Rafael, CA 94901.

12. Two studies note that many patients have effectively used hypnosis to relieve warts. See R. H. Rulison, "Warts: A Statistical Study of 921 Cases," *Archives of Dermatology and Syphilology*, vol. 46 (1942), pp. 66–81; and M. Ullman, "On the Psyche and Warts. II: Hypnotic Suggestion and Warts," *Psychosomatic Medicine*, vol. 22 (1960), pp. 68–76.

13. N. Whitehead et al., "Megaloblastic Changes in Cervical Epithelium: Association of Oral Contraceptive Therapy and Reversal with Folic Acid," *Journal of
the American Medical Association*, vol. 226 (193), pp. 1421–24; J. N. Orr, "Localized Deficiency of Folic Acid in Cervical Epithelial Cells May Promote
Cervical Dysplasia and Eventually Carcinoma of the Cervix," *American Journal
of Obstetrics and Gynecology*, vol. 151 (1985), pp. 632–35; J. Lindenbaum et al.,
"Oral Contraceptive Hormones, Folate Metabolism, and Cervical Epithelium,"
American Journal of Clinical Nutrition (Apr. 1975), pp. 346–53; S. L. Romney et
al., "Plasma Vitamin C and Uterine Cervical Dysplasia," *American Journal of
Obstetrics and Gynecology*, vol. 151, no. 7 (1985), pp. 976–80; S. L. Romney et al.,
"Retinoids in the Prevention of Cervical Dysplasia," *American Journal of Ob-
stetrics and Gynecology*, vol. 141, no. 8 (1981), pp. 890–94; S. Wassertheil-Smaller
et al., "Dietary Vitamin C and Uterine Cervical Dysplasia," *American Journal of
Epidemiology*, vol. 114, no. 5 (1981), pp. 714–24; C. LaVecchia et al., "Dietary
Vitamin A and the Risk of Invasive Cervical Cancer," *International Journal of
Cancer*, vol. 34 (1985), pp. 319–22; P. Ramsnamy and R. Natarajan, "Vitamin B$_6$
Status in Patients with Cancer of the Uterine Cervix," *Nutrition and Cancer*, vol.
6 (1984), pp. 176–80; E. Dawson et al., "Serum Vitamin and Selenium Changes in
Cervical Dysplasia," *Federal Proceedings*, vol. 43 (1984), p. 612.

14. L. Koutsky et al., "Underdiagnosis of Genital Herpes by Current Clinical and
Viral-Isolation Procedures," *New England Journal of Medicine*, vol. 326, no. 23
(1992), pp. 1533–39.

15. H. C. Taylor, "Vascular Congestion and Hyperemia," *American Journal of
Obstetrics and Gynecology*, vol. 57, no. 22 (1949), p. 22; and M. E. Kemeny et al.,
"Psychological and Immunological Predictors of Genital Herpes Recurrence,"
Psychosomatic Medicine, vol. 52 (1989), pp. 195–208.

16. M. A. Adefumbo and B. H. Lau, "Allium Sativum (Garlic): A Natural Antibiotic," *Medical Hypothesis*, vol. 12, no. 3 (1983), pp. 327–37.

17. There are a number of brands of garlic on the market: Kyolic (by the Wakunga
Company) and Garlicin (by Murdock) are two that Women to Women often
recommends.

18. Not all products labeled "tea tree oil" are equally effective. At Women to
Women we use Melaleuca oil or Melagel from the Melaleuca Company; see also
Richard Bruse, *Melaleuca: Nature's Antiseptic*, 1989, Sunnyside Health Center,
8800 S.E. Sunnyside Rd., Suite 111, Clackamus, Oregon 97015; tel. (503)
654-8225.

19. G. Eby, "Use of Topical Zinc to Prevent Recurrent Herpes Simplex Infection:
Review of Literature and Suggested Protocols," *Medical Hypothesis*, vol. 17
(1985), pp. 157–65; G. T. Terezhabny et al., "The Use of a Water-Soluble
Bioflavonoid Ascorbic Acid Complex in the Treatment of Recurrent Herpes
Labialis," *Oral Surgery, Oral Medicine, and Oral Pathology*, vol. 45 (1978), pp.
56–62; G.R.B. Skinner, "Lithium Ointment for Genital Herpes," *Lancet*, vol. 2
(1983), p. 288; E. F. Finnerty, "Topical Zinc in the Treatment of Herpes Simplex," *Cutis* (Feb. 1986), p. 130.

20. R. S. Griffith et al., "Multicentered Study of Lysine Therapy on HSV Infection," *Dermatologica,* vol. 156 (1978), pp. 157–67; McCane et al., article in *Cutis,* vol. 34 (1984), p. 366; D. D. Schmeisser et al., "Effect of Excess Lysine on Plasma Lipids in the Chick," *Journal of Nutrition,* vol. 113 (1983), pp. 1777–83; D. J. Thein and W. C. Hurt, "Lysine as a Prophylactic Agent in the Treatment of Recurrent Herpes," *Oral Surgery,* vol. 58 (1984), pp. 659–66; J. H. DiGiovanni and H. Blank, "Failure of Lysine in Frequently Recurrent Herpes Simplex Infection," *Archives Dermatology,* vol. 120 (1984), pp. 48–51.

21. M. H. Antoni and K. Goodkin, "Host Moderator Variables in the Promotion of Cervica Neoplasia—I. Personality Facets," *Journal of Psychosomatic Research,* vol. 32, no. 3 (1988), pp. 327–38; and K. Goodkin et al., "Stress and Hopelessness in the Promotion of Cervical Epithelial Neoplasia to Invasive Squamous Cell Carcinoma of the Cervix," *Journal of Psychosomatic Research,* vol. 30, no. 1 (1986), pp. 67–76.

22. It is important to know the laboratory to which your Pap smear is sent. The skill level of the pathologists at our hospital is very high, and I can speak to them personally about any abnormality that arises and obtain further samples from the patient as necessary.

23. M. D. Schauberger et al., "Cervical Screening with Cervicography and the Pananicolaou Smear in Women with Genital Condylomata," *Journal of Reproductive Medicine,* vol. 36, no. 2 (Feb. 1991), pp. 100–2.

24. J. D. Oriel, "Sex and Cervical Cancer," *Genitourinary Medicine,* vol. 64 (1988), pp. 81–89; C. LaVecchia, A. Decarli, A. Fasoli et al., "Oral Contraceptives and Cancer of the Breast and of the Female Genital Tract: Interim Results of a Case-Control Study," *British Journal of Cancer,* vol. 54 (1986), p. 311; J. J. Schlesselman, "Cancer of the Breast and Reproductive Tract in Relation to Use of CC's," *Contraception,* vol. 40 (1989), p. 1.

25. Pap smears are taken even after the cervix has been removed in a hysterectomy. This is especially important for women who have had a prior history of an abnormal Pap smear.

26. Therapeutic touch, a system of healing with the hands, has been very well studied, and its beneficial effects have been well-documented by Delores Kreiger, a registered nurse, at Columbia University. Marcelle Pick of Women to Women has studied with Dr. Kreiger.

27. I feel that chlamydia *may* also be a normal inhabitant of the vagina in some women and that it may cause problems only when there's an imbalance. Chlamydia is like the buzzard flying around the dying calf, as far as I'm concerned, though many of my colleagues would disagree.

28. Gardiner-Caldwell SynerMed, "The Role of Reduced Regimens in the Management of Vulvovaginitis," *Medical Monitor,* vol. 1, no. 1 (Apr. 1991), available from Gardiner-Caldwell SynerMed, P.O. Box 458, Califon, NJ 07830.

29. Mary Ryan Miles, M.D., Linda Olsen, M.D., Alvin Rogers, Ph.D, "Recurrent Vaginal Candidiasis: Importance of an Intestinal Reservoir," *Journal of the American Medical Association,* Oct. 24, 1977.

30. Mary Ryan Miles, M.D. et al. (see note 29).

31. D. Stewart et al., "Psychosocial Aspects of Chronic, Clinically Unconfirmed Vulvovaginitis," *Obstetrics and Gynecology,* vol. 76, no. 5, part 1 (Nov. 1990), pp. 852–56.

32. S. Mathur et al., "Anti-ovarian and Anti-lymphocyte Antibodies in Patients with Chronic Vaginal Candidiasis," *Journal of Reproductive Immunology,* vol. 2 (1980), pp. 247–62.

33. I am not an authority on AIDS and I do not treat AIDS patients at this time. I am aware, however, of several individuals who have reversed their HIV status from positive to negative through employing the measures discussed in Part Three of this book. See Note 35 for references.

34. Caroline Myss, *AIDS, Passageway to Transformation,* (Walpole, MA: Stillpoint Publications, 1985).

35. Niro Markoff, who went from HIV positive to HIV negative, now teaches internationally. Her story and her teaching are available in *Why I Survive AIDS* (New York: Simon and Schuster, 1991). Bob Owen, *Roger's Recovery from AIDS* (Cannon Beach, OR: Davar Press, 1987) also documents a case of reversal from HIV positive to HIV negative. It is available by writing Davar Press, P.O. Box 1100, Cannon Beach, OR 97110.

36. A tape of this panel presentation can be ordered from the American Holistic Medical Association (AHMA 4101 Lake Boone Trail, Suite 201, Raleigh, NC 27607; tel. (919) 787-5181.) See also Laurence Badgley, *Healing AIDS Naturally* (San Bruno, CA: Human Energy Press, 1987); available from Human Energy Press, Suite D, 370 West San Bruno Avenue, San Bruno, CA 94066.

Chapter 10: Breasts

1. In the nineteenth century, the unusual case history studies of Herbert Snow linked breast and uterine cancer with a history of a "troubled mind and chronic anxiety." Particularly evident in the women he studied was the loss of a significant relationship as the precipitating factor in the manifestation of a tumor. See Herbert Snow, *The Proclivity of Women to Cancerous Disease* (London, 1883).

   In this century, M. Tarlau and M. A. Smalheiser found that the typical pattern for women with breast cancer was that their father had been absent psychologically; for women with cervical cancer, the father had been absent due to death or desertion. See M. Tarlau and M. A. Smalheiser, "Personality Patterns in Patients with Malignant Tumors of the Breast and Cervix," *Psychosomatic Medicine,* vol. 13 (1951), p. 117. They also found that women with breast cancer uniformly had negative feelings about their sexuality, had adapted by denying their sexuality, and often had negative feelings about heterosexual relations as such. Women with cervical cancer, by contrast, had less negative feelings about their sexuality. The breast cancer patients were much more likely to have remained in an unsatisfactory marriage, while many of the cervical cancer patients were divorced or had been married several times. See M. Tarlau and

M. A. Smalheiser, "Personality Patterns in Patients with Malignant Tumors of the Breast and Cervix," *Psychosomatic Medicine,* vol. 13, p. 117 (1951).

A study by Bacon and colleagues found that many women with breast cancer frequently were unable to discharge or deal appropriately with their anger, aggressiveness, or hostility. Often these women covered up such feelings with a facade of pleasantness. Women with breast cancer frequently responded with "denial and unrealistic sacrifice" to resolve hostile conflict with their mothers. See C. L. Bacon et al., "A Psychosomatic Survey of Cancer of the Breast," *Psychosomatic Medicine,* vol. 14, no. 6 (1952), pp. 453–59.

See also C. B. Bahnson, "Stress and Cancer: The State of the Art," *Psychosomatics,* vol. 22, no. 3 (1981), pp. 207–20.

2. Sandra Levy et al., "Perceived Social Support and Tumor Estrogen Progesterone Receptor Status as Predictors of Natural Killer Cell Activity in Breast Cancer Patients," *Psychosomatic Medicine,* vol. 52 (1990), pp. 73–85.

3. A. Bremond, G. Kune, and C. Bahnson, "Psychosomatic Factors in Breast Cancer Patients: Results of a Case Control Study," *Journal of Psychosomatic Obstetrics and Gynecology,* vol. 5 (1986), pp. 127–36.

4. K. W. Pettingale et al., "Serum IgA Levels and Emotional Expression in Breast Cancer Patients," *Journal of Psychosomatic Research,* vol. 21 (1977), p. 395.

5. In my entire career, I have diagnosed only one cancer this way that would otherwise have been missed. Since the cytology lab fee is $70 to $90 for this service, sending fluid on every breast cyst has not been deemed "cost effective." Most of my patients want it done, however, just to be sure.

6. V. L. Ernster et al., "Effects of Caffeine-Free Diet on Benign Breast Disease: A Randomized Trial," *Surgery,* vol. 91, no. 3 (1982), pp. 263–67; C. Boyle et al., "Caffeine Consumption and Fibrocystic Breast Disease: A Case Control Study," *Journal of the National Cancer Institute,* vol. 72, no. 5 (1984), pp. 1015–19; J. P. Minton et al., "Caffeine, Cyclic Mastalgia and Breast Disease," *Surgery,* vol. 86 (1979), pp. 105–9; J. P. Minton, "Caffeine and Benign Breast Disease," letter to the editor, *Journal of the American Medical Association,* vol. 254, no. 17 (1985), pp. 2408–9; and F. Lubin et al., "A Case Control Study of Caffeine and Methylxanthines in Benign Breast Disease," *Journal of the American Medical Association,* vol. 253, no. 16 (1985), pp. 2388–92.

7. J. K. Pye et al., "Clinical Experience of Drug Treatments for Mastalgia," *Lancet,* vol. 2 (1985), pp. 373–77.

8. R. S. London et al., "The Effect of Alpha-Tocopherol on Premenstrual Symptomatology," *Cancer Research,* vol. 41 (1981), pp. 3811–13; R. S. London et al., "The Effect of Alpha-Tocopherol on Premenstrual Symptomatology," *Cancer Research,* vol. 41 (1981), pp. 3814–16; R. S. London et al., "The Effect of Alpha Tocopherol on Premenstrual Symptomatology: A Double-Blind Study," *Journal of American College Nutrition,* vol. 3 (1984), pp. 351–56; R. S. London et al., "The Role of Vitamin E in Fibrocystic Breast Disease," *Obstetrics/ Gynecology,* vol. 65 (1982), pp. 104–6; A. A. Abrams, "Use of Vitamin E for

Chronic Cystic Mastitis," *New England Journal of Medicine*, vol. 272 (1965), pp. 1080–81.

9. B. A. Eskin et al., "Mammary Gland Dysplasia in Iodine Deficiency," *Journal of the American Medical Association*, vol. 200 (1967), pp. 115–19.

10. Gina Kolata, "Breast Cancer Screening Under 50: Experts Disagree if Benefit Exists," *The New York Times* (Dec. 14, 1993), p. C-1; W. Gilbert Welch and William Black, "Advances in Diagnostic Imaging," *New England Journal of Medicine*, vol. 328 (Apr. 1993), pp. 1237–43; M. Nielson et al., "Breast Cancer and Atypia Among Young Middle-Aged Women: A Study of 110 Medical-Legal Autopsies," *British Journal of Cancer*, vol. 56 (1987), pp. 814–19; An unpublished autopsy study with similar findings was done at Cook County Hospital in Chicago. Personal communication with Kate Havens, M.D.

11. National Center for Health Statistics, *Vital Statistics of the United States, 1987*, vol. 2, *Mortality, Part A*, DHHS publication no. (PHS) 90–1101 (Washington, DC: U.S. Government Printing Office, 1990).

12. The following chemicals have been implicated: the pesticides DDT, heptachlor, and atrazine, several polycyclic aromatic hydrocarbons (PAHs), petroleum byproducts, dioxin, and polychlorinated biphenyls (PCBs). See also Janet Raloff, "Ecocancer: Do Environmental Factors Underlie a Breast Cancer Epidemic?" *Science News*, vol. 144 (July 3, 1993), pp. 10–13.

13. P. Buell, "Changing Incidence of Breast Cancer in Japanese-American Women," *Journal of the National Cancer Institute*, vol. 51 (1973), pp. 1479–83; L. Kinlen, "Meat and Fat Consumption and Cancer Mortality: A Study of Strict Religious Orders in Britain," *Lancet* (1982), pp. 946–49; W. Willett et al., "Dietary Fat and Risk of Breast Cancer," *New England Journal of Medicine*, vol. 316, no. 22 (1987).

14. M. H. Holl et al., "Gut Bacteria and Aetiology of Cancer of the Breast," *Lancet*, vol. 2 (1971), pp. 172–73; R. E. Hughes, "Hypothesis: A New Look at Dietary Fiber in Human Nutrition," *Clinical Nutrition*, vol. 406 (1986), pp. 81–86.

15. H. Adlercreutz et al., "Dietary Phytoestrogens and the Menopause in Japan," *Lancet*, vol. 339 (1992), pp. 1233; H. P. Lee et al., "Dietary Effects on Breast Cancer Risk in Singapore," *Lancet*, vol. 337 (May 18, 1991), pp. 1197–1200.

16. J. Michnovicz and H. Bradlow, "Altered Estrogen Metabolism and Excretion in Humans Following Consumption of Indole-3-Carbinol," *Nutrition and Cancer*, vol. 16 (1991), pp. 59–66.

17. K. P. McConnell et al., "The Relationship Between Dietary Selenium and Breast Cancer," *Journal of Surgical Oncology*, vol. 5, no. 1 (1980), pp. 67–70.

18. B. Goldin and J. Gorsbach, "The Effect of Milk and Lactobacillus Feeding on Human Intestinal Bacterial Enzyme Activity," *American Journal of Clinical Nutrition*, vol. 39 (1984), pp. 756–61. Lactobacillus acidophilus inhibits Beta glucuronidase, the fecal bacterial enzyme responsible for deconjugating liver-conjugated estrogen.

19. T. T. Kellis and L. E. Vickery, "Inhibition of Human Estrogen Synthetase (Aromatase) by Flavonoids," *Science*, vol. 255 (1984), pp. 1032–34. The bioflavonoids compete for estrogen as a substrate in fat metabolism.

20. R. R. Brown et al., "Correlation of Serum Retinol Levels with Response to Chemotherapy in Breast Cancer," *American Journal of Obstetrics and Gynecology,* vol. 148, no. 3, pp. 309–12.

21. S. Seely and D. F. Horrobin, "Diet and Breast Cancer: The Possible Connection with Sugar Consumption," *Medical Hypotheses,* vol. 3 (1983), pp. 319–27; K. K. Carroll, "Dietary Factors in Immune-Dependent Cancers," in M. Winick, ed., *Current Concepts in Nutrition,* vol. 6, *Nutrition and Cancer* (New York: John Wiley and Sons, 1977), pp. 25–40; S. K. Hoeh and K. K. Carroll, "Effects of Dietary Carbohydrate in the Incidence of Mammary Tumors Induced in Rats by 7, 12-dimethylbenzanthracene," *Nutrition and Cancer,* vol. 1, no. 3 (1979), pp. 27–30.

22. L. Rosenberg et al., "Breast Cancer and Alcoholic Beverage Consumption," *Lancet,* vol. 1 (1982), p. 267.

23. I. Kato et al., "Alcohol Consumption in Cancers of Hormone Related Organs in Females," *Japan Journal of Clinical Oncology,* vol. 19, no. 3 (1989), pp. 202–7.

24. W. Willett et al., "Dietary Fat and the Risk of Breast Cancer," *New England Journal of Medicine,* vol. 316 (1987), pp. 22–28.

25. S. Narod et al., "Familial Breast-Ovarian Cancer Locus on Chromosome 17q12q23," *Lancet,* vol. 338 (July 13, 1991), pp. 82–83.

26. Sonia Johnson, *Wildfire: Igniting the She-volution* (Albuquerque, NM: Wildfire Books), p. 38.

27. Breast cancer, in the conventional sense, can recur any time. Approximately 80 percent of women diagnosed with the disease eventually die from it. That is why no conventional doctor would consider Monica "cured." They would say that she is "in remission." Whatever one calls it, I like the way she looks and is living her life.

28. Anthony Sattilaro and Tom Monte, *Living Well Naturally* (Boston: Houghton Mifflin, 1984). Dr. Sattilaro, who is an anesthesiologist and is head of Methodist Hospital in Philadelphia, healed his own prostate cancer through a macrobiotic diet after failing to improve from standard, conventional therapy. His story has inspired many people.

29. Michio Kushi, *The Book of Do-In: Exercise for Physical and Spiritual Development* (Tokyo: Japan Publications, 1979).

30. Joan Borysenko, *Guilt Is the Teacher: Love Is the Lesson* (New York: Warner Books, 1991).

31. A. R. Staib and D. R. Logan, "Hypnotic Stimulation of Breast Growth," *American Journal of Clinical Hypnosis* (Apr. 1977), and R. D. Willard, "Breast Enlargement Through Visual Imagery and Hypnosis," *American Journal of Clinical Hypnosis* (Apr. 1977). A taped program called *Natural Breast Enlargement* is available from P.O. Box 1358, Glendora, CA, tel. (818) 963-3108.

Chapter 11: Our Fertility

1. I recently met a woman OB/GYN physician from China who told me she had performed twenty thousand abortions in her career. In China, only one child per couple is allowed—sometimes not even one. Abortion is commonly used

for birth control. If a couple has more than one child, the parents may lose a job or be subject to other sanctions. As a result, Chinese couples now selectively abort female fetuses, and now an entire generation of young men do not have enough women their age for wives—a fact that, although it is tragic, seems a cruel kind of justice.

2. Carroll Smith-Rosenberg, *Disorderly Conduct: Visions of Gender in Victorian America* (New York: Oxford University Press, 1986).

3. In a society in which there is so much incest and rape, sexual behavior is often distorted, starting in childhood. Any woman who has recovered from sexual abuse will tell you that having multiple sexual partners and sexual "acting out" are among the consequences of sexual abuse. I'm not blaming these women. I'm merely suggesting that we need to start the healing process somewhere.

4. Smith-Rosenberg, *Disorderly Conduct,* p. 218 (see note 2).

5. Gladys McGarey, *Born to Live* (Phoenix, AZ: Gabriel Press, 1980), p. 54.

6. R. Hatcher, et al., *Contraceptive Technology* (New York: Irvington Publishers, Inc., 1991).

7. M. K. Horwitt et al., "Relationship Between Levels of Blood Lipids, Vitamins C, A, E, Serum Copper, and Urinary Excretion of Tryptophan Metabolites in Women Taking Oral Contraceptive Therapy," *American Journal of Clinical Nutrition,* vol. 28 (1975), pp. 403–12; K. Amatayakul, "Vitamin Metabolism and the Effects of Multivitamin Supplementation in Oral Contraceptive Users," *Contraception,* vol. 30, no. 2 (1984), pp. 179–96; and J. L. Webb, "Nutritional Effects of Oral Contraceptive Use," *Journal of Reproductive Health,* vol. 25, no. 4 (1980), p. 151.

8. My introduction to the true scope of science backing natural family planning came when I heard Dr. Joseph Stanford speak at the 1993 annual meeting of the American Holistic Medical Association in Kansas City, Kansas. The research that is cited in this section was graciously provided to me by Dr. Stanford who currently teaches in the Department of Family and Preventive Medicine, The University of Utah, 50 North Medical Drive, Salt Lake City, Utah 84132.

9. The rhythm method relies on calendar estimates of the fertility period rather than physiologic signs of fertility. It is much less reliable than the methods discussed in the text.

10. Observation of vaginal mucus discharge to determine time of fertility was originally developed by two physicians, John and Evelyn Billings. Hence, this method is sometimes referred to as the Billings method.

11. T. W. Hilgers, A. I. Bailey, and A. M. Prebil, "Natural Family Planning IV. The Identification of Postovulatory Infertility," *Obstetrics and Gynecology,* vol. 58, no. 3 (1981), pp. 345–50.

12. T. W. Hilgers, "The Medical Applications of Natural Family Planning: A Contemporary Approach to Women's Health Care" (Omaha, NE: Pope Paul VI Institute Press, 1991); T. W. Hilgers, "The Statistical Evaluation of Natural Methods of Family Planning," *International Review of Natural Family Planning,* vol. 8, no. 3 (Fall 1984), pp. 226–64; J. Doud, "Use-Effectiveness of the

Creighton Model of NFP," *International Review of Natural Family Planning,* vol. 9, no. 54 (1985).

13. Thomas Hilgers, et al., "Cumulative Pregnancy Rates in Patients with Apparently Normal Fertility and Fertility-Focused Intercourse," *The Journal of Reproductive Medicine,* vol. 37, no. 10 (Oct. 1992), pp. 864–66.

14. Quote taken from lecture handout of J. Stanford, Annual Meeting of the American Holistic Medical Association, March 13, 1993. Study cited is in T. W. Hilgers, "The Medical Applications of Natural Family Planning," op. cit. (1991).

15. G. Freundl et al., "Demographic Study on the Family Planning Behavior of the German Population: The Importance of Natural Methods," *International Journal of Fertility,* vol. 33 (1988), suppl. pp. 54–58.

16. H. Klaus, "Natural Family Planning: A Review," *Obstetrics and Gynecology* survey, vol. 37, no. 2 (Feb. 1982), pp. 128–50; T. W. Hilgers, A. M. Prebil, "The Ovulation Method-Vulvar Observations as an Index of Fertility/Infertility," *Obstetrics and Gynecology,* vol. 53, no. 1 (Jan. 1979), pp. 12–22; World Health Organization, "A Prospective Multicentre Trial of the Ovulation Method of Natural Family Planning. I. The Teaching Phase," *Fertility and Sterility,* vol. 362 (Aug. 1981), pp. 152–58.

17. T. W. Hilgers, G. F. Abraham and D. Cavanagh, "Natural Family Planning. I. The Peak Symptom and Estimated Time of Ovulation," *American Journal of Obstetrics and Gynecology,* vol. 52, no. 5 (Nov. 1978), pp. 575–82.

18. Material for this section obtained from Dr. Joseph Stanford.

19. J. F. Cattanach and B. J. Milne, "Post-Tubal Sterilization Problems Correlated with Ovarian Steroidogenesis," *Contraception,* vol. 38, no. 5 (1988); J. Donnez, M. Wauters, and K. Thomas, "Luteal Function After Tubal Sterilization," *Obstetrics and Gynecology,* vol. 57, no. 1 (1981); and M. M. Cohen, "Long-Term Risk of Hysterectomy After Tubal Sterilization," *American Journal of Epidemiology,* vol. 125 (1987).

20. I. Gerhard et al., "Prolonged Exposure to Wood Preservatives Induces Endocrine and Immunologic Disorders in Women," *American Journal of Obstetrics and Gynecology,* vol. 165, no. 2 (Aug. 1991), pp. 487–88; and P. Thompkins, "Hazards of Electromagnetic Fields to Human Reproduction," *Fertility and Sterility,* vol. 53, no. 1 (Jan. 1990), pp. 185.

21. A. Stagnaw-Green et al., "Detection of At Risk Pregnancy by Means of Highly Sensitive Assays for Thyroid Autoantibodies," *Journal of the American Medical Association,* vol. 269, no. 11 (Sept. 19, 1990), pp. 1422–25; and O. B. Christiansen et al., "Autoimmunity and Spontaneous Abortion," *Human Reproduction* [Denmark], vol. 4, no. 8 (1989), pp. 913–17.

22. Ellen Hopkins, "Tales from the Baby Factory," *The New York Times Magazine* (Mar. 15, 1992).

23. Karl Menninger, "Somatic Correlations with the Unconscious Repudiation of Femininity in Women," *Journal of Nervous and Mental Disease,* vol. 89 (1939), p. 514; Therese Benedek and Boris Rubenstein, "Correlations Between Ovarian Activity and Psychodynamic Processes: The Ovulatory Phase," *Psychosomatic*

Medicine, vol. 1, no. 2 (1939), pp. 245–70; and A. Mayer, "Sterility in Women as a Result of Functional Disturbance," *Journal of the American Medical Association,* vol. 105 (1935), p. 1474.

24. Therese Benedek et al., "Some Emotional Factors in Infertility," *Psychosomatic Medicine,* vol. 15, no. 5 (1953), pp. 485–98.

25. Havelock Ellis, *Studies in the Psychology of Sex* (Philadelphia: Davis and Co., 1928); T. H. Van de Veld, *Fertility and Sterility in Marriage* (New York: Covici-Fried, 1931).

26. D. Levy, "Maternal Overprotection," *Journal of Psychiatry,* vol. 2 (1939), p. 563; R. P. Knight, "Some Problems Involved in Selecting and Rearing Adopted Children," *Bulletin of Menninger Clinic,* vol. 5 (1941), p. 65.

27. T. E. Mandy and A. J. Mandy, "Psychosomatic Aspects of Infertility," *International Journal of Fertility,* vol. 3 (1958), p. 287; H. R. Cohen, "The Psychosomatic Factor in Infertility," *International Journal of Fertility,* vol. 6 (1961), p. 396; and A. W. McLeod, "Some Psychogenic Aspects of Infertility," *Fertility and Sterility,* vol. 15 (1969), p. 124.

28. H. F. Dunbar, *Emotions and Bodily Changes* (New York: Columbia University Press, 1935), p. 595; R. L. Dickerson, "Medical Analysis of 1000 Marriages," *Journal of the American Medical Association,* vol. 97 (1931), p. 529; and C. C. Norris, "Sterility in the Female Without Gross Pathology," *Surgery, Gynecology, and Obstetrics,* vol. 15 (1912), p. 706.

29. D. H. Hellhammer et al., "Male Infertility, Relationships Among Gonadotropins, Sex Steroids, Seminal Parameters, and Personality Attitudes," *Psychosomatic Medicine,* vol. 47, no. 1 (1985), pp. 58–66.

30. Niravi Payne can be contacted by writing 100 Remsen, Brooklyn, NY 11201 or telephoning (800) 666-HEALTH or (718) 625-4802.

31. E. Dewan, "On the Possibility of a Perfect Rhythm Method of Birth Control by Periodic Light Stimulation," *American Journal of Obstetrics and Gynecology,* vol. 99, no. 7 (Dec. 1, 1967), pp. 1016–19. See also notes for Chapter 5, "The Menstrual Cycle."

32. E. R. Gonzalez, "Sperm Swim Singly after Vitamin C Therapy," *Journal of the American Medical Association,* vol. 20 (1983), p. 2747; T. R. Hartoma et al., "Zinc, Plasma Androgens, and Male Sterility," letter to the editor, *Lancet,* vol. 3 (1977), pp. 1125–26; M. Igarashi, "Augmentative Effects of Ascorbic Acid upon Induction of Human Ovulation in Clomiphene Ineffective Anovulatory Women," *International Journal of Fertility,* vol. 22, no. 3 (1977), pp. 68–73; and D. W. Dawson, "Infertility and Folate Deficiency," case reports, *British Journal of Obstetrics and Gynaecology,* vol. 89 (1982), p. 678.

33. J. Hargrove and E. Guy, "Effect of Vitamin B_6 on Infertility in Women with Premenstrual Tension Syndrome," *Infertility,* vol. 2, no. 4 (1979), pp. 315–22.

34. D. E. Stewart et al., "Infertility and Eating Disorders," *American Journal of Obstetrics and Gynecology,* vol. 163 (1990), pp. 1196–99.

35. Alan DeCherney, quoted in *The New York Times Magazine.*

36. Hopkins, "Tales from the Baby Factory" (see note 22).

37. A. Blau et al., "The Psychogenic Etiology of Premature Births," *Psychosomatic Medicine*, vol. 25 (1963), p. 201; Robert J. Weil, "The Problem of Spontaneous Abortion," *American Journal of Obstetrics and Gynecology*, vol. 73 (1957), p. 322.

38. Robert J. Weil and C. Tupper, "Personality, Life Situation, Communication: A Study of Habitual Abortion," *Psychosomatic Medicine*, vol. 22, no. 6 (1960), pp. 448–55.

39. Weil and Tupper, "Personality" (see note 38).

40. E. R. Grimm, "Psychological Investigation of Habitual Abortion," *Psychosomatic Medicine*, vol. 24, no. 4 (1962), pp. 370–78.

41. R. L. VandenBergh, "Emotional Illness in Habitual Aborters Following Suturing of Incompetent Cervical Os," *Psychosomatic Medicine*, vol. 28, no. 3 (1966), pp. 257–63.

42. Lucia Cappachione, *The Wisdom of Your Other Hand* (North Hollywood, CA: Newcastle Publishing Co., 1990).

43. For more information write Whitney Oppersdorff at the following address: RR #2, Box 606, Lincolnville, ME 04849.

44. Union of Concerned Scientists, 26 Church Street, Cambridge, MA 02238; telephone (617) 547-5552.

Chapter 12: Pregnancy and Birthing

1. U.S. Department of Health, Education, and Welfare, the National Center for Health Statistics, *Wanted and Unwanted Births by Mothers 15–44 Years of Age: United States, 1973* (Washington, DC: U.S. Government Printing Office, 1973); advance data from *Vital and Health Statistics*, no. 9 (Aug. 10, 1977); National Institutes of Health, Institute of Child Health and Human Development, research reports (Nov. 1992), available from NICHD Office of Research Reporting, building 31, room 2A312, National Institutes of Health, Bethesda, MD 20892; tel. (301) 496-5133; M. D. Muylder et al., "A Woman's Attitude Toward Pregnancy: Can It Predispose Her to Preterm Labor?" *Journal of Reproductive Medicine*, vol. 37, no. 4 (Apr. 1992); R. Newton and L. Hunt, "Psychosocial Stress in Pregnancy and Its Relationship to Low Birth Weight," *British Medical Journal*, vol. 288 (1984), p. 1191.

2. G. Berkowitz and S. Kasl, "The Role of Psychosocial Factors in Spontaneous Preterm Delivery," *Journal of Psychosomatic Research*, vol. 27 (1983), p. 283; R. Newton et al., "Psychosocial Stress in Pregnancy and Its Relation to the Onset of Premature Labour," *British Medical Journal*, vol. 2 (1979), p. 411; A. Blau et al., "The Psychogenic Etiology of Premature Births: A Preliminary Report," *Psychosomatic Medicine*, vol. 25 (1963), p. 201.

3. V. Laukaran and C. Van Den Berg, "The Relationship of Maternal Attitude to Pregnancy Outcomes and Obstetric Complications: A Cohort Study of Unwanted Pregnancies," *American Journal of Obstetrics and Gynecology*, vol. 139 (1981), p. 956; R. McDonald, "The Role of Emotional Factors in Obstetric Complications," *Psychosomatic Medicine*, vol. 30 (1968), p. 222; M.D. De

Muylder, "Psychological Factors and Preterm Labour," *Journal of Reproductive Psychology*, vol. 7 (1989), p. 55.

4. R. Myers, "Maternal Anxiety and Fetal Death," in L. Zichella and P. Pancheri, eds., *Psychoneuroendocrinology and Reproduction* (New York: Elsevier, 1979).

5. E. Muller-Tyl and B. Wimmer-Puchinger, "Psychosomatic Aspects of Toxemia," *Journal of Psychosomatic Obstetrics and Gynecology*, vol. 1, nos. 3–4, (1982), pp. 111–17; C. Ringrose, "Psychosomatic Influence in the Genesis of Toxemia of Pregnancy," *Canadian Medical Association Journal*, vol. 84 (1961), p. 647; and A. J. Copper, "Psychosomatic Aspects of Pre-eclamptic Toxemia," *Journal of Psychosomatic Research*, vol. 2 (1958), p. 241.

6. R. L. McDonald, "Personality Characteristics in Patients with Three Obstetric Complications," *Psychosomatic Medicine*, vol. 27, no. 4 (1965), pp. 383–90.

7. Katz et al., "Catecholamine Levels in Pregnant Physicians and Nurses: A Pilot Study of Stress and Pregnancy," *Obstetrics and Gynecology*, vol. 77, no. 3 (Mar. 1991), pp. 338–41.

8. Judith Levitt, *Brought to Bed: Childbearing in America, 1750–1950* (New York: Oxford University Press, 1988).

9. R. Sosa et al., "The Effect of Supportive Companions on Perinatal Problems, Length of Labor, and Mother-Infant Interaction," *New England Journal of Medicine*, vol. 303 (1980), pp. 597–600; M. H. Klaus, J. H. Kennell, S. S. Robertson, and R. Sosa, "Effects of Social Support During Parturition in Maternal and Infant Mortality," *British Medical Journal*, vol. 293 (1986), pp. 585–87; M. H. Klaus, J. H. Kennell, G. Berkowitz, and P. Klaus, "Maternal Assistance and Support in Labor: Father, Nurse, Midwife, or Doula?" *Clinical Consultation in Obstetrics and Gynecology*, vol. 4 (Dec. 1992).

10. F. T. Kapp et al., "Some Psychological Factors in Prolonged Labor Due to Inefficient Uterine Action," *Comparative Psychiatry*, vol. 4 (1963), p. 9; L. Gunter, "Psychopathology and Stress in the Life Experience of Mothers of Premature Infants," *American Journal of Obstetrics and Gynecology*, vol. 86 (1963), p. 333; A. Davids and S. Devault, "Maternal Anxiety During Pregnancy and Childbirth Abnormalities," *Journal of Psychosomatic Medicine*, vol. 24, (1972), p. 464.

11. J. J. Oat et al., "Characteristics and Motives of Women Choosing Elective Induction of Labor," *Journal of Psychosomatic Research*, vol. 30, no. 3 (1986), pp. 375–80.

12. Cited in Gayle H. Peterson, *Birthing Normally: A Personal Approach to Childbirth* (Berkeley, CA: Mindbody Press, 1981), appendix 2, pp. 181–99. See also Lewis Mehl, Gayle Peterson et al., "Complications of Home Delivery: Analysis of a Series of 287 Deliveries from Santa Cruz, California," *Birth and Family Journal*, vol. 2, no. 4 (1975), pp. 123–31; and Gayle Peterson, Lewis Mehl, et al., "Outcome of 1146 Elective Home Births," *Journal of Reproductive Medicine*, vol. 19, no. 3 (1977), pp. 281–90.

13. Data are from the Houston Healthcare Coalition, Houston, Texas (1986); Personal communications with Dr. Bethany Hays.

14. Luthy Shy et al., "Effects of Electronic Fetal Heart Rate Monitoring, As Compared with Periodic Auscultation, on the Neurologic Development of Premature Infants," *New England Journal of Medicine* (Mar. 1, 1990).

15. S. Gardner, "When Your Patient Demands a C-Section," *OBG Management*, (Nov. 1991).

16. Wilcox et al., "Episiotomy and Its Role in the Incidence of Perineal Lacerations in a Maternity Center and a Tertiary Hospital Obstetric Service," *American Journal of Obstetrics and Gynecology*, vol. 160 (1989), pp. 1047–52.

17. Data are from Watson Bowes, "Should Routine Episiotomy Be Performed Routinely in Primiparous Women?" *Ob/Gyn Forum*, vol. 5, no. 4 (1991), pp. 1–4.

18. P. Shiono et al., "Midline Episiotomies: More Harm than Good," *American Journal of Obstetrics and Gynecology*, vol. 75, no. 5 (May 1990), pp. 765–70.

19. Walker et al., "Epidural Anesthesia, Episiotomy, and Obstetric Laceration," *American Journal of Obstetrics and Gynecology*, vol. 77, no. 5 (May 1991), pp. 668–71.

20. James Thorpe et al., "The Effect of Continuous Epidural Anesthesia on Cesarean Sections for Dystocia in Primiparous Patients," *American Journal of Obstetrics and Gynecology* (Sept. 1989); H. Kaminski, A. Stafl, and J. Aiman, "The Effect of Epidural Analgesia on the Frequency of Instrumental Obstetric Delivery," *American Journal of Obstetrics and Gynecology*, vol. 69, no. 5 (May 1987); L. Fusi, P. J. Steer, M. J. A. Maresh, and R. W. Bears, "Maternal Pyrexia Associated with the Use of Epidural Analgesia in Labour," *Lancet* (1989), pp. 1250–52.

21. Jeanne Achterberg, *Woman as Healer* (Boston: Shambhala, 1990), p. 126.

22. Known as the McRoberts Maneuver, this can be demonstrated by bringing your legs up into a "squatting position" while lying on your back.

23. Membranes rarely rupture from pelvic examinations. Perhaps mine did because of an unusual umbilical cord insertion on the membranes, known as a villamentous insertion. Or maybe they were just ready to go!

24. As we will see, being "distracted" in the middle of a process as important as labor may not be the best approach.

25. Vicki Noble, *Shakti Woman* (San Francisco: Harper and Row, 1992).

Chapter 13: Motherhood: Bonding with Your Baby

1. Marshall H. Klaus and John H. Kennell, *Maternal-Infant Bonding* (St. Louis: C. V. Mosby Company, 1976).

2. Marshall Klaus and John Kennell, *Parent-Infant Bonding* (C.V. Mosby Company: St. Louis, MO, 1982).

3. Stephanie Field, *Science News*, vol. 127 (Dec. 9, 1985).

4. Actually, the first studies on putting babies in incubators were done on premature babies who weren't expected to live and who therefore had been "discarded" by their mothers. Martin Cooney, a pioneer in neonatal care, put a group of these infants in incubators and toured with them, even to the Chicago

World's Fair, where he had an attraction called "Live Babies in Incubator"; its receipts were second only to those of Sally Rand the Fan Dancer. Once he got the babies to a certain weight, he tried to give them back to their mothers, but the mothers didn't want them, having formed no emotional tie with them. This information is from Klaus and Kennell, *Maternal/Infant Bonding.*

5. George Dennison, "Unnecessary Circumcision," *Female Patient,* vol. 17 (July 1992), p. 13.

6. Data on the effects of circumcision are available from the Circumcision Resource Center, attn. Ronald Goldman, P.O. Box 232, Boston, MA 02133; tel. (617) 523-0088.

7. E. E. Ziegler et al., "Cow's Milk Feeding in Infancy: Further Observations on Blood Loss from the Gastrointestinal Tract," *Journal of Pediatrics,* vol. 116 (1990), pp. 11–18.

8. Frank Oski, *Don't Drink Your Milk* (Syracuse, NY: Mollica Press, 1983), available from Teach Services, Route 1, Box 182, Brushton, NY 12916; tel. (800) 367-1844.

9. A. Lucas et al., "Breast Milk and Subsequent Intelligence Quotient in Children Born Preterm," *Lancet* (Feb. 1, 1992), pp. 261–64.

10. Ellen Goodman, "Search for Father Dominating Lives," *Portland Press Herald* (Apr. 10, 1992), syndicated from *Boston Globe.*

11. Nancy McBrine Sheehan, 11 Fox Run, East Sandwich, MA 02537; used here with the author's permission.

Chapter 14: Menopause

1. Quoted in Tamara Slayton, *Reclaiming the Menstrual Matrix: Evolving Feminine Wisdom—A Workbook* (Petaluma, CA: Menstrual Health Foundation, 1990), p. 39.

2. Slayton, *Reclaiming,* p. 41 (see note 1).

3. Slayton, *Reclaiming,* p. 41 (see note 1).

4. Jerilynn Prior, "Critique of Estrogen Treatment for Heart Attack Prevention: The Nurses Health Study," *A Friend Indeed,* vol. 8, no. 8 (Jan. 1992), pp. 3–4.

5. Emily Martin, "Medical Metaphors of Women's Bodies: Menstruation and Menopause," *International Journal of Health Services,* vol. 18, no. 2 (1988). This article originally appeared as chap. 3 in Emily Martin, *The Woman in the Body: A Cultural Analysis of Reproduction* (Boston: Beacon Press, 1987).

6. C. Longscope, R. Hunter, and C. Franz, "Steroid Secretion by the Postmenopausal Ovary," *American Journal of Obstetrics and Gynecology,* vol. 138 (1980), pp. 564–68; C. Longscope, C. Bourget, and C. Flood, "The Production and Aromatization of Dehydroepiandrosterone in Postmenopausal Women," *Maturitas,* vol. 4 (1982), pp. 325–32.

7. C. Longscope, W. Jaffe, and G. Griffing, "Production Rates of Androgens and Oestrogens in Post-Menopausal Women," *Maturitas,* vol. 3 (1981), pp. 215–23.

8. C. B. Coulam, S. C. Adamson, and J. F. Annegers, "Incidence of Premature Ovarian Failure," *American Journal of Obstetrics and Gynecology,* vol. 67, no. 4 (1986).

9. M. des Moraes Ruehsen et al., "Autoimmunity and Ovarian Failure," *American Journal of Obstetrics and Gynecology,* vol. 112, no. 5 (1972); T. Miyake et al., "Acute Oocyte Loss in Experimental Autoimmune Oophoritis as a Possible Model of Premature Ovarian Failure," *American Journal of Obstetrics and Gynecology,* vol. 158, no. 1 (1988); "Evidence of Autoimmune Etiology in Some Premature Menopause," *ObGyn News* (Nov. 1985); M. Leer, B. Patel, M. Innes, and D. P. Cameron, "Secondary Amenorrhea Due to Autoimmune Ovarian Failure," *Australia and New Zealand Journal of Obstetrics and Gynecology,* vol. 20 (1980), pp. 177–79; Hurlimann J. Gloor, "Autoimmune Oophoritis," *American Journal of Clinical Pathology,* vol. 81 (1984), pp. 105–9; and C. B. Coulam, "Premature Gonadal Failure," *Fertility and Sterility,* vol. 38 (1982), p. 645.
10. L. L. Doyle et al., "Human Luteal Function Following Hysterectomy as Assessed by Plasma Progestin," *American Journal of Obstetrics and Gynecology,* vol. 110 (1971); N. Siddle, P. Sarrel, and M. Whitehead, "The Effect of Hysterectomy on the Age of Ovarian Failure: Identification of a Subgroup of Women with Premature Loss of Ovarian Function and Literature Review," *Fertility and Sterility,* vol. 47, no. 1 (1987).
11. I. Cohen and L. Speroff, "Premature Ovarian Failure: Update," *Obstetrics and Gynecologic Survey,* vol. 47, no. 3 (1981).
12. T. T. Hung et al., "Artificially Induced Menstrual Cycle with Natural Estradiol and Progesterone," *Fertility and Sterility,* vol. 51, no. 6 (1989).
13. From an essay by Ann Wright, quoted in Ann Voda, Myra Dinnerstein, and Cheryl R. O'Donnell, eds., *Changing Perspectives on Menopause* (Austin: University of Texas Press, 1982).
14. Data cited in Judith K. Brown and Virginia Kerns, eds., *In Her Prime: A New View of Middle-Aged Women* (Amherst, MA: Bergin and Garvey, 1985).
15. Vicki Noble, *Shakti Woman* (Harper San Francisco, 1992).
16. Susun Weed, *Menopausal Years: The Wise Woman's Way: Alternative Approaches for Women 30–90* (Woodstock, NY: Ash Tree Publishing, 1992), available from Ash Tree Publishing, P.O. Box 64, Woodstock, NY 12498.
17. Weed, *Menopausal Years* (see note 16).
18. Raul Ruz and Walter Stamm, "A Controlled Trial of Intravaginal Estriol in Post-Menopausal Women with Recurrent Urinary Tract Infections," *New England Journal of Medicine,* vol. 329, no. 11 (Sept. 9, 1993), pp. 753–56.
19. Jerilynn Prior et al., "Progesterone and the Prevention of Osteoporosis," *Canadian Journal of Ob/Gyn and Women's Health Care,* vol. 3, no. 4 (1991), pp. 178–83.
20. The U.S. National Center for Health Statistics, *Health and Nutritional Examination Survey* (HANES 1 Survey), conducted between 1971 and 1975, showed a high prevalence (6 to 18 percent) of abnormally low cortical bone density in women. See also J. Mangaroo, J. H. Glasser, W. Roht, and A. S. Kapadia, "Prevalence of Bone Demineralization in the United States," *Bone,* vol. 6 (1985), pp. 135–39.
21. W. A. Wallace, "The Increasing Incidence of Fractures of the Proximal Femur:

An Orthopaedic Epidemic," *Lancet*, (1983), p. 1413; and editorial, "More People Are Fracturing More Bones More Often," *Nutritional Review*, vol. 49 (1991), p. 25.

22. L. Avioli, "Osteoporosis: A Growing National Health Problem," *Female Patient*, vol. 17 (Sept. 1992), p. 84.

23. M. E. Farmer, L. R. White, J. A. Brody, and K. R. Bailey, "Race and Sex Differences in Hip Fracture Incidence," *American Journal of Public Health*, vol. 74 (1984), pp. 1374–80.

24. R. A. Owen, L. J. Melton, J. C. Gallaher, and B. L. Riggs, "The National Cost of Acute Care of Hip Fractures Associated with Osteoporosis," *Clinical Orthopedics*, vol. 150 (1980), p. 175.

25. M. Hernandez-Avila et al., "Caffeine, Moderate Alcohol Intake, and Risk of Fracture of the Hip and Forearm in Middle-Aged Women," *American Journal of Clinical Nutrition*, vol. 54 (1991), pp. 157–63.

26. D. E. Nelson, R. W. Suttin, J. A. Langois, C. A. DeVito, and J. A. Stevens, "Alcohol as a Risk Factor for Fall Injury Events Among Elderly Persons Living in the Community," *Journal of Geriatric Society*, vol. 40 (1992), pp. 658–61.

27. J. M. Gertner, "Pregnancy as a State of Physiologic Absorptive Hypercalcinuria," *American Journal of Medicine*, vol. 81 (1986), pp. 451–56.

28. M. Sowers et al., "A Prospective Evaluation of Bone Mineral Change in Pregnancy," vol. 77, no. 6 (June 1991), pp. 841–45.

29. J. C. Prior, "Spinal Bone Loss and Ovulatory Disturbances," *New England Journal of Medicine*, vol. 323 (1990), pp. 1221–27; R. Marcus et al., "Menstrual Function and Bone Mass in Elite Women Distance Runners," *Annals of Internal Medicine*, vol. 102 (1985), pp. 158–63; C. E. Cann, M. C. Martin, and R. B. Jaffe, "Decreased Spinal Mineral Content in Amenorrheic Women," *Journal of the American Medical Association*, vol. 25, no. 5 (Feb. 3, 1984), pp. 626–29; J. S. Lindberg, M. R. Powell, Hund, et al., "Increased Vertebral Bone Mineral in Response to Reduced Exercise in Amenorrheic Runners," *Western Journal of Medicine*, vol. 146 (1987), pp. 39–42.

30. Part of the reason for this focus is that natural progesterone and even synthetic progestin are generic drugs that cannot be patented. It currently costs about $3 million to get a new drug approved for use by the FDA. If a drug company cannot expect to make a profit on a particular drug, it makes no sense for it to do the necessary studies. This is another reason that so many "natural" remedies have not been studied nearly as well as drugs have. See also J. C. Prior et al., "Progesterone as a Bone-Tropic Hormone," *Endocrine Reviews*, vol. 11 (1990), pp. 386–98; and G. R. Snow and C. Anderson, "The Effect of 17 Beta Estradiol and Progestogen on Trabecular Bone Remodeling in Oophorectomized Dogs," *Calcification Tissue*, vol. 39 (1986), pp. 198–205.

31. J. McCann, N. Horwitz, "Provera Alone Builds Bone," *Medical Tribune*, (July 22, 1987), pp. 4–5; H. I. Abdalla, D. M. Hart, D. Purdee, et al., "Prevention of Bone Mineral Loss in Postmenopausal Women by Norethisterone," *Obstetrics*

and Gynecology, vol. 66 (1985), pp. 789–92; R. Lindsay, D. M. Hart, D. Purdee et al., "Comparative Effectiveness of Estrogen and a Progestogen on Bone Loss in Post Menopausal Women," *Clinical Science Molecular Medicine,* vol. 54 (1978), pp. 93–95; Dequeker and DeMuyider, "Longterm Progestogen Treatment and Bone Remodeling In Premenopausal Women: A Longitudinal Study," *Maturitas,* vol. 4 (1982), pp. 309–13; B. L. Riggs, J. Jowsey, P. J. Kelly et al., "Effect of Sex Hormones in Bone in Primary Osteoporosis," *Journal of Clinical Investigation,* vol. 48 (1969), pp. 1065–72.

32. John R. Lee, "Osteoporosis Reversal: The Role of Progesterone," *Clinical Nutritional Review,* vol. 10 (1990), pp. 884–89; J. R. Lee, "Is Natural Progesterone the Missing Link in Osteoporosis Prevention and Treatment," *Medical Hypotheses,* vol. 35 (1991), pp. 316–18; J. R. Lee, "Osteoporosis Reversal with Transdermal Progesterone," *Lancet,* vol. 336 (1990), p. 1327.

33. C. C. Johnston, S. Slemenda, and L. J. Melton, "Clinical Use of Bone Densitometry," *New England Journal of Medicine,* vol. 324, no. 16 (Apr. 1991), pp. 1105–9.

34. This program was originally developed and tested by Dr. John Lee. As presented here, it also includes my additions.

35. F. H. Nielsen et al., "Effects of Dietary Boron on Mineral, Estrogen, and Testosterone Metabolism in Post-menopausal Women," *Federation of American Societies for Experimental Biology Journal,* vol. 1 (1987), pp. 394–97; J. U. Reginster et al., "Preliminary Report of Decreased Serum Magnesium in Postmenopausal Osteoporosis," *Magnesium,* vol. 8, no. 2 (1989) pp. 106–9; F. H. Nielsen, "Studies on the Relationship Between Boron and Magnesium Which Possibly Affects the Formation and Maintenance of Bones," *Magnesium Trace Elements,* vol. 9, no. 2 (1990), pp. 61–91.

36. J. R. Willson, "Sexuality in Aging," in J. J. Sciarra, ed., *Gynecology and Obstetrics* (Philadelphia: Harper and Row, 1987), pp. 1–12.

37. G. A. Bachmann, "Correlates of Sexual Desire in Postmenopausal Women," *Maturitas,* vol. 7, no. 3 (1985), p. 211; cited in David Youngs, "Common Misconceptions About Sex and Depression During Menopause: A Historical Perspective," *Female Patient,* vol. 17 (Apr. 1992), pp. 25–28.

38. J. Pfenninger, "Sex and the Maturing Female," *Mature Health* (Jan.-Feb. 1987), pp. 12–15; and William Masters and Virginia Johnson, *Human Sexual Response* (Boston: Little, Brown and Co., 1966), pp. 117, 238.

39. Mantak Chia and Maneewan Chia, *Cultivating Female Sexual Energy: Healing Love Through the Tao* (Huntington, NY: Healing Tao Books, 1986); available from Healing Tao Books, 2 Creskill Place, Huntington, NY 11743.

40. Personal communication with Dr. Alan Gaby, a specialist in nutritional medicine.

41. J. K. Meyers, M. M. Weissman, and G. L. Tischler, "Six-Month Prevalence of Psychiatric Disorder in Three Communities," *Archives General Psychiatry,* vol. 41 (1984), p. 959.

42. McKinley, McKinlay, and Bramblilla, "Health Status and Utilization Behavior

Associated with Menopause," *American Journal of Epidemiology,* vol. 125 (1987), p. 110.

43. Marian Van Eck McCain, *Transformation Through Menopause* (Amherst, MA: Begin and Garvey, 1991).

44. Marguerite Holloway, "The Estrogen Factor," *Scientific American* (June 1992).

45. Lecture notes from Grand Rounds presentation, Maine Medical Center (June 20, 1990).

46. L. Bergkvist, H. O. Adami, L. Persson et al., "The Risk of Breast Cancer After Estrogen and Estrogen-Progestin Replacement," *New England Journal of Medicine,* vol. 321 (1989), pp. 293–97.

47. Siller-Arenas et al., "Menopausal Hormone Replacement Therapy and Breast Cancer: A Meta-Analysis," *Obstetrics and Gynecology,* vol. 79, no. 2 (Feb. 1992); G. A. Colditz et al., "Prospective Study of Estrogen Replacement Therapy and Risk of Breast Cancer in Postmenopausal Women," *Journal of the American Medical Association,* vol. 264 (1990), pp. 2648–52.

48. R. D. Gambrell, Jr., "Complications of Estrogen Replacement Therapy," in D. P. Swartz, ed., *Hormone Replacement Therapy* (Baltimore, MD: Williams and Wilkins, 1992), Chapter 9.

49. Alan Gaby, *Preventing and Reversing Osteoporosis* (Rocklin, CA: Prima Publications, 1994), p. 139 of manuscript.

50. In fact, some data indicate that estrogen treatment may increase the risk for heart disease, not prevent it.

51. Jerilynn Prior, letter to the editor, "Postmenopausal Estrogen Therapy and Cardiovascular Disease," *New England Journal of Medicine,* vol. 326, no. 10 (1992), pp. 705–7.

52. H. Aldercreutz et al., "Dietary Phyto-oestrogens and the Menopause in Japan," *Lancet,* vol. 339 (1992), p. 1233.

53. C. A. B. Clemetson, S. J. DeCarol, G. A. Burney, T. J. Patel, N. Kozhiashvili et al., "Estrogens in Food: The Almond Mystery," *International Journal of Gynecology and Obstetrics,* vol. 15 (1978), pp. 515–21; S. O. Elakovich and J. Hampton, "Analysis of Couvaestrol, a Phytoestrogen, in Alpha Tablets Sold for Human Consumption," *Journal of Agricultural Food Chemistry,* vol. 32 (1984), pp. 173–75.

54. L. Zussman et al., "Sexual Response after Hysterectomy-Oophorectomy: Recent Studies and Reconsideration of Psychogenesis," *American Journal of Obstetrics and Gynecology,* vol. 140, no. 7 (Aug. 1, 1981), pp. 725–29.

55. Henry Lemon et al., "Reduced Estriol Excretion in Patients with Breast Cancer Prior to Endocrine Therapy," *Journal of the American Medical Association,* vol. 196 (1966), pp. 1128–36.

56. H. H. Wotiz, D. R. Beebe, E. Muller, "Effect of Estrogens on DMBA-Induced Breast Tumors," *Journal of Steroid Biochemistry,* vol. 20 (Rp. 1984) pp. 1067–75; H. M. Lemon, "Estriol Prevention of Mammary Carcinoma Induced by 7, 12-Dimethylbenzanthracene and Procarbazine," *Cancer Research,* vol. 35 (1975), pp. 1341–53; Henry Lemon, "Pathophysiologic Considerations in the Treat-

ment of Menopausal Patients with Oestrogens; The Role of Oestriol in the Prevention of Mammary Carcinoma." *Acta Endocrinologica*, suppl, vol. 233 (1980) pp. 17–27.

57. H. M. Lemon, H. H. Wotiz, L. Parsons, and P. J. Mozden, "Reduced Estriol Excretion in Patients with Breast Cancer Prior to Endocrine Therapy," *Journal of the American Medical Association*, vol. 196 (1966), pp. 1128–36.

58. L. Speroff, "The Breast as an Endocrine Target Organ," *Contemporary Obstetrics and Gynecology*, vol. 9 (1977) pp. 69–72; and P. D. Bulbrook, M. C. Swain, and D. Y. Wang et al., "Breast Cancer in Britain and Japan: Plasma Oestradiol-17B Oestrone, and Progesterone, and Their Urinary Metabolites in Normal British and Japanese Women," *European Journal of Cancer*, vol. 12 (1976) pp. 725–35.

59. IpC, "Dietary Vitamin E Intake and Mammary Carcinogenesis in Rats," *Carcinogenesis*, vol. 3 (1982), pp. 1453–56.

60. R. S. London, et al., "Endocrine Parameters and Alpha-Tocopherol Therapy of Patients with Mammary Dysplasia," *Cancer Research*, vol. 41 (1981), pp. 3811–13.

61. L. Speroff. See note 58.

62. Dr. Lemon's study was unpublished by itself but is reported in Alvin Follingstad, "Estriol, The Forgotten Hormone," *Journal of the American Medical Association*, vol. 239 no. 1 (Jan. 2, 1978) pp. 29–30. See also, Henry Lemon, "Clinical and Experimental Aspects of the Anti-Mammary Carcinogenic Activity of Estriol," *Frontiers of Hormonal Research*, vol. 5 no. 1 (1977), pp. 155–73; and Henry Lemon, "Oestriol and Prevention of Breast Cancer," *Lancet*, vol. 1, no. 802 (Mar. 10, 1973), pp. 546–47.

63. V. A. Tzingounis, M. F. Aksu and R. B. Greenblatt, "Estriol in the Management of the Menopause," *Journal of the American Medical Association*, vol. 239 (1978), pp. 1638–41.

64. R. Punnonen, S. Vilsak, and L. Rauramo, "Skinfold Thickness and Long-Term Postmenopausal Hormone Therapy," *Maturitas*, vol. 4 (Apr. 5, 1984), pp. 259–62.

65. A. L. Kirkengen, P. Andersen, E. Gjersoe, G. R. Johannessen, N. Johnsen, E. Bodd, "Oestriol in the Prophylactic Treatment of Recurrent Urinary Tract Infections in Postmenopausal Women," *Scandinavian Journal Primary Health Care*, (June 10, 1992), pp. 139–42; and G. M. Heimer, D. E. Englund, "Effects of Vaginally-Administered Oestriol on Postmenopausal Urogenital Disorders: a Cytohormonal Study," *Maturitas*, vol. 3 (Mar. 14, 1992), pp. 171–79; and C. S. Iosif, "Effects of Protracted Administration of Estriol on the Lower Urinary Tract in Postmenopausal Women," *Archives of Gynecology and Obstetrics*, vol. 3, no. 251 (1992), pp. 115–20; and M. van Haaften, G. H. Donker, A. A. Haspeis, J. H. Thijssen, "Oestrogen Concentrations in Plasma, Endometrium, Myometrium, and Vagina of Postmenopausal Women, and Effects of Vaginal Oestriol (E3) and Oestradiol (E2) Applications," *Journal of Steroid Biochemistry*, vol. 4A (October 1989), pp. 647–53.

66. V. A. Tzingounis, see note 63, p. 1638.

67. As with natural progesterone, I suspect that its under-utilization in this country is related to the politics and economics of the pharmaceutical industry.

68. P. Stumf, "Estrogen Replacement Therapy: Current Regimens." In D. P. Swartz, ed., *Hormones Replacement Therapy* (Baltimore, MD: Williams and Williams, 1992), p. 183. Cited in Alan Gaby.

69. Personal communication with Dr. Jonathan Wright, and also Alan Gaby, *Preventing and Reversing Osteoporosis* (Rocklin, CA: Prima Publications), pp. 145–46.

70. J. Hargrove et al., "Menopausal Hormone Replacement Therapy with Continuous Daily Oral Micronized Estradiol and Progesterone," *Obstetrics and Gynecology,* vol. 73, no. 4 (Apr. 1989), pp. 606–12.

71. Dr. Isaac Schiff, lecture at Maine Medical Center (June 1990).

72. Susun Weed, from an introductory flyer for *Menopausal Years, The Wise Woman's Way* (Woodstock, NY: Ash Tree Publications, 1992).

73. Clarissa Pinkola Estes, "The Dancing Grandmas," *Common Boundary* (Mar.-Apr. 1993), pp. 38–41.

Chapter 15: Steps for Healing

1. Leslie Kussman, personal communication (May 6, 1992), before filming *Harbour of Hope,* a documentary about those who have healed from chronic or terminal illness. For information write Aquarius Productions, 31 Martin Road, Wellesley, MA 02181; tel. (617) 237-0608.

2. Joe Dominguez and Vicki Robin, *Your Money or Your Life* (New York: Viking, 1992); and Joe Dominguez, "Transforming Your Relationship with Money and Creating Financial Independence," brochure; write to New Road Map Foundation, P.O. Box 15981, Seattle, WA 98115.

3. Exercise adapted from a workshop author participated in with Annie Gill O'Toole. Annie Gill O'Toole is the author of the book *Choosing Life*, which contains many other helpful exercises for achieving health. Available from Lighthouse, International, 24 Wilson Street, Unit #3, Marlborough, MA 01752.

4. At one of my workshops a black woman from Atlanta told me that her women's group simply calls this deep work "the process." She had never heard of Anne Wilson Schaef or her work.

5. Anne Wilson Schaef, mixed intensive, Hermet, CA (Oct. 1987).

6. Naomi Wolf has documented the tragic aspects of this in *The Beauty Myth* (New York: Morrow, 1990).

7. Michael Marron, *Instant Makeover Magic* (New York: Rawson Associates, 1983).

8. Pythia Peay, "The Presence of Angels," *Common Boundary* (Jan.-Feb. 1991), p. 31.

9. Frances Scovell Shinn, *The Game of Life and How to Play It* (Marina del Rey, CA: DeVorss and Co., 1925).

10. Patricia Reis, author of *Through the Goddess* (Freedom, CA: Crossing Press,

1991), worked with us at Women to Women for four years, teaching us the deep patterns held in women's psyches and bodies.

11. K. Vogel and Vicki Noble, *The Motherpeace Round Tarot Deck* (U.S. Games Systems, Inc., 1983).

12. Vicki Noble, *Motherpeace: A Way to the Goddess Through Myth, Art, and Tarot* (Harper San Francisco, 1983).

13. An in-depth approach to this is available in Vicki Noble, *Shakti Woman* (Harper San Francisco, 1992).

14. Interview with Natalie Goldberg, by Cat Saunders, *The Sun,* Chapel Hill, NC, 1991, p. 9.

15. For more information, write to the Proprioceptive Writing Center, P.O. Box 83333, Portland, ME 05102; tel. (207) 772-1847.

16. Natalie Goldberg, *Writing Down the Bones* (New York: Bantam, 1987); Natalie Goldberg, *Wild Mind* (New York: Bantam, 1990).

17. "Rediscovering the Wild Woman," interview with Clarissa Pinkola Estes, by Peggy Taylor, *New Age Journal* (Dec. 1992), pp. 60–65.

18. Dream incubation is adapted from the work of Patricia Reis.

19. Peter Rutter, *Sex in the Forbidden Zone* (Los Angeles: Jeremy Tarcher).

20. Anne Wilson Schaef, *Beyond Therapy, Beyond Science* (Harper San Francisco, 1992).

21. Boston Women's Health Book Collective, *The New Our Bodies, Ourselves,* (New York: Simon & Schuster Inc., 1984); Riane Eisler, *The Chalice and the Blade: Our History, Our Future* (Harper San Francisco, 1988).

22. Stephen Levine, *Guided Meditations, Explorations and Healings* (New York: Doubleday, 1991), p. 324.

23. David Ehrenfeld, *The Arrogance of Humanism* quoted in Richard Sandor, "The Attending Physician," *Sun,* vol. 4 (Sept. 1991), p. 4.

24. Quoted in Jerry Hicks and Esther Hicks, *A New Beginning,* parts I and II; available from P.O. Box 106, Boerne, TX; tel. (210) 755-2299.

Chapter 16: Getting the Most Out of Your Medical Care

1. Norman Cousins, *Anatomy of an Illness as Perceived by the Patient* (New York: Bantam, 1979), pp. 49–50.

2. H. Benson et al., "The Placebo Effect: A Neglected Asset in the Care of Patients," *Journal of the American Medical Association,* vol. 232, no. 12 (June 23, 1975); A. B. Carter, "The Placebo: Its Use and Abuse," *Lancet,* (Oct. 17, 1973), p. 823; B. Blackwell et al., "Demonstration to Medical Students of Placebo Responses and Non-Drug Factors," *Lancet,* vol. 2 (June 1972), p. 1279; S. Wolf, "The Pharmacology of Placebo," *Pharmacological Review,* vol. 2 (1959), p. 698; H. K. Beecher, "The Powerful Placebo," *Journal of the American Medical Association,* vol. 159 (1955), pp. 1602–6.

3. Karl-Hendrick Robert, interview, "That Was When I Became a Slave," special issue: Making It Happen: Effective Strategies for Changing the

World, *In Context,* no. 28, Spring 1991, Bainbridge Island, Washington, p. 13.

4. The sense of the word *heroic* in this context is from the philosophy of Susun Weed, a wise woman herbalist who associates the heroic tradition with allopathic medicine.

5. *Gentle Visions: A Pre-operative Relaxation Program,* 1991, 1992. For more information or to order write to Healing Images, P.O. Box 2972, Framingham Center Station, Framingham, MA 01701.

6. One summer, while climbing Mount Katahdin, I ran a stick through my shin. Not only did it hurt, it left an ugly gash that I knew would leave a scar. I grieved for my leg, even as my brother joked, "What do you care? You're not a model—you don't need your legs to look good for anything."

Chapter 17: Nourishing Ourselves with Food

1. K. Johnson and T. Ferguson, *Trusting Ourselves: The Sourcebook of Psychology for Women* (New York: Atlantic Monthly Press, 1990), p. 371.

2. Susie Orbach, *Fat Is a Feminist Issue* (New York: Berkley Books).

3. Mary Catherine Bateson, *Composing a Life* (New York: Plume, 1989), p. 200.

4. Statistics from Kerry O'Nell, "*The Famine Within* Probes Women's Pursuit of Thinness," review of Katherine Gilday's film *The Famine Within,* in *Christian Science Monitor* (Aug. 31, 1992).

5. L.K.G. Hsu, "The Treatment of Anorexia Nervosa," *American Journal of Psychiatry,* vol. 143 (1986), p. 573.

6. J. E. Mitchell, M. C. Seim, E. Clon, et al., "Medical Complications and Medical Management of Bulimia," *Annals of Internal Medicine,* vol. 71 (1987).

7. Bob Schwartz, *Diets Don't Work* (Houston, TX: Breakthrough Publishing, 1982).

8. The scenario of the overachieving, driven adolescent girl is a setup for anorexia. It's estimated that 50 percent of prep school girls are bulimic or anorexic to some extent. Marion Woodman's *Addiction to Perfection: The Still Unravished Bride* (Toronto, Canada: Inner City Press, 1982), is a beautiful exploration of the depth issues represented by eating disorders.

9. "Obesity: The Cancer Connection," editorial, *Lancet,* vol. 1 (1982), p. 1223.

10. J. B. Wyngaarden, L. H. Smith, and S. Bennett, *Cecil's Textbook of Medicine,* 19th ed. (Philadelphia: W. B. Saunders, 1992).

11. M. Mackensie, "A Cultural Study of Weight: America vs. Western Samoa," *Radiance,* vol. 3, no. 3 (Summer/Fall 1986), pp. 23–25; cited in Johnson and Ferguson, *Trusting Ourselves* (see note 1).

12. Johnson and Ferguson, *Trusting Ourselves,* p. 370 (see note 1).

13. V. J. Felitti, "Long-Term Medical Consequences of Incest, Rape, and Molestation," *Southern Medicine Journal,* vol. 84 (1991), pp. 328–31; I. Cleary-Merker: "Childhood Sexual Abuse as an Antecedent to Obesity," *Bariatrician* (Spring 1991), pp. 17–22, and (Summer 1991), pp. 11–16; and D. A. Drossman, J. Leserman, G. Nachman, et al., "Sexual and Physical Abuse in Women with Func-

tional or Organic Gastrointestinal Disorders," *Annals of Internal Medicine*, vol. 113 (1990), pp. 828–33.

14. L. Lissner et al., "Variability of Body Weight and Health Outcomes in the Framingham Population," *New England Journal of Medicine*, vol. 324 (1991), pp. 1839–44. It appears that the constant weight fluctuations are dangerous in and of themselves.

15. During medical school, one of the surgeons I studied with performed intestinal bypass surgery on women (and men) who were morbidly obese. Though they lost weight quickly, post-operational many were unable to adjust to their new size and continued to think and feel fat.

16. Geneen Roth, *Why Weight? A Guide to Breaking Free from Compulsive Eating* (New York: Plume, 1989).

17. Martin Katahn and Jamie Popo-Cordie, *The T-Factor Diet* (New York: Bantam Books, 1989), is an excellent primer, with recipes as well as fat gram listings.

18. R. A. Anderson and A. S. Koslovsky, "Chromium Intake, Absorption, and Excretion of Subjects Consuming Self-Selected Diets," *American Journal of Clinical Nutrition*, vol. 41 (1985), pp. 1177–83.

19. W. Mestz et al., "Present Knowledge of the Role of Chromium," Federal Proceedings, vol. 33, pp. 2275–80.

20. At Women to Women we are currently using Sportron Power Pack, a combination of herbs and minerals. This product has helped some women safely rehabilitate their metabolism, when used in combination with a sound diet and exercise program.

21. Liz Gunner, "Alcoholism and Eating Disorders," *Nutrition and Dietary Consultant* (May 1987), p. 14; available from 1641 Sunset Road, B-117, Las Vegas, NV 89119.

22. Phyllis Havens, R.D., L.D. personal communication.

23. Fowkes et al., "Serum Cholesterol, Triglycerides, and Aggression in the General Population," *Lancet*, vol. 340 (Oct. 24, 1992), pp. 995–98.

24. Alexander Schauss, *Diet, Crime, and Delinquency* (Berkeley, CA: Parker House, 1980).

25. Saul Miller, *Food for Thought: A New Look at Food and Behavior* (New York: Prentice-Hall, 1979).

26. Though the concepts of yin and yang make a great deal of intuitive sense to me, they can be used addictively. Silly discussions of questions like "Am I too yin or too yang?" or "Is a carrot more yin than a parsnip?" can go on and on.

27. U.S. Department of Health, Education and Welfare, Public Health Service, *Healthy People*, publication no. 79-55071 (Washington, DC: U.S. Government Printing Office, 1979); B. R. Goldin et al., "Estrogen Excretion Patterns and Plasma Levels in Vegetarian and Omnivorous Women," *New England Journal of Medicine*, vol. 307 (1982), pp. 1542–47; R. Bavalve et al., "Vegetables Inhibit in Vivo, the Mutagenicity of Nitrite Combined with Nitrosable Compounds," *Mutation Research*, vol. 120 (1983), p. 145; U.S. Academy of Sciences, *Diet,*

Nutrition, and Cancer (Washington, DC: National Academy Press, 1982); Maine Vegetarian Resource Groups, c/o Shari Greenfield, RFD, Box 194, Belfast, ME 04915; tel. (207) 338-1861; P. Hill, "Environmental Factors and Breast and Prostate Cancer," *Cancer Research,* vol. 41 (1981), p. 3817; S. Gorbach, "Estrogens, Breast Cancer, and Intestinal Flora," *Review Infectious Disease,* vol. 6, suppl. 1 (1984) p. S85; B. Goldin, "Effect of Diet on Excretion of Estrogens in Pre- and Post-Menopausal Women," *Cancer Research,* vol. 41 (1981), p. 3771; and A. H. Follingstad, "Commentary: Estriol, The Forgotten Estrogen," *Journal of the American Medical Association,* vol. 239, no. 1 (1978), pp. 29–38.

28. A thorough discussion of yin and yang is beyond the scope of this book. I refer you to the writings of Michio Kushi, especially *The Book of Macrobiotics* (Tokyo: Japan Publications, 1986).

29. See the extensive bibliography of the medical literature in *Diet, Nutrition, and Cancer,* pp. 73–105 (see note 27).

30. B. MacMahan et al., "Urine Estrogen Profiles in Asian and North American Women," *International Journal of Cancer,* vol. 14 (1974), pp. 161–67; L. E. Dickinson et al., "Estrogen Profiles of Oriental and Caucasian Women in Hawaii," *New England Journal of Medicine,* vol. 291 (1974), pp. 1211–13; D. A. Snowden, letter to the editor, *Journal of the American Medical Association,* vol. 3, no. 254 (1985), pp. 356–57; D. W. Cramer et al., "Dietary Animal Fat and Relationship to Ovarian Cancer Risk," *Obstetrics and Gynecology,* vol. 63, no. 6 (1984), pp. 833–38; T. McKenna, "Pathogenesis and Treatment of Polycystic Ovary Syndrome," *New England Journal of Medicine,* vol. 318 (1988), p. 558; and D. Polson, "Polycystic Ovaries—A Common Finding in Normal Women," *Lancet,* vol. 1 (1988), p. 870.

31. P. Hill, "Diet, Lifestyle and Menstrual Activity," *American Journal of Clinical Nutrition,* vol. 33 (1980), p. 1192.

32. A. Sanchez, "A Hypothesis on the Etiologic Role of Diet on the Age of Menarche," *Medical Hypotheses,* vol. 7 (1981), p. 1339; and S. Schwartz, "Dietary Influences on the Growth and Sexual Maturation in Premenarchal Rhesus Monkeys," *Hormones and Behavior,* vol. 22 (1988), p. 231.

33. N. Boyd, "Effect of a Low-Fat, High-Carbohydrate Diet on Symptoms of Cyclical Mastopathy," *Lancet,* vol. 2 (1988), p. 128; D. Rose, "Effect of a Low-Fat Diet on Hormone Levels in Women with Cystic Breast Disease, I: Serum Steroids and Gonadotropins," *Journal of the National Cancer Institute,* vol. 78 (1987), p. 623; and D. Rose, "Effect of a Low-Fat Diet on Hormone Levels in Women with Cystic Breast Disease, II: Serum Radioimmunoassayable Prolactin and Growth Hormone and Bioactive Lactogenic Hormones," *Journal of the National Cancer Institute,* vol. 78 (1987), p. 627.

34. M. Woods, "Low-Fat, High-Fiber Diet and Serum Estrone Sulfate in Premenopausal Women," *American Journal of Clinical Nutrition,* vol. 49 (1989), p. 1179; D. Ingram, "Effect of Low-Fat Diet on Female Sex Hormone Levels," *Journal of National Cancer Institute,* vol. 79 (1987), p. 1225; and H. Aldercreutz, "Diet

and Plasma Androgens in Postmenopausal Vegetarian and Omnivorous Women and Postmenopausal Women with Breast Cancer," *American Journal of Clinical Nutrition*, vol. 49 (1989), p. 433.

35. Dean Ornish, "Can Lifestyle Changes Reverse Coronary Heart Disease?" Lifestyle Heart Trial, *Lancet*, vol. 336 (July 21, 1990), pp. 129–33.

36. D. Baird, "Medical Management of Fibroids," *British Medical Journal*, vol. 296 (1988), p. 1684; G. Abraham, "Nutritional Factors in the Etiology of the Premenstrual Tension Syndromes," *Journal of Reproductive Medicine*, vol. 28 (1983), p. 446; and J. Vaitukaitis, "Premenstrual Syndrome," *New England Journal of Medicine*, vol. 311 (1984), p. 1371.

37. Check to see if you have an East/West Center in your city. If not, call or write The Kushi Institute (address and phone number in Resource section).

38. John McDougall, *The McDougall Program: 12 Days to Dynamic Health* (New York: Plume, 1990), pp. 44–45.

39. Campbell's data cited in "More on the Dietary Fat and Breast Cancer Link: The Chinese Study," *NABCO News*, vol. 4, no. 3 (July 1990), pp. 1, 2; available from National Alliance of Breast Cancer Organizations (NABCO), 2nd floor, 1180 Avenue of the Americas, New York, NY 10036; tel. (212) 719-0154.

40. "Lean Beef Shown to Be as Healthy as Chicken and Fish," *Food Chemistry News*, vol. 32, no. 39 (1990), p. 6; cited in Jeffrey Bland, letter to the editor, *New England Journal of Medicine*, vol. 326, no. 3 (1992), p. 200.

41. Ann-Louise Gittleman, *Supernutrition for Women* (New York: Bantam, 1991).

42. J. A. Levy et al., *Basic and Clinical Immunology*, 4th ed. (Los Angeles, CA: Lange Medical Books, 1982), pp. 297–305; F. Price, "Theoretical Involvement of Vitamin B_6 in Tumor Initiation," *Medical Hypothesis*, vol. 15 (1985), pp. 421–28; and M. E. Poyduck et al., "Inhibiting Effect of Vitamin C and B_{12} on the Mitotic Activity of Acites Tumors," *Experimental Cell Biology*, vol. 47, no. 3 (1979), pp. 210–17.

43. M. S. Biskind, "The Effect of Vitamin B Complex Deficiency on the Inactivation of Estrone in the Liver," *Endocrinology*, vol. 31 (1942), pp. 109–14.

44. M. I. Botez, "Neurologic Disorders Response to Folic Acid Therapy," *Canadian Medical Association Journal*, vol. 15 (1976), p. 217.

45. "Subtle B_{12} Shortage May Be a Factor in Alzheimer's," *Brain/Mind Bulletin*, vol. 17, no. 7 (Apr. 1992); John Dommisse, article in *Medical Hypotheses*, vol. 34, pp. 131–40.

46. Macrobiotic foods such as tempeh and tamari contain vitamin B_{12}. Whether these cultured soybean products contain enough for all people is controversial. John McDougall points out that only twelve cases of documented B_{12} deficiency have been reported. But because of those, he recommends a B_{12} supplement (about 5 mcg. per day, only after you've been off *all* animal protein for three years or more). See McDougall, *McDougall Program* (see note 38); and Dan Seamans, "Eating for Optimum Health: Is There a Place for Animal Food in a Healthy Diet," interview with Ballantine and Doell, *Natural Health* (Nov.-Dec. 1992), p. 65.

47. Many traditional cultures, however, do consume some cheese, yogurt, and sheep or goat's milk.

48. Daniel Cramer et al., "Galactose Consumption and Metabolism in Relation to the Risk of Ovarian Cancer" *Lancet* (July 8, 1989).

49. Campbell is quoted in "More on the Dietary Fat and Breast Cancer Link," *NABCO News* (see note 39). "The Cornell-Oxford Project on Nutrition, Health, and Environment, known simply as 'the China Health Project' (CHP), draws from an array of large-scale surveys that began in 1983 to trace carefully the daily living habits of 6,500 Chinese in sixty-five counties widely dispersed across rural China. This study has been called 'The Grand Prix of epidemiology.'" Nathaniel Mead, "The Champion Diet," *East West* (Sept. 1990), p. 45.

50. William Manahan, *Eat for Health* (Tiburon, CA: H. J. Kramer), pp. 164–65. Dentists point out that the first place osteoporosis shows up is in the lower jaw, and that osteoporosis is linked with periodontal disease, the leading cause of adult tooth loss.

51. T. Colin Campbell, "Nutrition, Environment and Health Project; Chinese Academy of Preventive Medicine—Cornell-Oxford," reported in Mead, "Champion Diet," p. 46 (see note 49).

52. Bone metabolism also requires vitamin C, vitamin D, and a number of trace minerals including zinc, silica, copper, boron, and manganese. All of these substances, working synergistically, form bone.

53. L. Cohen and R. Kitzes, "Infrared Spectroscopy and Magnesium Content of Bone Mineral in Osteoporotic Women," *Israel Journal of Medical Science,* vol. 17 (1981), pp. 1123–25; L. Cohen et. al., "Magnesium Malabsorption in Post-menopausal Osteoporosis," *Magnesium,* vol. 2 (1983), pp. 139–43; L. Cohen et al., "Bone Magnesium, Crystallinity Index and State of Body Magnesium on Subjects with Senile Osteoporosis, Maturity Onset Diabetes and Women Treated with Contraceptive Preparations," *Magnesium,* vol. 2 (1983), pp. 70–75.

54. M. M. Linkswiler et al., "Calcium Retention of Young Adult Males as Affected by Level of Protein and Calcium Intake," *Transactions of the New York Academy of Science,* vol. 36 (1974), p. 333; R. A. Chander et al., "Effect of Protein Intake on Calcium Balance in Young Men Given 500mg Calcium Daily," *Journal of Nutrition,* vol. 104 (1974), pp. 695–700; and R. M. Walker et al., "Calcium Retention in the Adult Human Male as Affected by Protein Intake," *Journal of Nutrition,* vol. 102 (1972), pp. 1297–1302.

55. Jeffrey Bland, personal communication.

56. Jeffrey Bland, *How Do You Stand,* osteoporosis teaching program; available from HealthComm, Inc., Gig Harbor, WA 98335.

57. Jeffrey Bland, "The Calcium Pushers," *East/West* (1987); Jeffrey Bland, *The Bone Loss Seminar,* a tape series on preventing osteoporosis, available from HealthComm, Inc. (see note 56 for address).

58. Sources for this table are: U.S. Department of Agriculture, *Composition of Foods,* handbooks no. 8 and 456 (Washington, DC: U.S. Government Printing Office, 1963); J. A. Duke and A. A. Atchley, *Handbook of Proximate Analysis—*

Tables of Higher Plants (CRC Press, 1986); Leonard Jacobs, article in *East/West Journal* (May 1985); John Lee, "Osteoporosis Reversal: The Role of Progesterone," *International Clinical Nutrition Review,* vol. 10 (1990); Judith Cooper Madlener, *The Sea Vegetable Book* (New York: Clarkson N. Potter, 1977); Nutrition Search, Inc., John Kirschmann, dir. comp., *Nutrition Almanac,* rev. ed. (New York: McGraw-Hill, 1979); U.S. Department of Agriculture, *Nutritive Value of Foods,* handbook no. 72 (Washington, DC: U.S. Government Printing Office, 1971); Pedersen, *Nutritional Herbology* (Pedersen, 1987); and Maine Coast Sea Vegetables Co., Shore Road, Franklin, ME 04634.

The mineral waters are available from gourmet and liquor stores, if not from your local grocery store. Or call your local food distributor for sources.

59. These recipes are from Susun Weed, *Menopausal Years: The Wise Woman's Way: Alternative Approaches for Women 30–90* (Woodstock, NY: Ash Tree Publishing, 1992). A wide variety of sources are listed in Weed's *Healing Wise: A Wise Woman's Herbal* (Woodstock, NY: Ash Tree Publishing).

60. M. G. Enig et al., "Dietary Fat and Cancer Trends: A Critique," *Federal Proceeding,* vol. 37 (1978), pp. 2215–30.

61. G. Abraham, "Primary Dysmenorrhea," *Clinical Obstetrics and Gynecology,* vol. 21, no. 1 (1978), pp. 139–45.

62. J. F. Balch, *Prescription for Nutritional Healing* (New York: Avery Publications, 1990).

63. U. N. Das et al., "Benzo(a)pyrene and Gamma Radiation Induced Genetic Damage in Mice May Be Prevented in Mice by GLA but Not Arachidonic Acid," *Nutrition Research,* vol. 5 (1985), pp. 101–5.

64. D. Horrobin et al., "Omega 6 Fatty Acids May Reverse Carcinogenesis by Restoring Natural PGE-1 Metabolism," *Medical Hypotheses,* vol. 6 (1980), pp. 469–86; and J. J. Jarkowski and W. T. Cave, "Dietary Fish Oil May Inhibit Development of Breast Cancer," *Journal of the National Cancer Institute,* vol. 74 (1985), pp. 1145–50.

65. R. L. Swank et al., "Effect of Low Saturated Fat Diet in Early and Late Cases of Multiple Sclerosis," *Lancet,* vol. 336 (1990), pp. 37–39.

66. P. L. McLennon, "Reversal of Arrythmogenic Effects of Long-Term Saturated Fatty Acid Intake by Dietary N3 and N6 Polyunsaturated Fatty Acids," *American Journal of Clinical Nutrition,* vol. 51 (1990), pp. 53–58; D. Kim et al., "Dietary Fish Oil Added to Hyperlipidemic Diet for Swine Results in Reduction in Excessive Numbers of Monocytes Attached to Arterial Endothelium," *Atherosclerosis,* vol. 81 (1991), pp. 209–16; and C. J. Diskin et al., "Fish Oil to Prevent Intimal Hyperplasia and Thrombosis," *Nephron,* vol. 55 (1990), pp. 445–47.

67. For further reading, I recommend the bible on this subject: Udo Erasmus, *Fats and Oils* (Vancouver, B.C.: Alive Books) as well as Clare Felix's informative newsletter *The Felix Letter: A Commentary on Nutrition,* P.O. Box 7094, Berkeley, CA 94707.

68. S. Villance, "Relationship between Ascorbic Acid and Serum Proteins of the Immune System," *British Medical Journal,* vol. 2 (1977), pp. 437–38.

69. M. Alexander, et. al., "Oral B Carotene Can Increase the Number of OK T4 + Cells in Human Blood," *Immunology Letters,* vol. 9 (1985), pp. 221–24; W. C. Willet, G. Mac Mahon, "Diet and Cancer: An Overview," *New England Journal of Medicine,* vol. 310, no. 11 (1984), pp. 697–703; W. C. Willet, et al., "Prediagnostic Serum Selenium and the Risk of Cancer," *Lancet,* vol. 2 (1983), pp. 130–33; R. A. Winchurch, et. al., "Supplementary Zinc Restores Antibody Formation of Aged Spleen Cells," *European Journal of Immunology,* vol. 17, pp. 127–32.

70. Cox, et al. "Red Blood Cell Magnesium and Chronic Fatigue Syndrome," *Lancet,* vol. 337 (1991), pp. 757–60.

71. Ouchi, et al., "Effect of Dietary Magnesium on Development of Atherosclerosis in Cholesterol-Fed Rabbits," *Arterioclerosis,* vol. 10 (1990), pp. 732–37.

72. S. Belman, "Onion and Garlic Oil Inhibit Tumor Growth," *Carcinogenesis,* vol. 4, no. 8 (1983), pp. 1063–65.

73. I. Casoni, et al. "Changes in Magnesium Concentration in Endurance Athletes," *International Journal of Sports Medicine,* vol. 11 (1990), pp. 234–37.

74. MRC Vitamin Study Research Group, "Prevention of Neural Tube Defects. Results of Medical Research Council Vitamin Study," *Lancet,* vol. 338 (1991), pp. 131–37.

75. V. Sahakian, et al., "Vitamin B_6 Is Effective Therapy for Nausea and Vomiting in Pregnancy: A Randomized, Double-Blind Placebo Controlled Study," *Journal of Obstetrics and Gynecology,* vol. 78, (1991), pp. 33–36.

76. M. DeVos, "Articular Disease and the Gut: Evidence for a Strong Relationship Between Spondylarthropathy and Inflammation of the Gut in Man," *Acta Clinica Belgica,* vol. 45, no. 10 (1990), pp. 20–24. P. Jackson, et al., "Intestinal Permeability in Patients with Eczema and Food Allergy," *Lancet,* vol. 1 (1981), p. 1285.

77. D. N. Golding, "Is There Allergic Synovitis?" *Journal of the Royal Society of Medicine,* vol. 83 (1990), pp. 312–14; R. S. Panush, "Food Induced (Allergic) Arthritis: Clinical and Serological Studies," *Journal of Rheumatology,* vol. 17, no. 3 (1990), pp. 291–94; C. G. Graul, "Food Allergies and the Migraine," *Lancet,* (May 5, 1979), pp. 966–69; R. A. Finn et al., "Serum IgG Antibodies to Gliadin and Other Dietary Antigens in the Adult with Atopic Dermatitis," *Clinical Experimental Dermatology,* vol. 10, no. 3 (1985), pp. 222–28; I. Waxman, "Case Records of the MGH: A 59-Year-Old Woman with Abdominal Pain and an Abnormal CT Scan," *New England Journal of Medicine,* vol. 329, no. 5, pp. 343–49. For further information or a list of physicians familiar with treating this problem, write to Martin Lee, Great Smokies Laboratory, 18A Regent Park Blvd., Asheville, N.C. 28816.

78. Food allergy diagnosis is highly controversial within the conventional medical community and some allergists don't believe that it exists or that anything can be done about it.

79. IgE levels are known to be altered in diseases related to intestinal dysbiosis and food allergies. IgE is an immunoglobulin that is involved with the body's re-

sponse to outside elements such as pollen, animal danders, grass, wheat, etc., which are not usually harmful to our bodies. However, in those people who are chronically stressed either emotionally or physically, the IgE levels are elevated, creating the possibility for a hyperimmune response, which results in reactions to normally occurring environmental substances. In some people, the IgE levels are decreased, resulting in immunosuppression and therefore increased susceptibility to colds, etc.

80. T. Shirakawa et al., "Lifestyle Effect on Total IgE: Lifestyles Have a Cumulative Impact on Controlling Total IgE Levels," *Allergy,* vol. 46 (1991), pp. 561–69; I. Waxman, see note 77.

81. Data from *Brain/Mind Bulletin* (Dec. 1988).

82. Thomas Petros, article in *Physiology and Behavior,* vol. 41, pp. 25–30.

83. Statistics from ASH—Action on Smoking and Health, 2013H Street NS, Washington, DC 20006; tel: (203) 659-4310.

84. Data from Sheldon Ganberg, "Help for Nicotine Addiction Through Acupuncture," *Journal* (July 1991), pp. 1, 6.

85. B. Haglund et al., "Cigarette Smoking as a Risk Factor for Sudden Infant Death Syndrome," *American Journal of Public Health,* vol. 80 (1990), pp. 29–32.

86. R. A. Riemersma, et. al., "Risk of Angina Pectoris and Plasma Concentration of Vitamins A, C, E, and Carotene," *The Lancet,* vol. 337, pp. 1–5.

87. Ganberg, op. cit.; James S. Olms, M.D., of Ohio. *The American Journal of Acupuncture* (vol. 12, #4).

88. Interestingly breast milk contains 300 mg. of calcium per quart, while cow's milk contains 1200 mg. per quart. Yet the breast fed infant absorbs more calcium than the infant fed cow's milk. More isn't necessarily better. Source: Manahan, William, *Eat for Health,* H. J. Kramer, Inc. 1988, p. 164.

89. Frank Oski, *Don't Drink Your Milk* (Mollica Press, 1983); available from Teach Services, Route 1, Box 182, Brushton, NY 12916; tel. (800) 367-1844.

90. Martin Katahn and Jamie Popo-Cordie, *The T-Factor Diet* (Bantam Books, N.Y.) and *The T-Factor Fat Gram Counter* (New York: W. W. Norton and Co., 1989).

91. Jeff Woodward, *The Healing Power of Food: A Gourmet Cookbook for Lives in Transition* (Minneapolis: Traditional Cooking Arts, 1988); available from Traditional Cooking Arts, 5336 York Avenue South, Minneapolis, MN 55410; tel. (612) 929-2207.

92. Annemarie Colbin, *Food and Healing* (New York: Ballantine, 1987); Annemarie Colbin, *Book of Whole Meals* (New York: Ballantine, 1985); and Annemarie Colbin, *The Basics of Healthy Cooking,* videotape; available from Natural Gourmet Cookery School, 48 West 21st Street, Suite 202, New York, NY 10010; tel. (212) 645-5170.

93. Rick Perry, *Hurricane Kitchen* (Augusta, ME: Lance Tapley, 1988).

94. Kristina Turner, *The Self-Healing Cookbook* (Grass Valley, CA: Earthtones Press, 1987).

95. H. A. Jackson et al., "Aluminum from a Coffee Pot," *Lancet,* vol. 1 (1989), pp. 781–82.

96. G. Lubec et al. "Amino Acid Isomerization and Microwave Exposure," *Lancet,* vol. 2 (1987), pp. 1392–93.

97. J. S. Bland, Letter to the editor, *New England Journal of Medicine,* vol. 326, no. 3 (1992), p. 200.

98. Melvyn Morse, *Transformed by the Light.*

Chapter 18: The Power of Movement

1. David Spangler, lecture notes from conference entitled, Energy and Medicine: Intuition as a Prerequisite for 21st Century Medicine, Regents Park, London, Nov. 1991.

2. Brian Swimme, *The Universe Is a Green Dragon,* Bear and Company, 1983, p. 106.

3. Many of the following studies were found in R. A. Anderson, *Wellness Medicine* (Lynnwood, WA: American Health Press, 1987).

4. Body Bulletin, Rodale Press, Emmaus, PA, Jan. 1984.

5. Belloc and Breslow, "Relationship of Physical Fitness and Health Status," *Preventive Medicine,* vol. 1, no. 3 (1972), pp. 109–21.

6. R. J. Young, "Effect of Regular Exercise on Cognitive Functioning and Personality," *British Journal of Sports Medicine,* vol. 13, no. 3 (1979), 110–17; B. Gutin, "Effect of Increase in Physical Fitness on Mental Ability Following Physical and Mental Stress," *Research Quarterly,* vol. 37, no. 2 (1966), pp. 211–20.

7. M. S. Bahrke, "Exercise, Meditation, and Anxiety Reduction," *American Corr. Therapy Journal,* vol. 33, no. 2 (1979), pp. 41–44; J. W. Collingswood, and L. Willet, "The Effects of Physical Training Upon Self-Concept and Body Attitude," *Journal of Clinical Psychology,* vol. 27, no. 3 (1971), pp. 411–12.

8. R. Prince et al., "Prevention of Postmenopausal Osteoporosis: A Comparative Study of Exercise, Calcium Supplementation, and Hormone Replacement Therapy, [Journal], vol. 325, no. 17 (1991), pp. 1189–1204; J. F. Aloia et al., "Prevention of Involutional Bone Mass by Exercise," *Annals of Internal Medicine,* vol. 89, no. 3 (1978), pp. 351–58; Consensus Development Conference on Osteoporosis, National Institutes of Health, Washington, DC, 1989.

9. S. J. Griffin, and J. Trinder, "Physical Fitness, Exercise, and Human Sleep," *Psychophysiology,* vol. 15, no. 5 (1978), pp. 447–50.

10. J. Morgan et al., "Psychological Effects of Chronic Physical Activity," *Medical Science Sports,* vol. 2, no. 4 (1970), pp. 213–17.

11. Helmrich et al., "Physical Activity and Reduced Occurrence of Non-Insulin-Dependent Diabetes Mellitus," *New England Journal of Medicine,* vol. 325, no. 3, July 18, 1991.

12. J. Prior, "Conditioning Exercise Decreases Premenstrual Symptoms: A Prospective, Controlled 6-Month Trial," *Fertility and Sterility,* vol. 47, no. 402 (1987).

13. B. P. Worth et al., "Running Through Pregnancy," *Runner's World* (Nov. 1978), pp. 54–59.

14. My family still loves racing around outside. This works for them. My husband sometimes joins them in their heroic trips and I'm off the hook!

15. I have found that The Firm® aerobic work out with weights is very effective if you have the time to do it. Each work out lasts from 45 to 60 minutes and you can feel results in your body after only 5 or so workouts doing three workouts per week on average. To order a 5 minute video preview, call 1-800-THE FIRM. My favorites are volumes 4, 5, and 6. I'd recommend that you begin with vol 6.

16. H. H. Jones et al., "Humeral Hypertrophy in Response to Exercise," *Journal of Bone and Joint Surgery,* vol. 59, no. a2 (1977), pp. 204–8; N. K. Dalen, and E. Olsson, "Bone Mineral Content and Physical Activity," *Acta Ortho Scanda.* vol. 45, no. 2 (1974), pp. 170–74.

17. Putai, Jin, "Changes in Heart Rate, Noradrenaline, Cortisol, and Mood During Tai Chi," *Journal of Psychosomatic Research,* vol. 33, no. 2 (1989), pp. 197–206.

18. I'm a big fan of model-mugging—the training that helps women develop a strategy for surviving an attack.

19. Ann Ray Martin and Valerie Gladstone, "The Quickest Fixes," *Longevity,* (May 1991), pp. 48, 49.

20. R. Markus et al., "Menstrual Function and Bone Mass in Elite Women Distance Runners: Endocrine and Metabolic Features," *Annals of Internal Medicine,* vol. 102 (1985), pp. 158–63.

21. N. A. Rigotti et al., "Osteoporosis in Women with Anorexia Nervosa," *New England Journal of Medicine,* vol. 311 (1989), pp. 1601–5.

22. Nancy Lane, M.D. "Exercise and Bone Status," *Complementary Medicine* (May/June 1986).

23. L. L. Schweiger et al., "Caloric Intake, Stress, and Menstrual Function in Athletes," *Fertility and Sterility,* vol. 49 (1988), pp. 447–50.

24. B. L. Drinkwater et al., "Bone Mineral Density After Resumption of Menses in Amenorrheic Athletes," *Journal of the American Medical Association,* vol. 256, pp. 380–82; J. S. Lindbergh et al., "Increased Vertebral Bone Mineral in Response to Reduced Exercise in Amenorrheic Runners," *Western Journal of Medicine,* vol. 146, pp. 39–47.

Chapter 19: Healing Ourselves, Healing Our World

1. C. W. Birky, "Relaxed Cellular Controls and Organelle Heredity," *Science,* vol. 222 (1983), pp. 466–75; M. C. Corballis, M. J. Morgan, "On the Biological Basis of Human Laterality," *Journal of Behavioral Science,* vol. 2 (1978), pp. 261–336; Norman Geschwind and Albert Galaburda, "Cerebral Lateralization, Biological Mechanisms, and Pathology."

2. *The Burning Tree* is a documentary film that chronicles the burning of 9 million women and their sympathizers as witches during the Middle Ages. For more information, write to Donna Reed—Film maker, Direct Cinema, P.O. Box 10003, Santa Monica, CA 90410; tel. (310) 396-4774; (800) 525-4000. For more

information on this subject see Starhawk, *The Spiral Dance: A Rebirth of the Ancient Goddess* (Harper San Francisco, 1979).

3. Rupert Sheldrake, *The Presence of the Past: Morphic Resonance and the Habits of Nature* (London: Collins, 1988) and *A New Science of Life* (Boston: Houghton Mifflin, 1981). Sheldrake's theory concerns "morphic units," which can be regarded as forms of energy. "Although these aspects of form and energy can be separated conceptually they are always associated with one another. No morphic unit can have energy without form, and no material form can exist without energy." The characteristic form of a given morphic unit is determined by the form of previous similar systems that act upon it across time and space, in a process of "morphic resonance" through "morphogenic fields." This influence depends on the system's three-dimensional structures and patterns of vibrations.

For example, thousands of rats are trained to perform a new task in a laboratory in London. If Sheldrake's theory holds, then at a later time and in laboratories somewhere else, similar rats should be able to learn and carry out the same task more quickly. That's because the initial rats have changed the "morphogenic field" around rat learning. This effect should take place in the absence of any known physical connection or communication between the two laboratories.

Evidence that this effect actually occurs has been reported by Ager et al., "Fourth (final) Report on a Test of McDougall's Lamarckian Experiment in the Training of Rats," *Journal of Experimental Biology,* vol. 3 (1954), pp. 304–21.

4. *Ms.,* cover (Jan.-Feb. 1992).

5. Anne Wilson Schaef, *Meditations for Women Who Do Too Much,* daily calendar for May 15, 1992 (Harper San Francisco, 1990).

6. Audre Lorde, *Burst of Light* (Ithaca, NY: Firebrand Books, 1988), p. 131. According to her book, Lorde had metastases of breast cancer to her liver, diagnosed in 1984. In 1992, she was named the poet-laureate of New York State. Usually a tumor that has metastasized to the liver gives the person six months to live. Lorde lived for nine years after this diagnosis.

7. Annie Rafter, a registered nurse, is one of the original founders of Women to Women. When she was recently visiting from her present home in Santa Fe, she, Marcelle Pick, and I got together and did each other's exams and Pap smears. Dr. Bethany Hays, one of our newest additions, referred to this as a "Pap-a-rama"!

8. This thought had a bit of accuracy in it. Medical students are notorious for starting to experience the symptoms of the patients they are around when they're just learning about different diseases. My personal boundaries were not very well placed in the past, and I have "taken home" too much of what goes on in the office. Since I'm in the energy field associated with fibroids all day long and am quite empathetic with my patients, my energy field has undoubtedly been influenced by theirs—and I still have to take responsibility for this condition and learn and grow from it.

Index

A

Abnormal Pap smear. *See*
Pap smear, abnormal;
Cervical dysplasia.
Abortion, 42, 325–33
and fibroids, 192
and emotions, 328–31
on demand, 327
and PMS onset, 121
postabortion trauma, 328–
31
Abraham, 541
Abuse, childhood sexual, 4,
20, 28, 29, 42, 43, 58, 88,
127, 642
and chronic pelvic pain, 84
and disorders, 84
and energy system, 68–71
and fibroids, 185–86
and first chakra, 81
influence on adulthood,
70–72
and labor, 386
and relationships, 42
and sexuality, 229
and surgery, 561
memories of, 72, 642
Accidents, 26–27
Acetominaphen (Tylenol),
610
Achterberg, Jeanne, 27, 556
Acidophilus, lactobacillus,
305, 611
Acupuncture, 116, 137, 138,
166, 186, 317, 447, 530,
531, 557, 562, 651–52, 614
Acyclovir (Zovirax), 259
Addiction. *See* Addictive
characteristics; Addictive
system; Exercise

addiction; Food
addiction; Relationship
addiction; Self-abuse
addiction; Sex addiction
Addictive characteristics,
naming, 14–19
Addictive system, 3–24,
526–27, 557, 648
beliefs of, 7–12
and blame, 44
characteristics of, 10–11
and defensiveness, 13
and denial, 13
and dependency, 15
and menopause, 432
"nonliving" orientation of,
66
and physical destruction,
13
recovery from, 24, 71
and success, 154
and time, 310
Adenomyosis, 142, 561,
593–94. *See also*
Menstrual periods, heavy.
and heavy menstrual
periods, 141
and pelviscopic surgery,
165–66
Adhesions, 358
and pelviscopic surgery,
165–66
Adoption, 367–70
Advil (ibuprofen), 115, 143
Aerobic exercise, 583, 630–
31, 636
Aerobic weight training
630–31
Aggression, women's
potential for, 87

Aging. *See also* Menopause.
and exercise, 628–29
fear of, 433–36
and smoking, 614
androgen metabolism,
effect on, 438
AIDS, 229, 283–85, 301,
303. *See also* Immune
system; STDs.
Aikido, 632
Alcohol, 69, 251, 446
and osteoporosis, 452, 615
effects of excess
consumption of, 615
eliminating consumption
of, 615–16
Alcoholics Anonymous,
615, 655
Alcoholism, 318, 486, 533–
34, 567, 615
and breast cancer, 305
and cervical dysplasia,
269
and PMS, 128–29
Alexander technique, 632
Aloe vera gel, 560
Alpha waves, and exercise,
630
Amen, 136. *See also*
Progestin, synthetic.
Amenorrhea. *See* Menstrual
periods, absence of.
American Cancer Society,
263, 298, 301
American College of
Obstetrics and
Gynecology, 264, 298
American Holistic Medical
Association, 285, 545,
547

Anaprox (naproxen sulfate), 115, 116, 117, 143
Anatomy, importance of understanding, 499–500
Andrews, Lynn, 425
Androgens, 457–58, 459
  effect of age on metabolism of, 438
  during menopause, 436–38, 469
  ovaries, produced by, 197–98
Anemia, 141
Angel, guardian, 514–16
Anorexia nervosa, 11, 574, 634. *See also* Eating disorders.
Anovulation, 134. *See also* Menstrual cycle, without ovulation; PCO.
  and uterine cancer, 132
Antibiotics, 27, 243
  herpes, as treatment for, 259
  vaginitis, as cause of, 277
  overuse of, 610
Antibodies, 163
  against herpes, 256–57
Antibodies, antiovarian, 441. *See also* Menopause, premature.
Antioxidants, 265, 587, 608, 613. *See also* Nutritional supplements; Vitamins.
Apologizing, women and, 4
Archetypes, 85–87
  "hero," 86
  "mother," 86–87
  "prostitute," 86–87
  "rape," 85–87, 216
  and lower chakras, 85–86
Arnold, Roseanne, 567
Artificial breathing (endotracheal intubation), 8
Artificial insemination, 352
Astrology, 516
Augmentation mammoplasty. *See* Breast enlargement.
Autoimmune disorders, 35
  and intestinal dysbiosis, 610
  premature menopause as, 441
Autoimmunity
  and endometriosis, 35
  and infertility, 35

and premature menopause, 35
and vaginitis, 35
Aygestin (synthetic progestin), 133, 136, 143. *See also* Progestin, synthetic.

B
Bachmann, Gloria, 4, 84
Badgeley, Laurence, 285
Baker, Janine Parvati, 332, 333
Balch, Paulanne, 530, 573
Bateson, Mary Catherine, 569
BBT (basal body temperature), 339, 342–45, 354
Beans, as centering food, 587. *See also* Macrobiotic diet.
Beauvoir, Simone de, 5
Beliefs
  as biological constructs, 38
  changing, 39–40
  health-destroying, 38
  life expectancy, factor in, 27
  physicality of, 27, 35–40
  sorting through personal, 494–506
  and Tara Humara Indians, 435
Benedek, Therese, 102
Benign breast symptoms. *See* Breast pain; Breast lumps; Breast cysts; Nipple discharge.
Benign neoplastic cysts, 203. *See also* Ovarian cysts.
Benson, Herbert, 123
Bergkvist study, 466
Beta carotene, 255, 321, 456, 609, 613
Bifido factor, 280, 611
Bingeing 584–86. *See also* Food addiction.
Biofeedback, 31, 54, 55, 140, 392
Bioflavonoids, 143, 260, 305
Biopsy. *See* Breast biopsy; Cervical biopsy; Cone biopsy; Endometrial biopsy; Uterine biopsy.
Birth control pill. *See* Pill, birth control; Contraception.

Birth defects, and alcohol, 615
Birth, home, 410–13. *See also* Childbirth; Labor.
Birth power, reclaiming, 413
Birth technologies, 390–96
Birthing. *See* Childbirth; Labor.
Black currant seed oil. *See* Gamma linoleic acid; Essential fatty acids.
Blame
  as addictive characteristic, 10
  "blame walls," 45
  for illness, 44–45
  of men, 6
Bly, Robert, 33
Body
  listening to, 509–11, 649
  medical system attitudes toward, 8
  optimal functioning of, 59
  respecting, 511–14, 580
  trusting, 580
  as war zone, 7
Body weight
  "ideal," 573–74
  natural, 577–78
Body wisdom, 12, 31, 35, 44–45. *See also* Chakras; Emotions; Inner guidance.
  listening to, 8, 52–55, 62–63, 522–23
  and menstrual cycle, 144–48
  reclaiming, 3, 144–48
  women's greater access to, 33
Bodymind, 28–31
Bodywork, 531–32, 632
Bone densitometry, 453
Bone density, screening for, 453–54
Bone health, 454–56, 532, 602, 629. *See also* Calcium; Menopause; Osteoporosis.
  and menstrual periods, 131, 634–35
Borage oil. *See* Gamma linoleic acid; Essential fatty acids.
Boron, 456
Borysenko, Joan, 314
Boston Women's Fund, 654
Boston Women's Health Collective, 532

Bradley, Marion Zimmer, 235
Brain Sex 33
Breast abscess, 423
Breast augmentation. *See* Breast enlargement; Breast implants, silicone; Breast reconstruction.
Breast biopsy, 89, 298, 309, 310
Breast cancer, 50, 89, 96, 288, 293, 295, 303–14, 323, 544–45, 650. *See also* Breasts; Estrogen; Mammogram.
 and alcohol, 615
 and birth control pill, 109, 303
 and dairy food, 599
 and diet, 303–5, 591
 and environmental toxins, 303
 and ERT, 303, 466–67
 and estriol, 470–71
 and estrogen, 591, 592–93
 and fourth chakra, 288
 hereditary factors in, 173, 306–8
 and hyperestrogenism, 295, 304
 personality type for, 90, 288
 and Standard American Diet, 185, 592
 and vegetarian diet, 592
Breast colostrum (first milk), 415
Breast cysts, 96, 287, 293, 295
 and archetypes, 89
 and caffeine, 611
 diagnosis of, 295
 and Standard American Diet, 592
 treatment for, 295–97
 and vegetarian diet, 592
Breast disease, fibrocystic, 293–94
Breast enlargement, 287, 316. *See also* Breast implants, silicone; Breast reconstruction.
Breast-feeding, 322, 385
 versus formula-feeding, 420–24
Breast implants, silicone, 287, 314–21, 317, 318, 319
 healing program for, 320
Breast lumps, 89, 289–92,

293, 295. *See also* Lumpectomy.
 and mammograms, 300
 treatment for, 295–97
Breast pain (cystic mastalgia), 293
 treatment for, 295–97
Breast reconstruction, 314–16, 320
 following mastectomy, 323
Breast reduction, 321–22
Breast self-exam, 9, 289–92
Breast surgery, cosmetic. *See* Breast implants, silicone; Breast reconstruction; Breast reduction.
Breasts 96, 286–323. *See also* Breast cancer; Breast cysts; Mammary dysplasia; Mammogram.
 anatomy of, 289
 and caffeine, 293, 296
 cultural attitudes toward, 286–89, 315
 and diet, 296, 322
 and emotions, 297–98
 general care for, 322–23
 and hyperestrogenism, 293
 and nutritional supplements, 296
 and stress, 293
Buber, Martin, 41
Bulimia, 11, 354, 359, 574. *See also* Eating disorders.
Burns, George, 626
Burwell, Judith, 348
Butter and margarine, 606–8

C
C-section. *See* Cesarean section.
Ca-125 (screening test for ovarian cancer), 219
Caffeine, 42, 446, 567, 589, 611–12. *See also* Macrobiotic diet.
 and breasts, 293, 296
 and osteoporosis, 602
 and PMS, 121, 123
 and pregnancy loss, 362
Calcium, 599–600, 601–2, 609
 and cola drinks, 455, 602
 and epinephrine, 602
 foods high in, 603–6
 and osteoporosis, 452, 455–56, 599–602

Calendula ointment, 560
Campbell, T. Colin, 597, 599
Cancer, 87, 92. *See also* listings under specific organs.
 and chakras, 87
 and fibroids, 172
 personality types for, 88, 90, 288
Cannon, Joanne, 629
Castor oil packs (treatment), 116, 117, 135–36, 547, 557, 651. *See also* Immune system.
 for breasts, 297, 311, 320
 for DUB, 140
 for endometriosis, 166, 167
Cautery, 254, 265, 269. *See also* Cryocautery; Electrocautery.
Cayce, Edgar 135
Celibacy, 233, 238–39, 283
Centers for Disease Control, 285
Centripetal energy. *See* Earth's energy.
Cervical biopsy
 and HPV 250
Cervical cancer, 13, 97, 199, 255, 263, 272–74, 486
 and abnormal Pap smear, 262
 and archetypes, 89
 decline in death rate from, 264
 and emotions, 243, 244–45
 and herpes, 252
 and HPV, 248, 252
 personality type for, 90
 and smoking, 613
 symptoms of, 262
Cervical cap 337. *See also* Contraception.
Cervical cysts, 246
Cervical dysplasia, 19, 245, 261–72. *See also* Abnormal Pap smear; HPV.
 diagnosis of, 263
 and emotions, 243, 262
 and immune system, 249, 264–65
 and life stresses, 262
 nutritional treatment for, 255, 265–66
 symptoms of, 262
 treatments for, 265–66
Cervical erosion, 246, 294

Cervical intraepithelial neoplasia (CIN), 261
Cervical mucus, 341–42
Cervical os, 150
Cervicitis, 246, 261
and HPV, 250
Cervigraphy, 263–64
and HPV, 250
Cervix, 97, 150, 241–85
anatomy of, 245–48
cultural attitudes toward, 241–45
incompetent, 362–64
Cesarean section, 10, 391–93, 410, 413. See also Childbirth; Labor; Pregnancy.
and epidural anesthesia, 389
and fetal monitoring, 391–93
and herpes, 258–59
vaginal birth after, 393
Chakras, 73–92. See also Energy system; Female energy system.
first, 77, 80–82
second, 77, 82–85, 141–42, 152–53, 446
third, 77, 85, 199
fourth, 88–90, 526
fifth, 91
sixth, 91
seventh, 91–92
and depression, 445
and energy anatomy, 78–79
higher and lower, 75–92
and mind/body connection, 75
Chamberlain, Peter, 395
Chamberlain, Wilt, 229
Channeling, 557
Chemical irritants, as cause of vaginitis, 277
Chemotherapy, 8, 271, 309, 310, 311, 312, 313, 494, 508
and surgical menopause, 442
Chia, Mantak, 459
Childbirth. See also Labor; Motherhood; Pregnancy.
emotional changes caused by, 635
and PMS onset, 121
potential risk factors in, 388
Childrearing, 60, 170

Children, and healthy diet, 616–19
Chlamydia. See Vaginitis.
Cholesterol, 627
and estriol, 472
Chopra, Deepak, 39, 435
Chromium, 584
Chronic fatigue syndrome, 22, 156
and stress, 35
Circumcision, female, 71, 419
Circumcision, male, 418–20
Cleansing Your Dietary Intuition, 621
Cleocin (clindamycin), 279
Climacteric. See Menopause.
Clindamycin (Cleocin), 279
Clitoridectomy, 241, 419
Clomid (clomiphene citrate), 206, 218, 358–59
and DUB, 134
and premature menopause, 441–42
Codependence, 117, 309, 318, 527. See also Relationship addiction.
and PMS, 128–30
Coenzyme Q, 609
Cola drinks, 455
and osteoporosis, 602
Colbin, Annemarie, 622–23
Collagen, and estriol, 472
Colonoscopy, 534
Colostrum, 415
Colposcopy, 251, 264, 269
and HPV, 250, 251
Columnar epithelium, 150
Coming of Age Doll, 146
Communication styles, male and female, 33–34
Compulsive eating, 584–85
Conception, and emotions, 374–75
Condom, 336. See also Contraception.
Condylox (podofilox), 254
Condylomata acuminata, 250
Cone biopsy, 264, 265, 274
Conscious conception. See Contraception.
Contraception, 333–37. See also listings under specific methods.
methods compared, 336–37

Contraceptive sponge, 337. See also Contraception.
Cooking, 570–72, 621–24
Copulins, 112
Cornified epithelium, 447
Corpus luteum, 197. See also Luteal cysts.
Corticosteroids, and stress, 36
Cousins, Norman, 544
Cow's milk
effect on children, 617
effect on health, 598–99
effect on newborns, 421, 599
CPR (cardiopulmonary resuscitation), 8
Cramps, menstrual. See Menstrual cramps.
Creativity, 501–503
and ovarian cysts, 213–215
and ovaries, 195–96
Creighton Model Ovulation Method, 339, 340–41. See also Fertility awareness.
Crying
and menstrual cycle, 101
and release of toxins, 55
Cryocautery, 265
as treatment for HPV, 254
Crystals, 516
Cummings, e. e., 525–26
Cyclical nature, women's, 95, 97–194, 144, 148, 207, 518
Cystic and adenomatous hyperplasia, 132, 140, 330. See also Endometrium, excessive buildup of.
treatment for, 132–33
Cystic mastalgia. See Breast pain.
Cysts. See Benign neoplastic cysts; Breast cysts; Cervical cysts; Follicular cysts; Hemmorhagic cysts; Luteal cysts; Ovarian cysts.

D

D-alpha tocopherol. See vitamin E.
D&C (dilation and curettage), 36–37, 133, 140, 183, 328, 593
and fibroids, 171
Dairy food

and breast cancer, 599
and breasts, 313
effects on health of, 598–99
and endometriosis, 160, 166–67
and menstrual cramps, 114, 116, 117
and ovarian cancer, 217–19, 599
and PMS, 121, 123
and vaginitis, 277
as yang food, 587–624
Dalton, Katerina, 101
Danazol. *See* Danocrine sulfate.
Danocrine sulfate (Danazol), 166
and endometriosis, 163–64
Davis, M. E., 152
DeCherny, Alan, 361
Decreased libido. *See* Menopause, symptoms of.
Deep process work, 57
Defensiveness, as addictive characteristic, 11
Delivery. *See* Labor.
Dementia, and premature menopause, 441
Denial, 91
as addictive characteristic, 10
Dennison, George, 419
Dependency
as addictive characteristic, 11
and fourth chakra, 89
DepoProvera (synthetic progestin), 337, 338. *See also* Contraception.
Depression, 97, 486, 553, 632. *See also* Emotions.
and chakras, 445
and DUB, 133
and ERT, 464
and hot flashes, 445
in menopause, 460–61
as PMS symptom, 119
DES (diethylstilbesterol), 182, 364
DeVeaux, Alexis, 371
DHEA (dihydroepiandosterone), 459, 475
Diagnosis, intuitive, 59
Diaphragm, 336. *See also* Contraception.
Dickstein, Leah, 5

Diet, 567–69, 572–86. *See also* Dietary approach to healing; Dietary change; Food; Macrobiotic diet.
and breast cancer, 296, 304–6
and energy system, 586–87
and hyperestrogenism, 304
Diet, high-complex-carbohydrate, high-fiber, low-fat, 115, 123, 135, 142, 207, 320, 446, 454, 566–626
Diet, macrobiotic. *See* Macrobiotic diet.
Diet, Standard American. *See* Standard American Diet.
Diet, vegetarian. *See* Vegetarian diet.
Diet, weight-loss. *See* Weight-loss diet.
Dietary approach to healing, 553–55, 556, 557, 562, 566–626. *See also* Diet; Macrobiotic diet; Vitamins.
Dietary change, 63, 572–86. *See also* Diet; Dietary approach to healing; Food
Dietary fat, 584–85
and breast cancer, 305
hydrogenated, 587, 606–7
reducing consumption of, 583–84
Diethylstilbestrol (DES), 182, 364
Dihydroepiandosterone. *See* DHEA.
Dilation and curettage. *See* D&C.
Disease, as enemy, 7, 587
Dominguez, Joe, 502
Dossey, Barbara, 556
Dossey, Larry, 191
Douching, 241–42
Summer's Eve Medicated Douche, 277
Doughty, Susan, 586
Dow Chemical, 320
Dreams, 57–58
and alcohol consumption, 615
and fibroids, 188
and menstrual cycle, 99, 101

Dreamwork 523–25, 557
Drugs. *See* Addictive system.
Dryness, vaginal. *See* Vaginal dryness and thinning.
DUB (dysfunctional uterine bleeding), 133–41
alternative treatment for, 135–36
and birth control pill, 134
conventional treatment for, 134–35
and depression, 133
and emotions, 138–39
and endometrial hyperplasia, 134
and neurotransmitters, 133
Duerk, Judith, 95
Dysfunctional uterine bleeding. *See* DUB.
Dysmenorrhea. *See* Menstrual cramps.

E

Earth, 648–50
Earth's energy, 72–73, 74. *See also* Energy system; Female energy system.
Eating disorders, 567, 635
and childhood sexual abuse, 84
and infertility, 354–55
Eating, and hunger, 580–81
Eckhart, Meister, 374
Eclampsia, 377
Education, as factor in health, 27
Ehrenfeld, David, 540
Eisler, Riane, 532
Electrocautery, as treatment for HPV, 254
Embodied thinking. *See* Feminine intelligence.
Emerson, Ralph Waldo, 655
Emotional body, 572–73
Emotional cleansing. *See* Emotions, releasing.
Emotional incision and drainage. *See* Emotions, releasing.
Emotions, 12, 30, 42, 52–54, 495, 569–77, 586, 632. *See also* Endocrine system; Energy system; Immune system; Mind/body connection;

Nervous system.
  and abortion, 328–31
  and birth control pill, 111
  and breast cancer, 288, 323
  and breasts, 297–98
  and cervical cancer, 243,
    244–45
  and cervical dysplasia, 243,
    262
  and childbirth, 635
  and chronic pelvic pain,
    155
  and conception, 374–75
  controlled by intellect, 56
  and drugs, 56
  and DUB, 138–39
  and energy blockages, 69–
    71
  and estrogen, 102
  and herpes, 243
  and immune system, 317
  and infertility, 351–53
  and inner guidance, 31, 52,
    60–66, 506–9
  and irregular menstrual
    periods, 130
  and labor, 385–88
  and menstrual cycle, 99,
    102
  and miscarriage, 362–64
  negative, 63–64
  and ovulation, 102
  physical effects of, 19, 35
  and PMS, 125, 495
  and pregnancy, 375–78
  and progesterone, 102
  releasing, 6, 55, 56–57,
    192, 506–9, 557
  and Standard American
    Diet, 592
  suppression of, 35, 55, 56
  and surgery, 556–60, 561
  and uterine-ovarian
    function, 130
  and vaginitis, 243, 280–81
  and vegetarian diet, 592
  and venereal warts, 243
  and vulvar pain, 243
Endocervix, 150, 246, 264
Endocrine system, 19
  and endometriosis, 162–63
  and mind/body
    connection, 25
  receptor sites in, 29
  as source of
    neurochemicals, 30
  and suppressed emotions,
    35
Endogenous opiates, 36

Endometrial ablation 143
  and fibroids, 183
  as treatment for heavy
    menstrual bleeding, 143–
    44
Endometrial biopsy, 131,
    133, 134, 140, 644
  and fibroids, 171
Endometrial cancer, 463
  and birth control pill,
    109
Endometrial hyperplasia,
    132, 150. See also
    Endometrium, excessive
    buildup of.
  and DUB, 134
  treatment for, 132–33
Endometrioma, 357
Endometriosis, 19–20, 22,
    42, 157–68, 200, 486. See
    also Laparoscopy.
  and adenomyosis, 142
  autoimmune components
    of, 35
  as blocked energy, 84
  causes of, 158–59, 160,
    161–62
  as cause of infertility, 351
  and chronic pelvic pain,
    155, 158
  and dairy food, 160, 599
  diagnosis of, 159
  and diet, 591
  dietary treatment for, 166–
    67
  and estrogen production,
    166–67
  and fertility, 158, 160, 163
  and fibroids, 152, 158
  and heavy menstrual
    periods, 141
  hereditary factors in, 160–
    61, 173
  hormone treatment for,
    163–64
  neuroendocrine-immune
    connection, 162
  and pregnancy, 158
  and Standard American
    Diet, 592
  surgical treatment for, 165,
    166
  and vegetarian diet, 592
Endometriosis, internal. See
    Adenomyosis.
Endometriosis of the ovary,
    200, 202
Endometrium, 106. See also
    Endometrial hyperplasia;

Cystic and adenomatous
  hyperplasia.
  and estriol, 472
  excessive buildup of, 131–
    33
Endorphins, 107, 123
Energy blockages. See
  Energy system.
Energy field. See Energy
  system.
Energy, negative, 67
Energy system, 3, 25–27,
    78–79, 192, 508, 651. See
    also Chakras; Earth's
    energy; Female energy
    system; Life-energy;
    Morphogenic fields.
  blockages in, 69–71, 84,
    201, 530–31
  and breasts, 288
  and chakras, 73–74
  changing, 70–71
  and childhood sexual
    abuse, 68–72
  and diet, 546–87, 588
  and emotional body, 572–
    73
  energy flow, 69
  and fibroids, 186
  and forgiveness, 532–33
  and hot flashes, 445, 447
  leaks in, 68–72, 651
  and obsession, 68, 69–70
  and stress, 67–69
  and surgery, 564–65
  and tubal ligation, 347
  and vaginal, vulvar, and
    cervical problems 245
Epidural anesthesia, 394
  and cesarean section, 389
Epilepsy, autoimmune
  components of, 35
Epinephrine, and calcium
  loss, 602
Episiotomy, 12, 393–94,
    401. See also Labor.
  and vulvar warts, 252
Epithelial cancer, 218. See
  also Ovarian cancer.
Epithelium, cornified, 447
Epstein-Barr virus. See
  Chronic fatigue
  syndrome.
ERT (estrogen replacement
  therapy), 462–77, 494,
  555. See also Estrogen;
  Menopause; Progestin,
  synthetic; Osteoporosis;
  Phytoestrogens.

and brain changes, 468–69
and breast cancer, 303,
   466–67
choices in, 474–75
and FSH and LH, 468–69
and heart disease, 467
and hyperestrogenism, 468
medical system bias
   toward, 464–66, 467, 473
and menopausal sexuality,
   459
and natural progesterone,
   475–76
and osteoporosis, 453,
   454, 456, 462, 464
and surgical menopause,
   470
and synthetic progestin,
   475–76
as treatment for hot
   flashes, 446
as treatment for vaginal
   dryness and thinning,
   449
Erythromycin ointment,
   417
Essential fatty acids, 115,
   123, 135, 607
and carcinogens, 607
and menstrual cramps,
   607
and immune system, 607
Estes, Clarissa Pinkola, 15,
   194, 479, 523
Estrace (estradiol), 450, 474
Estraderm (estradiol), 474
Estradiol (E2) (Estrace,
   Estraderm), 198, 470–72,
   474
Estratest (estrogen and
   testosterone), 433, 459
Estriol (E3), 465, 470–72
and breast cancer, 470–71
and cholesterol, 472
and collagen, 472
and endometrium, 472
and osteoporosis, 472
and vaginal dryness and
   thinning, 450
Estrogen, 19, 107, 134. See
   also ERT; Estradiol;
   Estriol; Estrone;
   Hyperestrogenism;
   Menopause;
   Phytoestrogens.
and breast cancer, 591,
   592–93
choices in ERT, 474–75
cream, 449

deprivation of, and hot
   flashes, 444
and diet, 311
and dietary fat, 185
early loss of, 441
and emotions, 102
and endometriosis, 166
and environmental toxins,
   303
high levels of
   (hyperestrogenism), 135
and hormonal therapy, 164
and osteoporosis, 450,
   452–53
and PMS, 121
produced by ovaries, 197–
   98
quotient, 470–71
replacement therapy. See
   ERT.
synthetic. See DES.
and vaginal dryness and
   thinning, 447–48
Estrogen replacement
   therapy. See ERT.
Estrone (E1), 198, 470–72
and body fat, 304
Evening primrose oil. See
   Gamma linoleic acid;
   Essential fatty acids.
Examination, pelvic, 247–
   48, 548–51
Exercise, 124, 573, 628–30,
   638–39
and absence of menstrual
   periods, 634–35
addiction to, 633–34
aerobic, 583, 631–32, 636
choosing a program, 637
and menopause, 469
and osteoporosis, 452
weight bearing, 455

F

Fallopian tubes, and
   infertility 355. See also
   Ovaries, anatomy of;
   Tubal ligation.
Familial ovarian cancer. See
   Ovarian cancer, familial.
Faranoff, Dr., 416
Fear 283
of abandonment, 268
of aging, 433–36
of body, 510
of emotions, 12
of mammogram, 301
of natural processes, 11
of sexuality, 229

of shaman past, 646–47
of surgery, 558–60
Feldenkrais, 530, 633
Female body. See also
   Female energy system;
   Feminine intelligence;
   Natural cycles, women's.
denigration of, 11
wisdom of, 24
Female circumcision, 241,
   419
Female energy system, 67–
   92. See also Chakras;
   Energy system.
Feminine intelligence, 32–
   40, 519–25
and birth control pill, 112
and brain hemispheres,
   32–33
Feminism, and healing, 7
Fertility, 324–73
and orgasm, 352
and Earth's population,
   371
Fertility awareness, 336,
   338–45. See also
   Contraception.
Fertility drugs. See also
   Clomid; Pergonal.
and ovarian cancer, 219
Fetal monitoring, 391–93
Fibrocystic breast disease.
   See Breast disease,
   fibrocystic.
Fibroids, 22, 45, 84, 96,
   145, 151, 168–93, 522,
   550, 557, 561, 593–95,
   651–55
and abortion, 192
and abuse, 185–86
and adenomyosis, 142
as blocked energy, 84, 186
and cancer, 172
conservative treatment for,
   177–78
and dairy food, 599
degeneration of, 171, 184–
   85
and diet, 591
dietary treatment for, 185
and emotions, 84
and endometriosis, 152,
   158, 173–74
and energy system, 70
and GnRH agonists, 182
healing program for, 186–
   87
and heavy menstrual
   periods, 141

Fibroids (*continued*)
hereditary factors in, 172–73
hormone therapy for, 182
and hysterectomy, 178–80, 183, 189–91
and infertility, 174
and menopause, 184–85
and miscarriage, 174
myomectomy for, 181
and pelviscopic surgery, 165–66
and postabortion emotions, 329
and relationships, 84, 170, 187, 188–89, 191
and second chakra issues, 83, 84, 170
"seedling," 176
and Standard American Diet, 185, 592
and stress, 187
subserosal and submucosal, 170
symptoms of, 170–72
and ultrasound, 172
and vegetarian diet, 592, 593
and work issues, 153
Fimbria (ends of fallopian tubes), 149, 150
Fisher and Cleveland, 88, 90
Flagyl (metronidazole), 279
Flamm, Bruce, 393
Flaxseed oil. *See* Gamma linoleic acid; Essential fatty acids.
Folate, 354
Folic acid, 255, 265, 266
Follicle stimulating hormone. *See* FSH.
Follicular cysts, 201–202. *See also* Ovarian cysts.
Follicular phase. *See* Menstrual cycle.
Fonda, Jane, 633
Food addiction, 567, 574, 584–85. *See also* Bingeing; Food cravings.
ending, 578–79
Food allergies, 611
Food cravings, 572
and inner guidance, 579–80
Forceps delivery, 10
Forgiveness, 532–37
Fox, Matthew, 66
Free radicals, 606

Freud, Sigmund, 242, 286
FSH (follicle stimulating hormone), 98–100, 107, 296
and ERT, 468–69
during menopause, 439–41
Fundus (upper uterus), 149
Fuzzy thinking (in menopause), 461–62. *See also* Menopause, symptoms of.
distinguished from dementia, 441

G

Gaby, Alan, 466
Gamma linoleic acid, 114, 115, 123, 296
Gardnerella. *See also* Vaginitis.
and HPV, 250
Garlic, 609
as treatment for herpes, 259–60
Gaskin, Ina Mae, 405
Genital warts. *See* Warts, venereal.
George, Demetra, 99
George Washington School of Medicine, 136
Gittleman, Ann-Louise, 598
GnRH agonists
and endometriosis, 163–64
as treatment for fibroids, 182–83
Goals, setting lifetime, 542
Goddess, 517–19
Goethe, Johann Wolfgang von, 483
Goldberg, Natalie, 519, 523
Golden handcuff syndrome, and ovarian cancer, 217
Gonadotropin releasing hormone. *See* GnRH agonists.
Goodman, Ellen, 426
Gornick, Vivian, 647
Greer, Germaine, 24, 430
Guerin, Maude, 42

H

Hargrove, Joel, 476
Hay, Louise, 270
Hayden, Nora, 228
Hays, Bethany, 393, 403–5, 418

Healer. *See* Health care provider.
Healing. *See also* Dietary approach to healing; Surgery.
body's innate ability in, 56
contrasted with curing, 41–49
energy leaks, 69
and lower chakra wounds, 90–91
power of, 41–42
steps for, 485–542
Health care, getting the most out of, 544–65
Health care provider, 544–48
Healthy diet. *See also* High-complex-carbohydrate, high-fiber, low-fat diet; Macrobiotic diet; Vegetarian diet
and children, 616–19
types of, 596
Heart disease
and ERT, 467
and removal of ovaries, 215
Heart rate, target, 630–31
Hemispheres of brain, and feminine intelligence 32–33
Hemorrhagic cysts, 202–3. *See also* Ovarian cysts.
Herbs, 137, 166, 308, 446–47, 449, 469, 557, 560, 584
Herpes, 35, 42, 89, 97, 237, 243, 247, 256–61. *See also* Immune system.
and cervical cancer, 252
dietary supplements for, 260–61
dormancy of, 251–52
medications for, 259
nutritional treatment for, 259–60
as PMS symptom, 119
and pregnancy, 257–58
primary and secondary outbreaks, 256
transmission of, 257–58
types distinguished, 256
Herpes, genital, 10, 13, 18
Hesse, Lori, 5
High-complex-carbohydrate, high-fiber, low-fat diet, 115, 123, 135, 142, 207, 321, 446, 454,

566–626 *See also*
Macrobiotic diet.
Higher power, 14, 49, 514–
19
Highwater, Jamake, 3
History, personal, 485–92
Holistic medicine, 545–47
Home birth, 410–13
Home Health Products, 135
Homeopathy, 447
and fibroids, 186
and menopause, 469
Hormones. *See also*
Androgens; Estrogen;
Progesterone;
Testosterone.
and crying, 55
Hot flashes, 19–20, 42, 97,
130, 163, 444–47. *See also*
Menopause, symptoms
of.
causes of, 444
and depression, 445
as energy, 445
and ERT, 464
Houston, Jean, 32
HPV (human papilloma
virus), 248–56, 267
and cervical cancer, 248,
249, 252
diagnosis of, 250
dormancy of, 251–52
Human papilloma virus.
See HPV.
Hurricane Island Outward
Bound School, 623
Hydrogenated fat. *See*
Dietary fat.
Hyperestrogenism (high
estrogen levels), 135, 296.
See also Estrogen.
and breasts, 293
and breast cancer, 295, 304
and diet, 304, 591
and ERT, 468
Hyperprolactinemia (high
prolactin levels), 133
Hypertonic uterine inertia,
398
Hypnotism, 560
Hypoglycemia (low blood
sugar), and PMS, 129
Hysterectomy, 20, 42, 133,
140, 141, 143, 149, 151, 152,
178–80, 269, 469, 486,
556, 560, 561–62, 563,
594
effects of, 179–80
and endometriosis, 165

and fibroids, 174, 175, 184,
189–91
and heart disease, 180
and menopause, 180
and ovarian cancer, 219
and Pap smear, 264
and sexual response, 179–
89
and surgical menopause,
442
and urinary problems, 180
Hysterectomy-
oophorectomy, 179–80
Hysterosalpingogram, 174
Hysteroscopy, 183

I

Ibuprofen (Advil, Motrin),
143, 610
Illness, and blame, 44–45,
49
Immune system, 8, 9, 25,
29, 30, 35–36, 311, 444.
See also Castor oil packs;
Mind/body connection.
benefited by exercise, 629
and cervical dysplasia, 249,
264–65
and depression, 33
and emotions, 317
and endometriosis, 162–63
and essential fatty acids,
607
and food allergies, 611
and HPV, 249, 251, 252
and infertility, 351
and nutritional
supplements, 608–9
and pregnancy loss, 363
and STDs, 283–85
and vaginitis, 280
Immunosuppression, and
stress, 35–36
Implants. *See* Breast
implants, silicone.
In vitro fertilization. *See*
IVF.
Incest, 71, 88, 495
and chronic pelvic pain,
155
and first chakra issues, 81
and sexuality, 231
and vaginitis, 242
Incompetent cervix, 362–
64. *See also* Miscarriage.
Infante-Rivard, Claire, 363
Infertility, 57, 96, 167, 350–
67. *See also* Payne,
Niravi.

and artificial light, 354
autoimmune components
of, 35
and birth control pill, 354
causes of, 350–52
and eating disorders, 354–
55
and emotions, 351–53
and endometriosis, 160,
163, 351
and fibroids, 174
nutritional factors in, 354–
55
and relationships, 353
surgery techniques for,
564
and tubal problems, 355
Infibulation, 419
Infidelity, 281
Information-gathering,
531–32
Inner guidance, 14, 23, 24,
50–66, 514–19, 650. *See
also* Emotions; Energy
system; Female energy
system; Feminine
intelligence; Intuition.
and body wisdom, 31
and dietary change, 585–
86
and dreams, 57–58
and emotions, 31, 52, 60–
66, 506–9
and ERT, 476–77
and food cravings, 579–
80
and intuition, 59
and labor, 376, 378
and mammograms, 301
and menstrual healing, 103
and ovaries, 207
and ovarian cancer, 217
trusting, 12, 13, 21, 38, 50
Intercourse, frequent, as
cause of vaginitis, 276
Intercourse, painful
(dyspareunia), 237
International Childbirth
Education Association,
392
Intestinal biocultures, 280
Intestinal dysbiosis, 610
and vaginitis, 278
Intuition, 58–59, 649
and birth control pill, 108–
13
and exercise, 631
Intuitive diagnosis, 59
Iodine supplement, 297

Irritable bowel syndrome, 610–11
IUD (intrauterine device), 335, 336, 643–45. *See also* Contraception.
and infertility, 351
IVF (in vitro fertilization), 358–59

J

James, William, 31
Jesus, 640
Johnson, Dana, 61
Johnson, Karen, 566, 577
Johnson, Magic, 229
Johnson, Sonia, 7, 310, 648
Jones, Jenny, 315
Jujitsu, 632
Jung, Carl, 84

K

K-Y jelly, 448
Kaats, Gil, 584
Katahn, Martin, 621
Keeler, George, 34
Kegel's exercise, 235–36
Kennedy, John F. and Jacqueline, 65
Kennel, John, 416
Klaus, Marshall, 416
Klein, Luella, 324
Koilocytotic change, 269
Kübler-Ross, Elisabeth, 49, 365, 506
Kushi, Michio, 72, 587, 588. *See also* Macrobiotic diet.
Kussman, Leslie, 495

L

Labor, 384–91, 403
anesthesia in, 394
and childhood abuse, 386
dysfunctional, 96
and inner guidance, 376, 378
premature, 376–77
sterilization in, 395–96
Lahey Clinic, 500
Lamaze, 399, 402, 406, 407, 418
Landers, Ann, 230
Lane, Nancy, 634
Langer, Ellen, 40
Laparoscopy, 156, 159, 160, 167, 220, 357, 358. *See also* Endometriosis.
Large Loop Excision of Transformation Zone (LLETZ). *See* LEEP.

Laser treatment, 253, 265, 269
Laurel's Kitchen, 425
Lee, John, 165
LEEP (Loop Electrode Excision Procedure), 264, 265
for cervical dysplasia, 255
for wart removal, 255
LeGuin, Ursula, 532
Lemon, Harry, 470
Levine, Barbara, 511
Levine, Stephen, 57, 506, 537, 643
LH (luteinizing hormone), 98–103, 107, 296
and ERT, 468–69
during menopause, 436, 439–41
Life-energy, 502
Life expectancy, 27, 629
Light, artificial, and infertility, 354
Light therapy, 136
and osteoporosis, 452
for PCO, 207
for PMS relief, 124
Linoleic acid. *See* Gamma linoleic acid.
Lipotropic factors, 185
Lithium succinate ointment, 260
Longevity (magazine), 633
Loop Electrode Excision Procedure. *See* LEEP.
Lorde, Audre, 225, 650
Low serum retinol, 305
Lumpectomy, 308, 309, 310
Lupron 163, 182–83. *See also* GnRH agonists.
Luteal cysts, 202–3. *See also* Corpus luteum; Ovarian cysts.
Luteal phase. *See* Menstrual cycle.
Luteinizing hormone. *See* LH.
Lysine, as treatment for herpes, 260–61

M

Mackensie, Margaret, 577
Macrobiotic diet, 72, 185–86, 188, 237, 573, 587–624. *See also* High-complex-carbohydrate, high-fiber, low-fat diet; Vegetarian diet.
healing effects of, 588–95

and protein, 595–97
Macrobiotics. *See* Macrobiotic diet.
Magnesium, 114, 455, 560, 585, 600, 607, 609
and endometriosis, 167
and fibroids, 185
and osteoporosis, 452
and PMS, 122
Magnetic resonance imaging. *See* MRI.
Malpractice suit, 546
Mammary dysplasia, 471
Mammograms, 295, 298–303
Marron, Michael, 513
Martial arts, 632
Massage, 166, 186, 313, 530, 588
Mastectomy, 308, 309, 310, 323. *See also* Breast cancer.
Masters and Johnson, 457
Matter-energy continuum, 67–72. *See also* Energy system.
McCain, Marian Van Eck, 461
McClellan, Myron, 507
McDonald, Evy, 496
McDonald's, 590, 609
McDougall, John, 597
McGarey, Gladys, 135, 331
McKinlay, Sonja, 460
McNoll, Kenneth, 532
Mead, Margaret, 414
Meade, Michael, 33
Meal Plan for Self-Nurturance, 584
Meat, 566, 584, 585, 587–624
Meditation, 43, 92, 123–24, 137, 210, 447, 497, 516, 519, 521
on forgiveness, 537–39
Mefenamic acid (Ponstel), 143
Mehl, Lewis, 387
Melaleuca Company, 279
Melaleuca oil, as treatment for herpes, 259–60
Mellody, Pia, 282
Memories, prenatal and birth, 324
Menarche. *See* Menstrual periods, onset of.
Menopause, 11, 97, 130, 175, 436–42. *See also* Decreased libido; Fuzzy

thinking; Hot flashes;
Vaginal dryness and
thinning.
and androgen production,
436–38, 469
and breast cancer, 591
changes in menstrual cycle
in, 438–41
cultural attitudes toward,
430–36, 443–44
as deficiency disease, 198
and emotional stress, 443
and fibroids, 170
and fuzzy thinking, 461–
62
and hysterectomy, 180
and lunar information, 100
medicalization of, 432–36,
464–66
mood swings and
depression in, 460–61
self-care during, 477–79
sexuality in, 457–59
symptoms of, 442–50
Menopause, artificial. See
Menopause, surgical.
Menopause, natural. See
Menopause.
Menopause, premature,
441–42, 494, 508
as autoimmune disorder,
35, 441
and dementia, 441
Menopause, surgical, 438,
442
and ERT, 469–70
Menorrhagia. See
Menstrual periods, heavy.
Menses, Goddess, 147–48
Menses. See Menstrual
periods.
Menstrual cramps, 113–18,
142. See also Menstrual
cycle; Menstrual periods.
and birth control pill, 109
and dairy food, 114, 116,
599
dietary treatment for, 114–
15
distinguished from PMS,
113, 120
energy medicine for, 116
and essential fatty acids,
606–7
and PGF2 alpha, 114, 120
primary and secondary,
113
Menstrual cycle, 95, 97–
102, 104, 634. See also

Menstrual periods;
Natural cycles, women's.
and birth control pill, 108–
13
changes in, during
menopause, 438–41
and fertility awareness,
342–45
follicular and luteal
phases, 98–103
irregular, and
osteoporosis, 452
in native cultures, 103, 104,
147
without ovulation
(anovulatory cycle), 125
Menstrual cycle,
anovulatory, 125, 131
Menstrual Health
Foundation, 146
Menstrual periods, absence
of (amenorrhea), 96, 138.
See also PCO.
and bone loss, 634–35
and exercise, 634–35
and mind/body
connection, 205
and osteoporosis, 634–35
and PMS onset, 121
Menstrual periods, bleeding
between. See DUB.
Menstrual periods, end of.
See Menopause.
Menstrual periods, heavy
(menorrhagia), 96, 116,
141–44
and Standard American
Diet, 592
as symptom of fibroids,
170
and vegetarian diet, 592,
593
Menstrual periods,
irregular, 30–31, 96, 130–
31, 139–41. See also
DUB.
and alcohol, 615
and bone loss, 131
and menopause, 439
Menstrual periods, onset of
(menarche), 105
and breast cancer, 591
as rite of passage, 106,
144–48
Menstrual wisdom, 95, 98,
144–48
reclaiming, 104, 113, 144–
48
Menstruation. See

Menstrual cramps;
Menstrual cycle; listings
under Menstrual periods.
Menstruation, cultural
attitudes toward, 104–8
Mental efficiency, benefited
by exercise, 629
Metabolism, rehabilitating,
582–84
Metcalf, Linda Trichter,
519, 526
MetroGel (metronidazole),
279
Metronidazole (Flagyl,
MetroGel), 279
Microwave ovens, 624
Migraine headache, 53, 55
and intestinal dysbiosis,
610
as PMS symptom, 119
Milk. See Cow's milk.
Mind/body connection, 22
and body systems, 25
and chakras, 75
and energy fields, 26
and healing, 29
science of (PNI), 28
Miscarriage, 96, 130, 167,
362–64
and caffeine, 362
and emotions, 362–64
and fibroids, 174
and smoking, 613
and psychotherapy, 363
Molimina, 131
Montagu, Ashley, 66, 422
Moon, and female cycles,
97–100, 104, 518
Morning-after pill
(RU486), 328
Morphogenic fields, 646–
47
Mothering, 414–29
Motherpeace Tarot deck,
517, 652
Motrin (ibuprofen), 116, 143
MRI (magnetic resonance
imaging), 142
and fibroids, 174
Ms. (magazine), 649
Muir, Caroline and Charles,
226–27
Multimodal thinking. See
Feminine intelligence.
Multivitamin-mineral
supplement, 115, 123, 135,
143, 167, 185, 255, 266,
283, 311, 320, 354, 584,
585, 601

Myomectomy (removal of
    fibroids), 181, 560
Myss, Caroline, 71, 156,
    243, 348, 435, 651
    on abortion, 332
    on angels, 516
    on birthing, 384
    on breasts, 288
    on cancer, 310
    on chakras, 73–74, 75, 79,
        80, 87, 90
    on menstrual cramps and
        PMS, 113
    on fibroids, 169
    on hot flashes, 445
    on irregular periods, 130
    on menopause, 434–35,
        438
    on ovarian cysts, 209, 210
    on surgery, 561
    and victims, 530
    on tubal ligation, 347
    on tubal problems, 355

N

Nabothian cysts. See
    Cervical cysts.
Naproxen sulfate
    (Anaprox), 115, 116, 117,
    143
National Cancer
    Association, 293
National Cancer Institute,
    304
Native American healing,
    192
Natural family planning.
    See Fertility awareness.
Natural Gourmet Cookery
    School, 622–23
Natural menopause. See
    Menopause.
Natural progesterone. See
    Progesterone, natural.
Nature, and spirituality,
    518–519
Naturopathy, 447
Nautilus machine, 636
Navaho, 73, 443
Neonates, high-risk, 416
Nervous system, 19
    brain chemicals and
        receptor sites in, 29
    and endometriosis, 162–63
    and mind/body
        connection, 25
    stimuli processed by, 28
Neurochemicals, sources
    of, 29–30

Neuropeptides, 98–99
Neurotransmitters, 107
    and DUB, 133
New Cycle Company, 146
Newborns
    bonding with, 414–29
    importance of touching,
        414–18
Nipple discharge, 293, 294,
    295–97
Noble, Vicki, 412, 445, 517
Nonsteroidal anti-
    inflammatory drugs, 115,
    610
NordicTrack, 455, 636
Norepinephrine, 444
Norplant (synthetic
    progestin implant), 337,
    338. See also
    Contraception.
Nourishment, reframing,
    572–86
Nuprin, 115
Nutritional supplements,
    608–10. See also Calcium;
    Multivitamin-mineral
    supplement; Vitamins;
    Zinc.

O

O'Toole, Annie Gill, 503
OB/GYN, 546, 547
    attitude toward uterus, 151
    establishment and drug
        companies, 183
    conventional training in,
        10, 393, 397
Obesity, 576
    and childhood sexual
        abuse, 84
Obsession, and energy 68,
    69–70
Oil, cooking, 608
Oil of evening primrose.
    See Gamma linoleic acid;
    Essential fatty acids.
Oophorectomy, 179–80,
    469. See also Ovaries,
    removal of.
Orbach, Susie, 568
Orgasm, and fertility, 352
Ornish, Dean, 593
Ortho Pharmaceutical, 110
Oski, Frank, 421, 617
Osteopathy, 530
Osteoporosis, 450–56, 599–
    600
    and alcohol, 602, 615
    and caffeine, 602

and calcium, 599–602
and colas and root beer,
    602
and ERT, 462
and estrogen, 450, 452–53
and estriol, 472
and exercise, 634
and martial arts, 632
and muscle weakness, 631
and natural progesterone,
    453, 454
and removal of ovaries,
    198, 215
and smoking, 602, 614
and Standard American
    Diet, 592
and synthetic progestin,
    463
and vegetarian diet, 592
Ovarian cancer, 88, 96, 199,
    215–24
    and birth control pill, 109
    causes of, 216, 217–19
    conventional treatment
        for, 222–23
    diagnosis, 219–20
    and dairy food, 599
    and diet, 217, 591
    hereditary factors in, 173
    and hysterectomy, 218
    rapid growth rate of, 217
    and second chakra issues,
        216
    and socioeconomic status,
        217
    and Standard American
        Diet, 592
    and tubal ligation, 218,
        347
    and vegetarian diet, 592
Ovarian cancer, familial.
    See Ovarian cancer,
    hereditary factors in.
Ovarian cysts, 19, 96, 154,
    201–204, 357, 504, 546,
    550, 557, 562–63. See also
    Ovarian cancer; PCO.
    and cancer, 203
    hereditary factors in, 173
    and menstrual cycle, 196–
        201
    and second chakra issues,
        212
    and stress, 42
    surgery for, 210–11
    symptomatic functional,
        201–204
    and work issues, 153, 212–
        13

Ovarian energy, 154, 194–
96, 458–59
Ovarian growths, benign,
distinguished from
cancer, 199
Ovarian wisdom. See
Ovarian energy.
Ovaries, 96, 194–224. See
also Menopause.
anatomy of, 196–201
and androgens, 204
endometriosis of, 200, 202
and energy blockage, 84
enlarged, 135
functions in aging, 197–98,
215–16
and hormones, 197–98
and life stresses, 199–201,
205
during menopause, 436–
38
and non-Western
traditions, 198
and osteoporosis, 198
postmenopausal functions,
197–98
and second chakra, 83
and smoking, 614
Ovaries, removal of
(oophorectomy), 20, 197,
215–16, 220, 504
during other pelvic
surgery, 221–22
and surgical menopause,
442
and testosterone
production, 438
and tubes, 42
Overeaters Anonymous,
528, 580, 585
Overweight 568
and DUB, 134
as health risk, 576
and menstrual cycle, 635
and PMS, 122
Ovulation, 130, 196, 206.
See also Menstrual cycle;
Ovaries.
and emotions, 102
and infertility, 351
Ovulation Method. See
Fertility awareness.
Oxytocin, 421, 443

P

Paladin, Linda, 556
Pap smear, 9, 548, 549, 550
as diagnostic tool, 263
false negative rate, 263

history of technique, 263
recommended screening
interval, 264
Pap smear, abnormal, 21,
27, 43, 77, 244, 274, 501,
522. See also Cervical
dysplasia.
and smoking, 613
and cervical cancer, 262
Papanicolaou, George, 263
Parton, Dolly, 513
Patriarchy
as addictive system, 5–6
religions of, 5, 516
view of female body, 4,
10–12
view of success and failure
of, 373
Pauling, Linus, 455
Payne, Niravi, 163, 353,
361
PC muscle, 248, 551
in sex technique, 235–36
PCO (polycystic ovaries),
205–7
and amenorrhea, 205
and infertility, 206–7
and Standard American
Diet, 592
treatment for, 206–7
and vegetarian diet, 592
Peay, Pythia, 514
Pelvic examination, 247–48,
548–51
Pelvic organs, and second
chakra, 79
Pelvic pain, chronic, 19, 20,
22, 29, 42, 58, 142, 155–
57, 330
causes of, 155
and childhood sexual
abuse, 84
and endometriosis, 155,
158
Pelvic pressure, as
symptom of fibroids, 171
Pelviscopic surgery, 165–66
Pergonal (fertility drug),
218, 358
Perimenopausal, 174–75,
433
Peritoneum, 161
Perry, Rick, 623
Pert, Candace, 25, 29
Peterson, Gayle, 387
PGF2 alpha (hormone)
and menstrual cramps,
114–15, 120
and PMS, 120

Physician. See Health care
provider.
Phytoestrogens, 470–72
Pick, Marcelle, 270, 586
Piezoelectric effect, 632
Pill, birth control, 316. See
also Contraception.
and B vitamins, 265, 266,
335
and breast cancer, 303,
336
and cervical dysplasia, 265,
266, 336
as contraceptive, 335, 336,
338
and DUB, 134, 136
and emotions, 111
and endometriosis, 163
and female intelligence,
112
and infertility, 354
and intuition, 108–13
and ovarian cancer, 219
and PCO, 206
and menstrual cycle, 108–
13
and smoking, 134, 338
Pitocin, 398–99
Planetary healing, 648–50
Planned Parenthood, 230
Pliny the Elder, 104
PMS (premenstrual
syndrome), 22, 62, 96,
103, 118–29, 508
and birth control pill, 121
diagnosis and symptoms
of, 119–20
and emotions, 125, 495
and estrogen-progesterone
imbalance, 125
distinguished from
menstrual cramps, 113,
120
and lunar information, 100
and macrobiotic diet, 589
nutritional factors in, 121–
22
and prostaglandin
hormones, 120
and stress, 125
symptoms alleviated by
exercise, 629
Podofilox (Condylox), 254
Podophyllin, treatment for
HPV, 254
Polarity therapy, 186
Polycystic ovaries. See
PCO; Polycystic ovary
syndrome.

Polycystic ovary syndrome, 134–35. *See also* PCO.

Ponstel (mefenamic acid), 115, 143

Popo-Cordie, Jamie, 621

Postmenopausal bleeding, 130

Pre- and Perinatal Psychology Association, 332

Pregnancy, 96, 374–84
and age, 379–80
cultural attitudes toward, 375–80
ectopic, 202
and emotions, 375–78
and endometriosis, 158
and exercise, 629, 636
and fibroids, 173–74
and herpes, 257–58
and HPV, 252
loss of, 362–67
and nutritional supplements, 609
and smoking, 613
transforming power of, 380–84
teenage, 372

Premarin (estrogen cream), 433–34, 450, 466, 474

Premature menopause. *See* Menopause, premature.

Premenstrual syndrome. *See* PMS.

Prior, Jerrilyn, 432

ProGest cream (natural progesterone), 136, 138, 143, 165, 454

Progesterone, 107, 354, 380. *See also* Menopause; Menstrual cycle.
and corpus luteum, 197
and emotions, 102
and osteoporosis, 452–53
and ovaries, 197–98
and PMS, 121

Progesterone, natural, 124–26. *See also* ERT; Menopause; Progestone cream.
and DUB, 136
and endometrial hyperplasia, 133
and endometriosis, 165
in ERT, 475–76
and fibroids, 182, 184
and heavy menstrual periods, 143
and hot flashes, 446

and osteoporosis, 453, 454
and menopause, 469
and PMS relief, 124
distinguished from synthetic progestin, 124–25

Progesterone, synthetic. *See* Progestin, synthetic.

Progestin, synthetic, 124–25, 133–34, 337. *See also* Amen; Aygest; Contraception; ERT; Menopause; Provera.
and endometriosis, 163
in ERT, 475–76
and fibroids, 182, 184
and heavy menstrual periods, 143
and hot flashes, 446
injectable (as contraceptive method), 337, 338
and osteoporosis, 453, 463
and PCO, 206

Progestone cream (natural progesterone), 143

Prolactin, 133, 289, 294, 421, 443. *See also* Breasts; Motherhood.

Prostaglandin E series, 114

Prostaglandin F2 alpha. *See* PGF2 alpha.

Prostaglandin inhibitor, 143

Protein, need for, 597
consumption of, 597

Provera (synthetic progestin), 133, 136, 143, 206, 453, 463. *See also* Progestin, synthetic.

Prozac, 553–54

Psychoneuroimmunology. *See* PNI.

Psychotherapy, 526–30

Pubococcygeous muscle. *See* PC muscle.

PW (propioceptive writing), 519–22

R

Radiation (treatment), 8, 310

Radner, Gilda, 220

Rafter, Annie, 483, 529, 650

Rage, 649–50

Rainforest destruction, 566

Rape, 87, 88, 127
and sexuality, 231
and shame, 88

RAST (test for food allergies), 611

RDA (recommended daily allowance), 600, 608

Receptors, in nervous system, 29

Recommended daily allowance. *See* RDA.

Recovery movement, 528

Reduction mammoplasty. *See* Breast reduction.

Redwine, David, 158, 161, 162

Reiki treatment, 188, 530

Reis, Patricia, 41, 147, 231, 517

Reiter, Robert, 84

Relational thinking. *See* Feminine intelligence.

Relationship addiction, 13, 18, 189, 318, 527, 570, 652
as form of control, 14
and fourth chakra, 89
and PMS, 127–29

Relationships, 496, 526–27
and chakras, 82–85, 89
and childhood trauma, 42
and chronic pelvic pain, 155
and fibroids, 84, 170, 187, 188–89, 191
and heavy menstrual periods, 141–42
and infertility, 353
and labor, 387
and ovarian cysts, 200
and ovarian cancer, 216
and shame, 88
and uterus, 153
and vulva, vagina, and cervix problems, 242, 245

Relaxation, 447
as benefit of exercise, 629

Relaxation Response, 123–24

Replens, 448

Reproductive organs, and second chakra, 79

Responsibility for illness, 45

Rhythm method of contraception. *See* Fertility awareness.

Rich, Adrienne, 519

Robert, Karl-Hendrick, 554

Robin, Vicki, 502

Rolfing, 530

Roosevelt, Eleanor, 508

Rosenthal, Marge, 147

Roth, Geneen, 580

RU487. *See* Morning-after pill.
Rubenstein, Boris, 103
Ruble, Diane, 102
Rutter, Peter, 527

S

Sadker, Myra and David, 5
Sagan, Leonard, 27
Salpingo-oophorectomy, bilateral. *See* Menopause, surgical.
Sattilaro, Anthony, 313
Schaef, Anne Wilson, 4, 16–17, 50, 138, 270, 426, 496, 507, 525, 528, 555, 638, 640–41
  on addiction, 6
  on addictive system, 66
  on dependency, 15
  on rage, 549
  on romance addiction, 514
Schauss, Alexander, 586
Schwartz, Bob, 576
Schweitzer, Albert, 565
SCJ (squamocolumnar junction), 150, 246, 263, 264
Scott-Maxwell, Florida, 485
Seasonal affective disorder (SAD), 122
Selenium, 122, 255, 296, 304–5, 609
Self-abuse addiction, 638
Self-acceptance, benefited by exercise, 629
Self-acknowledgment, 503–5
Self-esteem, 283
  as factor in health, 27
  heightened by exercise, 629
  and sexuality, 228
  and third chakra, 77, 85
Sesame oil, 448
Sex addiction, 13, 127
Sex and Love Addicts Anonymous (SLA), 127, 189, 268
Sexual freedom, 326
Sexuality, tantric, 226
Sexuality, women's, 225–40
  and abuse, 229
  anatomy of, 225–26
  cultural conditioning about, 228–32
  and fears, 229
  and guilt, 242, 244
  and hysterectomy, 179–80

and incest, 231
  lesbian, 229
  in menopause, 457–59
  and nature, 234–40
  and rape, 231
  reclaiming, 232–40
  and religion, 231–32
  and second chakra, 445
  and self-esteem, 228
  Taoist practices, 235
  techniques, 235–36
  and vaginitis, 242, 243
Sexually transmitted disease. *See* STDs.
Shamanism, 646–48
  and abortion, 332
  and "soul retrieval," 68
Shame, 88
  and energy dysfunction, 88
Shaw, Farida, 430
Shealy, Norman, 75, 79, 286
Sheehan, Nancy McBrine, 428
Sheldrake, Rupert, 646–47
Shiatsu, 588
Shinn, Frances Scovell, 515
SIDS (sudden infant death syndrome), and smoking, 613
Siegel, Bernie, 8, 48, 270, 422, 515
SIL (squamous intraepithelial lesion), 261, 265
Silver nitrate, 417
Slayton, Tamara, 146, 431–32
Sleep
  benefited by exercise, 629
  deprivation, and hot flashes, 445
Smith-Rosenberg, Carroll, 327, 328
Smokers Anonymous, 614
Smoking, effects of, 612–15
  and HPV, 251
  and osteoporosis, 452, 455, 602
Spangler, David, 515, 627, 639
Spermicidal foam, 336. *See also* Contraception.
Spirituality, 514–19
Spock, Benjamin, 419
Squamocolumnar junction. *See* SCJ.
Squamous epithelium, 150, 246

Squamous intraepithelial lesion. *See* SIL.
Squamous metaplasia, 246
Standard American Diet, 596, 618–19
  benefits and risks, 587, 592, 593
  and menarche, 591
  and menopause, 591
Stanford, Joseph, 338, 339
Stanton, Elizabeth Cady, 232
STDs (sexually transmitted diseases), 13, 31, 283–85
Steinem, Gloria, 650
Stillbirth, 364–67
Strang High Risk Center, 306
Stress, 67–68, 651
  and androgens, 436
  and breasts, 293
  and chronic fatigue syndrome, 35
  and chronic pelvic pain, 155
  and corticosteroid levels, 36
  and DUB, 135
  effect on ovaries and uterus, 199
  and exercise addiction, 634
  and fibroids, 187
  and herpes, 35, 42
  and hot flashes, 447
  and HPV, 249
  and immunosuppression, 35–36
  and infertility, 351
  and menopause, 443
  and menstrual cramps, 114, 117
  and osteoporosis, 452
  and ovarian cysts, 42
  and ovarian functioning, 205
  and PMS, 125
  and pregnancy loss, 363
  reduction, 116, 123, 137
  and vaginitis, 277, 280
  and venereal warts, 42
  and vulvar problems, 243
Sugar, 69, 305, 445, 584–85
  addiction, 567
  and PMS, 121, 123
  as yin food, 587–624
Superdophilus, 280

Surgery, 552–55, 555–65
and energy system, 564–
65
preference of medical
system for, 8
Surgery, pelviscopic, 165–
66
Swimme, Brian, 539, 628
Symptoms as messages, 496
Synarel (GnRH agonist),
163–64, 182–83
cost of, 164
Synthetic progesterone. See
Progestin, synthetic.

T

Tai chi, 313, 632, 637
Tamoxifen, 471–72
and breast cancer, 592–93
Tannen, Deborah, 33
Tara Humara Indians, 435,
628
Tarot, Motherpeace deck,
517
TCA (trichloroacetic acid),
254, 265
as treatment for HPV, 254
Technologies, birth, 390–96
Testosterone, 438, 459
Therapeutic touch, 8, 188,
270, 530–31, 644
Therapeutic sound, 175
Thinness, cultural attitudes
toward, 511–12, 573–77,
633–34
Thinning, vaginal. See
Vaginal dryness and
thinning.
Thomas, Caroline, 71
Thomas, Lewis, 92
Tims, Bill, 624
Toxemia, 377–78
Treatment, choosing, 552–
55
Trichloroacetic acid. See
TCA.
Trichomonas. See Vaginitis.
Triestrogen, 475
Tubal ligation, 321, 337,
345–47. See also
Contraception; Fallopian
tubes.
and energy system, 347
laparoscopic, 159
and ovarian cancer, 219,
347
and PMS onset, 121
and surgical menopause,
442

unipolar electrocautery,
121
Tums, 602
Tupperwrite, C., 362
Turner, Kristina, 623
Twelve-step program, 37–
38, 127, 129, 189, 496,
528, 530, 532

U

Ultrasound (sonogram), 135
and fibroids, 174, 177
Urethral thinning, 448
Urinary frequency, 448
and caffeine, 611
as symptom of fibroids,
171–72
Urinary tract infection, 237,
610
Uterine biopsy, 36, 642
Uterine cancer, 36, 88
and chronic anovulation,
132
and Standard American
Diet, 592
and vegetarian diet, 592
Uterine energy, 154
Uterine lining. See
Endometrium.
Uterus, 96, 149–93
attitude of medical system
toward, 151–52
and chakras, 83, 152–53,
199
energy anatomy of, 152–
54
and hysterosalpingogram,
174
and life stresses, 199
as "low heart," 88

V

Vagina, 97, 241–85
anatomy of, 245–48
cultural attitudes toward,
241–45
Vaginal discharge, 275–76
Vaginal dryness and
thinning, 447–50, 458,
464. See also Menopause,
symptoms of.
causes of, 447
diagnosis of, 447
and estrogen, 447–48
estrogen treatment for,
449–50
herbal treatment for, 449
lubrication treatment for,
448–50

visualization treatment
for, 449
Vaginal infection. See
Vaginitis.
Vaginal intraepithelial
neoplasia (VIN), 267
Vaginitis, 13, 19, 42, 58, 231,
247, 275–83, 447, 533,
582
autoimmune components
of, 35
causes of, 276–78
and dairy food, 599
diagnosis of, 278
and douching, 279–80
and emotions, 243, 280–81
and guilt feelings over
sexuality, 242
and HPV, 250
and incest, 242
and intercourse, 244
and intestinal dysbiosis,
610
and macrobiotic diet, 589
medications for, 279
and sexuality, 243
symptoms of, 276
Valium, 122, 633
Vasectomy, 337. See also
Contraception.
Vegan diet, 596
Vegetables, as centering
food, 587–624
Vegetarian diet, 584. See
also Macrobiotic diet.
benefits and risks, 593
and menarche, 591
and menopause, 591
and protein, 595–98
and vitamin B$_{12}$, 591, 598
Venereal warts. See Warts,
venereal.
Virginity, 233
Visualization, 449, 557
Vitamins, 63. See also
Multivitamin-mineral
supplement.
vitamin A, 143, 255, 296,
305, 456, 609, 613
B vitamins, 114, 115, 121,
167, 185, 265, 266, 354,
468, 560, 585, 598, 607,
609
vitamin C, 114, 122, 143,
255, 260, 305, 354, 448,
455, 508, 560, 607, 608,
613
vitamin D, 456, 600
vitamin E, 115, 122, 250,

255, 296, 446, 471, 560,
609
Vogel, Karen, 517
Vulva, 97, 241–285
anatomy of, 245–48
cultural attitudes toward,
241–45
Vulvar cancer, 21
and smoking, 613
Vulvar dampness, as cause
of vaginitis, 277
Vulvar pain
and emotions, 243
and HPV, 250
Vulvovaginitis. *See*
Vaginitis.

W

Walker, Alice, 241
Walker, Barbara, 232, 242
Wants, determining, 61–
63
Warts, venereal, 19, 89, 97,
247, 247–56. *See also*
HPV.
and emotions, 243
and episiotomy, 252
and stress, 42
Weed, Susun, 446–47, 449,
478
Weight control, 567
Weight gain, reasons for
wanting, 579

Weight-loss diet
and healthy diet, 582
mentality, 573–77
Weight loss, reasons for
wanting, 579
Weight, natural
and Standard American
Diet, 592
and vegetarian diet, 592
Weight training, aerobic,
631–32
Weighted vaginal cones (sex
technique), 236
Weightlifting, 639
Weil, Andrew, 614
Weil, Robert J., 362
Welch, H. Gilbert, 301
Whole grains, as centering
food, 587–600
Wicca, 59
Willet, W., 305
Wilson, Robert, 462
Wisdom years. *See*
Menopause.
Withdrawal (contraceptive
method), 337. *See also*
Contraception.
Witnessing, 90–91
Wolf, Naomi, 322, 427
Women to Women, 503,
529, 531, 547–48, 584,
586, 610, 643
Confidential Health

Inventory of, 488–92
mutual support in, 18–
19
and therapy, 527
Women, Western cultural
attitudes toward, 3–24
Women-only settings, 528–
29
Wonder, Stevie, 49
Woodward, Jeff, 622
World Health
Organization, 455, 600
World Watch Institute, 5
Wright, Ann, 443
Wright, Jonathan, 475
Wynder and Gori, 304

Y

Yeast infection, 257. *See
also* Vaginitis.
and HPV, 250
Yeast-free diet, 611
Yeast-Gard, 279
Yoga, 237, 313, 588, 632,
636, 637

Z

Zen Buddhism, 313
Zinc, 354, 609
Zinc picolinate, 560
Zinc sulfate, 260
Zovirax (acyclovir), 259
Zuckerman, S., 130

About the Author

Christiane Northrup, M.D., is a holistic physician and member of the Natural Healing Advisory Board. She is a former president of the American Holistic Medical Association. In 1986, along with three other practitioners, she opened Women to Women in Yarmouth, Maine, to address the specific health concerns of women. She is a popular, internationally sought-after speaker.